PRINCIPLES AND APPLICATIONS IN AUDITORY EVOKED POTENTIALS

Other books of interest from the Longwood Division of Allyn and Bacon

Handbook of Auditory Evoked Responses
James W. Hall III
ISBN: 0-205-13566-8

Audiometric Interpretation: A Manual of Basic Audiometry, Second Edition
Harriet Kaplan, Vic S. Gladstone, and Lyle L. Lloyd
ISBN: 0-205-14753-4

Toward a Psychology of Deafness: Theoretical and Empirical Perspectives
Peter V. Paul and Dorothy W. Jackson
ISBN: 0-205-14112-9

Understanding Digitally Programmable Hearing Aids
Robert E. Sandlin (editor)
ISBN: 0-205-14845-X

Orientation to Deafness
Nanci A. Scheetz
ISBN: 0-205-13438-6

Acoustical Factors Affecting Hearing Aid Performance, Second Edition
Gerald A. Studebaker and Irving Hochberg
ISBN: 0-205-13778-4

Diagnostic Audiology
John T. Jacobson and Jerry L. Northern (editors)
ISBN: 0-205-13559-5

The Auditory Brainstem Response
John T. Jacobson (editor)
ISBN: 0-205-13549-8

PRINCIPLES AND APPLICATIONS IN AUDITORY EVOKED POTENTIALS

Edited by

JOHN T. JACOBSON

Professor and Director
Division of Audiology
Department of Otolaryngology—Head and Neck Surgery
Eastern Virginia Medical School
Norfolk, Virginia

ALLYN AND BACON

Boston   London   Toronto   Sydney   Tokyo   Singapore

Series Editor: Mylan Jaixen
Editorial Assistant: Susan Hutchinson
Cover Administrator: Suzanne Harbison
Manufacturing Buyer: Megan Cochran
Editorial-Production Service: Walsh Associates
Cover Designer: Suzanne Harbison

Copyright © 1994 by Allyn and Bacon
A Division of Simon & Schuster, Inc.
160 Gould Street
Needham Heights, Massachusetts 02194

Library of Congress Cataloging-in-Publication Data

Principles and applications in auditory evoked potentials / edited by John T. Jacobson.
    p.   cm.
   Includes bibliographical references and index.
   ISBN 0-205-14846-8 (hard cover)
   1. Auditory evoked response. I. Jacobson, John T., 1943–
   [DNLM: 1. Evoked Potentials, Auditory. 2. Audiometry, Evoked Response.
   3. Brain Stem—physiology. WV 272 P9565 1993]
RF294.5.E87P75   1993
617.8—dc20
DNLM/DLC
for Library of Congress   93-11128
                                        CIP

Printed in the United States of America

10 9 8 7 6 5 4 3 2   99 98 97 96 95

As a graduate student, I became intrigued and fascinated by the clinical and research activities of George E. Lynn. Dr. Lynn was always on the frontier of central auditory investigation and was one of the first professionals to bridge the gap between audiology and other medical disciplines. Over the years, we became colleagues and friends and my respect and memory for his dedication to audiology remains. I will always be grateful for his contribution, "Auditory Brainstem Response in Upper Brainstem Lesions," in the 1985 version of The Auditory Brainstem Response. *The untimely death of Dr. Lynn in 1986 has left a void in our profession. This book is dedicated to his memory.*

CONTENTS

PREFACE

With the publication of *The Auditory Brainstem Response* in 1985, the first primary text dedicated to a specific subclassification of auditory evoked potentials became reality. At the time the book was conceived, these short-latency evoked potentials were receiving such attention that the demands of clinical interest and implementation had far outgrown the current available literature. Thus, there was an attempt to provide a textbook that would provide both a literary source which focused on the role of the auditory brainstem response (ABR) in clinical settings and offered a comprehensive description of the current state of knowledge in ABR measurement. As in life, timing is an all important factor. The publication of *The Auditory Brainstem Response* and the need of the professional community were by no means coincidental.

By the late 1970s and early 1980s, the clinical energies of audiologists and other related hearing health care professionals who were interested in the area of auditory evoked potentials (AEPs) were focused on ABR measurement. Today, through the efforts of both research and clinical investigation, there has been an exponential increase in the knowledge and application of all subclassifications of auditory evoked potentials. The clinical benefits of our increased efforts have had a direct impact in both diagnostic accuracy and patient care management. As a result, a routine audiologic test battery, in addition to behavioral and immittance audiometry, also incorporates, in many cases, a series of auditory evoked potentials to clarify both peripheral and central integrity of the entire auditory pathway. The comprehensive use of AEPs has added significantly to our appreciation of difficult-to-test and other non-cooperative patients.

Because of the rapidly changing clinical dynamics seen in our profession, to simply update *The Auditory Brainstem Response* would have been an injustice to our current knowledge and application of auditory evoked potentials. This book clearly addresses that deficiency. Whereas this book is designed around the framework of *The Auditory Brainstem Response*, it goes considerably beyond in both depth and area.

Principles and Applications in Auditory Evoked Potentials embraces each AEP classification from electrocochleography and the ABR to more central auditory measures including the cortical and endogenous responses (P300) and brain mapping. *Principles and Applications in Auditory Evoked Potentials* focuses on clinical applications and the diagnostic evaluation and is intended to meet the needs of practicing clinicians who are striving to keep abreast of current AEP practice and also to serve as a textbook for graduate study in audiology, otolaryngology, neurology and other related disciplines.

As one might imagine, this task is no small undertaking. Therefore, selection of contributing authors was critical. Each author was chosen based on reputation in the field, expertise in a specific area, and recognized clinical excellence. Their writing reflects a comprehensive knowledge and an ability to report that information succinctly. To each, this editor is greatly indebted not only for their contribution, but also their suggestions, comments, and encouragement.

This textbook is divided into four primary sections. In Section I, *Foundations*, four chapters are devoted to the basic fundamentals of AEPs. Chapter 1, Prelude to Auditory Evoked Potentials, offers an introduction to the area of AEPs and their clinical applications. Chapter 2, Neural Generators of Auditory Evoked Potentials, reviews the anatomy and physiology of the auditory system and the neural generators. In Chapter 3, Signal Processing and Analysis, technical aspects of AEPs are addressed. Chapter 4, Stimulus Calibration in Auditory Evoked Potential Measurements, concludes this section with a description of stimulus calibration and data acquisition techniques. Section I emphasizes the facts, principles, and assumptions which underlie AEP measurement and clinical use.

In Section II, *Auditory Aspects*, five chapters address individual AEP components that are commonly used in clinical practice. Electrocochleography, The Normal Auditory Brainstem Response and Its Variants, The Auditory Middle Latency Response, The Slow Vertex Potential: Properties and Clinical Applications, and Cognitive Auditory Responses offer a sequential review of AEPs as they ascend the auditory pathway. These chapters are basic to each subclassification as well as to the remaining auditory and neurologic applications found thereafter. The final two additional chapters in this section, Effects of Peripheral Hearing Loss on the Auditory Brainstem Response, and Electrophysiologic Measures of Frequency-Specific Auditory Function, describe the evaluation and diagnosis of the peripheral auditory system and related pathology.

Section III, *Pediatric Assessment*, is devoted primarily to the pediatric application of the ABR. Chapters include Neurodevelopment and Auditory Function in Preterm Infants, Newborn and Infant Auditory Brainstem Response Applications, Neonatal Intensive Care Units: Impact on Hearing Screening, and Newborn Hearing Screening. It is clear that the ABR has changed the way we evaluate infants and children and that message is eloquently described within this section.

In Section IV, *Neurotologic Disorders and Management*, five chapters are devoted to the investigation of neural integrity of the auditory pathway. Chapters include Auditory Brainstem Response Measures in Acoustic Nerve and Brainstem Disease, Evoked Potentials in Multiple Sclerosis and other Demyelinating Diseases, Neurophysiologic Intraoperative Monitoring, Auditory Evoked Response in Acute Brain Injury and Rehabilitation, and Brain Mapping of Auditory Evoked Potentials. Unquestionably, the use of AEPs in a neurotologic context has bridged the gap of interdisciplinary communication. The final chapter, Auditory Evoked Potential Testing Strategies, is a synopsis of how AEPs can be clinically synthesized in the best interest of patient care.

I would like to express my appreciation to Dr. Alan Salamy and his colleagues who allowed me to modify and reproduce an illustration they submitted which is found in their chapter. This adapted illustration also appears on the front cover of this textbook. To Bio-logic Systems Corp. I am indebted for their support of the color brain mapping illustrations that appear in this text. Finally, to Claire and Seth who again tolerated my impatience, I will always be grateful.

JOHN T. JACOBSON

ABOUT THE EDITOR

John T. Jacobson is currently Professor and Director, Division of Audiology, Department of Otolaryngology—Head and Neck Surgery, Eastern Virginia Medical School, Norfolk, Virginia.

He is a member of the National and State Professional Hearing and Speech Associations, the American Auditory Society, the Association for Research in Otolaryngology, and the American Academy of Otolaryngology, Head-Neck Surgery. He is also a founding charter member of the American Academy of Audiology and Editor-in-chief of *Audiology Today*, the Bulletin of the Academy.

Jacobson has published articles and book reviews, contributed book chapters, and edited three texts, including the latest, *Principles and Applications in Auditory Evoked Potentials*. At present, he is editing a special issue on "Heredity and Other Childhood Auditory Deficits" in the *Journal of the American Academy of Audiology*.

Jacobson has presented at the state, national, and international level, and his primary clinical interests are in the areas of sensory evoked potentials, monitoring techniques, pediatrics, newborn auditory screening, and audiologic correlates of neurotology. These topics extend into the academic arena where he actively participates in lectures, seminars, and workshops.

CONTRIBUTING AUTHORS

Jaynee Butcher
The Veterans Administration Medical Center
Ann Arbor, MI

Susan E. Denson
University of Texas Medical School—Houston
Houston, TX

Andrée Durieux-Smith
Children's Hospital of Eastern Ontario
Ottawa, Ontario

John D. Durrant
Department of Otolaryngology
University of Pittsburgh
Pittsburgh, PA

Jos Eggermont
University of Calgary
Calgary, Alberta

Lynnette Eldredge
University of California, San Francisco
San Francisco, CA

John Ferraro
University of Kansas Medical Center
Kansas City, KS

Cynthia Fowler
Veterans Administration Medical Center
Long Beach, CA

Michael Gorga
Boys Town Institute for Communication Disorders in
Children
Omaha, NE

James W. Hall III
Vanderbilt University School of Medicine
Nashville, TN

Daniel P. Harris
Healthcare Rehabilitation Center
Austin, TX

Martyn Hyde
Mount Sinai Hospital
Toronto, Ontario

Claire A. Jacobson
Eastern Virginia Medical School
Norfolk, VA

Gary P. Jacobson
Henry Ford Hospital
Detroit, MI

John T. Jacobson
Eastern Virginia Medical School
Norfolk, VA

James F. Jerger
Baylor College of Medicine
Houston, TX

Robert W. Keith
University of Cincinnati Medical Center
Cincinnati, OH

Paul R. Kileny
University of Michigan Medical Center
Ann Arbor, MI

Nina Kraus
Northwestern University
Evanston, IL

Cynthia J. Lynn
Private Practice
Austin, TX

Therese McGee
Northwestern University
Evanston, IL

Aage R. Møller
University of Pittsburgh School of Medicine
Pittsburgh, PA

Michelle Morris
Hospital of the University of Pennsylvania
Philadelphia, PA

Stephen T. Neely
Boys Town Institute for Communication Disorders in Children
Omaha, NE

John K. Niparko
University of Michigan Medical Center
Ann Arbor, MI

Terrey Oliver Penn
Arkansas Department of Health
Little Rock, AR

Terence W. Picton
University of Ottawa
Ottawa, Ontario

Nabih Ramadan
Henry Ford Hospital
Detroit, MI

Roger A. Ruth
University of Virginia Health Science Center
Charlottesville, VA

Alan Salamy
University of California, San Francisco
San Francisco, CA

Daniel M. Schwartz
Neurophysiology Associates, Inc.
Newtown Square, PA

Brad A. Stach
Georgetown University Medical Center
Washington, DC

David R. Stapells
Albert Einstein College of Medicine
Bronx, NY

Laszlo Stein
Northwestern University
Evanston, IL

Bruce A. Weber
Duke University Medical Center
Durham, NC

PART ONE

FOUNDATIONS

CHAPTER 1

PRELUDE TO AUDITORY EVOKED POTENTIALS

JOHN T. JACOBSON

This chapter offers a summary of auditory evoked potentials (AEPs), their basic principles and clinical auditory and neurotologic applications. This overview focuses on the fundamentals and suppositions that underscore AEP measurement and their clinical use. Because of the nature of this book, introductory statements are elementary in their description and preparatory to more detailed and comprehensive accounts of the numerous AEP applications found in subsequent chapters.

This chapter contains a review of AEP generation and their clinical emergence. Introductory statements are followed by a cursory description of the historical development of AEP recordings, clinical importance and a general narrative of the various AEP classifications and nomenclatures. The basic concepts of neuroelectric activity and its effects on AEP recording follow. The final section is devoted to AEP measures in auditory and neurotologic assessment and general patient methodology. This book expands on the original text, *The Auditory Brainstem Response* (1985).

OVERVIEW

In the absence of sensory stimulation, the central nervous system (CNS) generates spontaneous, random neuroelectric activity. These neural events can be recorded using surface (cup/disk) or needle electrodes *on* or *in* the scalp and comprise the electroencephalogram (EEG). In addition, it is also possible to record neural activity that is related to specific types of sensory stimulation and through technical manipulation, extract those events from ongoing EEG activity; it is within this basic neurophysiologic premise that rests the fundamental essence of clinical AEP investigation.

The recording of these sensory evoked potentials (SEP) is based on the assumption that there is an exact temporal relationship that exists between the presenting sensory stimulation and the resulting neural response patterns. During SEP recordings, random EEG activity is many magnitudes larger than most SEPs and tends to obscure the measured SEP response of interest. As a result, in clinical SEP assessment, EEG activity may be considered unwanted *noise* and acts only to degrade the signal-to-noise ratio (SNR) of the neural event. The use of computers has virtually eliminated these problems by extracting the evoked potential from the EEG activity through an *averaging* process. With additional filtering and other differential recording techniques, SEPs can be routinely monitored in clinical environments in the assessment of auditory and neurotologic evaluation (see Hyde, Chapter 3, *Signal Processing and Analysis,* for a detailed description of signal averaging and recording techniques).

Although this book focuses on auditory stimuli as the primary generating signal source, visual and somatosensory stimuli (electrical stimulation to specific nerve sites) are also acceptable forms of sensory stimulation. When all three are used in clinical assessment, multimodality SEPs may provide the most reliable and valid clinical diagnoses in certain pathologies and patient populations. There are many excellent books on visual and somatosensory evoked potentials; however, due to the focus of this book on AEPs, neither modality will be discussed further.

Auditory evoked potentials can be recorded from

many sites in and around the ear and scalp. When recorded from the scalp, AEPs represent the contribution of incalculable neural events that arise from many discrete and multi-contributed neural generating sites along the auditory pathway from the cochlea to the cerebral cortex. It is from these basic concepts that have emerged the numerous clinical AEP applications that are discussed throughout this book. Whether other undiscovered AEP applications exist is not so much a matter of speculation but rather a matter of discovery as a consequence of future clinical investigation and technical improvements.

The past decade has brought forth considerable change in the methods and techniques that audiologists, neurophysiologists, neurotologists, and other medical disciplines evaluate patients who present with auditory and neurotologic complaint. Inspired by technologic advances and improved electrophysiologic measurement, the application of SEPs has become a primary component in the assessment and diagnosis of auditory disorders. Thus, this multidisciplinary approach to AEPs has provided a unique diagnostic dimension that has crossed clinical interprofessional boundaries.

Today, through manufacturing efforts, dedicated instrumentation has made the recording of AEPs a relatively simple and inexpensive investment. Concurrently, there have also been demonstrated improvements in the efficiency of patient care and test sensitivity. A fundamental motive for the clinical popularity of these objective electrophysiologic measures is their diagnostic correlation to behavioral and radiologic observation. As described in detail throughout, auditory, neurotologic, neurologic and cognitive AEP applications have become accepted protocol, particularly in difficult-to-test and other non-responding patient populations. For example, non-cooperative patients who were previously diagnostically problematic, benefit from objective and accurate AEP assessment in the confirmation of residual hearing. Further, the recording of AEPs has also had profound impact in the ability to establish functional integrity of the auditory tract within the peripheral and central nervous system. As such, AEPs have also gained rapid acceptance because of their ability to objectively detect, localize, and monitor auditory and neurologic deficits. Thus, clinical facilities unable to provide such expertise and services have added these

electrophysiologic measurements to the clinical neurophysiologic armamentarium.

Here, two caveats remain. First, although no obvious response is required from the patient during most AEP recordings, minimal cooperation is required. For example, the adult patient must remain relatively immobile and under certain circumstances, perform simple tasks. The infant should be tested in natural sleep or with the administration of sedation. The child must rest quietly. Recent evidence suggests that for some tests (the middle latency response in young infants and children), even levels of sleep must be monitored in order to predict accurate test results (see Kraus et al., Chapter 7, *The Middle Latency Response*). Thus, patient status is an important clinical consideration.

A second caveat to consider is that a great deal of knowledge and experience is required to accurately identify and interpret abnormal AEP recordings. Once records are obtained, subjectivity becomes inherent in every evaluation. As is the case in any subjective assessment, the key to proper test analysis is the development of a substantial normative data base, extensive hands-on experience, a consistent approach to data interpretation and a willingness to admit to an inconclusive outcome. It is hoped that this book will succeed in providing sufficient clinical information to answer many of the questions that the reader may have while simultaneously raising a number of queries for future study.

HISTORICAL PERSPECTIVE

The monitoring of spontaneous EEG activity generated from the CNS and recorded from the human scalp was first described by Berger (1929). This pioneering effort was followed by the work of Loomis, Harvey, and Hobart (1938), who first reported alterations in human EEG patterns brought about by the introduction of sensory stimulation. This process of extracting stimulus-related neuroelectric events from ongoing EEG activity set the stage for future clinical development in various aspects of SEP measurement.

In stimulus-related response measures, the spontaneous EEG voltage exceeds that of all types of AEPs. As a consequence, technical modifications have focused on a means of eliminating unwanted physiologic noise from the recorded response. To this end, several attempts have been made to extract the evoked potential from the recorded EEG pattern (Dawson, 1951, 1954; Geisler, Frishkopf, and Rosenblith, 1958). To date, the process of *averaging* has been the most successful in this pursuit. Clark (1958) and Clark, Goldstein, Brown, Molnar, O'Brien, and Zieman (1961) developed the principles of algebraic summation of neuroelectric events elicited by stimulus synchronization (time-locked repetition). This mathematical operation functions through a process of analog-to-digital conversion whereby EEG voltage is converted and expressed as a numerical value (binary system). During the conversion process, recorded neuroelectric information is maintained and the SNR remains constant so long as the sampling rate is adequate.

Because evoked potentials are predicated on event-related stimuli, they assume a constant time relationship to the presentation of the signal onset; in contrast, the ever-present unwanted noise (EEG activity) is random. Theoretically, noise has no time relationship to stimulus onset and thus evoked potentials can be extracted from the noise of the random EEG activity. Regardless of the process, however, the resulting response will always be contaminated to some degree by residual noise (Picton, Linden, Hamel, and Maru, 1983). Hence, the necessity for further SNR improvement techniques is required (see Hyde, Chapter 3, *Signal Processing and Analysis*).

Davis, Davis, Loomis, Harvey, and Hobart (1939) initially described the results of a series of cortical AEPs obtained from alert and sleeping humans. Their observations showed that with the introduction of repeatable auditory stimuli, small but consistent changes in raw EEG tracings were recorded. These AEPs were most robust when recorded from the vertex, thus the commonly used designation, the "V" or vertex potential. These *slow* or *late* potentials (see the Classification section in this chapter) were consistently observed in the latency range of 50 to 200 milliseconds (ms).

Following the discovery of the cortical AEPs from the human scalp, clinical interest began to concentrate on the refinement of technical and procedural variables. During this era, three additional AEPs, the compound cochlear nerve-action potential (AP) (Ruben, Sekula, Bordley, Knickerbocker, Nager, and Fisch, 1960; Teas,

Eldredge, and Davis, 1962), the middle latency response (MLR) with a latency around 20 to 60 ms (Goldstein and Rodman, 1967; Mendel and Goldstein, 1969) and the auditory cognitive evoked potential with a latency exceeding 250 ms (Walter, Cooper, Aldridge, McCallum, and Winter, 1964) were being successfully explored. Each response has significantly contributed to the overall understanding of evoked potentials. The reader is encouraged to review the historical summary of evoked potential evolution in greater detail in Davis (1976), Hall (1992), Gibson (1978), Moore (1983), and Reneau and Hnatiow (1975).

The most recent electrophysiologic procedure to dominate clinical auditory practice has been the auditory brainstem response (ABR). In reviewing pertinent literature, the ABR should be considered an outgrowth of research activity conducted in the exploration of the cochlear microphonic (CM), the compound action potential (AP), and the cortical response. Early investigations of the CM and AP involved the use of invasive techniques not readily available in the clinic setting. As a consequence, alternative procedures to surgical recording methods and their use of invasive needle electrodes took precedence. Among those investigating noninvasive electrode placement were Sohmer and Feinmesser (1967), who offered the first account of evoked potentials generated from the brainstem. They reported a series of four wave components, the first two waves comprise the N_1-N_2 complex of the acoustic nerve AP. The latter two waves were of questionable origin and it was surmised that the responses were either repetitive firing of the acoustic nerve or neural discharge patterns from the brainstem pathway. While later confirmed (Sohmer and Feinmesser, 1973), it was the seminal work of Jewett (1970) and colleagues (Jewett and Romano, 1972; Jewett, Romano, and Williston, 1970; Jewett and Williston, 1971) that definitively identified and described the origin of the far-field scalp-recorded ABR. In a humorous and informative commentary, Jewett (1983) discusses his first encounter with the brainstem response while recording cortical activity in anesthetized animals. Convinced that these responses found "at the far left of the display screen" (p. xxv) were artifacts, his investigative pursuits were restricted to informal seminars and discussions. After a relatively quiescent period, collaborative interest in the brainstem response resumed; the results of the investigations produced the now renowned series of previously cited publications by Jewett and co-workers.

It is interesting to note that within the past five years, there has been a reemergence of interest in the clinical use of the compound cochlear-nerve action potential. This technique commonly called *electrocochleography* (ECochG) has gained popularity with the application of ear canal and tympanic membrane electrodes. The use of ECochG has expanded into routine clinical use and in the operating room for the monitoring of retrocochlear pathology (see Ferraro and Ruth, Chapter 5, *Electrocochleography*).

This chapter is not intended to describe in detail the historical events that have led to the current status of the AEPs. Specific information is contained in each chapter of this book in a precise and sequential order. Suffice it to say that the AEP evaluation has embraced most clinical auditory and neurotologic investigation. Finally, evoked potentials have also become a reliable clinical tool in neurology and have expanded into the area of cognitive behavior. Comprehensive reviews of historical AEP development are found in Fria (1980), Hall (1992), Moore (1983), and Spehlmann (1985).

CLASSIFICATION

Description

Auditory evoked potentials comprise a continuum of neuroelectric events that are generated along the entire length of the auditory pathway. Under conventional recording conditions, as many as 15 AEPs have been identified within the first 500 ms post-stimulus onset (Picton, Hillyard, Krauz, and Galambos, 1974; Picton, Woods, Baribeau-Braun, and Healey, 1977). The underlying physiologic principle is that whereas evoked potentials may be measured independently (i.e., ECochG, ABR, MLR, SVP, P300, etc.), they coexist within the stimulated auditory pathway. Clinically, it is a matter of determining the latency epoch of importance and then selecting a methodology that will extract the particular response of inquiry from other neuroelectric activity.

AEP waveforms resulting from an *averaging* process disclose a series of wave components (peaks and troughs) that are described by their amplitude and latency characteristics. *Latency* is the time interval between a reference point and some feature (usually a specific peak of the AEP). The *amplitude* of a response can be measured from the voltage baseline to the wave peak, or from the peak of a wave and its following trough. The units of measure for latency and amplitude are usually milliseconds (ms) and microvolts (µV), respectively.

The stimulus-dependent AEPs used in clinical application and described throughout this book are either receptor potentials originating from within the cochlea, or neurogenic potentials from the acoustic nerve and/or neuron populations within the auditory central nervous system. Although AEPs may be caused by activation of muscles of the head and neck (myogenic activity), such responses are of little clinical interest unless they interfere with the AEP recording.

There are two primary receptor potentials that are generated from the sensory end-organ. They consist of the cochlear microphonic (CM) and the summating potential (SP). The CM is considered to be a neuroelectric analog of the auditory stimulus since it faithfully reproduces the signal input. The CM has no measurable latency delay to the presentation of the signal onset and it is thought to represent basal region outer hair cell activity. The CM has no physiologic threshold. The SP is seen as a negative DC voltage shift which lasts the duration of the input signal. As with the CM, the SP is thought to reflect outer hair cell activity. Whereas the CM has little clinical significance, comparative changes in the SP have become useful in the objective detection of certain end-organ disorders (see Ferraro and Ruth, Chapter 5, *Electrocochleography*).

The origins of neurogenic potentials arise from the acoustic nerve and multiple neural sites within the auditory CNS. They result from synchronized neural discharge patterns and graded post-synaptic potentials and are of significant clinical interest. The following is a general classification of neurogenic AEPs.

Currently, without any formally standardized AEP terminology, several classifications systems have been used. The two most familiar approaches employed in clinical practice refer to the "site-of-generation" and the "response-latency". For example, in Davis (1976), responses are expressed in order of their response-latency epoch (defined as a specific time frame) as follows: *first* (cochlear microphonic, summating potential and acoustic nerve response: 0–2 ms); *fast* (acoustic nerve and auditory brainstem response: 2–10 ms); *middle* (thalamus and auditory cortex: 8–50 ms); *slow* (primary and secondary areas of the cerebral cortex: 50–300 ms); and *late* (primary and association areas of cerebral cortex: 300+ ms). It is critical to recognize that the brainstem response and cortical or vertex "V" potential reflect the *presumed* sites of neural activity; thus, terms are often interchanged in the context of discussion.

There are some instances in which the "time-frame" is favored over other classifications. Take for instance, the *middle latency response* (MLR), which likely has both thalamic and cortical contributions. This response is almost exclusively referred to by its location in time; that is, described between the *fast* (e.g., *ABR*) and *slow* (e.g., *cortical*) latency response epochs.

Often, the presumed site of neural generation of a particular AEP tends to take precedence over other classifications. Thus, the term *auditory brainstem response* is more common than the term *fast* or *short-latency* response. Ironically, the presumption about response origin may not be absolute. For example, the first two ABR wave peak components are generated from the auditory nerve and not the brainstem (Møller, 1981; Møller and Jannetta, 1982). A summary of receptor and neurogenic potentials is presented in Table 1.1. For an expanded account of various classification systems the reader is encouraged to review Davis (1976), Hall (1992), Jacobson and Hyde (1985), and Picton and Fitzgerald (1983).

Wave Nomenclature

Within each designated latency epoch, AEP wave components have their own nomenclature. Each wave may be identified by its order in a sequence, its latency, polarity, or some reported combination. For example, a *polarity-latency* reference to a specific ABR component might be P_6, designating a scalp-positive peak with a latency of about 6 ms. The terms N_{90} and P_{300} are similar examples of designations for cortical responses. Ex-

amples of *polarity-order* component designation are N_1, for the acoustic nerve response (the numeral indicates that it is the first negative wave), or as in the MLR components: P_a, N_a, P_b, etc. As stated, any particular AEP component can be referred to in a number of ways, causing some confusion. Thus, one particular ABR peak has been called wave V (order) by Jewett and Williston (1971), N_4 (polarity-order) by Thornton (1975), and P_6 (polarity-latency) by Davis (1976). Remember that neither the order nor the latency designation is free from clinical misinterpretation. For example, as a consequence of technical and/or patient-related variables, in any series of wave components, peaks that are not present can upset the order designation. Depending on stimulation, acquisition parameters and pathology, the ABR wave designation P_6 may occur at any latency from 5 to 15 ms or more.

Another method of description involves a stimulus-response relationship. Responses have been classified as transient, sustained, or perceptual, reflecting the feature of the stimulus which is critical for response generation (Picton et al., 1977). The stimuli used for most AEP measures are clicks, brief tone pips, or tone bursts (see Gorga and Neely, Chapter 4, *Stimulus Calibration in Auditory Evoked Potential Measurements*). A transient response is evoked by a rapid change in the stimulus such as its onset or offset. In contrast, a prolonged stimulus may evoke a sustained response which lasts for the duration of the signal.

If the intent of the signal is to evoke a transient response such as an ECochG, then it makes little sense to use a long lasting stimulus. Recall, only the beginning (or the end) of the stimulus is effective in synchronized response production. However, if the aim is to generate a sustained response, then the stimulus must be of sufficient length to allow the sustained AEP to develop clearly. Perceptual response generation usually requires the use of a stimulus paradigm which imposes some cognitive significance onto the stimulus, such as in a discrimination task. Perceptual responses are thought to be related to the *meaning* of the stimulus and are limited to cognitive response measures (see Butcher, Chapter 9, *Cognitive Auditory Response*).

To illustrate this descriptive classification, Figure 1.1 presents a series of three separate response tracings

TABLE 1.1. AEP Classification Systems and Descriptions

Common Name	Physiologic Description	Anatomy Source	Latency Epoch	Latency Range	Stimulus-Response	Electrode-Response
Cochlear microphonic (CM)	Receptor	Hair cells	First	0	Sustained	Near-field
Summating potential (SP)	Receptor	Hair cells	First	0	Sustained	Near-field
Action potential (AP)(N_1, N_2) (ECochG)	Neurogenic	Auditory nerve	First	~2	Transient	Far-field
Auditory brainstem response (ABR) (I to VII)	Neurogenic	Auditory nerve Brainstem	Fast	<10	Transient	Far-field
Slow-negative (SN_{10})	Neurogenic	Brainstem	Fast	~10	Transient	Far-field
Frequency following response (FFR)	Neurogenic	Brainstem	Fast	Tone duration	Sustained	Far-field
Middle latency response (MLR)(No, Po, Na, Pa, Nb, Pb)	Neurogenic	Thalamus	Middle	8–50	Transient	Far-field
Slow-vertex potential (SVP) (P_1, N_1, P_2, N_2)	Neurogenic	Cerebral cortex (primary and association)	Late	50–300	Transient	Far-field
Late positive component (P_{300})	Neurogenic	Cerebral cortex (primary and association)	Late	250–350	Perceptual	Far-field
Cognitive negative variation (CNV)	Neurogenic	Cerebral cortex (association)	Late	300^+	Perceptual	Far-field

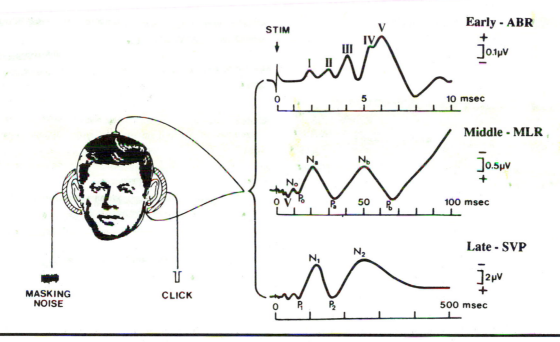

FIGURE 1.1.   Schematic representation of exogenous AEP wave component nomenclature. Three latency epochs are illustrated: 1) Early, 2) Middle and 3) Late. Modified with permission from the Publisher. Spehlmann, R. (1985). *Evoked potential primer: Visual, auditory, and somatosensory evoked potentials in clinical diagnosis*, p. 196. Boston: Butterworth.

representing different time bases from the periphery to the primary auditory cortex. The Jewett and Williston (1971) order nomenclature (I to VII) is used for the ABR, polarity with alphabetical order subscripts is used for MLR (Mendel and Goldstein, 1969) and polarity with numerical order subscripts is used for cortical responses (Davis and Zerlin, 1966). Thus, one must regard these nomenclatures merely as means of providing a labeling scheme for wave components. Each clinician must choose a classification system and recognize that other infrastructures exist.

Electrodes

Two additional points of possible confusion involve the terms given to electrodes and their relationship with the morphology of AEP traces. In bipolar recordings, three or four electrodes are applied to the scalp and are commonly referred to as the *active*, *reference*, and *ground*. These terms are misleading and do not accurately represent the underlying neural activity. For example, most short-latency AEP measures are based on neural synchronized discharges from subcortical levels. These electrical fields generated from caudal regions of the auditory mechanism are transmitted within a *volume conductive* medium of extracellular fluid and tissue. Thus, any electrode located on the scalp and remote from the generated electric field will potentially register neural activity causing the label *reference* (suggesting a nonactive or indifferent electric site) to be inaccurate.

Two sets of alternative electrode terms have gained clinical acceptance. They are *positive* and *negative* related to electrode input at the preamplifier stage and *noninverting* and *inverting* describing amplifier function. The third electrode is the *ground* or, more appropriately, the *common* electrode. The primary responsibility of the differential preamplifier is to amplify the resulting neural activity after a process of polarity reversal has occurred at the inverting electrode. The degree of internal noise cancellation is called the *common-mode rejec-*

tion ratio and is described fully in Hyde, Chapter 3, *Signal Processing and Analysis.*

Convention

For the most part, clinics in North America subscribe to a vertex-positive convention displayed in an upward direction. In contrast, there is a tendency for European and Scandinavian centers (a neurophysiologic influence) to reverse this directional pattern; that is, positivity is plotted downward. This direction in polarity is controlled by reversing electrode input at the preamplifier stage. See Schwartz et al., Chapter 6, *The Normal ABR and its Variants,* for a comprehensive description of ABR classifications and wave convention.

THE AUDITORY BRAINSTEM RESPONSE

Because a significant portion of this book is devoted to the ABR and its clinical application, the following discussion focuses on the ABR.

Description

The ABR is considered a far-field recording by virtue of the fact that monitoring electrodes attached to the scalp are distant from the site of the neural activity. In the adult patient, the ABR latency epoch consists of five to seven wave peaks measured within the first 10 to 15 ms following stimulation. In the healthy newborn and young infant population, due to a number of physiologic variables, the response usually consists of three replicable wave peaks (I, III, and V) whose latency and amplitude differ from adult values (Jacobson, Morehouse, and Johnson, 1982). Figure 1.2 presents a series of ABR traces obtained from a normal infant and an adult. Recording differences in the two series of ABR traces are readily observed.

The designated time interval of the brainstem response is usually based on the number of identifiable wave components, pathologic considerations, and technical variables. For instance, lesions of the acoustic nerve and auditory brainstem (see Part Four, *Neurotologic Disorders and Management,* in this book) may modify latency, diminish, or totally eliminate wave peak amplitude and

thereby change the expected number of wave peaks and their component morphology. Technical aspects will also affect the latency epoch. Factors include electrode placement, stimulus polarity, rate, filtering characteristics and stimuli, all of which may influence the latency, amplitude and morphology of the brainstem response. For instance, transient stimuli are used most often in evoked potential study because of their ability to initiate the neural synchronization of certain cell types whose onset discharge patterns are necessary in short-latency and MLR production. Stimuli that elicit ABR wave components have a relatively stable intersubject latency as a function of intensity (e.g., wave V = ~5.8 ms at 60 dB nHL). However, even in a normal ear, a change in the auditory signal (e.g., low-frequency tone pips having a longer signal envelope) will prolong the wave V latency to 13–15 ms at low signal intensity levels.

Wave nomenclature

There are several methods of identifying ABR wave peak components. Throughout this book, the order-sequence described by Jewett and Williston (1971) has been adopted to identify individual waves. This nomenclature, which uses Roman numerals (I–VII) to designate wave peaks, is the most commonly found classification system in the literature and is the least subject to misinterpretation. For example, in the absence of all waves other than wave V, it still remains wave V, not wave I because it is the first and only wave identified. The reader should be aware that other wave designations exist and are found in the literature (e.g., in the neurophysiology literature, P_5 substitutes for wave V). See Schwartz et al., Chapter 6, *The Normal ABR and its Variants,* for an indepth description of wave nomenclature.

PRINCIPLES OF NEUROELECTRIC ACTIVITY

Portions of this section have been adapted from Jacobson and Hyde (1985).

During routine clinical AEP evaluation, recorded electrical activity is the contribution of multiple neural generator sites. Single cell recordings are never monitored because practitioners do not place electrodes in,

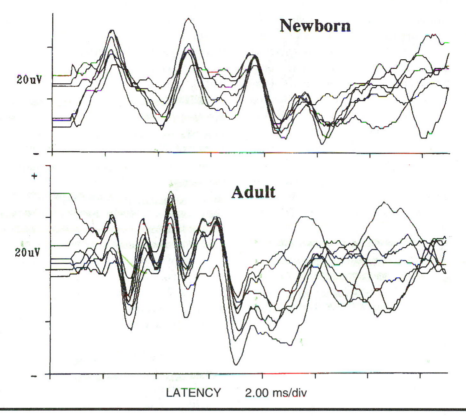

FIGURE 1.2. A series of 6 auditory brainstem response (ABR) waveforms, each obtained from the same ear of a term newborn (top) and that of an adult (bottom). Each trace represents the sum of 2000 click stimuli at 60 dB nHL.

on, or near individual neurons. Single-unit electrical events are rapidly attenuated in surrounding extracellular space and are unmeasurable at more than a few millimeters distance from the source. How then is it possible to record subcortical activity using surface electrodes placed on the scalp? The answer rests in the principle of neural *synchronization.* In order to understand this basic premise, it is necessary to discern the relationships between neuroelectric activity in the peripheral and central nervous system and the responses that are registered by recording electrodes that are distant from the neural generating sites. The following section describes the basic principles of neuroelectric activity in clinical AEP evaluation.

When individual neurons are simultaneously stimulated and each neuron contributes a minute but similar electrical event at a recording electrode, the overall result is the sum of all of the single-unit neuronal contributions. The importance of this statement is that *similar* events occur from each of the active neural sources and the recording electrode must *recognize* an electric field of the same shape at the same time. Once this criteria is established, the components augment one another and produce a measurable neuroelectric response field. If identical voltage patterns are simultaneously produced and their synchronization is exact, the summed result will closely resemble the neuroelectrical contribution of each active source. In practice these requirements are rarely met since it is difficult to excite multiple neurons at exactly the same time.

If all neuroelectric contributions were similar, but not exactly synchronized, the result at the recording electrode will tend to be *smeared* over time; that is, the result would be a reduction in voltage and a broader response spectrum than if the synchronization was exact. For example, a change in wave morphology is often observed when monitoring a multiple sclerosis patient with demyelination where synchronization within the pathway may not be exact. Next, consider the reverse condition; that is, temporal synchronization was exact, but the contributing neuroelectric fields were different. Under these circumstances, the recording of neural activity becomes problematic. If for instance, the polarity of neural activity were continually reversed, the resulting response may be canceled. Therefore, neural synchronization is only one condition necessary for recording activity at a remote electrode. Suffice it to say, it is difficult to make precise inferences about what occurs in an active neuronal population on the basis of what is seen at a distant electrode. Thus, in reality, the precision of diagnostic prognostication must be tempered by the chosen technique and the recording parameters used to manipulate neuroelectric activity.

Volume Conduction

The relationship between the neuroelectrical source fields and the recorded potentials can be extremely complex. Source fields are generated within a conducting medium comprised of extracellular fluid and many types of tissue. Such a medium is said to be a *volume conductor,* and its electrical properties can profoundly affect the spatial distribution of recorded electric potentials.

Neuroelectric Distribution

The requirement that the electrode should *recognize* similar activity from many active neural sources has implications for both spatial and temporal distribution. Because neuroelectric field strength declines rapidly with distance, the closer the spatial grouping of neural activity, the better the summation and activity at the electrode. For example, in the recording of cortical AEPs, the neural sources are post-synaptic potentials in the dendritic fields of many cortical cells that are arranged in layers parallel to the cortical surface. A sensory stimulus might excite thousands of cells, but this may not be clearly effective at the electrode unless the active cells were in close proximity to each other; that is, in approximation to the recording electrode.

The CM potential, recorded from the middle ear promontory, is a good example of the relationship of temporal and spatial generator distribution at a recording electrode. The CM is primarily associated with outer hair cell activity distributed along the length of the cochlea. At each point, the CM waveform reflects the time course of the local displacement of the basilar membrane. The electrode is closer to the basal aspects of the cochlea and therefore, the neural contributions are larger at the base than at the apex. As a traveling wave is hydrodynamically propagated rapidly down the length of the basilar membrane, it excites hair cells as it passes over them. Each cell will generate a damped oscillatory electrical response that is a potential contributor at the electrode. The velocity of the traveling wavefront is greatest at the base and declines toward the apex. Thus, the temporal synchronization of the neural activity is most efficient in the basal region. Activity from more remote apical sources will be more broadly distributed in time and their oscillations will have a greater tendency to cancel one another. The overall result is that the CM waveform seen by the electrode is strongly weighted toward outer hair cell activity in the basal (high frequency) region.

Synchronization

Two additional factors are important in connection with synchronization of neural activity. They are the *duration* of the time course of the neural fields and the *total number* of simultaneously contributing neural elements. When recording *gross* (remote from the active neural units) neuroelectric activity generated from the auditory periphery, the observed neural events are the compound cochlear-action potentials and post-synaptic potentials. These events are of brief duration and require a brief and effective stimulus to create synchronization. The *click* is the stimulus of choice since it is produced by a transducer with a rectangular voltage pulse which is capable of exciting large numbers of cells. This stimulus is most often used in short-latency AEPs and other nonfrequency specific AEPs.

In contrast, neuroelectrical source fields of longer duration do not necessitate precise synchronization. Here, the importance of excitation is less because the effects of temporal smearing are reduced. The general rule of thumb is that the more rostral the generating response, the less synchronization is needed. For example, temporal synchronization is less critical for cortical *late* AEPs. Potential sources for the MLR and the SVP are likely to be synaptic and dendritic electric fields which have longer time courses. In addition, because of neural multiplicity of the auditory pathway, small numbers of peripheral cells can elicit activity in large numbers of central cells. Thus, the need for a rapid stimulus onset is less. As such, pure tones having longer signal envelopes can be used for cortical AEP monitoring. Pure tone stimuli also have the advantage of greater frequency specificity thus fulfilling one clinical AEP prerequisite, that of audiometric approximation from objective measures. Finally, the second factor of synchronization is the total number of active neural elements, which must be large in order to meet clinical requirements. These numbers are never small and are relative to the response of interest. Generally, the more peripheral the response, the greater the number of synchronized neural discharge firing is required. See later in this chapter (Clinical Applications) and, Hyde, Chapter 8, *The Slow Vertex Potential,* for a summary of the clinical use of the cortical response.

The preceding discussion applies to an electrical field at a remote recording electrode at any one point in time. Unfortunately, the clinical measurement of AEPs is the result of a change in potential over a designated period of time. What is ultimately recorded is the result of creation, and the movement and decay of a complex structure of shifting electrical charges. This is all taking place within the head, a structure which is extremely varied in its physical and electrical properties (volume conductor). Given the previous examples, any specific inference about underlying neuronal activity on the basis of gross AEPs recorded from the scalp or within the ear is extremely complex and often problematic. However, favorably, it is not necessary to entirely understand a phenomenon in order to make

empirical use of it. Although restricted to imprecise and tentative statements about AEP origins, their usefulness as clinical correlates has been conceded by even the most skeptical.

CLINICAL APPLICATIONS

During the past two decades, there has been a dramatic increase in the efficiency of specialized audiologic test procedures in auditory, central processing, and neurotologic diagnoses. In today's clinical environment, individual tests are closely scrutinized with regard to their performance characteristics. The validity of a test, measured by the proportion of confirmed results, strongly influences its use and longevity. Improvements in technology and instrumentation, specific test selection in site-of-lesion analysis, and the inclusion of the test battery have all contributed to the overall improved accuracy of diagnostic evaluation and prediction.

With the role of the electrophysiologic test battery expanding to provide increased precision of peripheral and central deficits, the clinician can no longer be content with a test that simply provides a relatively high degree of sensitivity; that is, the ability of a test to correctly identify patients with auditory or neurotologic abnormalities. To improve diagnostic accuracy, a test must go beyond sensitivity as a measure of test validity. A test must also be accountable in terms of identifying patients with normal auditory function (i.e., specificity). The following section describes various AEP procedures and applications that can be applied in routine clinic environments.

Auditory Evoked Potentials in the Clinical Setting

Why have auditory evoked potentials gained such credibility as a routine clinical test procedure when conventional behavioral audiometry is available? Certainly one answer frequently cited is that AEPs offer an objective assessment of specific patient populations that are difficult, if not impossible, to test by any other means. By accepting this supposition, we endorse the premise that AEPs are both reliable and valid. If not, then our dependency on AEPs as a clinical measure is indefensible.

In clinical AEP application, one of the primary objectives must be to reconstruct the pure tone audiogram objectively. Depending on the purpose of the examination and the degree of specificity required, a number of AEPs can be used to equate behavioral audiometry. In such a pursuit, each AEP has its own set of merits and limitations. The selection and sequence of tests are usually governed by patient symptomology, clinical purpose, intended goals, and by the results obtained at each stage of the evaluation process.

A second, but no less important objective, is to determine the functional integrity of the auditory system. Again, several AEPs can be used to identify and localize disorders of the peripheral and central nervous system. It is this latter neurotologic application that has provided a common ground for various health related disciplines. Perhaps more than any other component, function integrity of the auditory system is of clinical interest to a wide spectrum of professionals who have come to rely on information gained from AEP evaluation in the management of undiagnosed patients.

Although these goals are sometimes elusive because of any number of uncontrolled variables and unforeseen circumstances, they are attainable. As in routine conventional audiometric evaluation, the battery approach, or cross-check principle is also applicable with AEPs. Specific clinical issues relative to individual AEPs are discussed in subsequent chapters. The following is an introduction to auditory and neurotologic AEP applications.

TEST STRATEGY

Auditory Assessment

Ideally, the AEP evaluation is used to confirm auditory sensitivity objectively following questionable or unobtainable behavioral threshold estimates in difficult-to-test populations such as the multiply handicapped, the neurologically impaired, the infant or non-cooperative young child, or the functional patient. For any given patient, one AEP procedure is likely to be optimal as the first (screening) stage of evaluation. Depending on the problems encountered and test results, other AEP options may be indicated. Individual tests in the AEP battery must be used as part of a coherent, goal-directed strategy (Picton and Smith, 1978). No single procedure is the answer for all patients, and the procedures must be made to fit the patient, not vice versa.

Consider the patient who is passively cooperative and awake. The *slow vertex potential* is probably the most useful procedure for detailed audiometry. This method is well validated and has excellent frequency specificity. The procedure is relatively insensitive to neuropathy and conventional pure tone stimuli and contralateral masking can be used. For most medical-legal and suspected functional cases, the SVP is an acceptable procedure and will give adequate results. If however, the SVP does not address all concerns, either from obvious causes such as difficulty in response recognition due to highly rhythmic EEG activity, or the responses do not define a clear threshold, then an alternative such as the MLR should be considered. See Hyde, Chapter 8, *The Slow Vertex Potential,* and Kraus et al., Chapter 7, *The Auditory Middle Latency Response.*

If the patient is uncooperative or too active, testing under sedation or general anesthesia will probably be necessary. The SVP is not reliable under these conditions and the ECochG or ABR is probably the most appropriate test. If the patient is likely to fall asleep, as in a neonate, these short-latency evoked potentials are the first choice. Most neonates and infants under 6 months of age can be induced to sleep quite readily. This becomes progressively more difficult with older infants, and there is a point when sedation or general anesthesia is required. Generally, clinicians achieve good results with sedation; however, on occasion, testing under sedation (e.g., usually with the administration of chloral hydrate) can be time consuming and ineffective. For example, there exists a small group of infants and children that become *hyperactive* to sedation. Unfortunately, predicting specific populations, or for that matter, individuals, is difficult at best. For the most part, these patients are the exception rather than the rule. If short-latency thresholds are unclear in a sleeping patient, the MLR is an alternative. The MLR has limitations, however, and in children and infants, the levels of sleep should be monitored for accurate test results (see Kraus et al., Chapter 7, *The Auditory Middle Latency Response*).

The last resort is general anesthesia. Testing under general anesthesia has the advantage that excellent EEG conditions are guaranteed. The down side is that the use of general anesthesia is only available under medical supervision, it may be difficult to coordinate the patient's schedule with the operating room and other hospital personnel. Finally, it usually occurs at an increased expense to the patient.

In the presence of significant brainstem neurotologic disorder, thresholds are difficult to predict since data acquisition may be affected by the disorder. Clinically abnormal ABR waveforms that are obtained at suprathreshold stimulus levels must be verified by some other AEP technique. Here, ECochG is useful because the cochlear nerve response can be clearly recorded with little chance of compromise due to neurotologic disease. Of course, this assumes that other pathology has not affected the peripheral auditory system. ECochG requires general anesthesia in children, whereas the cooperative adult is testable with local anesthesia (transtympanic electrode) or without (ear canal or tympanic membrane electrode). See Ferraro and Ruth, Chapter 5, *Electrocochleography*, for a summary of ECochG techniques using various electrode types.

For each AEP technique, the problems that may occur and the procedures for solving them may be uniquely different and often complicated. Certainly, the AEP battery demands diverse and considerable expertise. Testing methodologies must be highly adaptive, and the clinician must determine when to limit the objectives and how to achieve reliable interpretation of test results. See Stach et al., Chapter 21, *Testing Strategies in Auditory Evoked Potentials,* for a summary of AEP test synthesis.

Neurotologic Investigation

The second major application of AEPs is the detection and localization of disorders affecting the cochlear nerve, brainstem pathway, and more rostral levels, including the auditory cortex. Any disorder that disrupts neural synchrony can depress, delay, or abolish AEP waveform components (see Jacobson et al., Chapter 16, *Auditory Brainstem Response Measures in Acoustic Nerve and Brainstem Disease*). Some types of retrocochlear disorders, such as acoustic tumors, commonly present with auditory and/or vestibular symptoms, and such cases are usually referred for AEP evaluation via the otolaryngologist, neurosurgeon, or neurologist. For other disorders, such as multiple sclerosis, referral may be from the neurologist or primary care/attending physician.

The first AEP method to be proposed as a part of the test battery for acoustic tumor detection was transtympanic ECochG. Changes in the cochlear nerve response were noted in the presence of tumors, but these were difficult to distinguish from the effects of changes in the cochlear SP which also contributed to the overall AEP waveform. During the past two decades, ECochG has largely been replaced by ABR techniques for identification of lesions within the posterior cranial fossa. Interestingly, ECochG has recently regained clinical interest as a tool for more detailed examination of cochlear function and has emerged as a useful adjunct to ABR techniques when the latter are difficult to interpret. Specifically, the relationships between the SP and the AP response amplitude offers insight into cochlear endolymphatic abnormalities and potential perilymph fistulae. Also, new advances in ECochG recording techniques from the ear canal have added a new dimension to clinical investigation (see Ferraro and Ruth, Chapter 5, *Electrocochleography*). Whereas transtympanic needle placement has seen little popular acceptance in North America, probably more as a result of the medical-legal climate rather than any intrinsic deficiency, it has found new support in the operating room in the monitoring of retrocochlear pathology, particularly the acoustic neuroma and other lesions of the posterior fossa (see Kileny and Niparko, Chapter 18, *Neurophysiologic Intraoperative Monitoring* and, Ferraro and Ruth, Chapter 5, *Electrocochleography*). Here, the robust recording amplitude of the AP (analogous to wave I of the ABR), is used as a benchmark from which neural conduction time may be measured.

At present, the ABR technique has been the most promising of all AEPs in the investigation of retrocochlear disease. Such demonstrated acceptance has occurred because ABR waveforms are fairly similar across individuals and are highly stable and reproducible in any single individual. Of all AEPs they appear least affected by attention, sleep, medications, and most other metabolic factors. Also, the ABR reflects neural integrity in a well organized pathway which traverses vital regions of the brain. The apparent, though somewhat surprising correspondence between successive ABR waves and increasing rostral sites in the auditory mechanism gives a limited but useful ability to localize sources of abnormality. At present, it is not possible to identify the specific type of brainstem abnormality from the ABR waveshape. But as more accurate information about ABR generators becomes available, and as testing protocols and interpretative methods become more sophisticated, improvements can be expected in the precision of clinical investigations (see Jacobson et al., Chapter 16, *Auditory Brainstem Response Measures in Acoustic Nerve and Brainstem Disease*).

In more general neurologic investigations, AEPs are part of a larger battery of evoked potential tests of the peripheral and central nervous system. These typically include visual and somatosensory evoked potential measures. The development of a comprehensive and integrated multimodality evoked potential test battery is an important challenge in clinical neuroscience.

AEPs are used as an electrophysiologic tool that can reveal normal or abnormal neural function, as opposed to the analysis of structure, which is the domain of radiology. AEPs are a complementary evaluative modality and their noninvasive character and relatively low cost underlie their established role in neurotology and neurologic investigation. AEPs have proven valuable in the following areas: detection of acoustic tumors and other space-occupying lesions in the posterior cranial fossa, detection of more rostral lesions in the brainstem (see Jacobson et al., Chapter 16, *Auditory Brainstem Response Measures in Acoustic Nerve and Brainstem Disease*), refining diagnosis of demyelinating diseases such as multiple sclerosis (see Keith and Jacobson, Chapter 17, *Evoked Potentials in Multiple Sclerosis and other Demyelinating Diseases*), differentiating structural from metabolic causes of coma (see Hall and Harris, Chapter 19, *Auditory Evoked Potentials in Acute Brain Injury and Rehabilitation*), assessing abnormal maturation or degeneration of the auditory pathways (see Salamy et al., Chapter 12, *Neurodevelopment and Auditory Function in Preterm Infants*), monitoring neural function during brain surgery (see Kileny and Niparko, Chapter 18, *Neurophysiologic Intraoperative Monitoring*), and providing electrophysiologic correlates of various disorders of higher brain function (see Jacobson, Chapter 20, *Brain Mapping of Auditory Evoked Potentials*).

The Patient

The status of the patient's electromyogenic activity is an important factor when testing. Activity associated with gross movements, such as jaw clenching or high levels of muscle tension arising from anxiety is a major source of difficulty, especially with the ABR and MLR. The myogenic noise energy lies mainly in the 50 to 250 Hz range, which overlaps strongly with the ABR and MLR recording bandwidths. Such activity can change the noise levels by more than an order of magnitude, ultimately having an effect on the averaging requirements and averaged response.

Controlling the patient's emotional and physical state can be the most critical factor in achieving a clinically useful test. ABR and MLR tests are best performed with the patient lying supine to reduce neck muscle tension. As stated earlier, sleep, sedation, and general anesthesia are useful ways of further reducing muscle activity, so long as they do not affect the response. The MLR is slightly altered by these sedating maneuvers, and the SVP is more strongly affected. This latter test is most reliable with the patient awake, alert and sitting. The SVP, with its recording bandwidth in the 1 to 15 Hz range, is less affected by myogenic activity but is degraded by low frequency artifacts arising from movement of electrode leads or from high impedance electrode-skin interface. This response is also obscured by classical EEG rhythms, especially the alpha rhythm (8 to 13 Hz). This rhythm is reduced if the eyes are open, and more so with visual fixation, so having the patient read during this test is helpful.

Experience suggests that it is best to communicate with referring colleagues and discuss what should and should not be told to scheduled patients. For example, patients will arrive more manageable if they are informed that they are going to be seen for hearing confirmation or to measure the function of the auditory system objectively rather than to *rule out* the possibility of a *tumor*. Even in the best of circumstances, there are times when adult patients arrive for testing with high anxiety levels that produce artifacts which interfere with testing. At this point, the administration of a mild sedative such as diazepam is a viable option, assuming that administration is not medically contraindicated.

Test Environment

The patient's environment is usually an electrically shielded, acoustically isolated enclosure. Sometimes, testing in more adverse environments such as an operating room or an intensive care unit is unavoidable with consequential limitations due to ambient sound levels and electrical interference. Power line interference at 60 Hz is a common problem, especially for ABR and MLR recordings. Special filters (notch filters) can suppress this type of interference but can severely distort the response waveform. By choice, it is best to locate and solve the source of the problem. Often the source is found in poor or unequal electrode impedance or unnecessary proximity to electrical powerleads. In any case, it is important to ensure that the stimulus repetition rate is not an exact integer submultiple of the number 60, so that the interference is not locked in time to the averaging process. See Kileny and Niparko, Chapter 18, *Neurophysiologic Intraoperative Monitoring* and Hall and Harris, Chapter 19, *Auditory Evoked Responses in Brain Injury and Rehabilitation* for an account of AEP recordings under adverse conditions.

AUDITORY BRAINSTEM RESPONSE

This section is devoted to the use of specific ABR clinical applications.

Role of ABR

Although more than two decades old, the ABR remains the most recent electrophysiologic procedure to be integrated into the AEP test battery. The development of the ABR has focused on two principal areas of clinical application: 1) the evaluation and diagnosis of the peripheral auditory system and related pathology, and 2) the determination of the neural integrity of the acoustic nerve and caudal levels of the brainstem pathway (Hecox and Jacobson, 1984).

The test performance of the ABR in clinical practice has achieved a relatively high degree of validity. This is especially evident in the diagnosis of retrocochlear lesions where it is not unexpected to find hit rates of ABR abnormality exceeding 95%, whereas false-positive rates are usually less than 10% (Eggermont, Don, and Brackman, 1980; Glasscock, Jackson, Josey, Dickins, and Wiet, 1979; Selters and Brackman, 1979; Terkildsen, Osterhammel, and Thomsen, 1981). See Jacobson et al., Chapter 16, *Auditory Brainstem Response Measures in Acoustic Nerve and Brainstem Disease*, for an account of the operating characteristics of ABR in retrocochlear pathology.

The high-risk infant population is another group for which the ABR has a proven track record of test efficiency. Although there are a number of complicating issues in neonatal testing, including middle ear effusion, transient neurologic deficits, correct gestational age estimates, and appropriate follow-up services, the predictive rate of the ABR is superior to all other newborn test procedures (see Jacobson and Hall, Chapter 13, *Applications in Newborn and Infant Auditory Brainstem Responses*, and Weber and Jacobson, Chapter 15, *Newborn Hearing Screening*). It follows that in special populations and in the study of certain neurotologic disease, the ABR has established itself as the evaluative electrophysiologic tool of choice demonstrated by practical clinical application and superior overall test performance.

The following comments are limited to the use of a click stimuli for ABR evaluation. Recall that for more frequency specific information, tone pips or tones bursts are routinely used. In Stapells et al., Chapter 11, *Electrophysiologic Measures of Frequency-Specific Auditory Function,* these authors provide an excellent summary of alternative signal source generation and its correlation to audiometric data. Additionally, Fowler and Durrant, Chapter 10, *Effects of Peripheral Hearing Loss on the Auditory Brainstem Response,* detail the precautions of test interpretation when either conductive, sensory hearing loss, or both, are present.

Auditory Assessment

In the assessment of residual auditory sensitivity, a primary objective of the ABR is to identify, as accurately as possible, the patient's hearing status. This is normally accomplished in one of two ways. The first involves the monitoring of the evoked response while systematically decreasing the stimulus intensity until the presence of a brainstem response is no longer replicated. Typically, the absolute latency of each wave peak is measured and compared to some established data base. In ABR, the wave V peak component is most often used to estimate threshold. The resulting estimated difference between the electrophysiologic and behavioral thresholds is noted. Thresholds are dependent on pathologic conditions and technical parameters used in ABR measurement. Due to these variables, the two thresholds are unlikely to be identical. The electrophysiologic threshold is about 10 dB elevated in adults and approximately 10 to 15 dB elevated in the infant population when compared to psychophysical estimates. Figure 1.3 is an illustration of ABR threshold results in an adult subject with normal auditory sensitivity and no evidence of neurotologic insult.

The second method applies an input-output function as a means of assessing auditory sensitivity. In the case of the ABR, this usually describes the relationship between the stimulus intensity and the latency of the brainstem response. This is known as the latency-intensity function and involves a comparison of wave V latencies (most frequently used peak amplitude al-

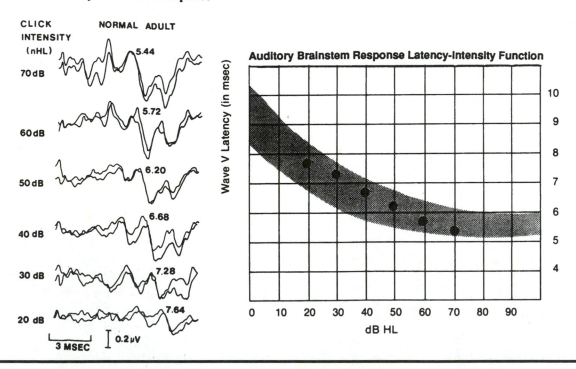

FIGURE 1.3.   A series of ABR traces obtained from a normal hearing adult subject. The latency-intensity function is plotted based on the latency of wave V.

though other waves can also be compared) at several intensity levels to an established normative data base. The result is a slope function measured in milli- or microseconds per decibel. Although somewhat variable, the adult slope function is about 0.04 ms/dB with a range of 0.03 to 0.06 ms/dB (Galambos and Hecox, 1978). The advantage of the latency-intensity function is that it provides a standard from which site-of-lesion determination may be evaluated. Deviations of greater than 0.06 ms/dB are indicative of sensory pathology, whereas slope functions of 0.03 ms/dB or less suggest primarily high-frequency hearing loss (Hecox and Jacobson, 1984). For slope functions that parallel but are offset in latency, conductive pathology is suspect. Figure 1.3 plots a latency-intensity function based on the ABR traces in the same figure. An accurate estimate of auditory sensitivity can be made based on: 1) the presence of a repeatable wave peak; 2) the latency of a response; and 3) the plotted latency-intensity configuration.

Neurotologic Investigation

The second major application of the ABR and perhaps the most significant in its role as a diagnostic tool is the identification of neurotologic disease. As cited, the sensitivity of the ABR to predict eighth nerve and brainstem lesions has been uncanny. This ability has not been exclusively limited to space-occupying lesions but also encompasses demyelinating and degenerative diseases and vascular lesions. The ABR is also used in the examination of high-risk neurologically impaired newborns confined to the neonatal intensive care nursery. Finally,

neurologic application of the ABR is being used with growing interest as an intraoperative monitoring technique and in comatose and other neurologically compromised patients.

Implicit in clinical neurotologic application is the understanding that any evoked potential will reveal only functional abnormality and not specific pathologic locus. In addition to the complexity of the brainstem pathway, the size, number, and impingement of the lesion at any particular point will influence the resulting response. Further it is important to recall that any peripheral abnormality will affect the interpretation of the neurotologic assessment. Therefore, it is imperative to know the status of the peripheral mechanism and its influence on the brainstem response prior to judgmental inference about the neurotologic condition.

SUMMARY

From this brief overview it can be seen that AEP techniques and their clinical applications have become an integral part of the audiologic, neurotologic, and other central test batteries. As instrumentation improves and clinical applications broaden to other disciplines, there will be an ever increasing demand on clinical service and skill level. The ease with which AEPs can be performed should not, however, fool the naive. AEPs must be respected, conducted and interpreted by knowledgeable professionals. Their variability, subjectivity, and sophisticated instrumentation do not lend themselves to use by the casual operator.

REFERENCES

Berger, H. (1929). Uber das elektroenkephalogram des menschen. *Archives für Psychiatrie und Nervenkrankheiten, 87*, 527–570.

Clark, W. A., Jr. (1958). *Average response computer (ARC-1).* Quarterly Progress Report No. 49. Research Laboratory of Electronics, Massachusetts Institute of Technology. Cambridge, MA: MIT Press.

Clark, W. A., Jr., Goldstein, M. H., Jr., Brown, R. M., Molnar, C. E., O'Brien D. F., and Zieman, H. E. (1961). The average response computer (ARC): A digital device for computing

averages and amplitudes and time histograms of electrophysiological responses. *Transactions of IRE, 8*, 46–51.

Davis, H. (1976). Principles of electric response audiometry. *Annals of Otology, Rhinology, and Laryngology, 85*, Supplement 28.

Davis, H., Davis, P. A., Loomis, A. L., Harvey, E. N., and Hobart, G. (1939). Electrical reactions of the human brain to auditory stimulation during sleep. *Journal of Neurophysiology, 2*, 500–514.

Davis, H. and Zerlin, S. (1966). Acoustic relations of the

human vertex potential. *Journal of the Acoustical Society of America, 39*, 109–116.

Dawson, G. D. (1951). A summation technique for detecting small signals in a large, irregular background. *Journal of Physiology, 115*, 2P-3P.

Dawson, G. D. (1954). A summation technique for the detection of small evoked potentials. *Electroencephalography and Clinical Neurophysiology, 6*, 65–84.

Eggermont, J., Don, M., and Brackman, D. (1980). Electrocochleography and auditory brainstem electric responses in patients with pontine angle tumors. *Annals of Otology, Rhinology, and Laryngology, Supplement 75*.

Fria, T. J. (1980). The auditory brainstem response: Background and clinical applications. *Maico Monographs in Contemporary Audiology, 2*, 1–44.

Galambos, R. and Hecox, K. (1978). Clinical application of the auditory brainstem response. *Otolaryngologic Clinics of North America, 11*, 709–722.

Geisler, C. D., Frishkopf, L. S., and Rosenblith, W. A. (1958). Extracranial responses to acoustic clicks in man. *Science, 128*, 1210–1211.

Gibson, W. P. R. (1978). *Essentials of clinical evoked response audiometry.* New York: Churchill Livingstone.

Glasscock, M., Jackson, C., Josey, A., Dickins, J., and Wiet, R. (1979). Brainstem evoked response audiometry in clinical practice. *Laryngoscope, 89*, 1021–1034.

Goldstein, R. and Rodman, L. B. (1967). Early components of averaged evoked responses to rapidly repeated auditory stimuli. *Journal of Speech and Hearing Research, 10*, 697–705.

Hall, J. W. III. (1992). *The handbook of auditory evoked responses.* Boston, MA: Allyn and Bacon.

Hecox, K. and Jacobson, J. T. (1984). Auditory evoked potentials. In J. L. Northern (ed.), *Hearing disorders.* Boston: Little, Brown.

Jacobson, J. T. and Hyde, M. (1985). An introduction to auditory evoked potentials. In J. Katz (ed.), *Handbook of clinical audiology.* Baltimore: Williams & Wilkins.

Jacobson, J. T., Morehouse, C. R., and Johnson, M. J. (1982). Strategies for infant auditory brainstem response assessment. *Ear and Hearing, 3*, 263–270.

Jewett, D. L. (1970). Volume conducted potentials in response to auditory stimuli as detected by averaging in the cat. *Electroencephalography and Clinical Neurophysiology, 28*, 609–618.

Jewett, D. L. (1983). Introduction. In E. Moore (ed.), *Bases of auditory brain-stem evoked responses.* New York: Grune & Stratton.

Jewett, D. L. and Romano, M. N. (1972). Neonatal development of auditory system potentials from the scalp of rat and cat. *Brain Research, 36*, 101–115.

Jewett, D. L., Romano, M. N., and Williston, J. S. (1970). Human auditory evoked potentials: Possible brain stem components detected on scalp. *Science, 167*, 1517–1518.

Jewett, D. L. and Williston, J. S. (1971). Auditory evoked far fields averaged from the scalp of humans. *Brain, 94*, 681–696.

Loomis, A., Harvey, E., and Hobart, G. (1938). Disturbances of patterns in sleep. *Journal of Neurophysiology, 1*, 413–430.

Mendel, M.I. and Goldstein, R. (1969). Stability of the early components of the averaged electroencephalic response. *Journal of Speech and Hearing Research, 12*, 351–361.

Møller, A.R. (1981). Latency in the ascending auditory pathway determined using continuous sounds: Comparison between transient and envelope latency. *Brain Research, 207*, 184–188.

Møller, A.R. (1982). Signal processing in the auditory system and how it may relate to binaural hearing. *Scandinavian Audiology, Supplement 15*, 65–79.

Moore, E. (ed.), (1983). *Bases of auditory brain-stem evoked responses.* New York: Grune & Stratton.

Picton, T. W., and Fitzgerald, P. G. (1983). A general description of the human auditory evoked potentials. In E. J. Moore (ed.), *Basis of auditory brainstem evoked responses* (141–156). New York: Grune & Stratton.

Picton, T. W., Hillyard, S. H., Krauz, H. J., and Galambos, R. (1974). Human auditory evoked potentials. 1. Evaluation components. *Electroencephalography and Clinical Neurophysiology, 36*, 179–190.

Picton, T. W., Linden, R. D., Hamel, G., and Maru, J. T. (1983). Aspects of averaging. *Seminars in Hearing, 4*, 327–340.

Picton, T. W. and Smith, A.D. (1978). The practice of evoked potential audiometry. *Otolaryngologic Clinics of North America, 11(2)*, 263–82.

Picton, T. W., Woods, D. L., Baribeau-Braun, J., and Healey, T. (1977). Evoked potentials audiometry. *Journal of Otolaryngology, 6*, 90–118.

Reneau, J. P. and Hnatiow, G. Z. (1975). *Evoked response audiometry: A topical and historical review.* Baltimore: University Park Press.

Ruben, R. J., Sekula, J., Bordley, J. E., Knickerbocker, G. G., Nager, G. T., and Fisch, U. (1960). Human cochlear responses to sound stimuli. *Annals of Otology, Rhinology, and Laryngology, 69*, 459–476.

Selters, W. and Brackman, D. (1979). Brainstem electric response audiometry acoustic tumor detection. In W. House and C. Luetje (eds.), *Acoustic tumors*. Baltimore: University Park Press.

Sohmer, H., and Feinmesser, M. (1967). Cochlear action potentials recorded from the external ear in man. *Annals of Otology, Rhinology, and Laryngology, 76*, 427–438.

Sohmer, H. and Feinmesser, M. (1973). Routine use of electrocochleography (cochlear audiometry) in human subjects. *Audiology, 12*, 167–173.

Spehlmann, R. (1985). *Evoked potential primer: Visual, auditory, and somatosensory evoked potentials in clinical diagnosis*. Boston: Butterworth.

Teas, D.C., Eldredge, D.H., and Davis, H. (1962). Cochlear responses to acoustic transients: an interpretation of the whole-nerve action potentials. *Journal of the Acoustical Society of America, 34*, 1438–1459.

Terkildsen, K., Osterhammel, P., and Thomsen, J. (1981). The ABR and MLR in patients with acoustic neuromas. *Scandinavian Audiology, Supplement 13*, 103–108.

Thornton, A.R.D. (1975). The diagnostic potential of surface recorded electrocochleography. *British Journal of Audiology 9*, 7–13.

Walter, E.G., Cooper, R., Aldridge, V.J., McCallum, W.C., and Winter, A.L. (1964). Contingent negative variation: an electric sign of sensorimotor association and expectancy in the human brain. *Nature, 203*, 380–384.

CHAPTER 2

NEURAL GENERATORS OF AUDITORY EVOKED POTENTIALS

AAGE R. MØLLER

Potentials that are related to a transient sound can be recorded from electrodes placed on the scalp during a period as long as 500 ms after the onset of the sound. The aim of this chapter is to present a contemporary review of our understanding of the origin of these potentials, i.e., which anatomical structures generate these potentials.

TYPES OF AUDITORY EVOKED POTENTIALS AND THEIR USES

The auditory evoked potentials that are clinically useful can be separated into three types on the basis of their latencies: 1) short-latency potentials are cochlear potentials called electrocochleographic (ECoG) potentials and auditory brainstem responses (ABR), which occur within the first 10 ms after the presentation of a transient stimulus; 2) middle-latency potentials, called middle-latency responses (MLR), which occur at latencies from 10 to 50 (or 100) ms; and 3) long-latency potentials, called event-related potentials (ERP), which occur at latencies between 100 and 300 (or 500) ms.

Auditory evoked potentials with latencies up to 50 ms (ABR and MLR) are essentially a result of the progressive propagation of auditory neural activity through the ascending auditory pathway, including the ear and the auditory cortex. These potentials can be observed by recording from electrodes placed on the surface of the head, and they represent complex transformations of the summation of the electrical fields of many nerve fibers and nerve cells. Long-latency potentials (ERP) are generated by numerous higher brain centers that receive input from the auditory system.

During the past decade we have seen an increase in the use of ABR in making otoneurologic diagnoses (see other chapters in this book) (Chiappa, 1983). In addition, ABRs are being used increasingly intraoperatively to monitor the function of the auditory nerve for the purpose of reducing the risk of neurologic deficits in neurosurgical operations in which the auditory nerve is being manipulated. Monitoring of ABR has also been found to be useful in neurosurgical operations in which there is a risk of compressing the brainstem (Møller, 1988a), as well as in patients in whom trauma has occurred to the head (Hall and Hargadine, 1985; Jacobson, 1985). Middle-latency responses (MLR) have only recently begun to be used to aid in neurologic diagnoses (Musiek et al., 1984a); at present MLR are seldom monitored intraoperatively. Long-latency auditory evoked potentials (ERP) have been used in studies of higher brain functions (Regan, 1989).

Recently, the function of the auditory nervous system has been studied using recordings of the magnetic field that is generated by neural activity in higher auditory centers, and that can be recorded by placing sensitive magnetometers outside the head (Weinberg et al., 1987; Hari and Ilmoniemi, 1986). There are indications that the characteristics of this recorded magnetic activity may provide information of clinical use if equipment can be developed to record these events reliably and practically in the clinical setting.

For any type of auditory evoked potentials to be useful clinically, we must know the anatomical origin of the various components of the recorded potentials and how various pathologies affect these potentials. To understand how the far-field potentials that can be recorded from electrodes placed on the scalp are generated, however, we must first consider the electrical activity that is generated by single nerve fibers and nerve cells, as well as the potentials that can be recorded from nerves, fiber tracts, or nuclei through electrodes placed in direct contact with the structures in question.

Electrical Activity in the Auditory Nervous System

A microelectrode placed on a single nerve fiber or nerve cell in a nucleus can record the electrical activity in that fiber or cell. This activity appears as neural discharges or spikes, but the potentials that can be recorded from the surface of a nerve or a nucleus with a gross electrode are the summation of the neural discharges generated in a large number of individual nerve fibers or nerve cells. When recorded from a nerve, such potentials are known as compound action potentials (CAPs). Assuming that the waveforms of all single-unit discharges are identical, the waveform of a CAP is the convolution between the sum of the distribution of nerve impulses in the nerve fibers that contribute to the response and the waveform of a single neural discharge (Goldstein, 1960). The responses that are generated by nuclei are more complex than those generated by nerves and fiber tracts and they have two main sources: *dendrites*, which usually produce relatively slow potentials; and the cell bodies that, when discharging, produce sharp electrical impulses (as do nerve fibers). The gross responses that originate from cell discharges are known as *somaspikes*.

Essentially, all structures of the ascending auditory pathway from the auditory nerve to the various fiber tracts and nuclei produce distinct near-field potentials when they are activated by a transient sound. What these near-field potentials contribute to the far-field potentials, however, depends not only on the magnitude of the near-field potentials but also on a number of other factors. Thus, the far-field potential that results from propagated activity in a *long nerve* seems to depend to a large extent on these two factors: 1) whether the nerve has a straight course or is bent (Gardi et al., 1987; Chimento et al., 1987); and 2) the electrical conductivity of the surrounding media (Lueders et al., 1983).

For the far-field potential produced by a *nucleus*, on the other hand, the relationship to the near-field potential depends to a great extent on the internal organization of the nucleus. Thus, a nucleus in which the dendrites have a uniform orientation (open field) produces a strong far-field potential, whereas an equally activated nucleus in which the cell bodies are in the center and the dendrites are organized in such a way that they point in all directions (closed field) will produce small far-field potentials (Lorente de No, 1947*b*) (Figure 2.1). However, the near-field potentials that can be recorded by placing an electrode directly on the exposed surface of a nucleus will show little difference in these two types of nuclei. Comparison between the near-field and the far-field potentials of different nuclei of the ascending auditory pathway has shown that some of these nuclei contribute little to the far-field potentials (ABRs), despite the fact that a large response can be recorded from their surfaces (Møller and Burgess, 1986). While dendrites in the cortex point in nearly the same direction, so that they are likely to have a large far-field, there may be differences in the far-field potentials recorded from the cortex, depending on how large an area of the cortex is activated synchronously. We will present some detailed results from

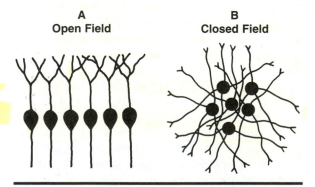

FIGURE 2.1.   Two different types of organizations of cells in a nucleus. A: Open field. B: Closed field. (Modified from Lorente de No, 1947*b*.)

such studies later in this chapter and discuss the cause of that phenomenon and the implications for the use of ABRs in clinical diagnosis.

Identification of the Neural Generators of Auditory Evoked Potentials

The fundamental reason that it is possible to separate the contributions to the far-field response from different structures in the ascending auditory pathway is that the nerve tracts and nuclei of the pathway are activated in succession in response to a transient stimulus. This means that, in general, the contributions made to the response by different structures in the pathway appear in the far-field potentials as components that are separated in time—that is, these components appear with different latencies. This generalization does not hold true in every case, however. Due to the complexity of the ascending auditory pathway, which includes pronounced parallel processing of auditory information, contributions from different structures to a certain transient stimulus may appear with the same latency, and the contributions from such sources become indistinguishable in a far-field recording.

Essentially three different methods have been used to identify the neural generators of auditory evoked potentials. One is based on simultaneous recording from electrodes placed on the scalp and different structures of the auditory nervous system when they become exposed during neurosurgical operations or during stereotactic procedures. The intracranially recorded potentials are then correlated with the far-field potentials.

The second method makes use of pathologies that are known to affect specific structures of the ascending auditory pathway. A prerequisite for the use of this method is that both the location and the extension of the pathology is known so that it can be related to the deviations from normal in the far-field evoked potentials. Recordings in animals and animal experiments in which controlled lesions are made in specific areas of the auditory pathway have been used to study and compare the recorded (near-field) responses and far-field responses.

In addition, three-dimensional recording techniques have been used to identify dipole sources using a Lissajous

presentation of the results. However, this method does not allow unique identification of the individual sources of specific components of far-field evoked potentials (Gardi et al., 1987; Chimento et al., 1987; Pratt et al., 1985; Scherg and von Cramon, 1985).

All of these methods have shortcomings that are important to consider when evaluating the results of studies in which these methods are used. Thus, as Arezzo et al. (1979) pointed out, it is not possible to identify with certainty the intracranial sources of the various components of the far-field potentials recorded from the surface of the scalp by comparing latencies of the near-field potentials with latencies of the various components of the far-field potentials. Potentials from other sources may have the same latency, and their contributions to the surface-recorded potential may thus be indistinguishable from the contributions of the structure in question. Also, a source may generate weak far-field potentials, even though strong potentials can be recorded when an electrode is placed directly on the structure.

The use of changes in far-field potentials caused by pathologies has the shortcoming that the anatomical extent of a lesion can seldom be assessed accurately, and it is not usually known how much a radiologically identifiable lesion reduces the function of the structure in question. Finally, there is a problem with the use of animal experiments designed to assess the generators of auditory evoked potentials due to the uncertainty in translating data from one species to another. One important such difference between animals commonly used in experimental research and man is head size, but there are other possible differences.

AUDITORY BRAINSTEM RESPONSES (ABRs)

Auditory Brainstem Responses (ABRs) are the potentials that appear during the first 10 ms after a transient stimulus. When recorded in the traditional clinical way—differentially between an electrode placed at the vertex and one placed on the ipsilateral mastoid (or earlobe)—the ABRs in man typically consist of five vertex-positive peaks. In many subjects, however, a clear sixth peak can be seen to follow the fifth peak.

These peaks are usually labeled by Roman numerals, a system introduced by Jewett and Williston (1971). This system of labeling peaks in the ABR is inconsistent with conventions for labeling other sensory evoked potentials. A positive peak in other evoked potentials is usually labeled "P" followed by a number that represents the peak's normal latency value; a negative peak is labeled "N" followed by a number that represents the peak's normal latency value.

Although both the electrodes in the configuration are usually used to record ABR record auditory evoked potentials, the vertex electrode may be regarded as the (most) active electrode, and many times ABRs are displayed with vertex positivity as an upward deflection as is found throughout the remainder of this book. In this chapter, however, we will follow the convention used for other evoked potentials—and, indeed, most neuroelectric potentials—namely, showing negativity at the active electrode as an upward deflection.

The exact waveform of the recorded ABR is affected by the filters used in the recordings. Since the clinically most important feature of the ABR is the latencies of the different peaks, we, in our own clinic as well as for research purposes, routinely use aggressive filtering, not only to attenuate noise but also to enhance individual peaks (Møller and Møller, 1985; Møller, 1988a,b). We can perform such filtering without causing any shift in time of the peaks by using zero-phase digital filters (Møller, 1988b). The use of digital filtering avoids problems that occur with electronic filters, such as errors in the form of uneven shifts in the locations of the various peaks caused by the fact that most electronic filters have a phase shift that is not a linear function of the frequency (Doyle and Hyde, 1981; Boston and Ainslie, 1980).

As mentioned above, the far-field potentials recorded from the ear and the auditory nervous system in the brainstem are thought to be mainly of two types: 1) summations of the neural discharges of many nerve fibers in nerves and fiber tracts or nerve cells (soma-spikes), and 2) potentials generated by dendrites. Potentials of the first type are dependent upon a precise time-locking of the neural discharges in individual nerve fibers to the time pattern of the stimulus sound (phase-locking). These potentials are most prominent

in response to transient sounds such as click sounds or short tonebursts with fast rise times, and they appear as sharp peaks in the far-field potentials.

The second type of potential is the slow potential. These potentials are much less dependent on the synchrony of firing and, therefore, are less dependent on the transient nature of the stimulus. However, such slow potentials may be attenuated by filtering the recorded potentials and they may also be less prominent in a far-field recording because they are generated by nuclei that have a more-or-less closed field.

Anatomical Basis of ABR

The interpretation of ABRs is complicated by the complexity of the ascending auditory pathway: the auditory system is more complex than other sensory systems and there are several connections between the left and right sides (Moore, 1987a,b; Jungert, 1958; Morest et al., 1973). The main nerve tracts and nuclei of the auditory system are outlined in Figure 2.2. What is shown schematically in Figure 2.2 is, however, only one part of the ascending auditory pathway—the lemniscal system. There is a parallel system, the extralemniscal system, which is more diffuse and less well understood both anatomically and physiologically than the lemniscal system. The extralemniscal pathway is located in the core of the brainstem and its contribution to auditory evoked potentials is unknown.

The lemniscal pathway has four main relay nuclei between the ear and the auditory cortex. The auditory nerve fibers terminate in the cochlear nucleus complex, that mainly contains second-order neurons but also contains neurons of higher order. Three fiber tracts ascend from the cochlear nucleus: 1) the stria of Monakow, which is located most dorsally and which terminates largely in the nucleus of the contralateral-lateral lemniscus and the inferior colliculus; 2) the stria of Held, which is located medially, and 3) the ventral stria (trapezoidal body). All three striae make connections with the numerous subnuclei of the superior olivary complex (Figure 2.2B).

The superior olivary complex contains mainly third-order neurons and serves as the first relay nucleus

(A)

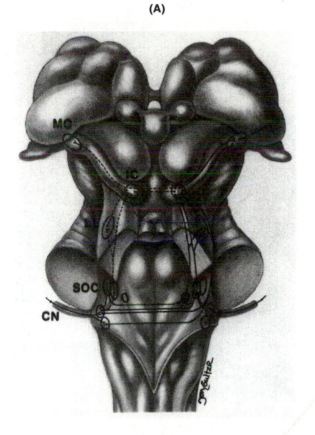

(B)

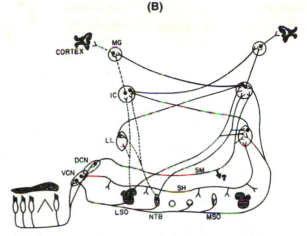

FIGURE 2.2. (A) Illustration of how the main auditory nuclei and fiber tracts are located in the brain. CN: cochlear nucleus; SOC: superior olivary complex; IC: inferior colliculus; MG: medial geniculate. (from Møller, 1988a.) (B) Schematic drawing of the ascending auditory pathway. VCN: ventral cochlear nucleus; DCN: dorsal cochlear nucleus; SO: superior olivary complex; TB: trapezoidal body; SM: stria of Monakow (dorsal stria); SH: stria of Held (intermediate stria); LL: lateral lemniscus; IC: inferior colliculus; MG: medial geniculate body (from Møller, 1983b).

that receives input from both ears. From the superior olivary complex, connections are made to the inferior colliculus via the lateral lemniscus, mostly by neurons that receive their input from the opposite ear. Some fibers leaving the cochlear nucleus, however, reach the nucleus of the ipsilateral lateral lemniscus. Fibers leaving the inferior colliculus reach the thalamic auditory relay nucleus (medial geniculate body) via the brachium of the inferior colliculus. The primary auditory cortex receives its input from this nucleus.

We shall, in the following section, discuss the different potentials that can be recorded from the cochlea, the auditory nerve, and the nuclei and nerve tracts of the ascending auditory pathway. We will then show how these potentials relate to the ABRs recorded by the conventional methods used in clinical studies.

Electrical Potentials of the Ear and the Auditory Nerve

Several different sound-evoked potentials can be recorded from the *cochlea*: the cochlear microphonic (CM), the summating potential (SP), and the compound action potential (CAP) (Dallos, 1973; Møller, 1983b). These potentials can be recorded from an electrode placed on the round window or from various types of electrodes placed inside the cochlea. The CM and the SP appear in response to sound stimulation with essentially no delay, whereas the initial components of the CAP appear with a latency of about 1 ms when elicited by a broadband click sound. Sounds of different types will evoke all three potentials, but each potential is most clearly seen in response to a particular type of sound. Thus, the CM is best seen in response to pure tones of relatively low frequency, the SP is best elicited by tones of high frequency, and the CAP is best seen in response to transient sounds such as clicks or tonebursts with rapid rise. In small animals such as cats, guinea pigs, and rats, the CAP that can be recorded from the cochlea shows two negative peaks (N_1 and N_2) (Figure 2.3A): the earliest one (N_1) is believed to represent the synchronized discharges in many auditory nerve fibers, and the latter one (N_2) is believed to represent the discharges of nerve cells in the cochlear nucleus (Fisch and Ruben, 1962; Møller, 1983a). Potentials of similar waveforms can be recorded from the exposed *auditory nerve* in small animals.

In man, however, the potentials recorded from the cochlea (promontorium or round window) (Figure 2.3B) mainly consist of a single negative potential that is essentially lacking the N_2 component seen in the potentials recorded from small animals (Elberling, 1976; Eggermont, 1974; Spoor et al., 1976). The lack of a clear second negative (N_2) component in the human cochlear CAP is probably a result of the longer distance in man between the recording site and the cochlear nucleus compared to that in small animals in which the cochlear nucleus is located very close to the cochlea. The auditory nerve in man is about 2.5 cm long (Lang, 1981), while in the animals usually used in studies of the auditory system the auditory nerve is only about 0.5 cm long.

When the human response to transient sounds is recorded from the exposed intracranial portion of the eighth nerve with a monopolar electrode, it appears as a triphasic wave. The triphasic waveform of the response obtained when recording the near-field potential from a long nerve represents the second derivative of the action potential of a single nerve fiber (Lorente de No, 1947a). The earliest deflection in this triphasic wave is a small, positive deflection, which is followed by a large negative peak that in turn is followed by a smaller positive deflection (Møller and Jannetta, 1981; Hashimoto et al., 1981; Spire et al., 1982; Møller et al., 1981a,b, 1982, 1988a) (Figure 2.3).

The potentials recorded from the intracranial portion of the human auditory nerve decrease in amplitude and their latencies increase when the stimulus intensity is decreased (Figure 2.4), which is similar to what is seen in animals. The earliest components of the potentials recorded from the eighth nerve near the porus acusticus have shorter latencies than do those recorded

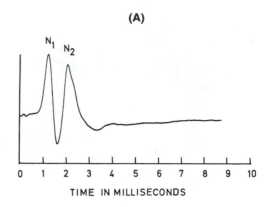

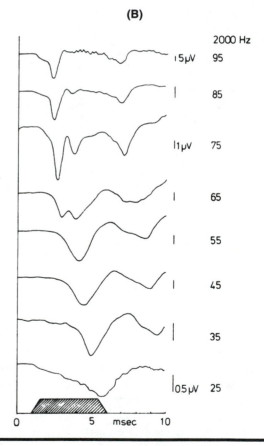

FIGURE 2.3. Compound action potentials recorded from the round window of a rat (from Møller, unpublished) (A) and from the promontorium of a human subject with normal hearing; (B) negativity down (from Eggermont et al., 1976).

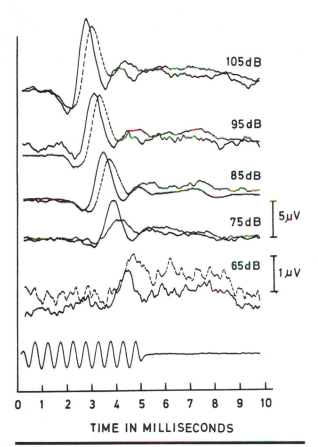

105 dB

95 dB

85 dB

75 dB   5 μV

65 dB   1 μV

0 1 2 3 4 5 6 7 8 9 10

TIME IN MILLISECONDS

FIGURE 2.4. Recordings made from the auditory nerve of a patient undergoing a neurosurgical operation in which the eighth nerve was exposed. The results obtained at different stimulus intensities are shown in decibels above normal human hearing threshold. The sound stimuli were 2000 Hz tonebursts of 5 ms duration presented through an insert earphone. Solid lines represent responses from a location slightly more distal on the nerve than the responses represented by dashed lines (from Møller and Jannetta, 1981).

from the nerve at a location near the brainstem. This indicates that these potentials represent propagated neural activity that is subjected to neural delay, and not volume-conducted potentials from, for instance, the ear.

The latency of the negative peak in the response from the intracranial portion of the auditory nerve at a position halfway between the porus acusticus and the

brainstem in patients with normal hearing is slightly more than 3 ms when the stimulus is short bursts of a 2000 Hz tone at 100 dB above normal hearing threshold (Møller et al., 1981a; Møller and Jannetta, 1981). The latency of the response to click sounds at an intensity similar to that used clinically is 2.58 ms for rarefaction clicks and 2.69 ms for condensation clicks (average of 14 patients) (Møller et al., 1988), thus slightly shorter than the latency of the response to 2000 Hz tonebursts. This is about 1 ms longer than the N_1 that can be recorded from the round window of the human cochlea (Elberling, 1976; Eggermont, 1974), a difference that represents the time it takes for the neural impulses to pass from their origin at the auditory nerve in the cochlea to the recording site on the intracranial portion of the auditory nerve. This distance is about 2 cm, and the delay of 1 ms thus corresponds to a conduction velocity of about 20 m/s. This correlates well with the conduction velocity of 20 to 40 m/sec expected from a nerve, such as the auditory nerve in man, composed of fibers with a diameter of 2 to 4 μ (Engstrom and Rexed, 1940; Lazorthes et al., 1961). More recently, Spoendlin and Schrott (1989) found that the diameter of nerve fibers in the human auditory nerve increases with age and so does the range of fiber diameters. In young children the distribution of the diameters of the cochlear nerve fibers has a sharp maximum around 2.5 μm.

Relationship of Cochlear and Auditory Nerve Potentials to ABRs

Comparison of the potentials recorded directly from the intracranial portion of the eighth nerve with ABRs recorded intracranially from electrodes placed on the vertex and the earlobe shows that the auditory nerve potential recorded from the proximal end of the auditory nerve appears with about the same latency as does peak II of the ABR (Figure 2.5) (Møller et al., 1981a,b, 1982; Møller and Jannetta, 1983c; Spire et al., 1982; Møller et al., 1988). Because the auditory nerve in man is a long nerve, it gives rise to two separate peaks in the ABR, while in animals it is much shorter and therefore only one peak can be discerned in the far-field response. Thus, while peak I in the ABR in man, as well

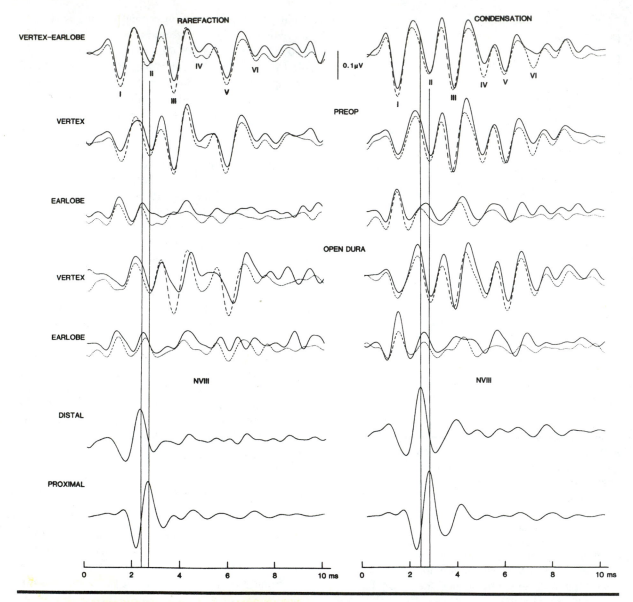

FIGURE 2.5. Recordings obtained in a patient who had a compression of the eighth nerve by a blood vessel near the porus acusticus. The stimuli were rarefaction clicks (115 dB Pe SPL) presented at a rate of 18 pps. The upper calibration refers to the recordings from electrodes placed on the scalp. The amplitude of the compound action potentials recorded from the auditory nerve varied from 20 to 50 μV, depending on the degree of shunting from cerebrospinal fluid (from Møller et al., 1988).

as in small animals, is generated by the distal portion of the auditory nerve, there is evidence that the origin of peak II in man is the proximal portion of the auditory nerve (Møller et al., 1981a,b; Møller and Jannetta, 1981, 1982a; Møller et al., 1988), while in small animals it is most likely generated in the cochlear nucleus (Fisch and Ruben, 1962; Møller, 1983a). The results of recent experiments thus show that there is a fundamental difference between the far-field potentials generated by the auditory nerve in man and those generated by the auditory nerve in small animals: whereas the results of earlier experiments in animals were thought to show that the origin of the second vertex-positive peaks in the ABR in man is secondary neurons located in the cochlear nucleus (Buchwald and Huang, 1975; Huang and Buchwald, 1977; Achor and Starr, 1980a,b; Britt and Rossi, 1980; Rossi and Britt, 1980) or that the cochlear nucleus at least plays a role in the generation of this peak (Hashimoto et al., 1981), the results of recent studies (Møller et al., 1988) confirm that it is the portion of the eighth nerve close to the brainstem that generates peak II in the human vertex ABR recording. The interpretation from intracranial recordings that the auditory nerve in man generates two separate peaks in the ABR (I and II) has been supported by other studies using different techniques (Scherg and von Cramon, 1985).

The question of how a long nerve can generate stationary peaks in the far-field potentials is not completely resolved, but the results of several investigations show that the electrical conductivity of the surrounding media plays an important role in the generation of far-field peaks from propagated activity in a (long) nerve (Kimura et al., 1983, 1984; Lueders et al., 1983). Others (Chimento et al., 1987; Jewett, 1987) have shown that the waveshape of a far-field potential generated by a long nerve is related to whether the nerve has a straight course or is bent.

In conclusion, the results of experiments in small animals such as the cat cannot directly explain the origin of the early components in the human ABR. The important anatomical differences between the animal that is being studied and man, particularly the difference in the lengths of their auditory nerves, must be taken into account for the results of animal experiments to be used appropriately in determining the neural generators of the ABR in man.

The way ABRs are traditionally recorded is not optimal for the purpose of relating the different components of the ABR to specific intracranial sources. This is because the ABRs recorded in the traditional way represent the difference between the potentials recorded from electrodes placed at two locations—the vertex and the mastoid—with both electrodes recording a response to an acoustic stimulus. The responses recorded by two such electrodes are different, so the ABR recorded differentially between two such electrodes will be a combination of two auditory evoked potentials. As the potentials that are recorded from two locations are slightly shifted in time, the resulting ABR will have peaks with latencies different from the latencies of peaks in the potentials recorded at either of the two electrode locations (Terkildsen et al., 1974; Møller et al., 1988) (Figure 2.6). This adds uncertainty to the identification of the neural generators of the different components of the ABR.

The use of a noncephalic reference,[1] which makes it possible to study the contributions from the vertex electrode and the earlobe electrode separately, has led to more precise information about the contribution from the intracranial portion of the auditory nerve (Møller and Jannetta, 1984; Møller et al., 1988). These results have supported the finding that it is the intracranial portion of the auditory nerve, specifically the portion of the audi-

---

[1]Noncephalic references are used to record selectively from certain locations on the scalp. If no potentials are recorded by the reference electrode to auditory stimulation, this implies that all auditory potentials are true responses to auditory stimulation. Much work has been devoted to analyzing such situations, and it has been found that placement of reference electrodes at any place on the body outside the head is equivalent to placing the reference electrode for the recording in a plane through the neck. There is thus no difference in the auditory evoked potentials picked up by reference electrodes placed at various locations on the body. Secondly, it has been debated whether any noncephalic reference can be regarded as being totally "silent" with regard to picking up auditory potentials. Another unrelated finding is that a noncephalic reference will pick up interference signals, such as biologic potentials from muscles, particularly the heart muscles, and also externally generated electrical interference, to a much greater extent than will cephalic references.

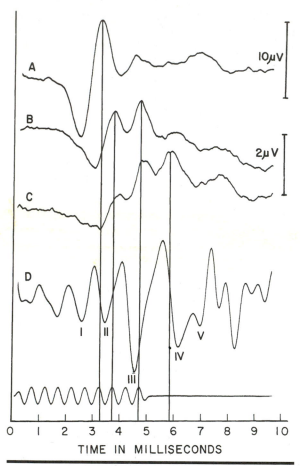

FIGURE 2.6. Comparison between potentials recorded at different locations on the auditory nerve and brainstem from a patient undergoing a microvascular decompression operation for hemifacial spasm. (A) Recording from the eighth nerve near the porus acusticus. (B) Similar recording made near the entrance of the eighth nerve into the brainstem. (C) Recording made from a location on the brainstem about 4 mm medial and rostral to the entrance of the eighth nerve that is assumed to overlie the superior olivary complex. (D) ABR recorded simultaneously from scalp electrodes. The stimuli were 2000 Hz tonebursts of 5 ms duration presented with an interstimulus interval of 150 ms. The recording bandpass for the potentials recorded intracranially was 3 to 3000 Hz, and the ABR were digitally filtered to enhance the peaks (from Møller and Jannetta, 1984).

tory nerve that is close to the brainstem (proximal portion), that is the generator of peak II in conventionally recorded human ABRs (Møller et al., 1988).

The example in Figure 2.5 shows that the vertex electrode recorded early, high-amplitude components of the ABR. More often, however, earlier components of recordings from the vertex have smaller amplitudes, and peaks V, VI, and VII are more prominent. In recordings from the earlobe the first three or four peaks usually have the largest amplitudes, while peaks V, VI, and VII have relatively low amplitudes.

The mean latencies of the peaks of potentials recorded intracranially varied from patient to patient, as did the latencies of the peaks in the potentials recorded from electrodes placed on the scalp, but the mean values illustrated in Table 2.1 show a good agreement between the latency of peak II and the negative peak in the potentials recorded directly from the intracranial portion of the auditory nerve.

Potentials Generated by the Cochlear Nucleus and Superior Olivary Complex

The cochlear nucleus is located near the entrance of the eighth nerve into the brainstem, and it is relatively larger in small animals than in man, where it is pushed caudally by the inferior cerebellar peduncle. This location in man makes it difficult to gain direct access to the cochlear nucleus for recording during neurosurgical operations. Potentials recorded from the vicinity of the cochlear nucleus, such as from the brainstem at the point where the eighth nerve enters, contain a slow, negative potential that follows a sharp, negative peak (Figure 2.6); a second negative peak is seen about 1 ms after the first negative peak. This second negative peak is most likely generated by second-order auditory neurons located in the cochlear nucleus, while the slow potential is probably generated by dendrites in the cochlear nucleus (Møller and Jannetta, 1982a). The latency of the second peak remains unchanged while its amplitude increases (Figure 2.6,A,B) as the recording site is moved towards the brainstem, indicating that this second negative potential represents potentials that are conducted passively to the recording electrode from a stationary source, and it is reasonable to assume that the source of this second

TABLE 2.1. Latencies of positive peaks in the recording from the vertex and those of the negative peaks in the recording from the earlobe obtained after the patient was anesthetized, but before the beginning of the operation, compared with latency values of the negative peaks in the recording from the intracranial portion of the eighth nerve. Also shown are the latencies of the vertex-positive peaks in differential recordings from the vertex and earlobe made after the patient was anesthetized, but before the beginning of the operation (from Møller et al., 1988).

PT	DX*	Click polarity	Vertex (pos. peaks)			Earlobe (neg. peaks)			N VIII Dist/mid (neg. peaks)		N VIII Prox. (neg. peaks)		Vertex-earlobe (vertex pos. peaks)			
			I	II	III								I	II	III	V
1	DPV	Rare	1.56	2.84	3.76	1.44	2.40	4.16		3.92	2.84	4.12	1.48	2.80	3.80	5.98
		Cond	1.60	2.76	3.72	1.48	2.44	3.80		4.40	2.72	4.60	1.52	2.64	3.76	5.92
2	DPV	Rare	1.64	2.84	3.80	1.24	2.32	3.32		3.56	2.76	4.56	1.60	2.68	4.04	6.52
		Cond	1.84	2.60	4.08	1.36	2.84	3.36			2.80	5.36	1.40	2.64	4.50	6.60
3	DPV	Rare	1.96	3.00	3.92	1.76	2.72	4.40		3.96	3.12	4.48	1.80	2.80	4.20	6.04
		Cond	2.00	3.04	3.96	2.00	2.76	4.20		4.08	3.08	4.48	1.80	3.04	4.08	6.12
4	DPV	Rare	2.32	2.92	4.20	1.12	2.60	3.48		3.28	2.96	3.76	1.92	2.60	4.24	6.04
		Cond	2.04	3.08	4.04	1.04	2.80	4.28		3.96	3.24	4.40	2.08	2.92	4.08	6.32
5	DPV	Rare	1.72	2.80	3.76	1.52	2.52	3.80		3.72	2.96	4.24	1.56	2.60	3.80	5.76
		Cond								4.12						
6	DPV	Rare	2.16	3.04	3.80	1.68	2.64	4.32	2.64	4.04	3.00	4.40	1.68	2.60	4.28	5.84
		Cond	2.24		4.12	1.88	3.08	3.60	2.80	4.04	3.32	4.68	1.92	3.04	3.64	6.38
7	DPV	Rare	1.80	2.72	3.72	2.08	3.88		2.36	4.36			1.80	2.68	3.76	5.96
		Cond	1.76	2.80	3.76	1.60	2.68	3.92	2.60	3.88			1.72	2.80	3.80	6.08
8	TN	Rare	1.60	2.80	3.64	1.60	2.24	3.12	2.68	4.12			1.60	2.80	4.04	5.64
		Cond	1.64	2.80	3.72	1.68	2.48	3.88	2.56	3.80			1.64	2.80	3.72	5.56
9	TN	Rare	2.00	3.04	3.96	1.76	2.72	4.52	3.20	4.56			1.84	2.76	4.00	6.00
		Cond	2.00	3.00	4.08	2.16	3.08	4.28	3.36	4.88			2.04	3.04	4.24	5.92
10	TN	Rare	1.64	2.68	3.68	1.80	2.32	3.36	2.52	3.80			1.88	2.48	3.68	5.96
		Cond	1.80	2.72	3.76	1.76	2.56	3.44	2.48	3.84			1.80	2.60	3.80	5.88
11	HFS	Rare	1.64	3.28	4.08	1.80	2.76	4.44	2.60		2.80	3.56	1.76	3.20	4.12	6.24
		Cond	1.92	3.12	3.92	1.68	2.68	4.48	2.80		2.68		1.72	2.92	4.00	6.04
12	DPV	Rare	1.56	2.88	3.64	1.60	2.56	4.20	2.68	3.84	3.08	3.80	1.60	2.56	3.60	5.80
		Cond	1.76	2.72	3.92	1.68	2.36	3.16	2.84	4.08	3.04	4.20	1.72	2.52	3.84	6.04
13	DPV	Rare	1.60	2.92	3.92	1.52	2.36	4.56	2.64	4.32	2.96	4.52	1.56	2.96	3.96	5.92
		Cond	1.52	2.96	4.00	1.56	2.72	4.56	2.72	4.04	2.96	4.32	1.56	2.92	4.04	5.92
14	HFS	Rare	1.88	3.04	4.00	1.52	2.56	4.12			3.00	4.48	1.80	2.92	3.96	6.00
		Cond									3.04	4.40				
Average rare			1.79	2.91	3.85	1.60	2.61	3.98	2.58	3.96	2.97	4.23	1.71	2.75	3.96	5.98
Average cond			1.84	2.87	3.92	1.66	2.71	3.91	2.69	4.10	3.02	4.59	1.74	2.82	3.96	6.07
S.D. rare			0.23	0.15	0.16	0.23	0.39	0.49	0.70	0.31	0.29		0.13	0.18	0.20	0.20
S.D. cond			0.20	0.17	0.14	0.28	0.22	0.44	0.27	0.36	0.23	0.33	0.19	0.18	0.24	0.26

*DPV = disabling positional vertigo; HFS = hemifacial spasm; TN = trigeminal neuralgia.

negative peak is located in the brainstem (Møller and Jannetta, 1982a, 1983a).

These results were confirmed and enlarged upon after evaluation of intracranial recordings made in a patient who was operated upon for a tumor of the fourth ventricle. In this patient it was possible to obtain direct access to the medial side of the cerebellar peduncle and, thus, to the cochlear nucleus or its vicinity (Møller and Jannetta, 1983b). Recordings from this location showed a potential with a large, negative peak (Figure 2.7), the latency of which was similar to peak III of the ABR (Figure 2.7C).

While it is relatively easy to record the evoked potentials from the superior olivary complex in animals, it is difficult to record from this complex of nuclei in man. The superior olivary complex in man is a small nucleus, the cells of which are scattered through a wide region of the brainstem (Moore, 1987a,b). The only way it has been possible to record from these nuclei in man is to place a recording electrode on the lateral surface of the brainstem when this area becomes exposed in neurosurgical operations that involve the cerebellopontine angle (Møller and Jannetta, 1984). Recordings made from this location on the lateral surface of the brainstem, which is presumed to overlie the superior olivary complex, are dominated by a negative peak, the latency of which is about 1 ms longer than that of the second negative peak in the recording made near the brainstem (Figure 2.6C) (which was assumed to be the response from the cochlear nucleus). A peak with the same latency, but with a much smaller amplitude, can also be seen in the recording from a location where the eighth nerve enters the brainstem (root entry zone) (Figure 2.6B). The fact that this third peak rose in amplitude when the recording electrode was moved from the REZ to a location on the lateral side of the brainstem close to the superior olivary complex indicates that the superior olivary complex is likely to be the source of this third peak in the potentials that are recorded intracranially. This is further supported by the fact that the latency of this third peak is about 1 ms longer than that of the second negative peak, indicating that its source is third-order auditory neurons, which are known to be located mainly in the superior olivary complex, although presumably there are also third-

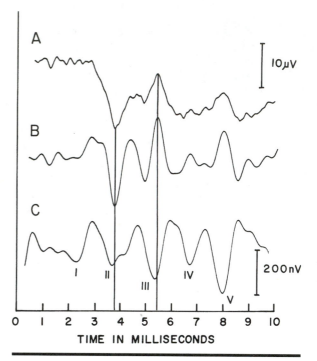

FIGURE 2.7.   Comparison of recordings from the vicinity of the cochlear nucleus and from the vertex made in a patient undergoing an operation to remove a tumor located in the fourth ventricle. (A) Recordings made from the cerebellar peduncle at a location medial to the cochlear nucleus and near the floor of the fourth ventricle. (B) The same recording after digital filtering. (C) Simultaneous recording of the ABR from an electrode placed on the vertex (with a noncephalic reference). The same recording after digital filtering. The stimuli were 2000 Hz tonebursts of 5 ms duration presented at 95 dB to the ipsilateral ear (from Møller and Jannetta, 1983b).

order neurons in the cochlear nucleus of man, as has been shown to be the case in animals.

Contributions to the ABR From the Cochlear Nucleus and Superior Olivary Complex

The finding that the large negative peak seen in the potentials recorded intracranially from the vicinity of the cochlear nucleus appears with the same latency as peak III of the ABR (Figure 2.6B and Figure 2.7) recorded simultaneously from scalp electrodes indicates that peak III of the ABR is generated mainly in the cochlear nucleus. On the basis of animal experiments, it was thought that peak III originated in the superior olivary complex, but the fact that an additional delay occurs in the auditory nerve in man and that peak III has a much larger amplitude than peak II supports the hypothesis that peak III in the human ABR is generated by a relatively large nucleus that has an orderly organization of its neurons, such as the cochlear nucleus.

Since the third peak in the potentials that are recorded intracranially from a location overlying the superior olivary complex has a latency that is close to that of peak IV in the ABR recorded simultaneously (Figure 2.6), this peak may be expected to be generated by the superior olivary complex. However, there is less clear correspondence between the near-field and the

far-field potentials in this case. Also, determination of the neural generators of peak IV is complicated by the fact that this peak is more variable than the other four of the five main peaks in the ABR. The fact that peak IV's latency is so close to that of peak V results in peak IV often appearing as a small peak riding on the slope of peak V. This makes it difficult to determine the latency of peak IV accurately. Furthermore, the far-field potentials of the superior olivary complex may be less well defined than the far-field potentials of other structures of the ascending auditory pathway because the nuclei of the superior olivary complex are dispersed in the brainstem. The fact that the major parts of the ascending auditory pathway cross the midline at this level, while some parts continue uncrossed toward higher auditory centers, may further contribute to temporal dispersion of the neural activity that is generated by these nuclei.

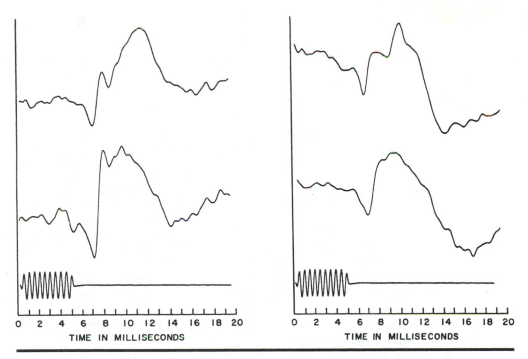

FIGURE 2.8. Recordings from the inferior colliculus or its vicinity obtained in patients undergoing neurosurgical operations. Negativity is shown as an upward deflection. The stimuli were 2000 Hz tonebursts of 5 ms duration presented to the contralateral ear (from Møller and Jannetta, 1982b).

Potentials Generated by the Lateral Lemniscus and the Inferior Colliculus

Typical potentials recorded from the inferior colliculus in man in response to contralateral sound stimulation are shown in Figure 2.8. A small positive peak is followed by a large and broad negative deflection on which several smaller peaks are riding. The sharp, initial positive potential is most likely generated by the lateral lemniscus as it enters the inferior colliculus, while the slow negative potential following this is likely a dendritic potential of the inferior colliculus (Møller and Jannetta, 1982b, 1983c; Hashimoto, 1982a).

Contribution to the ABR from the Lateral Lemniscus and the Inferior Colliculus

When our only information about the neural generators of the ABR was that learned from studies of animals, it was generally assumed that peak V in the ABR was generated in the inferior colliculus. The results of recordings made from the inferior colliculus in patients undergoing neurosurgical operations in which this structure becomes exposed have shown a more complex relationship between the ABR and the intracranially recorded potentials. Thus, the earliest component of the response from the inferior colliculus in man occurs with a latency equal to that of peak V in the ABR recorded from the scalp (Møller and Jannetta, 1982b, 1984) (Figure 2.9A).

When the potentials recorded directly from the inferior colliculus are compared to the ABRs recorded from the vertex using a noncephalic reference, both being recorded in such a way that low frequencies are preserved (Figure 2.9A), it is evident that the broad negative peak in the near-field response from the inferior colliculus has about the same latency as does the vertex-negative potential in the ABR (Møller and Jannetta, 1982b, 1983c). This slow vertex-negative component with a latency of about 10 ms was first described by Davis and Hirsh (1976), who named it SN_{10} (slow negative at 10 ms). They used this potential as a convenient indicator of auditory threshold.

Since the latencies of the slow component of the near-field response from the inferior colliculus and the

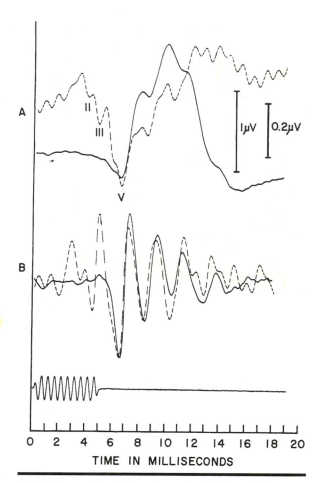

FIGURE 2.9.   Recordings from the inferior colliculus (solid lines) compared to recordings made simultaneously from the vertex using a noncephalic reference (dashed lines). (A) Recording bandwidth was 3 to 3000 Hz; response was zero-phase digitally lowpass filtered with a triangular weighting function 0.8 ms wide. (B) Same data as in A, but after attenuating the low-frequency components by zero-phase bandpass digital filtering. Lefthand calibration relates to the recording made intracranially, and the righthand calibration relates to the vertex recording (from Møller and Jannetta, 1983c).

far-field SN_{10} are about the same, it has been suggested that the neural generator of the SN_{10} may be the inferior colliculus (Møller and Jannetta, 1986). When assessing the contribution from a nucleus to the potentials that can be recorded from the scalp (far-field), it must be remembered that the fact that a component of the far-field potential is coincident in time with the potentials that are recorded directly from the nucleus is not sufficient to prove that the component of the far-field potential in question is generated by the nucleus. This is because the magnitude of the far-field potentials that are generated by a nucleus depends not only on the magnitude of the near-field potential but also on the internal organization of the nucleus (Lorente de No, 1947*b*).

When the slow component of the near-field potential that can be recorded from the human inferior colliculus is removed by bandpass filtering, a series of two to three peaks are seen to follow the initial positive peak, as shown in Figure 2.9B. The latencies of these sharp peaks have values that are close to the latencies of the positive peaks VI and VII of the ABRs recorded from the vertex using a noncephalic reference. These sharp peaks probably represent synchronized firing of neurons in the inferior colliculus, called somaspikes (Møller and Jannetta, 1983*c*). As noted at the beginning of this chapter, animal experiments have shown that the nucleus of the inferior colliculus can be ablated without affecting the far-field potentials noticeably, despite the large near-field potentials, thus questioning the contribution to the ABR from the inferior colliculus (Møller and Burgess, 1986).

Sources of Slow and Fast Components of the ABR

In discussions of the neural generators of peak V in the ABR, it is important to note that it has recently been recognized that the slow and fast components of the ABR may have different origins. Several investigators have studied these two components by separating ABR on the basis of their spectrum (Fullerton and Kiang, 1990; Hashimoto, 1982*a,b*; Møller and Jannetta, 1986).

Summary of Findings Regarding Neural Generators of the Human ABR

From our just completed comparison between intracranially recorded potentials in man and the far-field potentials recorded from scalp electrodes, we can say: peak I of the ABR originates exclusively from the dis-

tal portion of the eighth nerve; peak II originates mainly from the proximal portion of the auditory nerve, although there may be some small contribution from other, more distal portions of the auditory nerve; and peak III is mainly generated by the neurons in the cochlear nucleus, although it may also receive some small contribution from nerve fibers entering the cochlear nucleus. The neural generators of peak IV are uncertain, but they are probably third-order neurons, mostly those located in the superior olivary complex. This peak may also, however, receive contributions from neurons in the cochlear nucleus and the nucleus of the lateral lemniscus.

Other studies of the neural generators of ABRs in man that have been based on intracranial recordings have essentially obtained results similar to those just summarized (Hashimoto et al., 1981; Spire et al., 1982). Nevertheless, this interpretation, particularly regarding peaks III and IV, is only a generalization of the findings. There is no doubt that sources other than the cochlear nucleus and superior olivary complex also contribute to peaks III and IV of the ABR.

The neural generators of peak V are complex. The sharp vertex-positive portion of peak V is most likely generated by the termination of the lateral lemniscus in the inferior colliculus, and the vertex-negative slope of this peak, including the following slow, vertex-positive component, are likely to be dendritic potentials in the inferior colliculus, perhaps with contributions from the earliest somaspikes of the nucleus. Peak VI seems to be mainly generated by somaspikes of the inferior colliculus.

A schematic illustration of the way the neural generators of the ABRs in man are conceptualized is shown in Figure 2.10. This illustration is a simplified diagram of the main part of the ascending auditory pathway and indicates the main neural generators of the ABR. It is important to emphasize that the neural generators of peaks IV, V, VI, and VII are complex in that more than one anatomical structure contributes to each peak and that each anatomical structure contributes to *more* than one peak.

The contribution of the extralemniscal system to the far-field potentials is practically unknown, but the existence of such a contribution is known from the results of studies in which severance of the lateral lemniscus on both sides failed to eliminate responses from the auditory nerve to acoustic stimulation (Galambos and Sheatz, 1962; Osman and Galambos, 1967).

Differences Between Results Obtained in Man and Those Obtained in Experimental Animals

The results of studies in cats show that the auditory nerve is the generator of peak I, the cochlear nucleus is the generator of peak II, the superior olivary nucleus is the generator of peak III, the lateral lemniscus is the generator of peak IV, and the inferior colliculus is the generator of

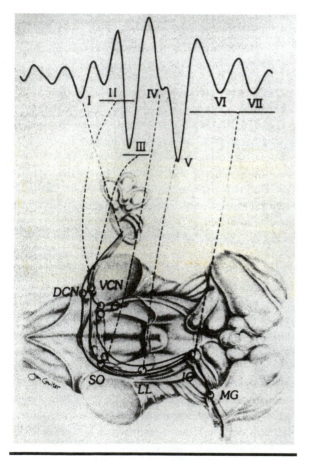

FIGURE 2.10. Schematic illustration of the neural generators of the ABR in man (Møller and Jannetta, 1984. In: J.T. Jacobson (ed.) *The Auditory Brainstem Response*, pp. 13–31. Austin, TX: PRO-ED, Inc.).

peak V in the cat (Buchwald and Huang, 1975). However, the results of studies on the origins of ABRs in small animals cannot directly be applied to man because of anatomical differences among species, specifically in the lengths of their auditory nerves; the auditory nerve is much longer in man (Lang, 1981, 1983) than it is in the cat and other small animals that are commonly used in such studies. This is a natural consequence of the fact that man has a larger head than such animals.

The most important effect on the ABR of the longer auditory nerve in man is that there is a considerably longer delay in the arrival of auditory information at the cochlear nucleus. In addition, there is evidence that man's longer auditory nerve results in the generation of two separate far-field peaks in the human ABR; in small animals, the auditory nerve only generates one peak. As a result of these anatomical differences, man has five main peaks in the ABR, while small animals only have four peaks in the ABR. Recently, however, it has been shown that peak I in the cat has two components when recorded using high-temporal resolution and a non-cephalic reference (Starr and Zaaroor, 1990). These two components were assumed to correspond to peak I and peak II in man on the basis of their latency difference and the length of the auditory nerve in the cat.

Although there is no evidence that the general organization of the human auditory system differs qualitatively from that of these small animals, there are differences in the nuclei of the ascending auditory pathway between primates and carnivores (Moore and Moore, 1971; Moore, 1987a,b). Whether these differences are sufficient to cause significant differences in the ABRs recorded from these species is not clear. The much longer distance from the recording electrode to the neural generators of the ABR in man compared with small animals is responsible for the much smaller amplitude of the potentials recorded from human subjects compared to those that can be recorded from small animals.

Effects of Pathology on Near-field and Far-field Potentials

The ways in which different components of the ABR are affected by various pathologic conditions are poorly understood. This hampers the use of ABR in topical diagnosis and it is also a source of uncertainty when we try to use information from patients with lesions of known location and extent to identify the neural generators of the ABR. Just because a patient has a lesion that is rather large (as shown by computerized axial tomography [CAT] scans or magnetic resonance imaging [MRI], for example) in the auditory nervous system does not necessarily mean that the particular region in which the lesion is located does not generate (or conduct) neural activity: a missing or distorted component of the ABR is not necessarily generated by the structure that appears radiologically abnormal. On the other hand, some lesions may not manifest themselves radiologically, but may cause abnormal neural function. For example, a lesion in a pathway that leads to a structure from which ABRs are recorded will affect the ABR recorded from that structure. Thus, if the component in the ABR that is assumed to be generated by the cochlear nucleus is normal but the following component, assumed to originate in the lateral lemniscus where it terminates in the inferior colliculus, is absent, a lesion may be affecting the entire lateral lemniscus and thus involve a relatively large part of the pons.

To use ABRs in intraoperative monitoring most efficiently to aid in making clinical diagnoses and to reduce the risks of neurologic deficits as a result of surgical manipulations, it is important to know not only the sources of the different components of the ABR, but also to know how different pathologic conditions and lesions affect the ABR and the CAP recorded from the eighth nerve. So far, a prolongation in the latencies of the various peaks of the ABR have been the dominating feature utilized in clinical diagnoses, but pathologies also affect the amplitude and waveform of the different components. These changes may be of importance if it was known how they are related to various pathologic conditions. From clinical experience we know that certain pathological conditions lead to prolongation of the latencies of the various peaks in the ABR, but while changes in the waveforms and amplitudes of various components of the far-field potentials are often noted as well, the clinical implications of these latter latency changes have not yet been identified.

The effects of acute lesions to the auditory nerve on the potentials that can be recorded from the eighth cra-

nial nerve have been studied both in animals and in patients undergoing neurosurgical operations, so we have gained some understanding of the effects of such injury on the potentials recorded directly from nerve tracts and nuclei (Sekiya and Møller, 1987a,b; Møller, 1988a). It is interesting to note that acute injury to the auditory nerve can result in either a prolongation of the latency of the potentials without major changes in the waveform, or in such radical changes in the waveform that the potentials become dominated by the initial positivity and there is more-or-less complete obliteration of the negative peak that dominates the normal response. Although the latter type of change can be assumed to be the result of a more-or-less complete conduction block at a location close to the recording site, the mechanism by which an injury causes an increase in latency is obscure.

The concomitant changes in the ABR (far-field potential) are more difficult to assess. An injury to the eighth nerve that results in a certain increase in latency of the early components would be expected to cause a similar increase in latency of later components; however, this is not always the case, and later components seem to be less affected than earlier components (Achor and Starr, 1980b; Sekiya and Møller, 1987a, 1988).

MIDDLE-LATENCY RESPONSES (MLRs)

Middle-latency responses (MLRs) are usually defined as potentials that can be recorded from electrodes placed on the scalp between 8 and 80 to 100 ms after the onset of a transient sound (Goldstein, 1973; Musiek et al., 1984a), although the middle-latency response has sometimes been defined as those potentials that occur between 10 and 50 ms after the onset of an acoustic stimulus. These potentials were first described by Geisler et al. (1958), and consist of three to four vertex-positive peaks (P_o, P_a, P_b, P_c) with latencies of about 12, 25, 50, and 75 ms and three negative waves (N_a, N_b, N_c) with latencies of about 16, 36, and 60 ms (Figure 2.11) (from Musiek et al., 1984a) that occur in response to a short toneburst. The waveform of the MLR is more likely than that of the ABR to be severely distorted by the electronic filters used to obtain the data (Scherg, 1982); this is because the MLR potentials are slower

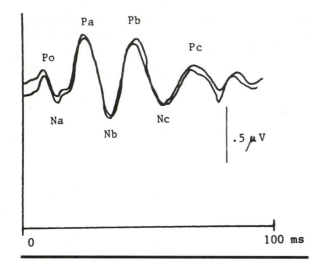

FIGURE 2.11.   Typical middle latency potentials (from Musiek et al., 1984*a*).

than the ABRs and their spectral content extends below the lower cutoff frequency (30 to 100 Hz) that is often used in evoked potential recording, which in turn may explain some of the variations in latencies of the different components reported from different studies.

Recording MLR: Clicks do not seem to yield as distinct a middle-latency response as do tonebursts. Myogenic response to relatively high-intensity sounds occurs with a latency in the range of the MLR (Kiang et al., 1963; Bickford et al., 1964), and Picton et al. (1974) listed the latencies of a series of such myogenic potentials. Bickford et al. (1964), Horwitz et al. (1966), and later Harker et al. (1977), however, showed that MLRs could be recorded in paralyzed (curarized) subjects and thereby proved that potentials of neurogenic origin with latencies of 10 to 100 ms do occur. This confusion as to the origin of these potentials discredited MLR potentials for a long time as valuable indicators of auditory function, and for a long time the main use of MLR potentials has been to determine the pure-tone threshold in patients who, for one reason or another, were unable to undergo conventional pure-tone audiometry (Musiek and Donnelly, 1983).

Ruhm et al. (1967), in recording from the exposed cortex in man, contributed evidence of the neural origin of the various components of the MLR by identifying

potentials that resembled those recorded from the scalp. These results were supported by a study by Picton et al. (1974) and studies by Celesia and co-workers (Celesia et al., 1968; Celesia and Puletti, 1969, 1971), who compared scalp and intracranial recordings and confirmed that the MLR is of neurogenic origin.

Since the issue of myogenic contamination has been clarified, interest has increased in using these potentials to aid in diagnosis of various types of neurologic problems. However, such applications require a great deal of knowledge about the neural generators of these potentials (Musiek et al., 1984*b*; Kraus et al., 1982).

Neural Generators of MLRs

Information about the origins of the MLR is sparse compared with what is known about the origins of ABR, but it is generally agreed that the neural components of these potentials are likely to originate from locations in the thalamus, the primary auditory cortex, and the association cortex. On the basis of its latency of about 25 ms, the P_a component could be expected to be generated by the primary auditory cortex. Studies of auditory evoked potentials in patients with cortical lesions (Kraus et al., 1982; Parving et al., 1980; Ozdamar et al., 1982) revealed that the latency and waveshape of P_a is unaffected by temporal lobe lesions involving the auditory cortex, but the amplitude of this peak is often reduced when such a lesion is present. The conclusion of these studies is that the MLR reflects, at least to some extent, activity in the auditory cortex.

One problem that arises when attempts are made to identify the generators of the MLR by studying patients with various lesions of the auditory nervous system is that cortical representation of sounds is strongly bilateral. Thus, a one-sided lesion may affect potentials recorded from the scalp relatively little because of contributions to the scalp-recorded potentials from the unaffected side. This may explain why an amplitude change (in P_a) is the major visible change in MLR of a unilateral cortical lesion. Naturally, lesions in the thalamus will have a more definite effect on the MLR than will cortical lesions, because lesions in the thalamus block input to the cortex (Kraus et al., 1982). As explained by Kraus et al. (1982), many patients who present with temporal lobe lesions have pathology in other parts of the auditory system as well, as evidenced by abnormal ABRs and/or abnormal results of audiologic testing.

Intracranial recordings made in patients undergoing neurosurgical procedures have been the source of most of our information about the origins of these MLR potentials. In a study of the cortical response, Ruhm et al. (1967) recorded directly from the exposed cortex and found a coincidence in time between a positive deflection with a latency of about 30 ms and the P_a in the MLR recorded from the vertex. However, other investigators (Celesia et al., 1968; Celesia and Puletti, 1971; Celesia, 1976) found a more complex and less direct relationship between the potentials that could be recorded from the scalp and those recorded intracranially from the exposed cortex.

Thus, Celesia and Puletti (1969) showed that the response from the exposed auditory cortex to acoustic stimulation in man has a polyphasic waveform, with the earliest identifiable components appearing with a latency of 13 ms in unanesthetized patients. This shows that any component of the MLR with a latency of 13 ms or longer could originate in the auditory cortex. In a patient who was studied under general anesthesia, prolonged latencies of the different components of the recorded potentials were noted. In addition to this initial surface-positive component, these investigators found two more positive peaks with latencies of 26.6 and 58.2 ms. Three well-defined negative peaks had latencies of 16.4, 58.2, and 105.8 ms. These values are close to the latencies of P_o (12 ms), N_a (16 ms), and P_a (25 ms) of the MLR, as given by Picton et al. (1974). As we have pointed out earlier in this chapter, such coincidence in latencies of intracranially recorded potentials and scalp-recorded potentials naturally does not constitute proof that the near-field potentials are the sources of the far-field potentials, particularly since they were not recorded in the same subjects. Hashimoto (1982a) found evidence that P_o and N_a originate in the midbrain region, and they confirmed that P_a and P_b are most likely generated by structures that are close to the primary auditory cortex.

The reason why different investigators obtained different latencies may partly be a result of their use of different filter settings. As mentioned above, the MLR is more affected by conventional electronic filtering than is the ABR (see Scherg, 1982), and the use of filters with different cutoff frequencies and different rates of rolloff may shift the peaks in time and therefore give rise to differences in the obtained latencies. In addition, the different components of the MLR are naturally affected by the stimulus parameters used, and since these vary among different investigators, it becomes an additional factor to the difference in results obtained by different investigators.

THE 40 HZ RESPONSE

The 40 Hz response is the nearly sinusoidal wave that can be recorded between the vertex and the ipsilateral mastoid in response to short tonebursts or clicks that are presented at a rate of about 40 stimuli per second (40 Hz) (Galambos et al., 1981). This response is assumed to be related closely to the MLR, because examination of the MLR reveals that the individual peaks merge when stimuli are presented at a rate near 40 Hz. As a result of this, the 40 Hz response appears as a long train of identical waves (Figure 2.12). Although the 40 Hz response can be regarded as a special variant of the MLR, its clinical importance warrants that its neural generators are considered separately.

Neural Generators of the 40 Hz Response

The generators of the 40 Hz response cannot be directly deduced from what is known about the generators of the MLR, because the MLR is defined for a much lower stimulus rate than is used to record the 40 Hz response. When the stimulus rate is increased beyond 3 stimuli per second, the waveform of the response changes, and essentially only a positive-negative wave is discernible. Naturally, these stimuli should elicit an ABR that could be expected to appear in the beginning of each tracing, but because the MLR and the 40 Hz response are usually recorded using a much lower high-frequency filter cutoff (lower setting of the lowpass filter) than is used to record ABRs (usually 500 Hz versus 3000 Hz), the ABR is usually not prominent in MLR recordings, ex-

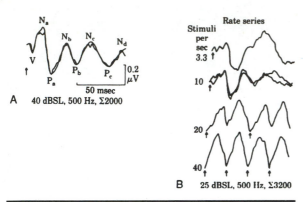

A   40 dBSL, 500 Hz, Σ2000

B   25 dBSL, 500 Hz, Σ3200

FIGURE 2.12. (A) Averaged responses to click stimuli presented at a rate of 10 pps. Peak V of the ABR is marked by "V" and traditional MLR waves are indicated "N_a, P_a, N_b, P_b, N_c, P_c, and N_d". (B) Effect of increasing stimulus rate from 3.3 to 40.0 pps (from Galambos et al., 1981).

cept for peak V of the ABR, which can often be recognized even with a filter setting of 500 Hz upper cutoff. At stimulus rates of 10 pps or higher the large negative peak with a latency of about 150 ms becomes attenuated and the response becomes dominated by a positive peak with a latency of about 25 ms (Figure 2.12). Evidence that the generator of the 40 Hz response is not the same as peak V of the ABR has been presented by Spydell et al. (1985).

The fact that tactile stimuli produce responses similar to the 40 Hz response has led to the suggestion that the 40 Hz potential is generated in the midbrain and/or by the thalamus as a more general expression of sensory activation (Galambos, 1982).

LONG-LATENCY POTENTIALS (EVENT-RELATED POTENTIALS, ERPs)

Long-latency auditory evoked potentials (also known as event-related potentials, ERPs) were the earliest of the auditory potentials to be discovered (Davis, 1939), but, paradoxically, the generators of these potentials are still the least well understood. ERPs are somewhat related to the so-called "K-complex," which are potentials that can be seen in the EEG of a subject at sleep in response to a tone, or any sound for that matter, when

the EEG is at low voltage or spindling (Loomis et al., 1938). It was in fact the discovery of the K-complex that led to the discovery of the long-latency auditory evoked potentials. In many ways the long-latency auditory evoked potentials resemble potentials evoked by other sensory modalities (Allison et al., 1977).

Long-latency auditory evoked potentials can be recorded from practically all locations on the scalp. When recorded from an electrode placed on the vertex in response to a transient sound (click or brief tone) in an awake subject, these potentials typically have a negative peak (N_1) with a latency of about 100 ms and a broad positive peak (P_2) at a latency of about 175 ms, followed by a second negative peak with a latency of about 280 ms. This last peak is known as the P_{300} (or P_3), and in contrast to components with shorter latencies, the P_{300} is dependent on cognitive factors and attention. It may appear as a response to a sound, but it can also be evoked by omitting a sound in a periodic train when the subject is given the task to count the omissions. A P_{300} also is present if a certain tone in a sequence of tones is replaced by a different tone and the subject is given the task of counting the tones that are different. If, however, the subject is asked to ignore omitted or different sounds, there is no P_{300}. Because it is evoked by activity in the brain itself, the P_{300} is often called an endogenous potential, in contrast to exogenous potentials, which are evoked by sound stimuli.

Neural Generators of Long-Latency Auditory Potentials

While it seems certain that the peaks in the short- and middle-latency (ABR and MLR) auditory potentials correspond to stages of information processing in the ascending auditory pathway, this relationship is not as clear for long-latency potentials, although it has been accepted and used to evaluate psychobiological functions (Donchin, 1979).

The 100-ms component of the ERP seems to be generated in the auditory cortex of the supratemporal plane (Vaughn and Ritter, 1969; Naatanen and Picton, 1987; Wikswo and Roth, 1988), and the P_{300} component seems to be generated by many different parts of the brain.

REFERENCES

Achor, L. and Starr, A. (1980*a*). Auditory brain stem responses in the cat: I. Intracranial and extracranial recordings. *Electroencephalography and Clinical Neurophysiology, 48,* 154–173.

Achor, L. and Starr, A. (1980*b*). Auditory brain stem responses in the cat. II. Effects of lesions. *Electroencephalography and Clinical Neurophysiology, 48,* 174–190.

Allison, T., Matsumiya, Y., Goff, G.D., and Goff, W.R. (1977). The scalp topography of human visual evoked potentials. *Electroencephalography and Clinical Neurophysiology, 42,* 185–197.

Arezzo, J., Legatt, A.D., and Vaughan, H.G. Jr. (1979). Topography and intracranial sources of somatosensory evoked potentials in the monkey: I. Early components. *Electroencephalography and Clinical Neurophysiology, 46,* 155–172.

Bickford, R.G., Jacobson, J.L., and Cody, D.T. (1964). Nature of average evoked potentials to sound and other stimuli in man. *Annals of the New York Academy of Sciences, 112,* 204–223.

Boston, J.R. and Ainslie, P.J. (1980). Effects of analog and digital filtering on brain stem auditory evoked potentials. *Electroencephalography and Clinical Neurophysiology, 48,* 361–364.

Britt, R. and Rossi, G. (1980). Neural generators of brain stem auditory evoked responses: Part I. Lesion studies. *Neuroscience Abstracts, 6,* 594.

Buchwald, J. and Huang, Ch. (1975). Far-field acoustic response: Origins in the cat. *Science, 189,* 382–384.

Celesia, G.G. (1976). Organization of auditory cortical areas in man. *Brain, 99,* 403–414.

Celesia, G.G. and Puletti, F. (1969). Auditory cortical areas of man. *Neurology, 19,* 211–220.

Celesia, G.G. and Puletti, F. (1971). Auditory input to the human cortex during states of drowsiness and surgical anesthesia. *Electroencephalography and Clinical Neurophysiology, 31,* 603–609.

Celesia, G.G., Broughton, R.J., Rasmussen, T., and Branch, C. (1968). Auditory evoked responses from the exposed human cortex. *Electroencephalography and Clinical Neurophysiology, 24,* 458–466.

Chiappa, K.H. (1983). *Evoked potentials in clinical medicine.* New York: Raven Press.

Chimento, T.C., Williston, J.S., Jewett, D.L., and Gardi, J.N. (1987). The 3-channel Lissajous' trajectory of the auditory brain-stem response. VIII. Isolated frog sciatic nerve in a volume conductor. *Electroencephalography and Clinical Neurophysiology, 68,* 380–385.

Dallos, P. (1973). *The auditory periphery.* New York: Academic Press.

Davis, P.A. (1939). Effects of acoustic stimuli on the waking human brain. *Journal of Neurophysiology, 2,* 494–499.

Davis, H. and Hirsh, S. (1976). The audiometric utility of brain stem responses to low-frequency sounds. *Audiology, 15,* 181–195.

Donchin, E. (1979). Event-related brain potentials: A tool in the study of human information processing. In H. Begleiter (ed.), *Evoked brain potentials and behavior,* pp. 13–88. New York: Plenum Press.

Doyle, D.J. and Hyde, M.L. (1981). Analogue and digital filtering of auditory brainstem responses. *Scandinavian Audiology (Copenhagen), 10,* 81–89.

Eggermont, J.J. (1974). Basic principles of electrocochleography. *Acta Otolaryngologica (Stockholm), 316,* (Supplement).

Eggermont, J.J., Spoor, A., and Odenthal, D.W. (1976). Frequency specificity of tone-burst electrocochleography. In R.J. Ruben, C. Elberling and G. Salomon (eds.), *Electrocochleography,* pp. 215–246. Baltimore, MD: University Park Press.

Elberling, C. (1976). Stimulation of cochlear action potentials recorded from the ear canal in man. In R.J. Ruben, C. Elberling, and G. Salomon (eds.), *Electrocochleography,* pp. 151–168. Baltimore, MD: University Park Press.

Engstrom, H. and Rexed, B. (1940). Uber die Kaliber Verhaltnisse der Nerven Fasern im N. Stato-acusticus des Menchen. *Zeitschrift für Mikroskopisch-Anatomische Forschung (Leipzig), 47,* 448–455.

Fullerton, B.C. and Kiang, N.Y.S. (1990). The effect of brainstem lesions on brainstem auditory evoked potentials in the cat. *Hearing Research, 49,* 363–390.

Fisch, U.P. and Ruben, R.J. (1962). Electrical acoustical response to click stimulation after section of the eighth nerve. *Acta Otolaryngologica (Stockholm), 54,* 532–542.

Galambos, R. (1982). Tactile and auditory stimuli repeated at high rates (30–50 per sec) produce similar event related potentials. *Annals of the New York Academy of Sciences, 388,* 722–728.

Galambos, R. and Sheatz, C. (1962). An electroencephalograph study of classical conditioning. *American Journal of Physiology, 203,* 173–184.

Galambos, R., Makeig, S., and Talmachoff, P.S. (1981). A 40-Hz auditory potential recorded from the human scalp. *Proceedings of the National Academy of Sciences, U.S.A., 78,* 2643–2647.

Gardi, J.N., Sininger, Y.S., Martin, W.H., and Jewett, D.L.

(1987). The 3-channel Lissajous' trajectory of auditory brain-stem response. VI. Effects of lesions in the cat. *Electroencephalography and Clinical Neurophysiology, 68*, 360–367.

Geisler, C.D., Frishkopf, L.S., and Rosenblith, W.A. (1958). Extracranial responses to acoustic clicks in man. *Science, 128*, 1210–1211.

Goldstein, M.H. Jr. (1960). A statistical model for interpreting neuroelectric responses. *Information and Control, 3*, 1–17.

Goldstein, R. (1973). Electroencephalic audiometry. In J. Jerger (ed.), *Modern developments in audiology*, pp. 407–433. New York: Academic Press.

Hall, J.W. and Hargadine, J.R. (1985). Sensory evoked responses in head injury. *Central Nervous System Trauma, 2*, 187–205.

Hari, R. and Ilmoniemi, R.J. (1986). Cerebral magnetic fields. *CRC Critical Reviews in Biomedical Engineering, 14*, 93–126.

Harker, L., Hosick, E., Voots, R., and Mendel, M.I. (1977). Influence of succinylcholine on middle component auditory evoked potentials. *Archives of Otolaryngology, 103*, 133–137.

Hashimoto, I., Ishiyama, Y., Yoshimoto, T., and Nemoto, S. (1981). Brainstem auditory evoked potentials recorded directly from human brainstem and thalamus. *Brain, 104*, 841–859.

Hashimoto, I. (1982a). Auditory evoked potentials from the human midbrain: Slow brain stem responses. *Electroencephalography and Clinical Neurophysiology, 53*, 652–657.

Hashimoto, I. (1982b). Auditory evoked potentials recorded directly from the human VIIIth nerve and brainstem: Origins of their fast and slow components. In P.A. Buser, W.A. Cobb, and T. Okuma (eds.), *Proceedings of the Kyoto Symposia, Electroencephalography and Clinical Neurophysiology, Supplement 36*, pp. 305–314. Amsterdam, The Netherlands: Elsevier Biomedical Press.

Horwitz, S., Larson, S., and Sances, A. (1966). Evoked potentials as an adjunct to the auditory evaluation of patients. *Proceedings of the Symposium on Biomedical Engineering, 1*, 49–52.

Huang, Ch. and Buchwald, J. (1977). Interpretation of the vertex short-latency acoustic response: A study of single neurons in the brain. *Brain Research, 137*, 291–303.

Hubbard, J.I., Llinas, R., and Quastel, D.M. (1969). Extracellular field potentials in the central nervous system. In *Electro-physiological analysis of synaptic transmission*, pp. 265–293. London: Edward Arnold Publishers.

Jacobson, J.T. (1985). An overview of the auditory brainstem response. In J.T. Jacobson (ed.), *The auditory brainstem response*, pp. 3–12. San Diego, CA: College Hill Press.

Jewett, D.L. (1987). The 3-channel Lissajous' trajectory of the auditory brain-stem response. IX. Theoretical aspects. *Electroencephalography and Clinical Neurophysiology, 68*, 386–408.

Jewett, D.L. and Williston, J.S. (1971). Auditory-evoked far fields averaged from scalp of humans. *Brain, 94*, 681–696.

Jungert, S. (1958). Auditory pathways in the brainstem: A neurophysiological study. *Acta Otolaryngologica (Stockholm) Supplement, 138*, 1–67.

Kiang, N.Y.S., Crist, A.H., French, M.A., and Edwards, A.G. (1963). Postauricular electrical responses to acoustic stimulation in human. *Massachusetts Institute of Technology RLE Quarterly Progress Report, 68*, 207–218.

Kimura, J., Mitsudome, A., Beck, D.O., Yamada, T, and Dickens, Q.S. (1983). Field distribution of antidromically activated digital nerve potentials: Models for far-field recordings. *Neurology, 33*, 1164–1169.

Kimura, J., Mitsudome, A., Yamada, T, and Dickens, Q.S. (1984). Stationary peaks from moving source in far-field recordings. *Electroencephalography and Clinical Neurophysiology, 58*, 351–361.

Kraus, N., Odzamar, O., Hier, D., and Stein, L. (1982). Auditory middle latency responses (MLRs) in patients with cortical lesions. *Electroencephalography and Clinical Neurophysiology, 54*, 275–287.

Lang, J. (1981). Facial and vestibulocochlear nerve, topographic anatomy and variations. In M. Samii and P.J. Jannetta (eds.), *The cranial nerves*, pp. 363–377. New York: Springer-Verlag.

Lang, J. (1983). *Clinical anatomy of the head*. New York: Springer-Verlag.

Lazorthes, G., Lacomme, Y., Ganbert, J., and Planel, H. (1961). La constitution du nerf auditif. *Presse Medicine, 69*, 1067–1068.

Loomis, A.L., Harvey, E.N., and Hobart, G.A. (1938). Distribution of disturbance patterns in human EEG with special reference to sleep. *Journal of Neurophysiology, 1*, 413.

Lorente de No, R. (1947a). Analysis of the distribution of action currents of nerve in volume conductors. *Studies of the Rockefeller Institute for Medical Research, 132*, 384–482.

Lorente, de No, R. (1947b). Action potential of the motoneurons of the hypoglossus nucleus. *Journal of Cell and Comparative Physiology, 29*, 207–287.

Lueders, H., Lesser, R., Hahn, J., Little, J., and Klem, G. (1983). Subcortical somatosensory evoked potentials to median nerve stimulation. *Brain, 106*, 341–372.

Møller, A.R. (1983a). On the origin of the compound action

potentials (N_1, N_2) of the cochlea of the rat. *Experimental Neurology, 80*, 633–644.

Møller, A.R. (1983*b*). *Auditory physiology*. New York: Academic Press.

Møller, A.R. (1988*a*). *Evoked potentials in intraoperative monitoring*. Baltimore, MD: Williams & Wilkins Co.

Møller, A.R. (1988*b*). Use of zero-phase digital filters to enhance brainstem auditory evoked potentials (ABRs). *Electroencephalography and Clinical Neurophysiology, 71*, 226–232.

Møller, A.R. and Burgess, J.E. (1986). Neural generators of the brain-stem auditory evoked potentials (ABRs) in the rhesus monkey. *Electroencephalography and Clinical Neurophysiology, 65*, 361–372.

Møller, A.R. and Jannetta, P.J. (1981). Compound action potentials recorded intracranially from the auditory nerve in man. *Experimental Neurology, 74*, 862–874.

Møller, A.R. and Jannetta, P.J. (1982*a*). Auditory evoked potentials recorded intracranially from the brainstem in man. *Experimental Neurology, 78*, 144–157.

Møller, A.R. and Jannetta, P.J. (1982*b*). Evoked potentials from the inferior colliculus in man. *Electroencephalography and Clinical Neurophysiology, 53*, 612–620.

Møller, A.R. and Jannetta, P.J. (1983*a*). Monitoring auditory functions during cranial nerve microvascular decompression operations by direct recording from the eighth nerve. *Journal of Neurosurgery, 59*, 493–499.

Møller, A.R. and Jannetta, P.J. (1983*b*). Auditory evoked potentials recorded from the cochlear nucleus and its vicinity in man. *Journal of Neurosurgery, 59*, 1013–1018.

Møller, A.R. and Jannetta, P.J. (1983*c*). Interpretation of brainstem auditory evoked potentials: Results from intracranial recordings in humans. *Scandinavian Audiology (Copenhagen), 12*, 125–133.

Møller, A.R. and Jannetta, P.J. (1984). Neural generators of the brainstem auditory evoked potentials (ABR). In: R.H. Nodar and C. Barber (eds.), *Evoked potentials II: The second international evoked potentials symposium* (held in Cleveland, Ohio, October 18–20, 1982), Chapter 14 (pp 137–144). Boston, MA: Butterworth Publishers, Inc.

Møller, A.R. and Jannetta, P.J. (1986). Simultaneous surface and direct brainstem recordings of brainstem auditory evoked potentials (BAEP) in man. In R.Q. Cracco and I. Bodis-Wollner (eds.), *Evoked potentials*, pp. 227–234. New York: Alan R. Liss, Inc.

Møller, M.B. and Møller, A.R. (1985). Auditory brainstem evoked responses (ABR) in diagnosis of eighth nerve and brainstem lesions. In M.L. Pinheiro and F.E. Musiek (eds.), *Assessment of central auditory dysfunction: Its*

foundations and clinical correlates, Chapter 4, pp. 43–65. Baltimore, MD: Williams & Wilkins, Co.

Møller, A.R., Jannetta, P.J., Bennett, M., and Møller, M.B. (1981*a*). Intracranially recorded responses from human auditory nerve: New insights into the origin of brain stem evoked potentials. *Electroencephalography and Clinical Neurophysiology, 52*, 18–27.

Møller, A.R., Jannetta, P.J., and Møller, M.B. (1981*b*). Neural generators of the brain stem evoked responses: Results from human intracranial recordings. *Annals of Otology Rhinology and Laryngology, 90*, 591–596.

Møller, A.R., Jannetta, P.J., and Møller, M.B. (1982). Intracranially recorded auditory nerve response in man: New interpretations of BSER. *Archives of Otolaryngology, 108*, 77–82.

Møller, A.R., Jannetta, P.J., and Sekhar, L.N. (1988). Contributions from the auditory nerve to the brainstem auditory evoked potentials (BAEPs): Results of intracranial recording in man. *Electroencephalography and Clinical Neurophysiology, 71*, 198–211.

Moore, J.K. and Moore, R.Y. (1971). A comparative study of the superior olivary complex in the primate brain. *Folia Primatology (Basel), 16*, 35–51.

Moore, J.K. (1987*a*). The human auditory brain stem: A comparative view. *Hearing Research, 29*, 1–32.

Moore, J.K. (1987*b*). The human auditory brain stem as a generator of auditory evoked potentials. *Hearing Research, 29*, 33–44.

Morest, D.K., Kiang, N.Y.S., Kane, E.C., Guinan, J.J., and Godfrey, D.A. (1973). Stimulus coding of caudal levels of the cat's auditory nervous system. II. Patterns of synoptic organization. In A.R. Møller (ed.), *Basic mechanisms in hearing*. New York: Academic Press.

Musiek, F.E. and Donnelly, K. (1983). Clinical applications of the (auditory) middle latency response—an overview. *Seminars in Hearing, 4*, 391–401.

Musiek, F.E., Geurkink, N.A., Weider, D.J., and Donnelly, K. (1984*a*). Past, present, and future applications of auditory middle latency response. *Laryngoscope, 94*, 1545–1552.

Musiek, F.E., Kibbe, K., Rackliffe, L., and Weider, D. (1984*b*). Auditory brainstem response I-V amplitude ratio in normal cochlear and retrocochlear ears. *Ear and Hearing, 5*, 52–55.

Naatanen, R. and Picton, T.W. (1987). The N_1 wave of the human electric and magnetic response to sound. *Psychophysiology, 24*, 375–425.

Osman, E. and Galambos, R. (1967). Activation of auditory cortex by clicks after bilateral lesions of the brachium and of the inferior colliculus. *Journal of the Acoustical Society of America, 42*, 512–514.

Ozdamar, O., Kraus, N., and Curry, F. (1982). Auditory brain stem and middle latency responses in a patient with cortical deafness. *Electroencephalography and Clinical Neurophysiology, 53*, 224–230.

Parving, A., Salomon, G., Elberling, C., Larsen, B., and Lassen, N.A. (1980). Middle components of the auditory evoked response in bilateral temporal lobe lesions. *Scandinavian Audiology (Copenhagen), 9*, 161–167.

Picton, T.W., Hillyard, S.A., Krausz, H.J., and Galambos, R. (1974). Human auditory evoked potentials. I. Evaluation of components. *Electroencephalography and Clinical Neurophysiology, 36*, 179–190.

Pratt, H., Bleich, N., and Martin, W.H. (1985). Three-channel Lissajous' trajectory of human auditory brain-stem evoked potentials. I. Normative measures. *Electroencephalography and Clinical Neurophysiology, 61*, 530–538.

Regan, D. (1989). *Human brain electrophysiology.* New York: Elsevier Press.

Rossi, G. and Britt, R. (1980). Neural generators of brainstem evoked responses. Part II. Electrode recording studies. *Neuroscience Abstracts, 6*, 595.

Ruhm, H., Walker E. Jr., and Flanigin, H. (1967). Acoustically evoked potentials in man: Mediation of early components. *Laryngoscope, 77*, 806–822.

Scherg, M. (1982). Distortion of middle latency auditory response produced by analog filtering. *Scandinavian Audiology (Copenhagen), 11*, 57–60.

Scherg, M. and von Cramon, D. (1985). A new interpretation of the generators of BAEP waves I-V: Results of a spatiotemporal dipole. *Electroencephalography and Clinical Neurophysiology, 62*, 290–299.

Sekiya, T. and Møller, A.R. (1987*a*). Cochlear nerve injuries caused by cerebellopontine angle manipulations. An electrophysiological and morphological study in dogs. *Journal of Neurosurgery, 67*, 244–249.

Sekiya, T. and Møller, A.R. (1987*b*). Avulsion rupture of the internal auditory artery during operations in the cerebellopontine angle: A study in monkeys. *Neurosurgery, 21*, 631–637.

Sekiya, T. and Møller, A.R. (1988). Effects of cerebellar retractions on the cochlear nerve: An experimental study on rhesus monkeys. *Acta Neurochirurgica (Wien), 90*, 45–52.

Spire, J.P., Dohrmann, G.J. and Prieto, P.S. (1982). Correlation of brainstem evoked response with direct acoustic nerve potential. In J. Courjon, F. Manguiere, and M. Reval (eds.), *Advances in neurology: Clinical applications of evoked potentials in neurology* (Volume 32), pp. 159–167. New York: Raven Press.

Spoendlin, H. and Schrott, A. (1989). Analysis of the human auditory nerve. *Hearing Research, 43*, 25–38.

Spoor, A., Eggermont, J.J., and Odenthal, D.W. (1976). Comparison of human and animal data concerning adaptation and masking of eighth nerve compound action potentials. In R.J. Ruben, C. Elberling, and G. Salomon (eds.), *Electrocochleography*, pp. 183–198. Baltimore, MD: University Park Press.

Spydell, J.D., Pattee, G., and Goldie, W.D. (1985). The 40-Hz auditory event-related potential: Normal values and effects of lesions. *Electroencephalography and Clinical Neurophysiology, 62*, 193–202.

Starr, A. and Zaaroor, M. (1990). Eighth nerve contributions to cat auditory brainstem responses (ABR). *Hearing Research, 48*, 151–160.

Terkildsen, K., Osterhammel, P., and Huis In't Veld, F. (1974). Far-field electrocochleography, electrode positions. *Scandinavian Audiology (Copenhagen), 3*, 123–129.

Vaughn, H.G. Jr. and Ritter, W. (1969). The sources of auditory evoked responses recorded from the human scalp. *Electroencephalography and Clinical Neurophysiology, 28*, 360–367.

Weinberg, H., Stroink, G., and Katila, T. (1987). *Biomagnetism.* New York: Wiley.

Wikswo, J.P. and Roth, B.J. (1988). Magnetic determination of the spatial extent of a single cortical current source: A theoretical analysis. *Electroencephalography and Clinical Neurophysiology, 69*, 266–276.

CHAPTER 3

SIGNAL PROCESSING AND ANALYSIS

MARTYN L. HYDE

INTRODUCTION

This chapter addresses some of the most important principles and techniques of signal processing and analysis that underlie the instrumentation and measurement procedures for many auditory evoked potentials (AEPs).

The primary technical problem is that AEPs occur concurrently with unwanted potentials from many other sources, both physiologic and nonphysiologic (see Table 3.1). Referring to the total measured potential as the activity, the AEP of interest as the signal, and all other potentials as noise, the problem is that the signal is much smaller than the noise. There is a sequence of what could be viewed as "basic" procedures, directed at increasing the signal-to-noise ratio (SNR) to the point at which an AEP, if present, could be detected and measured with sufficient accuracy for whatever clinical or research purpose is intended. Unless this fundamental goal is achieved, subsequent data manipulations and inferences are likely to be ineffective and incorrect. The basic procedures include differential recording and amplification, bandpass filtering, analog-to-digital conversion, amplitude-based artifact rejection, and simple time-domain averaging.

In recent years, it has become increasingly common to apply additional or more complex manipulations to AEP signal and noise data, usually oriented towards improving the efficiency, objectivity, or utility of the AEP measurements. This includes an increased emphasis on several types of multichannel recording and analysis. Such procedures for digital signal processing (DSP) and analysis are usually both computationally intensive and of greatest value if applied essentially in real time, as distinct from being applied at leisure to stored data. These developments have been fueled not so much by advances in fundamental knowledge as by increasing availability of affordable but substantial computing and graphical display power at the PC and workstation level.

This chapter will cover the basic procedures of AEP recording and analysis in some detail, and will outline some of the more advanced procedures. Although there is overlap with the material in the 1985 edition of

---

TABLE 3.1   Some components of electrical noise in AEP recordings.

PHYSIOLOGIC NOISE	NONPHYSIOLOGIC NOISE
Unwanted evoked potentials	Electromagnetically induced
Spontaneous EEG	potentials from:
Electromyogenic potentials	-radio-frequency broadcasts
-from the head and neck	-high-voltage equipment
-from the heart	-stimulus artifact radiation
-from other muscles	-50/60 Hz power line radiation
Corneoretinal potentials	Internal instrumentation noise
Electrodermal potentials	Electrode polarization

this text, this chapter is aimed at a slightly higher technical level. More mathematical material is given in the Appendix. A good, technical AEP primer is due to Spehlmann (1985). A useful and comprehensive text that gives additional background for many of the technical aspects discussed here is provided by Regan (1989). The classical, general sourcebooks on signal processing include Bendat and Piersol (1971), Oppenheim and Schafer (1975), and Beauchamp and Yuen (1979). For more depth on digital filters, see Hamming (1983). For a good, general presentation of time series methods, DSP fundamentals, and pattern recognition techniques, see Cohen (1986).

In the interests of brevity and consistency, terms such as auditory brainstem response (ABR) and middle latency response (MLR) will be used here. See Chapters 1 and 8 for further comments on AEP nomenclature.

MODELS OF AEP ACTIVITY

To understand the purpose and the potential effectiveness of many of the signal processing procedures to be described in this chapter, it will be helpful to start with consideration of a conceptual model of the recorded electrical activity. The early development of such a model will also provide a useful terminology with which to formulate and discuss the techniques and their limitations. Because much of the AEP measurement and analysis problem has to do with random variation, and with quantities that are not deterministic (that is, not predictable exactly), the most appropriate model of AEP data is a statistical one. An attempt will be made to relegate most formulae to the Appendix, but an appreciation of the basic principles and methods of statistical inference will be helpful for understanding some of the following material. For a good, general statistical primer, see Norman and Streiner (1986). For a more detailed, classical introduction to statistical methods, see Snedecor and Cochran (1980).

Independence of Signal and Noise

The most common and important data model is that the activity at any instant is the algebraic sum of statistically independent signal and noise components. This implies that the characteristics of the signal, such as its mean and variance, are unrelated to those of the concurrent noise, and vice versa. What is being addressed here is the properties of the hypothetical, underlying "population" of possible signal and noise time-histories, from which any observed time-history constitutes a single sample, or "realization". There are several ways in which the independence assumption can be violated. One example occurs when both the AEP of interest and a component of the noise are related to the stimulus, such as when recording conditions allow the target AEP to overlap temporally with another, unwanted AEP. This occurs commonly when the ABR is overlapped by the MLR, while averaging with stimulus repetition rates above about 20 per second and recording filter bandwidths extending below about 100 Hz. Here, the MLR constitutes "noise" with a nonzero mean, and it biases (distorts) the estimate of the ABR waveform. The potential result is confusion, because it is not clear what is the AEP of interest and what is not.

Other mechanisms that might compromise the signal and noise independence include the target AEP and the noise having common electrophysiologic sources, modulation of the AEP and the noise sources by common neurological systems, or inter-modulation of signal and noise, such as might arise from neural nonlinearities. These possibilities seem most probable for the slow vertex potential (SVP), because both the SVP and an important component of its associated noise, the sinusoidal EEG activity called the "alpha rhythm" (8–13 Hz), are generated cortically. Indeed, Sayers, Beagley, and Henshall (1974) concluded that the SVP and the ongoing EEG were not independent, and that the SVP represented some kind of temporal synchronization (phase-locking) imposed upon the ongoing EEG activity. This view was based upon the fact that if the signal and noise were, indeed, additively independent, the total energy of the activity (proportional to the square of its amplitude) should increase in the time region of the AEP. No such increase was found, so the additive model was rejected. This phase-locking model is still widely quoted, but was cast in doubt by Jervis, Nichols, Johnson, Allen, and Hudson (1983), who found energy in the response region that was consistent with the additive model.

For the ABR, the concept of independent signal and

noise has high face validity, but because of the lower SNR in comparison with the SVP, it is even more difficult to investigate the model properly. The main noise associated with the ABR is electrical activity from head and neck musculature, so it seems very probable that this AEP and its noise are independent. For the MLR, the noise is mainly myogenic and there is a history of confusion between the neurogenic and myogenic AEP components that overlap temporally between 10 ms and 100 ms latency; at the higher stimulus levels associated with elicitation of, say, post-auricular myogenic components, lack of independence is quite likely. At low stimulus levels, at which the MLR is neurogenic, the independence assumption is more reasonable.

Invariance of the Signal

The standard model also asserts that the signal (AEP) is identical following each stimulus in the train of stimuli that is used for averaging. There are many ways in which this may not be true, and they fall into two main classes: random and systematic AEP variation. The most popular concept of random variation is "latency jitter," wherein the elementary signals elicited by each individual stimulus during averaging differ by time increments that are randomly distributed (Woody, 1967). The effect of such jitter on the average AEP estimate would be to broaden peaks, decrease amplitudes and increase latencies (Sayers, Beagley, and Ross, 1979). Furthermore, changes in the amount of latency jitter could underlie some of the AEP amplitude and waveform changes that are associated with changes in stimulus parameters, or with neuropathy. For example, an increase in stimulus level might increase AEP amplitude simply by reducing jitter, or neuropathy might reduce AEP amplitude by increasing jitter. The important point is that it is unwise to assume that a simple correspondence exists between the average potentials that we are accustomed to examining, and the underlying, elementary potentials elicited by individual stimuli.

An alternative to random latency fluctuation is systematic latency trend across the stimulus set. Cumulative refractoriness of neural generators, for example,

might be expected to cause progressively increased AEP latencies, perhaps through altering the rate of post-synaptic summation in response generation pathways.

Whether or not there are latency changes, both random and systematic amplitude changes are also possible. Again, the best candidate mechanism is neural adaptation. For example, the ABR is essentially a sequence of overlapping compound action potentials, and sampling variations from stimulus to stimulus in the number and synchrony of the underlying contributory single-unit action potentials are inevitable; systematic trends over repeated stimuli are also possible, reflecting either passive (such as metabolic fatigue) or active (such as habituation) neural mechanisms. Note that spatial and temporal post-synaptic summation offer a plausible mechanism for correlation between amplitude and latency changes.

A useful technique for exploring systematic trend is that of the cumulative sum (cumsum, Glaser and Ruchkin, 1976), usually a plot of cumulating total amplitude as a function of the number of stimuli delivered, evaluated at some specific latency that often corresponds to a peak or trough in the final average. Figure 3.1 shows amplitude cumsums of the SVP that illustrate various kinds of changes over time that appear to be systematic, as opposed to random. It is not yet clear whether the cause of these changes is actually trends in elementary response amplitude, because similar changes might arise from trends in latency, or in both variables simultaneously. To clarify this would require the use of latency cumsums as well, and these are much more intensive computationally than amplitude cumsums, because of the need to recalculate the peak location for every new total number of stimuli.

Another approach to analysis of signal (AEP) variation was first reported for the SVP by Ritter, Vaughan, and Costa (1968). They presented many blocks of repeated stimuli, then averaged between blocks the records that were in the first, second, third, etc., position within each block. This revealed rapid, asymptotic changes in SVP amplitude and waveform within the first ten stimuli of the block. Of course, there would be changes in the first few stimuli for most transient AEPs recorded at clinically relevant stimulus repetition rates; for any particular averaging run, only the first AEP is totally unadapted. For the

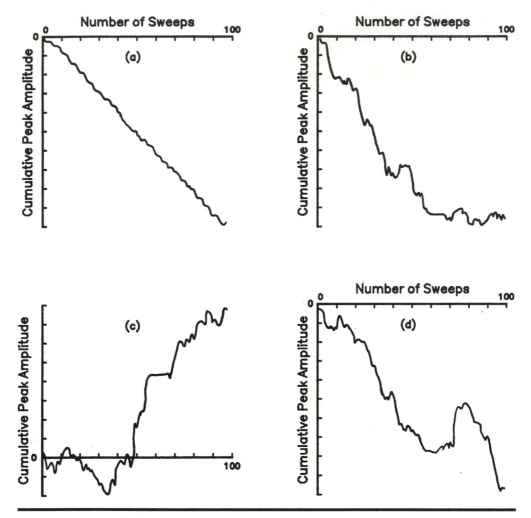

FIGURE 3.1. The elementary responses for each stimulus in an average may, or may not, be constant for each stimulus (sweep). The figure shows cumulative sums (cumsums) of peak amplitude at several post-stimulus times for the slow vertex potential (monaural 60 dB HL 500 Hz tone bursts at 1 per two seconds) in a normal adult. (a) Linear growth, consistent with the constant-response model, (b) initial linear growth asymptoting to zero growth, suggesting habituation, (c) zero initial growth, suggesting the opposite of habituation, and (d) variable and non-random growth.

ABR and MLR, because of the relatively large number of stimuli used per average, the overall average potential will tend to estimate the asymptotically adapted AEP; for the SVP, for which as few as 20 stimuli might be used, response changes over the first few stimuli might affect the average significantly.

Exploration of these putative response changes is analytically demanding and computationally intensive, especially for AEPs with small SNR (such as the ABR), because it is desirable to store and manipulate the data for every stimulus repetition. However, commercial neurophysiologic acquisition and analysis systems that are affordable but sufficiently fast and powerful have become available recently. In general, looking for random variation of amplitude or latency is much more difficult than exploring systematic trend, because of the low SNRs and the difficulty of distinguishing between signal and noise changes; meaningful analysis may be actually impossible for AEPs such as the ABR. As yet, there is a lack of unequivocal evidence that significant latency jitter, for example, occurs for the ABR, MLR or SVP, but the possibility certainly exists. Of course, a phenomenon may occur, and have consequences, without being easy to demonstrate. Several workers have accepted that random signal variation does occur, at least for some EPs of cortical origin; see the discussion by Regan (1989).

Stationarity of the Noise

The noise is usually assumed to be random and statistically stationary, that is, its statistical properties (mean, variance, etc.) do not change over time. Many kinds of nonstationarity are possible. The earlier example of ABR/MLR overlap is a case of nonstationarity of the mean noise that is locked in time to the stimulus, assuming that the MLR is to be regarded as noise, when the AEP of interest is the ABR. However, most nonstationarity is not time-locked. For example, it is well known that the variance of the noise can change dramatically over time: in ABR or MLR measurement, such a change occurs if the subject becomes uncomfortable or moves, generating higher levels of electromyogenic noise. For the SVP, the biggest concern is changes in the amplitude of the alpha rhythm, associated with drowsiness or eye closure. Another type of nonstationarity is the occasional, high-amplitude artifact, such as is due to a brief myogenic burst during ABR or MLR recordings, or a blink or sudden movement during SVP recordings.

Noise nonstationarity increases variability of the averaged activity, both within any given average and between averages. The former may lead to difficulty and error in AEP identification and measurement; the latter may lead to errors in forming inferences based on several averages, such as regarding AEP repeatability or the estimation of AEP threshold. The main weapon against transient artifacts is the amplitude-based artifact rejection system, described later. For the slower types of nonstationarity, one approach is to select the number of sweeps in each average in such a way as to compensate for changes between averages in the noise variance; for example, maintaining approximate proportionality between a measured noise variance estimate and the number of sweeps would tend to give constant variance of the averaged activity, which is desirable (Elberling and Don, 1984). This is most practicable if the averaging protocol is under computer control.

Independence of Noise Epochs

Another assumption in the standard AEP model is that the noise is statistically independent, at least from one stimulus to the next. This means that there should be zero correlation between the noise samples in any two successive analysis sweeps (windows, analysis intervals, epochs associated with individual stimuli). There will certainly be correlation between the successive noise samples within any given sweep, but that is another matter. For the ABR and MLR, the inter-sweep independence assumption is probably valid, except at stimulation rates that are so high that the successive windows either almost overlap, such as for a 20 ms tonepip ABR window in an infant and a stimulation rate approaching 50 per second, or actually do overlap, such as for the 40 Hz MLR. For the SVP, the independence assumption is usually false. The low-frequency EEG rhythms (especially alpha, 8–13 Hz, and theta, 4–7 Hz) can cause significant correlation between successive sweeps. Failure of the independence assumption can have a substantial effect on the effectiveness of averaging, because it tends to increase the amount of variability, both within and between averages.

Normality of Noise Distribution

It is usually assumed that the noise has a statistically normal (Gaussian) distribution of amplitude. This assumption is not strictly necessary for the validity of arguments such as the root-N law of averaging (see the Appendix), but normality is a desirable property for many reasons. It provides a relatively straightforward and well-understood basis for certain inferences or data manipulations that are dependent upon the distributional shape, such as for certain statistical automatic AEP detection procedures, or for setting appropriate artifact rejection limits. Another advantage is that if two variables are normally distributed, then if they are uncorrelated they are also statistically independent; this is not always true for non-normal distributions. Statistical independence of variables is itself desirable because the properties of combinations of independent variables can be derived easily from the properties of the individual variables.

Usually, the assumption of noise normality is well-founded, both for the primary recorded activity and for the averaged or summed activity. In both cases, this reflects the central limit theorem (Snedecor and Cochran, 1980), which states that any linear combination of random variables (such as a sum or average) will tend to be normally distributed, regardless of the distributions of the component variables. In the case of gross electrophysiologic activity, evoked or spontaneous, the linear combination arises implicitly from contribution to the overall activity by thousands of elementary events; for sums or averages, the linear combination is explicit. High-amplitude artifacts, such as eyeblink artifacts in SVP recording or myogenic bursts in ABR/MLR recording, represent extreme-value departures from the normal distribution, but they are usually removed by artifact rejection systems.

DIFFERENTIAL RECORDING AND AMPLIFICATION

The noise components in electrical activity on the head can be from about one to four orders of magnitude larger than the AEPs of interest. However, many noise components, especially those of nonphysiologic origin and those from distant muscle groups, such as from the heart or from gross limb movements, take similar values at various points on or near the head, at any point in time. In contrast, the scalp distribution (topography) of sensory evoked potentials usually shows marked variation across the head and neck (Picton, Hillyard, Krausz, and Galambos, 1974). Thus, by measuring not

absolute potentials but differences in potential at two or more points, usually both on the head, the noise components will at least partially cancel. Given appropriate electrode placements, the AEP components may not cancel, and may even be enhanced. In this way, the SNR can be increased massively.

The effects of differential recording, and the importance of recording electrode position, can be determined by considering the scalp amplitude topography of the signal and noise components. Each component has its own topographic distribution, which will evolve over time. The key to improving the SNR is to place the electrodes at sites where the signals differ as much as possible (ideally, of opposite polarity at the two sites), but the noise is as similar (positively correlated) as possible. Note that if an AEP were to radiate to the scalp in such a way that the potential at any instant were the same all over the head, then differential recording would not register it. Also, there is not necessarily a net gain from differencing; statistically, the act of subtracting two random variables increases the variance of the result, unless there is substantial positive correlation between the noise processes at the two sites of the differential pair.

There has been much more attention paid to scalp topography of the various AEPs than there has been to their associated noise processes, except in the case of the SVP, for which the noise mainly comprises the classical EEG and corneoretinal potentials, both of which have been mapped extensively. To address fully the problem of optimizing the SNR, topographic studies of the noise in the time domain would have to address matters such as the amplitude and autocorrelation function of the noise at various sites and the cross-correlation functions between sites; in the frequency domain, the pertinent measures include the power spectra and cross-spectral coherence functions. For the ABR and MLR, it is the topography and correlation structure of myogenic activity that is crucial; for the SVP, it is the properties of the alpha and theta rhythms.

For a single differential recording channel, three electrodes are required: the noninverting (positive), inverting (negative), and common (ground) electrodes. Terms such as "active" and "reference" are outdated and usually inappropriate, because both the noninverting and inverting electrodes are usually "active" in the sense that there is significant signal at both sites.

For single-channel AEP measurements, the non-inverting electrode is usually placed on the scalp vertex, at position Cz, in the 10–20 System of the International EEG Federation (Jasper, 1953; Regan, 1989), or high on the forehead in the midline (Fz). The forehead is not an efficient site for the SVP. Usually, the inverting electrode is in the periauricular region (mastoid, earlobe, external meatus) of the ear being stimulated, the stimulation being usually monaural, by supra-aural or insert earphone. The common electrode is often in the contralateral periauricular region. Such electrode montage allows registration of all the common waves in the ABR, MLR, and SVP, but is not necessarily optimal (in the amplitude sense) for any specific AEP component. For example, ABR wave V usually has the same polarity at the vertex and the mastoid ipsilateral to the stimulus, but is larger at the vertex, so partial cancellation occurs. This wave develops no significant amplitude at the neck, for example, so a larger net amplitude would be obtained with the inverting electrode at that site (Parker, 1981). However, the periauricular site is appropriate for recording ABR wave I, whereas the neck is not. For the SVP, the periauricular site need not be ipsilateral to be stimulated ear; this may also be true for the MLR and even for the ABR, for threshold measurement specifically, as long as ABR wave P2 (wave I) is of little interest.

Although differential amplification is a vital step in improving the SNR, it is very important not to forget that in the measurement and interpretation of the AEPs recorded in this way, we are dealing not with the actual potential at any single site, but with a potential difference. An obvious example is that ABR wave I is actually skin-negative in the periauricular region but is usually inverted relative to the vertex activity, whereas wave V is mainly vertex-positive. This differencing permits potentially misleading effects; for example, if natural anatomical variation, or certain stimulus parameters, or pathological changes, were to alter the topographic balance of potential registered at each of the differential sites, the observed (difference) AEP could increase, decrease, go to zero, or change sign. A zero resultant AEP

does not mean a zero actual scalp AEP, an increased resultant AEP could have been caused by a reduction in actual scalp AEP amplitude, and an apparent latency shift could have arisen from a sign change. For a more detailed discussion, see Regan (1989) and for a thorough exposition, see Nunez (1981).

If the noninverting and inverting electrodes were switched, all that would happen is that the difference waveform would be inverted. While it might seem perverse to upturn centuries of Cartesian geometry and plot the net voltage negative upwards, widespread inconsistency of practice lingers on. Debates about which way up AEPs should be plotted seem futile; what matters most is that in published reports it should be absolutely clear what is up, which is often not the case, in more ways than one.

Effectively, the differential preamplifier subtracts the activity at the inverting electrode from that at the noninverting electrode, and multiplies the difference by the gain factor, typically 10,000–50,000. The common electrode is required as an electrical reference point for the preamplifier, but the activity at the common site does not contribute significantly to the amplifier output. A measure of the preamplifier's ability to reject similar activity at both inputs is the common-mode rejection ratio, or CMRR. This is the ratio of amplifier output when a signal is presented to only one input, relative to the output when the same signal is presented to both inputs. Typical values for the CMRR exceed 80 dB; in voltage terms, this means that the output for activity common to both inputs (common-mode activity) will be more than 10,000 times smaller than for the single-input condition (20 dB per factor of 10).

The CMRR varies with frequency and is often tuned to be maximal for the most problematic noise source, such as 60 Hz power line interference. Periodic readjustment may be needed to maintain optimal values, especially on older equipment. Note that a 10 dB decrease in CMRR is roughly equivalent to tripling the common mode noise level at the preamplifier output, an increase that is likely to have a drastic effect on the accuracy of AEP measurements.

The electrical impedance of each electrode/skin interface is usually in the range of 1–10 kilohms, and because the preamplifier input impedance is of the order of megohms or higher, there will be negligible voltage drop across the interface (by Ohm's Law). Thus, the interface impedance has little effect on the AEP waveform itself. However, this impedance is important for two reasons. First, the size of the voltage developed at the amplifier input by an electric current source, such as electromagnetically induced noise current, is proportional to the source impedance; thus, high impedances can degrade the SNR not by affecting the signal, but by increasing the noise level. Stimulus artifact and 60 Hz power line pickup are examples of electromagnetically induced noise. Second, impedances may all be very good in absolute terms, such as less than 2 kilohms, but the CMRR of the preamplifier is degraded by any impedance asymmetry within the differential pair. The maximum CMRR obtainable is equal to twice the amplifier input impedance, divided by the absolute value of the difference in electrode impedances (Regan, 1989). Thus, if the amplifier impedance is 10 megohms, a 1 kilohm difference will limit the CMRR to 86 dB; a 2 kilohm difference will halve that CMRR to 80 dB, that is, will double the common-mode noise level. To put this in perspective, note that to halve a root-mean-square (RMS, equivalent to the standard deviation for normally distributed noise with zero mean) noise level requires a four-fold increase in the amount of averaging required to maintain a given measurement accuracy.

Differential amplification, in spite of being an important step in rendering the AEP detectable, is by no means sufficient. The main reason for this is that much of the physiologic noise that obscures the AEP is not identical at the noninverting and inverting electrodes; it is largely uncorrelated noise and its ability to obscure the signal is affected little by the differential action.

FILTERING

Introduction

Filtering is usually the next basic step in the effort to improve the SNR. Its general objective is to suppress preferentially those frequency components of the activity that contain particularly high amounts of noise

energy. The action of a filter can be expressed either in the time or the frequency domains (see the Appendix), but is easiest to conceptualize in the frequency domain. The effect at any frequency f is expressed by the filter transfer function, which has two parts: a modulus, which affects the amplitude of any input frequency component at f, and a phase shift, which alters the phase angle of that input frequency component. The modulus and the phase shift are functions of frequency, the modulus taking values between zero and unity, and the phase shift taking a wide range of values, positive or negative (in degrees or radians). The filter effects on the amplitude and phase of input frequency components are quite distinct; it is possible to have phase-shifting filters with unit modulus at all frequencies, filters with non-unit modulus and zero phase shift, and a huge variety of intermediate combinations of modulus and phase functions, depending on the precise design of the filter.

Filters can be implemented in analog or digital form; an analog filter is a physical device that operates on a continuously varying voltage-time input process that can take any real value, that is, it can take any value on the so-called real line, a continuum that extends between plus and minus infinity. The filter output is a similar type of process. In contrast, a digital filter is a numerical algorithm that operates on a sequence of numbers; the numbers can be real numbers, but usually they are discrete (taking only certain values), such as an integer sequence obtained by sampling and digitizing a continuous voltage-time process. The digital filter output is a modified numerical sequence. The filtering algorithm can be implemented by a general-purpose computer or by dedicated hardware.

Filter Designs

A useful concept is that of the ideal filter, which passes some input frequency components unchanged (in the pass band), but totally suppresses others (in the stop band). Common types of ideal filter moduli are shown in Figure 3.2, and include the low pass, high pass, band pass, and band stop types. In practice, such moduli can only be approximated by real filters, whether analog or digital; examples of this are also shown in the figure.

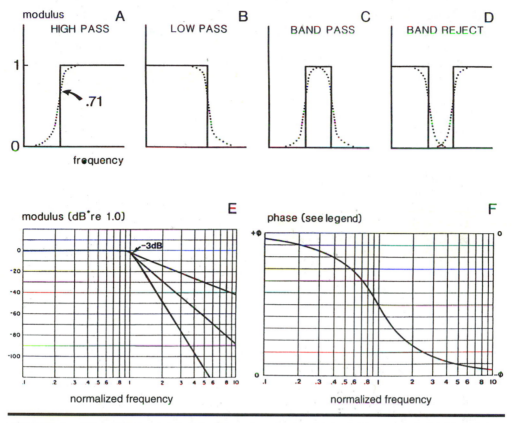

FIGURE 3.2.   (A) to (D) Some ideal (solid) and realizable (dotted) filter moduli. (E) Moduli for 12, 24, and 48, dB/octave Butterworth filters; note the linear rolloff on log-log axes, and the common 3 dB down point. The abscissa is *f/fc* for a low-pass filter, and *fc/f* for a high-pass filter, where *fc* is the cutoff (–3 dB) frequency. (F) The phase function for a Butterworth filter. The left-hand ordinate indicates positive phase shift (phase lead) for a high-pass filter; the right-hand ordinate indicates negative phase shift (phase lag) for a low-pass filter. Full scale is 180, 360 or 720 degrees, for 12, 24, and 48 dB/octave filters, respectively. The abscissa is *f/fc* for all cases.

Real filters have a frequency region (the transition band) where the modulus takes values intermediate between zero and unity.

There are many designs of each type of filter, distinguishable by the exact form of their transfer functions; some standard designs from the analog filter world are called Bessel (also known as maximally flat delay), Butterworth (maximally flat), Chebychev Types I and II, and elliptic (Cauer) filters, which terms relate to the underlying mathematical expressions (usually polynomials of various degrees) involved in the transfer function. These common designs differ in the manner in which they approximate the ideal modulus functions, and in the form of the phase shift function. For a given order of filter (first, second, etc.), which depends on the degree of the polynomial(s) in the transfer function, the rate of change of the modulus is usually a corresponding multiple of 6 dB per octave, well outside the passband. However, the details of the amplitude and phase behavior vary a great deal between filter designs.

Generally, there is a trade-off between the extent to which the modulus approximates the ideal, and the amount of nonlinearity of the phase function.

Effects of Filters

In an analog filter, the number of electronic components and the accuracy of component specifications required increase rapidly with the filter order; filters with order higher than eight (48 dB/octave cutoff) are unusual, and first, second, or fourth order filters (6, 12, or 24 dB/octave) are the most common in AEP work. While there is a tendency to think of filters as behaving almost ideally, the actual amount of attenuation achieved outside the passband is often quite small, especially for real filters with low order. For example, a 12 dB/octave high-pass filter with a cutoff frequency (–3 dB point) of 100 Hz will attenuate 60 Hz activity by a factor of only about three, and a 24 dB/octave filter with the same cutoff frequency will achieve a factor of about eight.

The extent to which filtering will improve the SNR depends primarily on the amount of overlap of the signal and noise spectra. If these spectra are identical, the filter may not alter the SNR at all. If, on the other hand, there is no overlap, an ideal filter would completely eliminate the noise and a real filter might also perform quite well, depending on its slope. For most AEPs, the signal and noise spectra overlap strongly, so the SNR enhancement achievable by filtering is modest. This issue has not been studied in sufficient depth for any AEP, so it is difficult to predict how effective a particular filter will be, or to specify filters that will be in some sense optimal for various recording situations.

One of the results of filtering signal and noise components that have overlapping spectra is that the filter alters the signal. It does this by two mechanisms: first, by attenuating certain signal frequency components, in frequency regions of significant response energy and less than unit filter modulus. The limiting case of attenuation is disappearance, and an example of the impact of this is that for several years it was widely believed that a low-frequency stimulus such as a 500 Hz tonepip did not evoke an ABR; then, Suzuki and Horiuchi (1977) obtained clear responses with wide

recording bandwidth, which disappeared when using the high-pass cutoff frequencies of 100 Hz or more that were customary for recording click ABRs.

The second mechanism by which a filter can alter, or distort, an input waveform is by changing the relative phase (and therefore, the relative timing) of its frequency components, even those not significantly attenuated. This effect, known as phase distortion, often dominates the changes in AEP waveform (see, for example, Boston and Ainslie, 1980; Doyle and Hyde, 1981a; Stapells and Picton, 1981; Kileny, 1983). Whether this distortion is important or not depends entirely on what use is being made of particular AEP features. If the specific goal of the measurement is solely AEP detection, which is often the case when estimating audiometric thresholds, phase distortion may not matter or may even improve response detectability. In contrast, for making inferences about the presence or absence of a retrocochlear lesion, there is usually a need for more detailed calculations involving latencies; here, the filter effects must be considered more carefully.

Some generalizations can be made about the distortions introduced by the high-pass and low-pass components of a bandpass filter. The low-pass filter will smooth out the high-frequency components, and will introduce a time lag in each frequency component. The lag at any frequency is equal to the rate of change of phase angle with frequency, at that point (that is, its first differential). If the filter phase function were linear over f, it is easy to deduce that the time lag would be constant over frequency, for all components of the input signal, so there would be no phase distortion; of the classes mentioned earlier, the Bessel filter approximates this most closely, and especially in the low-pass mode.

A high-pass filter will introduce time lead (that is, negative lag) by the same argument, and because high-pass filters often encroach more significantly on frequency regions that contain large amounts of response energy, their effects on the signal waveform are often more profound that those of commonly used low-pass filters. The effects are also more difficult to predict. In general, high-pass filtering will depress the amplitude of any given peak in the wide-band ABR, and will introduce an artifactual succeeding peak of opposite polarity. More severe filtering may abolish the wide-band peak, depress the succeeding peak, and induce a later artifactual peak of the same polarity as the original peak. These distortions can occur for all peaks in a sequence such as the ABR, and their summed effect can be quite complex, in terms of relating peaks in the filtered waveform to those in the wide-band waveform. Some examples of these effects are shown in Figure 3.3. On more than one occasion in the history of AEP applications, these distortions have confounded clini-

cal practice and research. An example was the investigation of the physiologic origin of waves that were purely a product of phase distortion.

In the classical world of analog filters, the choice among the filter designs usually depends on the relative importance of the modulus approaching the ideal, versus the phase distortion or time-domain ringing (an oscillatory response to impulsive excitation) associated with phase nonlinearity. A Bessel filter has the most linear phase function, but the onset of cutoff is very gradual. A

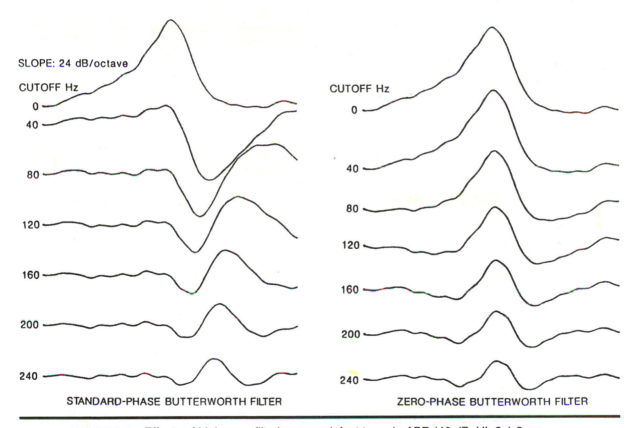

FIGURE 3.3.   Effects of high-pass filtering on an infant tonepip ABR (40 dBnHL 2-1-2 ms, 500 Hz tonepip, notch masking; window 25.6 ms). The top waveforms show the true response waveform, with recording bandwidth 1–1500 Hz; only a broad vertex-positive wave V peak is visible. The left-hand column shows the effect of increasing high-pass cutoff frequency for a regular 24 dB/octave Butterworth filter. Note the depression of wave V, development of an artifactual succeeding negative wave (SN_{10}), and a later positive wave, as well as the changes in peak latency. The right-hand column shows the results for the same filter moduli, but with zero phase shift. The two columns show the distortions introduced by the modulus alone (right) and the modulus plus phase effects (left).

Butterworth filter has moderate phase nonlinearity and a very uniform modulus in the passband, with a fairly rapid cutoff onset. A Chebychev Type I filter modulus exhibits constant-amplitude "ripple" (equiripple, typically less than 3 dB) in the passband, but has very rapid cutoff onset; the Chebychev Type II has a monotonic passband modulus, rapid cutoff onset and equiripple in the stopband. The elliptic filter has equiripple in both the passband and stopband, and for a given order of filter, it has the narrowest possible transition band. Both Chebychev and elliptic analog filters have relatively strong phase nonlinearity.

For creating a filtered masking noise, for example, phase may be relatively unimportant and the modulus behavior very important, so the Chebychev or elliptic designs might be favored. On the other hand, for improving the SNR of a transient wave packet such as an AEP, where distortion of the waveform is often unacceptable, the Bessel or the Butterworth designs are more common.

Digital Filters

For many reasons, the power and flexibility of digital filters are very much greater than those of analog filters. Any analog filter can be simulated digitally; it is a matter of developing the appropriate numerical algorithm. However, many digital filters exist that cannot be implemented in analog form. For example, consider a digital filter in which a section of the digitized activity is stored prior to manipulation by a numerical algorithm. It is possible, in such a filter that has memory, to run the stored activity backwards through the algorithm, that is, to reverse time, which is sometimes done to produce zero phase shift. Clearly, this is not possible in an analog filter, which usually operates on the input process as it occurs in real time. In the world of signal processing, even when an analog output is required, the power of digital filters is such that it is nowadays quite common to digitize the input process with an analog to digital converter (ADC), implement the filter numerically, then generate the desired continuous output via a digital to analog converter (DAC).

It is possible to design digital filters with a huge variety of modulus and phase characteristics, including the classical designs. It is a relatively straightforward matter to construct filters with zero phase shift, that cause no phase distortion, and this can be a major advantage in some AEP applications. The increasing availability of sophisticated digital filters offers many possibilities, some of which are being implemented in the latest commercial AEP instrumentation systems. See Marsh (1988) for an introduction to digital filtering of AEPs. For detailed technical information about digital filter design, see Cohen (1986), Hamming (1983), and Rabiner and Gold (1975).

At present, digital filtering is most commonly implemented after averaging, not before it as is the case for analog filtering. The averaging and filtering operations are both linear, which means that they commute, that is, their order is interchangeable. It is easier to digitally filter an average, rather than the primary activity, because the speed and volume of computation required are much less. An advantage of digital filtering after averaging is the ability to try out various, or multiple, filtering operations without altering the source data (the average). For example, the commonly available n-point smoothing (with n typically ranging from three to seven) is a simple digital filtering operation. It is increasingly common to be able to apply a wider variety of digital filters, so nowadays the main filtering operations for SNR enhancement are sometimes carried out after averaging. Also, it is even possible to remove digitally any phase distortion caused by prior analog filtering (Doyle and Hyde, 1981b).

There is almost always a need for at least a certain amount of analog low-pass filtering prior to the stage of analog to digital conversion (ADC), in order to prevent aliasing errors (described later) during the sampling process. Analog low-pass filtering for SNR enhancement may perform the anti-aliasing function as well, but even if most of the filtering for SNR enhancement is to be carried out digitally, the ADC must be preceded by an anti-aliasing analog low-pass filter. There is also usually a need for a certain amount of analog high-pass filtering before ADC, because without it, high-amplitude low-frequency noise excursions will trigger artifact rejection systems (see later) excessively and unnecessarily.

Wiener Filters

It was noted earlier that the degree to which filters will improve the SNR depends upon the spectra of the signal and noise. Classical filter designs permit only limited variations in filter parameters, often restricted to specifications of cutoff frequency and order. Also, such filters have transfer functions that are chosen a priori, and are not intimately dependent on the actual data to be filtered. More sophisticated digital filter designs, such as the so-called "Wiener" filter, can take account of signal and noise characteristics more explicitly. For a known, deterministic signal and known, stationary noise, the Wiener filter is a zero-phase digital filter that is optimal, in the sense that it produces a filtered process that estimates the true signal with minimum mean square error. The classical Wiener filter transfer function is the ratio of the known spectra of the signal (AEP) and noise. For most AEP measurements, the signal and the noise are both probably nonstationary, and certainly are also unknown in the sense that they must be estimated statistically from a sample. The Wiener approach can still be used, based upon certain signal and noise estimates, and this is called "a posteriori" Wiener filtering (Doyle, 1975). The average AEP estimate is usually the best approximation to the true AEP waveform, so the spectrum of this average essentially estimates the signal spectrum. The primary epochs (sweeps) of the source activity that are used for averaging are dominated by the noise process, which is why averaging is needed in the first place, so the average spectrum of the source activity provides an estimate of the noise spectrum. See de Weerd and Martens (1978), or the DSP texts cited earlier, for more detailed discussions of Wiener filtering technique.

An advantage of the estimated Wiener filter approach is that it takes detailed account of the signal and noise characteristics for the individual AEP measurement, and will tend to give smaller mean square signal estimation errors. However, this sensitivity to the noise conditions pertaining in the individual subject at any particular time, coupled with effects of sampling error, may result in unstable Wiener filter estimates, such that the Wiener approach may be least helpful when it is most needed, that is, when the SNR is very small

(Wastell, 1981). In principle, at least, sampling error in the estimation of the filter transfer function can lead to increased overall variation in AEP estimates that is potentially counterproductive (Doyle and Hyde, 1985). Also, many of the otoneurologic applications of AEPs depend upon specific waveform features, such as peak latencies and interwave intervals, the properties of which may not be optimized by approaches oriented towards minimization of mean square amplitude error. However, Dobie and Wilson (1990) showed recently that Wiener filtering improved ABR and 40 Hz MLR consistency within subjects, and lowered the visual detection thresholds for these AEPs. Further research oriented towards very specific AEP measures, measurement goals and test circumstances is required to determine fully the practical value of this filtering approach.

Time-variant Filters

All of the filters discussed up to this point have fixed parameters, that is, their transfer functions are constant over the duration of the AEP waveform to be filtered. It is also possible to design digital filters with transfer functions that evolve over time; these are time-variant filters (de Weerd, 1981). Almost any filter design can be implemented in a time-variant fashion; one approach is to divide the data to be filtered into a series of segments, and then apply a series of filters that have changing parameters. Time-variant filters are of most obvious interest when the signal itself has characteristics that change substantially over time; this might be the case for the full ABR wave sequence, for which there is a discernible trend to lower frequency activity later in the sequence. The MLR and SVP, however, do not usually exhibit such trends, so the value of time-variant filtering is limited with those AEPs.

Filter Optimization

The optimal choice of filter is far from straightforward. First, optimality will depend on the measurement goals, and the processing that is best for, say, AEP detection will probably not be the best for AEP estimation involving detailed measurement of waveform features. Here, being able to apply several digital filters nondestructively, to the average, may prove to be especially useful. Second, there is the need to account for both intra- and interindividual components of variation of both signal and noise, in relation to AEP detection and classification criteria. For example, a procedure that reduces intra-average or intrasubject variation of AEP estimates could actually increase inter-subject variation (through distortion, for example), with an overall deterioration in diagnostic accuracy. Third, there is the problem that "optimal" filtering in the individual subject may vary greatly over the wide range of possible pathology-induced changes in AEP waveform. It follows that an iterative approach, developing adaptive, outcome-specific filters might be required. Much further research is needed in this area.

Artifact Rejection Filters

While the usual goal of filtering is to increase the SNR in the actual data that will be averaged, it may be useful to apply a quite different filter to a parallel data channel, specifically in order to enhance noise components or artifacts. Such a channel could be used to trigger the artifact rejection operation for the main data channel (see later), or it might be possible to combine the two channels in such a way as to increase the net SNR. Such a method is sometimes used, albeit with electrode sites directed specifically at artifact pickup, to reduce eye movement artifact in the recording of late AEPs (Regan, 1989).

Notch Filters

Special analog filters designed to suppress specific noise components, notably 60 Hz power line pickup, are available in most commercial AEP systems. These are often called notch filters, a special case of the bandstop type. In the past, the notch filters commonly available caused considerable phase distortion, but the exact amount of distortion will depend on the precise notch filter phase characteristics. Prior to using any such filter clinically, the amount of distortion that it causes should be measured under the exact, intended

conditions of use. Generally, it is appropriate to caution that commonly available notch filters should be used only as a last resort in very adverse recording situations, such as may arise in buildings with wiring that is not in metal conduit. Moreover, even if better notch filters could be implemented, the occurrence of high levels of 60 Hz interference is often symptomatic of problems such as poor electrode contact, for which filtering is not usually the best answer. It should be noted that the impact of coherent, sustained noise components such as 60 Hz pickup depends strongly on the stimulus repetition rate, because time-domain averaging itself has some filtering characteristics (see later).

Whether the main noise is myogenic, as for the ABR and MLR, sinusoidal EEG rhythm, as in SVP recording, or nonphysiologic, as for 60 Hz power line pickup in any AEP measurement, noise problems should be addressed at the source, wherever possible, rather than by signal processing maneuvers. Thus, in ABR or MLR recording, high levels of myogenic activity are usually better tackled by trying to adjust the subject's posture, level of discomfort or anxiety, than by applying strong filtering or artifact rejection. Similarly, for SVP measurement, giving the subject a mid-session break can cause improvements in the noise levels that would be hard to match by a great deal of signal processing. It is useful to think of many of the signal processing operations at our disposal, such as filtering, artifact rejection, and averaging, as necessary evils to be used sparingly. There is a tendency to place undue reliance upon these techniques, when a little more attention to the subject and to the electrodes would be far more beneficial.

ANALOG-TO-DIGITAL CONVERSION (ADC)

Introduction

After differential amplification and initial analog filtering, the next steps in signal processing for SNR enhancement require that the activity be converted to digital form. This is a process of replacing a random process (the activity) that is continuous both in time and amplitude by a process that is discrete in both respects. The time domain is made discrete by the process of sampling the activity, usually uniformly, that is, at fixed intervals. The amplitude is made discrete by the process of quantization, which is the generation of an integer that approximates the (continuously variable) amplitude of the activity at each instant of sampling. The result is a discrete sequence (a time series) that represents the activity (see Figure 3.4A).

Sampling

The process of sampling a continuous time-history can be thought of as one of multiplying it by a series of equally spaced unit pulses. The main issue in sampling is the choice of sampling rate, that is, the number of samples per second, and this choice relates to whether all the information present in the continuous process is actually still present, albeit hidden, in the sampled process. Suppose a sampled sine wave is available and the problem is to work out what the frequency of the origi-

nal sine wave was. Now, consider any sine wave that is sampled at twice its frequency, at the zero crossings, say. It is apparent that there is no sinusoid of lower frequency that could give exactly the same pattern, but there are many of higher frequency that could, for example, the harmonics (see Figure 3.4B). It follows that, given some sample series, if it is known that the original sinusoid had a frequency of less than half the sampling rate, then its frequency is determined uniquely by the samples. However, if it could have had a higher frequency, there is the potential for confusion between possible options. Other ways of saying this are that if the sampling rate is not sufficient, then the samples do not define the original signal uniquely, or that there has been a loss of information due to the sampling. The usual, practical example of this loss of information is the stagecoach wagon wheel in the western movie. The camera frame speed is analogous to the sampling rate and is fixed; there is no problem representing the mo-

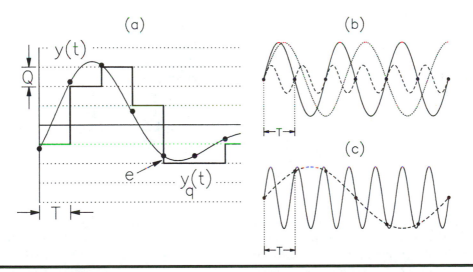

FIGURE 3.4.   (A) The sampling and quantization of a continuous waveform y(t) to yield a digitized output waveform yq(t). The sampling instants are indicated by dots, with sampling interval T. Q is the step size and e is a sampling error. (B) Information content of samples: the solid sinusoid is sampled at two samples per period; a higher frequency sinusoid such as an harmonic (dashed) could also give the same pattern of sample values (all zeros in this example), whereas any lower frequency sinusoid (dotted) could not. (C) Aliasing: sampling a sinusoid (solid) at less than the Nyquist rate (two samples per period) leads to illusory low-frequency energy (dotted) indistinguishable from genuine low-frequency energy that may be present in a complex signal with many component frequencies.

tion of the wheel, provided its actual rate of rotation is much lower than the frame speed. As it speeds up, the wheel can appear to rotate at any speed, even backwards, depending on the exact relationship of rotation and frame speeds, and then the rotation rate cannot be deduced with certainly from the apparent rate.

Suppose the process to be sampled is now a random time-history, such as might be obtained from a pair of scalp electrodes; generally, such a time-history will have many frequency components, such as might be revealed by Fourier analysis. The above argument about sampling sinusoids could be applied to every frequency component. It follows that the time-history can be sampled without loss of information, only if the sampling rate is at least twice the frequency of the highest-frequency component present. This is an informal approach to Shannon's sampling theorem, which states in effect that a band-limited signal of maximum frequency f (one with no energy above f) must be sampled at a rate of at least $2f$, in order to be deducible and, in fact, mathematically recoverable without error, from the sample series. The rate $2f$ is known as the Nyquist rate. The details of how the original signal is recovered from the samples are given in standard signal processing texts, and it involves convolution (see Appendix) with a $\sin x/x$ function.

If the sampling theorem is not satisfied, then the potential exists for confusing signal energy at several frequencies. This spectral confusion is called aliasing. Most commonly, there is some signal energy at above the Nyquist frequency because the low-pass filter that is supposed to prevent this (the anti-aliasing filter) has either too gradual a rolloff, or too high a cutoff frequency. What happens then is that the energy above the Nyquist frequency becomes mixed with the true components of the signal, causing measurement error. In the signal processing field, it is common to sample at from 2.5 to 10 times the cutoff frequency of the anti-aliasing filter, in order to avoid this problem.

A slightly more formal approach to the sampling problem is as follows. A band-limited process has a spectrum that actually extends from $-f$ to f, that is, it has width $2f$. It can be shown that the spectrum of the sampled process is that of the continuous process, but repeated at intervals of F, where F equals $1/T$ and T is the time between samples. It follows that the repeating spectra will overlap unless the sampling frequency F is greater than or equal to $2f$. Now, the spectrum of a process is the square of its Fourier transform and the time-domain and frequency-domain representations of the activity are Fourier transform pairs, that is, they are interconvertible and formally equivalent. Normally, any band-limited function of time has associated with it an unique Fourier transform, and the time function can be regenerated from the transform, by the process of inverse transformation. This is also true for the sampled process, provided the multiple images of the spectrum do not overlap. If they do, then energy from more than one image is mixed irrevocably and the 1:1 correspondence between the Fourier transform and the original time function is lost, so it cannot be recovered by inverse transformation.

The sampling theorem is rarely an issue in practical AEP recording, unless many channels of activity are being multiplexed to a single ADC; under these circumstances, the effective sampling rate for any one channel is the ADC rate divided by the number of channels, and this can become a concern if the number of channels is large. There is also a potential problem if all the channels are not sampled at the same instant, but sequentially, which can cause errors in those analyses that depend strongly on the exact temporal relationships between the activities in the various channels, such as in topographic or vectorial analyses (see later). It is preferable to use simultaneous sampling and a high-performance ADC, in sophisticated multichannel analyses.

For the more common types of AEP measurement, with small numbers of channels, the sampling theorem is rarely a concern because the activity is sampled at a sufficiently high rate that the time series closely resembles the waveform of the activity itself, for purposes of visual inspection; this practice leads to rates substantially higher than the Nyquist rate. For example, to produce a time series that adequately defines an ABR peak in response to a click stimulus of moderate intensity, a sampling rate of at least 10,000 Hz is required, yet there is little response energy above 2000 Hz. Effects of sampling at too low a rate for accurate, direct visualization are changes in apparent amplitude and latency of peaks.

Quantization

At each instant of sampling, the ADC generates an N-bit binary word that represents the input process. The number of distinct values that the word can take is two to the power N. The number of bits is commonly referred to as the resolution of the ADC. An eight-bit quantizer, for example, generates 256 distinct values, and if the input activity has an amplitude range from $-V$ to V, the quantization step is $V/128$. Thus, the entire input voltage range is mapped onto 256 output values, but the actual amplitude of the input process will rarely be exactly equal to any of the 256 possibilities; the resulting errors are quantization errors.

The quantization errors can be thought of as small random error terms that are added to the input process, to yield the quantized process (see Figure 3.4A). The variance of the sum of two independent processes is the sum of their variances, so the quantization errors add noise to the input process. To a good approximation, the statistical distribution of quantization error is uniform over any given quantization step. If a random variable is uniformly distributed over a range Q, then it is easy to show that its variance is $Q^2/12$ (Snedecor and Cochran, 1980). To put this error in perspective, suppose the activity has a standard deviation (SD) of ten microvolts at the subject's head. A preamplifier gain of 100,000 will give a signal of SD 1.0 V at the output. Let the anti-aliasing filter have unit gain, and the ADC have an input range from -5 V to 5 V, with eight-bit resolution. The quantization step size is about 0.4 microvolts at the head, so the quantization noise variance is about 0.013 microvolts squared, giving an SD of about 0.11 microvolts, about one percent of the total SD. This is not significant. For a much more detailed, general analysis of the statistics of quantization, see Cohen (1986).

The ADC output is the input to either summation or averaging, which has the effect of increasing the effective resolution. For example, if each of two quantities can take 256 distinct values, then their average can take 512 distinct values. Thus, an 8-bit ADC is sufficient for most average AEP measurements, and the quantization noise is negligible. Quite reasonable AEP waveform estimates after summing or averaging can be obtained with only a one-bit conversion, which is

equivalent to capturing only the sign of the input data (Hyde and Doyle, 1983; Picton, Linden, Hamel, and Maru, 1983), although there is substantial quantization noise for convertors with less than about four bits, in ABR recording (Picton, Hink, Perez-Abalo, Linden, and Wiens, 1984).

EDITING OR ARTIFACT REJECTION

The idea that a set of repeated measurements might contain "extreme values" or "outliers," values that are somehow corrupted and not representative of the bulk of the sample, is a familiar one in experimental science. Extreme values can cause substantial bias of sample statistics such as the sample mean and variance. There are many statistical approaches to such a situation, ranging from simple criteria for removing the outliers from the sample, through to the use of estimators that are less vulnerable (more "robust") to outliers than is the ordinary mean. Examples of such measures include various "trimmed" means and rank statistics such as the median. See Snedecor and Cochran (1980) for an introductory discussion of robust estimation.

The noise processes in a typical AEP measurement often exhibit high-amplitude events that are best considered to be outliers or artifacts. Sources include eye movement and electrode movement artifacts in SVP recordings, and electromyogenic artifacts in ABR and MLR recordings. If included in the subsequent summation or averaging, high-amplitude artifacts can bias the result in such a way as to mimic a genuine AEP waveform, or to suppress or distort the genuine AEP waveform. The impact of a single artifact depends on the value of N and the size of the AEP of interest; the smaller the N and the smaller the AEP, the larger the impact. For example, in an SVP measurement with an N of 50, a single artifact of size 50 microvolts contributes an average amplitude of one microvolt, which must be considered in relation to a typical size for the average SVP of about 5–10 microvolts at moderate stimulus levels, and 1–2 microvolts near threshold; the cause for concern is clear. In an ABR measurement with an N of 2000, the same single artifact would contribute 25 nanovolts to the average, not a major problem in itself, although the combined effects of a few such artifacts could easily bias significantly the estimate of the true ABR. Thus, it is common to apply acceptability conditions to the segments of EEG activity that are later to be summed or averaged. Usually, each digitized segment of primary activity is routed to a buffer array and tested for acceptability, before inclusion in the average.

The usual approach to acceptability testing is not necessarily the best one, but is easy to implement. Typically, the buffer array is tested for presence of amplitudes outside some acceptable range, and sweeps (arrays) that do not satisfy the criterion are discarded. If implemented with an appropriate criterion, even such a simple procedure can improve the accuracy of AEP measurements considerably, under conditions of sporadic high-amplitude noise levels, such as with subjects who are active, uncomfortable, or not entirely cooperative.

The correct management of artifact rejection criteria is not a simple matter, but it can have quite strong effects on the quality of averages. The most common fault is to set the rejection criterion at too large a value relative to the general amount of fluctuation in the activity, resulting in insufficient rejection. Conversely, the major drawback of using too small (sensitive) rejection criteria is that the time taken to achieve the target N is increased. If the noise were really stationary, the mean (or sum) array without any artifact rejection would be the most powerful and efficient estimator of the true signal waveform; any deletion or alteration of any value in the sample would result only in loss of information. Thus, artifact rejection does not usually improve the quality of well-behaved data. However, admitting artifact-laden sweeps, while increasing the N more rapidly, can degrade the precision of the final average substantially. Thus, there is a compromise to be found. There appears to have been little published formal analysis of this problem of optimizing artifact rejection levels. In the author's experience, an effective approach is to set the level so as to achieve between 5 and 10 percent rejected sweeps when the noise conditions are considered to be stable and satisfactory. For the price of a negligible increase in averaging time under good EEG conditions, considerable protection from the effects of transient or sustained noise nonstationarity can be gained by this means (see Figure 3.5).

In the event that the activity from a given subject does not show well-demarcated periods of low and high variance, the task is more difficult. If the noise level is sustained and higher than usual, the cause in ABR and MLR recordings is probably a steady level of myogenic activity, often seen in subjects who are tense and anxious. Here, there is no clear distinction between good and bad activity, it is all fairly bad. By far the best course of action is to improve the quality of the source data, perhaps by reassuring or moving the subject, or if necessary, by relaxant medication. The next best course is to set the rejection level to give at least 10% rejection, and increase the amount of averaging in an attempt to compensate for the increased noise variance. An undesirable but common course is to ignore the poor quality of the data and suffer the ensuing loss of accuracy, or worse still, to open up the rejection limits so as to speed up the acquisition of the desired number of sweeps.

As suggested earlier, the most effective artifact rejection strategy would be based on accurate and sensitive detection of significant noise events, but the prior filtering of the activity is intended to suppress noise components. Thus, artifact rejection systems might operate more effectively if their input were not the actual data to be averaged, but a parallel data stream that had been configured for the express purpose of artifact detection.

If the rejection system operates on the data channel that is subsequently to be summed or averaged, which is the usual state of affairs in current instrumentation, the choice of high-pass filter characteristics often has a strong effect on the proportion of sweeps that will be rejected; this is because low-frequency energy is often dominant, at least for ABR and SVP measurements. It is important to set the preceding high-pass filter such that much of the dynamic range within the artifact rejection limits is occupied by activity in the main spectral regions of the AEP energy. For example, insufficient high-pass filtering of SVP data can lead to the tester reducing system gain so as to avoid excessive triggering of artifact rejection by large, slow (less than 1 Hz) voltage drifts associated mainly with transcutaneous potentials or electrode polarization effects. The spectral peak of the SVP is at about 5 Hz, so the energy below 1 Hz is almost irrelevant, but if it is not filtered appropriately, its

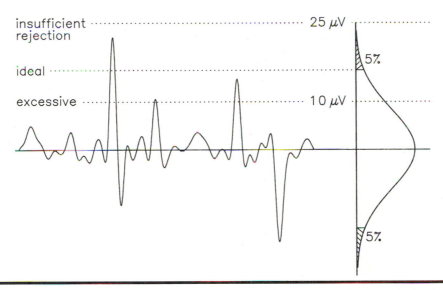

FIGURE 3.5. Amplitude-based artifact rejection can work well if the rejection criterion level is such that about 5–10% of "well-behaved" sweeps are rejected; see the EEG time-history and amplitude distribution (probability density function). Having to adjust the effective rejection criterion via the amplifier gain/sensitivity control (e.g., for 10 or 25 microvolt sensitivity) can cause insufficient rejection, leading to loss of measurement accuracy, or excessive rejection, leading to inefficient use of averaging time.

presence will lead to use of artifact rejection limits that are much too wide to deal effectively with more important artifacts in the 2 to 10 Hz range. A comparable argument applies to ABR recording.

It is regrettable that many current AEP instrumentation systems still fail to offer adequate control of the voltage level at which artifact rejection will occur. With systems in which rejection occurs simply at the ADC limits, the only way to control the effective rejection criterion level at the patient's head, which is what matters, is by altering the preamplifier gain. Gain steps are typically coarsely quantized, such as 10k, 20k, 50k, and so on, and this does not provide sufficiently fine adjustment. The typical result is that a strategy such as that proposed above is impossible, and that the effective rejection level is either much too high or much too low. This will have a tangible impact on the accuracy and efficiency of clinical AEP measurements, especially if threshold measurement is commonly the goal. The preferred AEP instrumentation systems allow re-

jection levels to be set at almost any value, such as a percentage of the full-scale display.

TIME-DOMAIN SUMMATION OR AVERAGING

The Root-*N* Law

Suppose that the activity conforms to the simple additive model discussed earlier. For each of N identical stimuli, let there be an associated digitized segment of primary activity (a sweep) that satisfies the artifact rejection criterion. Each sweep is synchronized (time-locked) to its associated stimulus, and comprises a time-series array of M values arising from regular sampling of the activity. The data for N sweeps then comprise a matrix with N rows and M columns. The operation of summation or averaging over N for each column creates the sum or average array of M elements.

For any column in the matrix, the SNR is usually defined as the ratio of root-mean-square (RMS) amplitudes of the signal (*s*) and the noise (*n*). It is shown in the Appendix that, regardless of whether the *N* sweeps are simply summed or are truly averaged, which requires a running division by the number of sweeps acquired at any point during the accumulation of the data matrix, the SNR in the sum or average array is the single-sweep SNR multiplied by the square root of *N*. It is important to note that the factor root *N* is based on statistical expectation (expected value) of the noise variance; the actual SNR obtained in practice, for any individual average, will exhibit sampling fluctuations.

The only important difference between summing and averaging lies in the visual appearance of the displayed result as the procedure progresses. If an AEP is present, then with summation, the response will appear to grow steadily relative to a noise background which also grows, but not as rapidly. For averaging, there is no impression of growth but, rather, one of gradual convergence to the final AEP estimate, as the noise variance in the average decreases. Hereafter in this chapter, the term "averaging" will be used exclusively.

The Number of Sweeps Required

Because averaging takes up most of the time in any AEP measurement session, and because the SNR in the average governs the accuracy of interpretive decisions, it is important to consider exactly how much averaging is needed. This is not a simple matter, but a ballpark figure for *N* can be derived easily. The bottom line on, say, an AEP determination for audiometric threshold estimation is a reliable decision about the presence or absence of response in a given average record. Of course, the average may still contain a lot of noise, it may even be entirely noise, so that decisions based on such records will be statistical ones having finite probability of error. Human observers looking at averaged records are comfortable making response detection decisions that have fairly low rates of false-positive detection; they require SNRs of about two or more before deciding with confidence that the AEP is present. This suggests that a putative response peak in the average must be about twice the size of the visually estimated standard deviation of the noise fluctuations in

the rest of the record. If the SNR in the average must be at least two, and the typical SNR in the elementary record is denoted as *R*, then the root-*N* law suggests that the number of sweeps required will be at least the square of (2/*R*). Typical values for *R* are 0.4 for the SVP, 0.1 for the MLR and 0.05 for the ABR, leading to requirements of 25, 400, and 1600 sweeps, respectively. However, these are just crude guidelines, and there are many factors that may influence the number of sweeps required in the individual case.

Even for a given AEP and purpose of measurement, it is not very reasonable to use a constant value of *N*. Suppose that one subject has on average twice the noise RMS of another, but that the AEPs are about the same size. This is perfectly plausible. To achieve similar levels of accuracy in detection decisions for the two subjects requires that the *N* be changed to compensate for the noise differences, about four times as many records being needed for the subject with the higher noise levels. To illustrate this, in a situation of fairly low EEG noise levels, averages of 2000 records are common practice for the ABR. For another subject whose noise level is twice as large, the continued use of 2000 sweeps per average is equivalent to the use of only 500 sweeps in the well-behaved case; few would consider that number to be adequate. This leads us to the reasonable conclusion that the greater the amplitude of the noise, the more averaging is required. Strictly speaking, the size of the AEP should also be taken into account.

Of course, there is an upper bound to the amount of averaging that can be accomplished in a feasible test time. The bottom line is that if the source data are of poor quality and test time is constant, something has to give; no amount of data processing will make a silk purse out of a sow's ear. In such situations, it is usually better to spend the available time getting a few large-*N* results that are reliable, rather than many that are not.

The use of large *N* may be less time-consuming than it appears, if a suitable stimulus repetition rate is used. There is a common tendency to use rates that are less than optimal. Whether for threshold or suprathreshold AEP measurements, a pertinent statistic to consider is a student *t*-like variable (Snedecor and Cochran, 1980) that is the ratio of the average AEP amplitude to the standard error of the noise in the average, as a function of stimulus repetition rate, given the constraint of constant averaging time. This quantity was called "efficacy" by Hyde and Blair (1981) and "efficiency" by Picton et al. (1983). To a greater extent than might be anticipated, loss of AEP amplitude due to adaptation is offset by the increased amount of averaging that can be done per unit test time. To a first approximation, it is worth considering the change from a stimulation rate A to a higher rate B if the ratio of expected AEP amplitude at B to that at A exceeds the square root of the ratio of interstimulus intervals for B over A. That is, other things being equal, it pays to double the rate if there would be less than about a 30% loss of AEP amplitude at the higher rate.

These arguments concerning the required N are not usually taken into account in clinical AEP testing, wherein the choice of N is rarely based on any quantitative rationale. The typical practice is to use a constant and somewhat arbitrary N for all averages, so the accuracy of AEP estimation or decision-making will vary inversely with the noise levels that occur. Unfortunately, current instrumentation rarely provides adequate information on which to base any quantitative strategy for selecting N. As systems become more sophisticated, it is to be hoped that data characteristics such as noise RMS will be extracted automatically, and either displayed in a helpful way to the tester or used in automatic control paradigms that guide the averaging to achieve consistent and known levels of accuracy, both for response detection decisions and for waveform description.

Part of the difficulty is that the specification of N is a non-trivial statistical problem that requires at least the specification of an explicit measurement precision goal, and such goals have not yet been formulated properly. However, as technology and automation impact more heavily on commercial AEP systems, more quantitative approaches will emerge. A good example is the approach proposed by Elberling and Don (1984, 1987), based upon the variance ratio measure known as Fsp, that adaptively predicts the number of sweeps needed to achieve a specified level of measurement accuracy.

More Complex Averaging Procedures

There are many modifications of the simple averaging procedure, or adjuncts to it, that are aimed mainly at further improvement in the SNR of the result. These procedures are usually computation-intensive and are not yet commonly implemented in commercial AEP systems. Two important techniques address variation of the signal over the set of rows in the data matrix, and nonstationarity of the noise over those rows. For a detailed and general analysis, see McGillem, Aunon, and Yu (1985). As mentioned earlier, the signal variation addressed most commonly is latency jitter, and the technique to deal with it is called latency-corrected averaging (Woody, 1967; Wastell, 1977; Regan, 1989). A typical algorithm for adaptive latency correction involves first storing every individual sweep and computing the simple average. Next, the cross-correlation function is determined between the average and every sweep; for any sweep, this involves computation of the correlation coefficient between the sweep and the average, for a set of time shifts between them, called lags. Lags can be positive or negative (time lead), and the set of correlation coefficients at the various lags comprises the cross-correlation function. If a maximum in that function occurs within some selected time range in the region of zero lag, the lag value at the maximum is assumed to approximate the amount of jitter for that sweep. The sweep is then time-shifted to set the jitter to zero. This procedure is followed for all sweeps, and then a new average is computed. This technique has been applied most frequently to EPs of cortical origin. The impact is a function of the primary SNR and, of course, the amount of jitter. Technical difficulties can arise at low SNR (Steeger, Herrman, and Spreng, 1983). It is not yet clear whether this latency-corrected averaging technique has any real clinical value in audiology, especially for AEPs caudal to the cerebral cortex. However, it is possible that pathophysiologic dysfunction that has no obvious effect on the simple average might manifest itself by causing AEP variation that is detectable by the latency-correction technique or some other, comparable approach.

Nonstationarity of the noise is, perhaps, a more concrete and familiar problem than latency jitter. The extreme example of it is the high-amplitude artifact that should trigger the artifact rejection system, if properly set. However, there is a certain range of noise variability that will pass through the rejection system and be incorporated into the average; some of this is just sampling variation, but actual nonstationarity of the noise variance may also occur. Two approaches to this problem will be discussed. The first involves computation of the cross-correlation between the average and every sweep, but only for zero lag. Then, a weighting value is assigned to each sweep, according to the size of the correlation coefficient, such that larger correlation is associated with higher weight. The effect is that sweeps that look like the average are assigned greater importance. It seems reasonable to expect that very noisy sweeps will tend to be downweighted by this procedure. A new average is then calculated, using the weighted sweeps. This approach can be applied to deal either with noise nonstationarity or with amplitude variation of single AEPs, or a combination of both. As demonstrated by Gasser, Mocks, and Verleger (1983), the accuracy of the weighted average can exceed that of the simple average. A possible concern with this kind of recursive estimation process would be the tendency for the weighted average to converge to patterns in the simple average that are not necessarily genuine AEPs.

Another technique of weighted averaging that is apparently free from such concerns of recursiveness uses the noise variance estimated within the primary sweeps as the basis for deriving the set of weighting coefficients; the higher the variance, the lower the sweep weight (Elberling and Wahlgreen, 1985).

If all the assumptions of the additive model discussed earlier were met, simple averaging would provide a statistically optimal estimate of the true AEP waveform. In that case, procedures such as weighted averaging would be not only unnecessary, but also would actually degrade the accuracy of estimation. Unfortunately, real AEP data are nonideal in many ways, and the search for robust estimation procedures that provide protection against violation of the assumptions of the simple, additive model, while retaining statistical precision of AEP estimation that is close to optimal, is an area of active investigation. Concomi-

tantly, the violation of assumptions itself offers potentially useful insights into AEP data that have not yet been fully explored and exploited.

A Frequency-domain View of Averaging

Most operations on time series data can be formulated as filtering operations, and time-domain averaging is no exception. Consider averaging that is time-locked to a fixed rate of stimulation, which is the most common situation in AEP measurement. The effect of averaging on a continuous sinusoidal input that has a frequency such that the averaging cycle time (the time between initiation of successive sweeps) is an integral multiple of the period of the sinusoid, is that of a filter with unit modulus; the averaging has no effect because the sinusoid is in phase, for each sweep. If, on the other hand, the averaging cycle time is an odd number of half-periods, there will be total cancellation of the sinusoid for even numbers of sweeps averaged, that is, the effective filter modulus is zero for any such input signal frequency. For intermediate frequencies, the modulus of the averaging filter takes values between zero and unity. In fact, for a cycle time of T seconds, time-domain averaging is a "comb filter" with the teeth (points of unit modulus) of the comb set at frequencies of $1/T$, $2/T$, $3/T$, and so on. For example, with a stimulus rate of 20 per second, T is 0.05 and the teeth are at 20, 40, 60, . . . Hz. The larger the number of sweeps, the sharper the teeth of the comb, that is, the more effective is the cancellation of frequencies other than the tooth frequencies. This property of time-domain averaging is well-known in the signal processing field (Dawson, 1953), and is easy to derive mathematically (see Figure 3.6).

Phase-locked Noise Components

For the root-N law of SNR enhancement by simple averaging to be valid, the noise must be a stationary random process. This is clearly untrue for such noise components as 60 Hz power line interference, and associated harmonics or periodic transients that can arise from exposed power lines and fluorescent lighting, for example. The impact of averaging with a fixed cycle

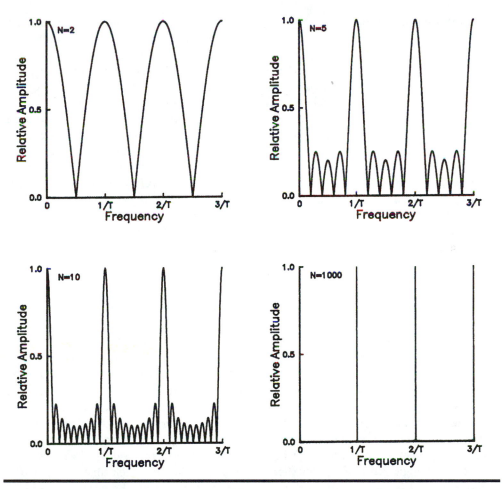

FIGURE 3.6. Time-domain averaging with a fixed stimulus repetition rate is equivalent to a comb filter in the frequency domain that passes without attenuation only those activity components with frequencies that are integer multiples of the repetition rate. The larger the number of sweeps averaged (N), the narrower the teeth of the comb. Comb filter moduli are shown for 2, 5, 10, and 1000 stimuli, where T is the stimulus repetition interval.

time (averaging period) on power line interference can be deduced from the comb filter concept; if 60 Hz or any of its major harmonics falls close to one of the comb teeth, the averaging could have little or no suppressive effect. Indeed, averaging with wide recording bandwidth and at a rate of 60 sweeps per second or an integer submultiple of that rate (30/s, 15/s, etc.) is a useful test for the presence of power line interference in the preamplifier output. To minimize the effects of

such coherent noise components, it is usually desirable to use stimulus repetition rates that tend to position the comb filter teeth well away from the major noise component frequencies, even to render such components identically zero if the rate is chosen such that the offending noise energy is located midway between two teeth. However, the presence of coherent noise and the effect of the chosen rate are not always theoretically obvious. The precise rates to be used in any clinical or research measurements must be checked in practice for absence of nonphysiologic noise.

A less obvious source of phase-coherent noise and violation of the root-N law is low-frequency EEG energy; high-amplitude alpha rhythms can be very problematic in SVP measurements (see Chapter 8). Although the degree of phase coherence between sweeps cannot be nearly as high for the alpha rhythm as it can be for power line pickup, the assumption of noise independence between sweeps can be strongly violated. At any point during averaging, constructive interference of high-amplitude, coherent alpha activity can build up rapidly over a few sweeps, so as to simulate or obscure genuine SVPs. Altering the stimulus repetition rate to promote phase cancellation in successive sweeps can be useful.

As noted earlier, a stimulus sequence itself can induce physiologic "noise" (unwanted activity) that is synchronized to the averaging cycle, and that can seriously distort the average, especially at stimulus repetition rates above about 35/s. In ABR recording, the postauricular myogenic response and the MLR are the main offenders; the latter phenomenon is precisely what underlies the recording conditions for the so-called 40 Hz event-related potential, which can be a significant source of ABR distortion. Its effects can be reduced by raising the high-pass filter cutoff frequency to 100 Hz or higher, which will attenuate the MLR. This is fine for otoneurologic ABR work, with high-intensity click stimuli, but is not feasible when it is desired to detect responses to near-threshold tonepip stimuli, especially at low tonepip frequencies. Here, the ABR energy distribution shifts to frequencies that are not much higher than those where the MLR is concentrated, and any filter that suppresses the MLR may then also affect the ABR quite strongly.

Use of Rapid Stimulus Sequences

Ordinarily, AEP recording conditions for transient AEPs are such that each sweep corresponds to a single stimulus delivery; the interval between stimulus onsets is greater than the sweep length, and the noise is assumed to be statistically independent, for successive sweeps. However, there are several procedures for which more than one stimulus is associated with each sweep, the most obvious example being the 40 Hz MLR. If it is assumed that 40 Hz has no special significance in excitation of the auditory cortex, such as resonance with some intrinsic thalamocortical cycle of excitation and inhibition, then the putative efficiency gain of the 40 Hz technique over, say, a conventional MLR recording (at, say, 11 stimuli/second) lies in the possibility of constructive interference (overlap) between the wave sequences evoked by the successive stimuli. The evoked potential is treated virtually as a steady-state phenomenon, and there is no attempt to recover any estimate of the non-overlapped AEP. The efficiency gain over the lower-rate approach lies in the increased response amplitude and its relatively simple, oscillatory form. Note that the actual rate of averaging is usually less than 40 Hz, because of the common use of window lengths that contain several response cycles (for example, 50 ms).

A very interesting class of techniques involves the use of very rapid and specially timed stimulus sequences (usually, but not necessarily, click stimuli) that are based upon what are known generically as m-sequences (Sutter, 1987). There are many types of m-sequence, including "maximum length" and Legendre sequences (Burkard, Shi, and Hecox, 1990). Expressed informally, the response of a system such as the cochlea and auditory brainstem pathways to a brief acoustic transient such as a click (that is, the ABR) is considered to represent the impulse response of the system (see the Appendix). The net response to a set of such stimuli presented very close together in time is assumed to be the sum of overlapping impulse responses to the individual stimuli. This net waveform may bear no obvious relationship to the waveform of the individual impulse responses (ABRs), but for a linear system, the impulse response can always be recovered by a deconvolution operation (see Appendix) applied to the average estimate of the overlapped, composite AEP. If the temporal structure of the stimulus pulse sequence has any of several specific forms, namely the m-sequences, very efficient algorithms that greatly reduce the computational load can be applied to recover the impulse response.

Use of maximum-length sequences for high-speed

ABR recordings was first proposed by Eysholdt and Schreiner (1982). The technique has subsequently been investigated in detail by Burkard and his colleagues, for the ABR (Burkard et al., 1990*a,b*). The m-sequence deconvolution method can be applied at effective stimulus repetition rates (interpulse intervals within the m-sequence) that are as high as 500 per second. However, the practical utility of this technique is not yet established. The need for more efficient procedures is acute, but the putative gain in recording efficiency through the use of very high stimulation rates may be offset by several factors such as loss of AEP waveform amplitude or temporal synchrony due to adaptation at very high stimulus rates, by the violation of the noise independence assumption and the root-*N* law, by increase in noise variance as a result of the linear combination operations inherent in the deconvolution, or by the development of strong system nonlinearities that confound the deconvolution.

Once again, however, it may be that the very phenomena that compromise one procedure offer new insight if viewed differently. For example, the m-sequence procedure can be conducted in such a way as to explicitly quantify certain aspects of system nonlinearity (Sutter, 1987). In general, a linear system can be completely specified by its impulse response function. Once that function is known, for example, then the output of the system can be predicted for any input whatsoever, because the output is simply the convolution of the input with the impulse response. A nonlinear system, on the other hand, must be characterized by a set of functions of which the impulse response is just the first and the simplest. These functions are most commonly known as the nth-order Wiener kernels or Volterra kernels of the system. It is probable that electrophysiologic elucidation of auditory system nonlinearities by this approach will turn out to be useful (Shi and Hecox, in press).

Alternatives to Time-domain Averaging

There are several ways to characterize the response of a noisy system other than by estimating its response to a transient stimulus by time-domain averaging. For example, the impulse response of a linear system can also be estimated by stimulating the system with continuous random noise, and cross-correlating the stimulus waveform with the output activity. See Dobie and Clopton (1980) and Dobie and Wilson (1988) for examples of this technique applied to AEPs. Other approaches that are intrinsically oriented towards the situation of rapid, almost continuous stimulation, and overlapped response as in the so-called steady-state paradigms, are based upon several varieties of Fourier analysis. See Regan (1989) and Picton, Vasjar, Rodriguez, and Campbell (1987) for more detailed discussion. The importance and clinical value of such methods in the audiologic and otoneurologic contexts are not yet clear. Approaches based on continuous stimulation may be more affected by stimulus artifact and by system nonlinearities such as adaptation, yet they may be more efficient and may tap clinically informative features of the adapted (more highly stressed) system state.

AEP DETECTION

To determine whether or not an AEP was genuinely present in some particular average record is often the main goal of the recording, as in estimation of hearing threshold; in all other applications, AEP detection is a prerequisite for further decision making. There are many procedures that can assist human judgment of response presence, or replace it with more objective evaluation.

Assistive Procedures

Some of these steps are quite obvious and are practiced commonly. First, it must be established that the data have been filtered appropriately, and this is often not the case; the ability to apply zero-phase digital filters after averaging can be very useful indeed to improve the detectability of the AEP. Also, it is quite common to require that a putative response waveform should be reproduced reasonably in at least two independent averages, especially near AEP threshold. Of course, doing more work will usually improve performance, so the real question is whether the accumulation of a single average of size *N* will lead to better or worse decisions than two of size *N*/2, or three of size *N*/3. This is not a simple problem and the answer is not clear. The author's impression is that a single average is formally best, but only if all the assumptions of the additive model are absolutely valid. In the real world, replication of averages (or splitting into subaverages) seems to be sometimes very helpful. Near threshold, a visual judgment criterion of response presence in at least two out of three subaverages can promote greater consistency of decisions.

Because noise nonstationarity is one of the main reasons why making reliable AEP detection judgments can be difficult, it makes little sense to place much reliance on conventional "no-stimulus" averages to provide noise estimates free from AEP. It is often much more effective to position the stimulus between about a quarter and halfway through the sweep, so as to obtain a sufficient prestimulus representation of the noise characteristics actually extant during the accumulation of the average. This is most helpful if the recording conditions are such that the immediate prestimulus period does not contain any AEP that is carried over across successive sweeps. A prestimulus epoch is particularly helpful in measurements of the SVP, to help assess the effects of bursts of high-amplitude alpha rhythm.

Another method is the so-called plus/minus (±) reference, in which a second average is simultaneously accumulated, but with the sign of the data reversed for half the records (Schimmel, 1967; Wong and Bickford, 1980). This is a helpful aid to subjective judgment, especially if suboptimal artifact rejection criteria were used and fairly large transient artifacts were admitted into the average. Any deflection present in both the regular average and the reference average cannot be response, according to the additive data model.

It is not obvious how best to accumulate the reference average. If it is done with sign alternation of every other sweep in the sequence, this will defeat the often-used alternation of stimulus polarity as a device for reducing stimulus artifact. More importantly, such a method will allow clear identification of single, isolated artifacts, but because of the sign alternation, it will not represent well those composite artifact clusters that are due to constructive interference of noise over several sweeps, a more common problem than isolated artifacts if the rejection levels have been set properly. The problems with changing the sign only once are that

it usually requires foreknowledge of the ultimate value of N and it will not provide good AEP cancellation if there is slow response variation over the stimulus set, such as might be due to adaptation. A reasonable compromise might be to change sign every ten percent of a conservative estimate of what N might be, but the author is unaware of any formal studies in this area.

A statistical curiosity that is counter-intuitive, but which is easy to derive and may be useful in the area of statistical response detection criteria, is that the ± reference average is statistically independent of its associated simple average, despite the common pool of data from which both are determined.

In recent years, the computing power needed to provide real-time analyses that can help optimize the test protocol (especially averaging) and assist response detection decision-making has become readily available (Ozdamar, Delgado, Eilers, and Widen, 1990). The limitation is now not so much technologic as methodologic. It is not clear exactly what to do. A potentially useful approach, though one not without its inherent assumptions and limitations, is that based on the variance-ratio measure Fsp (Elberling and Don, 1984), and such procedures are very recently becoming available in commercial AEP systems. It is to be hoped that there will be a increasing trend towards implementations of public-domain algorithms such as Fsp. This is in marked distinction to the use of proprietary data-processing or decision-making algorithms, which is counterproductive because of the likelihood of gimmickry and false claims of effectiveness, as well as the large amount of empirical work that is generated to quantify and validate their actual effect.

Objective Detection Methods

Objective, automated decision-making for AEP detection has been an area of active investigation for many years, the earliest efforts being directed at the SVP, but not necessarily restricted to it (Salomon, 1974; Schimmel, Rapin, and Cohen, 1974). This is a technically demanding area, and while as yet there is no procedure that is clearly optimal, there are large bodies of knowledge that can be brought to bear on the problem, especially from the domains of statistical decision theory and pattern recognition (McGillem, Aunon, and Childers, 1981; Cohen, 1986). There are many approaches to AEP detection (Hyde, 1976; Arnold, 1985), most of them statistical in nature, in contrast to rule-oriented "syntactic" methods (Cohen, 1986; Boston, 1989). The two classes of statistical approach are based on the time domain, with variance ratios (Schimmel, Rapin, and Cohen, 1974; Wong and Bickford, 1980; Don, Elberling, and Waring, 1984) and correlation between averages or with AEP template waveforms (Salomon, 1974; Weber and Fletcher, 1980; Mason, 1984; Mason and Barber, 1984), or on the frequency domain, with Fourier Transform phase variance (Beagley, Sayers, and Ross, 1979; Fridman, Zappulla, Bergelson, Greenblatt, Malis, Morrel, and Hoepner, 1984), a multivariate approach (Valdes-Sosa, Bobes, Perez-Abalo, et al., 1987), spectral coherence functions (Brillinger, 1978; Dobie and Wilson, 1989), and many more. The strengths and weaknesses of the various approaches are not yet completely clear. It is probable that no single method will be clearly preferable for all circumstances and all AEPs and that approaches requiring strong assumptions about the AEP data model will prove to be inappropriate. It is desirable that significance levels of tests for response detection should be accurate, and this can cause difficulty; time-domain approaches (such as *Fsp*) that are not multivariate have to deal with the problem that correlation between successive samples of the activity renders the effective statistical degrees of freedom in the activity much smaller than might be expected from the number of data points considered (Sayers, Ruggiero, and Feuerlicht, 1981). Frequency-domain approaches do not suffer from this particular difficulty, because the successive harmonics in the discrete Fourier Transform (Cohen, 1986) are statistically independent.

In general, it is to be expected that the detection problem will be most difficult to solve accurately for slow potentials, partly because of the relatively small numbers of sweeps that can be accumulated per stimulus condition, in practicable test times, and partly because of the coherent and non-stationary nature of low-frequency EEG noise. Whatever the AEP or detection technique under investigation, for a proper research solution it is necessary to address near-threshold stimulus conditions

and to apply analytic methods that take account of the effects of variation in detection decision criterion, such as the relative operating characteristic (Swets, 1988). Examples of this approach to AEP detection have been reported by Valdes-Sosa, Bobes, Perez-Abalo ct al. (1985) and Elberling and Don (1987).

MULTICHANNEL TECHNIQUES

The vast majority of AEP measurements and reports to date deal with one or two channels of activity, obtained with one or two differential electrode pairs. The time-history obtained from any pair only reveals potential differences that are developed along a directional axis intersecting the two electrode sites. This affords a restricted and possibly quite misleading view of the true, three-dimensional temporally evolving pattern of activity in the head. For example, if some pathophysiologic change in the site or orientation of AEP generator sources were to alter the scalp distribution of potential such that the two electrodes of a differential pair became isopotential, then there would be zero net AEP even though a large absolute AEP may actually exist. There are many other ways in which a single time-history may not capture, or may even misrepresent, the underlying electrical information.

There are several ways to try to capture a more detailed and informative picture of the gross evoked electric events within the head. The approaches differ in terms of whether the main focus is upon visualizing the temporal or spatial characteristics of the signal, in terms of the extent of assumptions required about AEP generator sources and the electrical properties of the head, and in terms of the volume of data (number of recording electrodes) that are needed. Some of the concepts are illustrated in Figure 3.7.

Joint Evaluation of Many Channels

The most direct approach to accessing more information about the underlying electrical events is to add more electrodes and apply to the resulting entire set of time-histories the same kinds of parametric analyses (such as, in terms of amplitudes and latencies) that are common in single-channel studies. An example of this

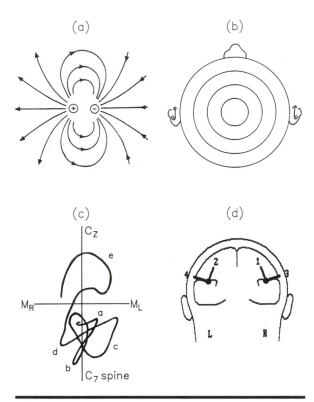

FIGURE 3.7. (A) The electric field pattern due to an electric dipole. (B) Scalp isopotential contours arising from a vertical AEP source equivalent dipole at the head center; several concurrently active dipoles can combine to yield a single, apparent (equivalent) dipole, and any entire scalp topographic map is predictable from only three quantities: the equivalent dipole magnitudes in the *x*, *y*, and *z* directions. (C) Dipoles cause potential differences at the scalp that can be expressed as voltage vectors in a three-dimensional space. The path traced in time by the vector endpoint is known as a three-component Lissajous' trajectory (3-CLT). The figure illustrates one view of a human 3-CLT from three electrode pairs (*X*: nasion-inion, *Y*: mastoid-mastoid, *Z*: vertex-neck). Five planar segments (a–e) are indicated. (D) Dipole source potential analysis uses constraints on possible source locations to help solve the "inverse problem" of deriving an unique, parsimonious set of generator equivalent dipoles from scalp potential measurements at many sites. The example in the figure shows two tangential (1,2) and two radial (3,4) dipoles in primary auditory cortex that predict very accurately the waveform of the slow vertex potential (50–200 ms).

with the ABR is the use of a vertex (or forehead) to contralateral mastoid channel to clarify the location of wave P6 (V) when waves P5 and P6 (IV and V) recorded ipsilaterally to the stimulus are fused into a broad peak of indeterminate latency. Another example is simultaneous evaluation of average AEPs from several points on the head so as to make inferences specifically from between-site comparisons, such as to detect inter-hemispheric asymmetries of middle or late potentials, in the exploration of cortical dysfunction. This approach, essentially combining the results of several, joint, single-channel analyses, is only viable with few channels. As the number increases, there is a combinatorial expansion and it becomes increasingly difficult to integrate the overall picture to extract meaningful inferences.

Topographic (Spatiotemporal) Analysis

One way of combining the information from many data channels is to represent it as a temporally evolving topographic contour map of potential, with isopotential (equipotential, isovoltage) contour lines or with gray scale or color coding of equipotential areas, to represent the distribution of potentials at any instant. This representation is very different from the joint multiple-channel approach, because it is the spatial distribution that is emphasized, not the temporal aspects. Time-series (waveform) information must be inferred either from separate inspection of selected averages or implicitly from changes throughout a series of topographic snapshots, taken at predetermined post-stimulus times or at times corresponding to the latencies of especially interesting peaks. It is within the capability of modern graphics workstations to represent topographic maps almost as movies, conveying more directly the underlying spatiotemporal information.

There is no doubt that topographic and spatiotemporal mapping can access much more *data* than is possible with one or two channels. The problem at present, especially in seeking clinical applications of these techniques, is to find the most effective ways of extracting the key *information* from the large volume of data that is generated. The issues are data reduction and goal-oriented measurement. A complication that can arise if there is an insufficient number of electrodes and data channels is inadequate spatial resolution; the algorithms that interpolate potential in order to derive isopotential contours or equipotential region boundaries cannot function properly with insufficient data, and the resulting contours may bear little resemblance to what would have been obtained with a sufficiently dense electrode array.

For further information about these spatio-temporal methods, with particular emphasis on the MLR, see Grandori, Comacchio, Martini, and Ravazzani (1990) and Kraus and McGee (1988, 1990).

Vector and Planar Analysis

To specify the location of a point in a three-dimensional space (3-space) requires three coordinates, usually specified in Cartesian (x, y, z) or polar (r, θ, ϕ) form. A vector is a quantity that posesses both magnitude and direction; for example, a line drawn from an origin to any point in a 3-space can represent a vector. The modulus (magnitude) of the vector is the length of the line, and can be derived from the size of its various components in the x, y, and z directions.

Under certain simplifying conditions, measurements of electric potential in three directions are both necessary and sufficient to specify completely an electric field in a 3-space such as the head. AEP measurements from three differential electrode pairs can be combined vectorially. For example, suppose the anteroposterior axis of the head from the nasion (nose) to the inion (occiput) is considered the x-axis, from mastoid to mastoid is the y-axis, and the vertex to neck is the z-axis. Then, the "true" AEP can be thought of as a three-dimensional vector that evolves in time, and the geometric projections of the vector modulus upon the x, y, and z axes would form the components of the vector in those three directions; thus, each component of the vector is a time-history recorded from one of the differential pairs. The regular vertex-mastoid derivation for the ABR, for example, would yield a mixture of the y and z components of an underlying vector ABR.

Throughout the time course of the AEP, the vector endpoint describes a trajectory (curve) in the 3-space. By appeal to elementary physics and the plotting of one voltage against another using oscilloscopes, such curves are often referred to as Lissajous' trajectories. For an exhaustive description of the three-component

Lissajous' trajectory (3-CLT) of the ABR, and related measures, see the collection of reports introduced by Jewett, Martin, Sininger, and Gardi (1987). For a recent, detailed review of the technique and its clinical promise, see Pratt, Martin, Kaminer, and Bleich (1990).

An ABR 3-CLT and its components are shown in Figure 3.7C. In principle, at least, the vector modulus represents a potentially useful way of combining the information in the three component channels, and of avoiding some of the limitations of the restricted view offered by single-channel, differential recording. Also, there is much more information in the 3-CLT than is revealed even by the vector modulus. For example, within certain time regions, the trajectory restricts itself to distinct planes (2-dimensional regions) in the 3-space (Williston, Jewett, and Martin, 1981). In the human click ABR, there are typically up to ten such planar segments (Sininger, Gardi, Morris, Martin, and Jewett, 1987), which may represent activity in distinct groups of nerve fibers. The quantification of these planar segments, such as by their latency and orientation, has been called planar analysis; it may provide a more sensitive and insightful representation of ABR activity than the conventional time-histories or than the 3-CLT vector modulus. Much further development is required to clarify the clinical and research utility of this approach.

Compared to spatiotemporal mapping, the 3-CLT method is at least superficially attractive, because it might provide a parsimonious representation of the overall, three-dimensional, spatiotemporal activity pattern that comprises the true AEP. Thus, a topographic pattern of potential that seems complicated might be summarizable in terms of just a few underlying variables, such as the direction and magnitude of the vector (see Figure 3.7B). The limitations of the vectorial approach relate to the validity of assumptions about the nature and location of the AEP sources, and about the electrical properties of the head. For example, the usual model is that there is only a single, overall AEP vector contributing to the scalp potentials at any point in time, and that vector is assumed to be located at the center of a head that has somewhat idealized geometric and electrical properties. This seems more reasonable for AEPs with deep intracranial sources such as the ABR, than for AEPs with superficial, cortical sources. However, vectorial measures may have empirical utility, regardless of the apparent validity of the associated models.

Dipole Source Potential Analysis

According to one simple model, the sources of scalp evoked potentials can be considered to be electrical dipoles in the head. A dipole comprises two equal and opposite electrical charges separated by some distance (see Figure 3.7A). The dipole orientation is reflected in the direction of the axis separating the charges. The so-called "dipole moment" is a vector that expresses the size and separation of the charges, and the orientation of the dipole. To emphasize the physiologic, anatomic and electrodynamic simplifications and abstractions inherent in the intracerebral source dipole model, especially the fact that concurrently active dipoles will tend to combine vectorially and appear as a single, overall dipole, these model sources are often called "equivalent dipoles." See Nunez (1981), Regan (1989) and Williamson and Kaufmann (1990) for more detailed explanations.

The head is usually modelled electroanatomically as a spherical, multi-layered (three-shell) volume conductor (Ary, Klein, and Fender, 1981). Any system of active dipolar sources within the head will produce some particular topographic pattern of potential on its surface. Given the dipole source parameters, namely their positions and dipole moments, it is a simple matter to compute the scalp potential distribution; this is known as the "forward" problem. It is not so easy to solve the inverse problem, that is, to derive the dipole source characteristics from the scalp potential topography, because many dipolar configurations may give rise to scalp topographies that are indistinguishable (Kavanagh, Darcey, Lehmann, and Fender, 1978). However, using a sufficient number of electrodes, and considering only those numbers and positions of dipoles that are physiologically and anatomically plausible, it is usually possible to derive a plausible source configuration that explains the observed scalp potentials with acceptable accuracy (see Figure 3.7D). See Scherg (1989) and Scherg and von Cramon (1990), for detailed descriptions of the technique, which typically involves the use of at least 12–16 electrodes, together

with sophisticated analysis software. The method has shed new light on the probable sources of several AEPs (Scherg and von Cramon, 1986; Scherg, Vajsar, and Picton, 1990; Scherg and von Cramon, 1990). Recently, software that can run on a PC-level workstation has become commercially available.

By indicating the probable number, position, orientation and strength of the set of equivalent dipole sources that underlie an observed pattern of scalp potential, the source analysis approach seems potentially more informative than either spatiotemporal mapping or the 3-CLT approach. The promise of being able to disentangle and examine the actual AEP source characteristics and time histories, as opposed to viewing the end result of their summation at the scalp, is considerable. Despite skepticism in some quarters, arising from the anticipated difficulties intrinsic in solving the inverse problem, the research utility of this technique is already established, and its clinical utility is an area of vigorous investigation. Limitations in clinical practise can be expected to arise from problems with poor SNR, constraints on recording time, and the effect of diverse pathophysiologic states on the validity of the constraining assumptions about the possible sources.

As usual, no single approach to multichannel AEP measurement and analysis is necessarily the most suitable for all AEPs and clinical measurement goals. For the ABR, the 3-CLT assumption of central source location is at least roughly satisfied, so a topographic ABR analysis may be relatively inefficient and a full ABR dipole localization may be overkill. For cortical AEPs, on the other hand, the 3-CLT method seems inappropriate, and the relative merits of mapping and source localization/source waveform analysis will depend mainly on their comparative validity and accuracy as tools for making specific clinical decisions.

CONCLUDING REMARKS

In recent years, there have been significant developments in several areas of AEP signal processing and analysis, as reflected in commercial EP systems. These developments have occurred mainly in the areas of digital filtering and various multichannel methods. These improvements have been spurred primarily by cost reductions in computer technology, especially in specialized DSP and graphics processors, as distinct from major conceptual advances. While the multichannel approaches have the potential to disentangle, at least partially, the complex and compound electrical events occurring at the scalp, much further research remains to be done to establish their clinical utility and a clear advantage over measurements with only a few, well-positioned electrode pairs. It is necessary to resist the impression that more data necessarily means more useful information and better clinical decisions.

Even in the latest commercial systems, there is sometimes a need for more attention to basic matters, such as variable artifact rejection limits, a sufficiently wide range of filter parameters, and the ability to route signals to external devices for additional processing. There is a tendency to offer potentially insufficient proprietary approaches, too few options, and too little flexibility for all but the most basic user.

As well as the continuing need for attention to signal processing fundamentals, there is an acute need for AEP systems to provide move advanced decision support in relation to test protocol control and interpretation of records. This applies strongly to common and relatively basic AEP applications involving one or two channels of data, and oriented towards estimation of the puretone audiogram or otoneurologic site-of-lesion inference. Some well-known tools, such as the ± reference, should by now be routinely available, and newer approaches such as Fsp are helpful. Whatever the application, the emphasis in clinical instrumentation systems should be upon use of published and proven algorithms with flexible, modular implementation, sensible default options, high ease of use, high customizability and good capacity for interfacing to more powerful technical workstations or for networking to administrative systems.

All in all, over the last decade, the pace of theoretical and practical advance in this field has been modest. Spatiotemporal maps, vectors, dipole localization, and statistical response detection algorithms were all being studied actively in the late 1960's, albeit using specialized laboratory AEP systems. There are several reasons for this limited rate of progress. Most of all, this area is one that requires good communication between persons with widely different skills: in clinical application, in analytic methods, and in development engineering. Also, there has not been sufficient high-quality, academic and clinical research in the area, nor is there a vast device market to provide much stimulus for proprietary research and development. Furthermore, the communication links between the various constituencies, such as scientists, clinicians, and instrumentation manufacturers, are generally less than ideal and are often parochial.

It is to be expected that matters will improve. Neuroelectric imaging with AEP data is demanding, in terms of data acquisition, number-crunching and graphical display power. Newer techniques pose demands that were almost unthinkable even as little as ten years ago. However, the computing power is now readily available at reasonable cost. Digital technology is flexible, and most of today's developments have to do with software, not hardware. The challenge, therefore, is not technologic, but technical. It is up to the clinical and scientific AEP communities to develop jointly clear measurement goals and innovative, effective techniques for test protocol control and clinical decision support.

APPENDIX

Averaging

Each individual sweep of the recorded bioelectric activity is modeled as the sum of a signal (the AEP) and a noise process (everything else), which can be written as:

$$x(t) = s(t) + n(t).$$

In terms of digitized time series, this becomes:

$$x(j) = s(j) + n(j),$$

where j is an integer in the range 1 to M, and represents the successive samples in each sweep. If N such records are collected, a matrix of N rows and M columns is developed, and any data point in the matrix can be represented as:

$$x(ij) = s(ij) + n(ij),$$

where the sweep index i goes from 1 to N.

If the signal is identical for each sweep, the index i can be dropped because $s(ij)$ depends only upon j, the position of the sample point in each sweep, thus:

$$x(ij) = s(j) + n(ij).$$

The i index is retained for the noise components, which are random and may differ in each sweep, as will the activity x.

The SNR for any elementary record is a ratio of the size of the signal and the noise. The signal changes with time, that is, with j, so the SNR must be specified at any particular value of j, such as one that corresponds to the latency of some important waveform feature. The SNR is defined more formally as the RMS ratio of signal and noise, and the RMS of a constant quantity is the quantity itself, so the RMS of $s(j)$ is $s(j)$. The noise $n(ij)$ is usually assumed to be taken from a population of values that is normally distributed (Gaussian) with mean zero and variance σ^2. This is true for any i and j, if the noise is stationary. The RMS value of $n(ij)$ equals its standard deviation σ, if the process has zero mean value.

At any j, therefore, the SNR in the elementary record is simply $s(j)/\sigma$.

Suppose $x(ij)$ is summed over i, for all values of j. This will produce an array of sums, denoted by $X(j)$, where:

$$X(j) = x(1j) + x(2j) + \ldots + x(nj),$$

that is, summing each column of the data matrix $[x(ij)]$. What is the SNR in this sum array? At any j, the size of the signal component is simply N times the value in each sweep, because the signal is identical at any j in all sweeps. Thus the signal RMS becomes $N \cdot s(j)$. With regard to the noise, statistical theory states that the variance of the sum of N independently and identically distributed random variables is the sum of their individual variances (Snedecor and Cochran, 1980), so the variance of the noise component at any j in the sum is $N \cdot \sigma^2$. The noise RMS is the standard deviation, which is the square root of the variance, so the noise RMS is $\sigma \cdot \sqrt{N}$. It follows that the SNR in the sum is $N \cdot s(j)/\sigma \cdot \sqrt{N}$, which equals $N \cdot s(j)/\sigma$; thus the SNR in the sum is N times the SNR in the elementary sweep.

Several commercial AEP systems merely sum the sweeps and display the scaled sum, but others actually divide the sum by the number of sweeps to date, producing and displaying a true running average. Both proce-

dures give exactly the same improvement in SNR, but the underlying statistical arguments change slightly. For true averaging, the SNR of the signal component in the average is $s(j)$, at any j, because the average value of a constant is that constant. The variance of the average of N independently and identically distributed random variables is the sum of the individual variances divided by N^2, that is, the variance of the average is $N \cdot \sigma^2/N^2$, which equals σ^2/N, so the RMS value is $\sigma/\sqrt{N}$. It follows that the SNR in the average record is $N \cdot s(j)/\sigma$, which is the same result as for summation.

Convolution

To understand several new methods of AEP analysis, it is increasingly necessary to be familiar with fundamental DSP operations such as convolution and its inverse, deconvolution. An informal explanation is given here. Convolution is a mathematical operation that involves forming a cross-product of two functions, usually functions of time or of frequency. For continuous variables, integration is involved, but for discrete series, summation is used. The discrete formulation for convolution of two time functions, denoted by $x(k)$ and $h(j)$, is:

$$y(k) = \sum x(k-j) \cdot h(j), j = 0,1,2, \ldots$$

where k and j are discrete time variables, $x(k)$ and $h(j)$ are the functions that are being convolved and $y(k)$ is the resulting time series. Thus, y is the convolution of x and h, and the operation is conventionally denoted by a star:

$$y(t) = x(t)*h(t).$$

The operation is shown in Figure 3.8A. In words, the result at any instant k in "actual" time is the weighted sum of cross-products of all previous values of the input with the weighting function $h(j)$. As the "dummy" time variable j increases, $x(k-j)$ is the input that occurred further and further back in time, but the sequence of values $h(j)$ evolves in the ordinary way, with time increasing. For every new value of actual time k, the entire process is repeated for all dummy times.

Now, a linear system is a system (a black box, perhaps) for which the output due to a sum of inputs equals the sum of the outputs for each input individually. Many systems are assumed to be linear; some re-

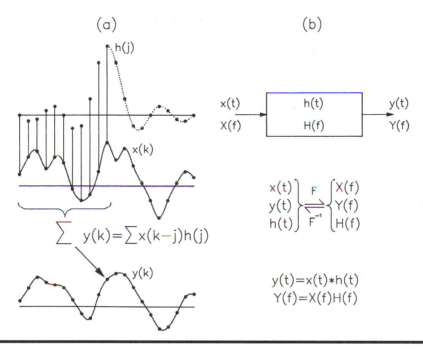

FIGURE 3.8.   (A) Convolution of a discrete (non-continuous) input time series *x(k)* with a discrete impulse response *h(j)*, to yield the output time series *y(k)*. The output at any time point *k* can be regarded as a sum of the input values going back in time from *k* by amounts *j*, each point being weighted by the impulse response value for that *j*. Because the impulse response goes to zero at large *j*, points in the distant past do not contribute to the output *y(k)*. The process is schematized by reflecting the digitized impulse response back in time about *x(k)*, with vertical lines showing cross-multiplication. (B) Block diagram and equations showing the operation of linear system in the time and frequency domains, including the impulse response function *h(t)* and the system transfer function *H(f)*, which are an example of a Fourier Transform pair, indicated by double arrows. Convolution in the time-domain (starred), as in figure part (A), is equivalent to multiplication in the frequency domain, and vice versa.

ally are, and some are approximately so. Any real, linear system (such as one of the filters discussed earlier) has an associated function that completely describes the system, and permits the system output to be derived from known system input. This so-called "impulse response" of a system is the time function obtained as output when the input is a special, idealized impulse of infinite height and zero width, but unit area, known as a Dirac delta function, or unit impulse. An acoustic click could be viewed as a (poor) approximation to a unit impulse. The impulse response of any system is

usually denoted as $h(t)$, and often has a damped, oscillatory form that goes to zero at large t. With a discrete time variable, the impulse response can be denoted as $h(j)$, where j represents discrete time.

For a linear system, the above convolution operation now takes on special meaning, because the output of the system at any time k is the convolution of the input with the impulse response. What it means is that the output right now, say, depends upon both the history of the input and the impulse response; input values in the recent past are likely to contribute a great deal to the output right now, because the impulse response is usually large at a small time interval after excitation by the unit impulse (small values of j). At large j, the impulse response will usually dwindle to zero, reflected in the convolution sum as a negligible contribution to the output right now from input events in the distant past (large j). In so far as any filtering operation can be expressed in terms of the impulse response of the filter, so the action of the filter can be conceptualized in terms of the convolution summation. Actual implementation of a digital filter is usually done by using techniques that are less intensive computationally.

The operation of deconvolution is the inverse process to convolution. It can be applied to linear systems in order to determine an unknown input, given known output and impulse response, or to determine an unknown impulse response, given known input and output. See Ozdamar and Delgado (1990), for an example of its use in neuronal source modelling for the ABR.

It is also worth noting that time-domain convolution of two functions is equivalent to multiplication of the Fourier Transforms of those functions, and vice versa. The Fourier Transform of the system impulse response is known as the system transfer function. The transfer function of a linear filter can be expressed in the form $H(f) = M(f)\exp\{-j\phi(f)\}$, where $M(f)$ is the modulus function, and $\phi(f)$ is the phase shift function. These relationships are indicated in Figure 3.8B.

REFERENCES

Arnold, S.A. (1985). Objective versus visual detection of the auditory brain stem response. *Ear and Hearing, 6*, 144–150.

Ary, J.P., Klein, S.A., and Fender, D.H. (1981). Location of sources of evoked scalp potentials: corrections for skull and scalp thicknesses. *IEEE Trans. Biomed. Eng. BME-25*, 447–452.

Beagley, H.A. (ed.) (1979). *Auditory investigation. The scientific and technical basis*. New York: Oxford University Press.

Beauchamp, K. and Yuen, C. (1979). *Digital methods for signal analysis*. London: Allen and Unwin.

Bendat, J.S. and Piersol, A. (1971). *Random data: analysis and measurement procedures*. New York: Wiley.

Boston, J.R. (1989). Automated interpretation of brainstem auditory evoked potentials: A prototype system. *IEEE Transactions on Biomedical Engineering, BME 36*, 528–532.

Boston, J.R. and Ainslie, P. (1980). Effects of analog and digital filtering on brainstem auditory evoked potentials. *Electroencephalography and Clinical Neurophysiology, 48*, 361–364.

Brillinger, D.R. (1978). A note on the estimation of evoked response. *Biological Cybernetics, 31*, 141–144.

Burkard, R., Shi, Y., and Hecox, K.E. (1990a). A comparison of maximum length and Legendre sequences for derivation of brain-stem auditory-evoked responses at rapid rates of stimulation. *Journal of the Acoustical Society of America, 87*, 1656–1664.

Burkard, R., Shi, Y., and Hecox, K.E. (1990b). Brain-stem auditory-evoked responses elicited by maximum length sequences: Effect of simultaneous masking noise. *Journal of the Acoustical Society of America, 87*, 1665–1672.

Cohen, A. (1986). *Biomedical signal processing. Volume I. Time and frequency domains analysis. Volume II. Compression and automatic recognition*. Boca Raton, FL: CRC Press.

Dawson, G.D. (1953). Autocorrelation and automatic integration. *Electroencephalography and Clinical Neurophysiology, Suppl 4*, 26–37.

de Weerd, J.P. (1981). A posteriori time-varying filtering of averaged evoked potentials. I. Introduction and conceptual basis. *Biological Cybernetics, 41*, 211–222.

de Weerd, J.P. and Martens, W.L. (1978). Theory and practice of a posteriori "Wiener" filtering of average evoked potentials. *Biological Cybernetics, 30*, 81–94.

Dobie, R.A. and Clopton, B.M. (1980). Auditory evoked responses obtained by cross-correlation: a preliminary report. *Otolaryngology Head and Neck Surgery, 88*, 797–802.

Dobie, R.A. and Wilson, M.J. (1988). Auditory responses to the envelopes of pseudorandom noise stimuli in humans. *Hearing Research, 36*, 9–20.

Dobie, R.A. and Wilson, M.J. (1989). Analysis of auditory evoked potentials by magnitude-squared coherence. *Ear and Hearing, 10*, 2–13.

Dobie, R.A. and Wilson, M.J. (1990) Optimal ("Wiener") digital filtering of auditory evoked potentials: Use of coherence estimates. *Electroencephalography and Clinical Neurophysiology, 77*, 205–213.

Don, M., Elberling, C., and Waring, M. (1984). Objective

detection of averaged auditory brainstem responses. *Scandinavian Audiology, 13*, 219–228.

Doyle, D.J. (1975). Some comments on the use of Wiener filtering for estimation of evoked potentials. *Electroencephalography and Clinical Neurophysiology, 38*, 533–534.

Doyle, D.J. and Hyde, M.L. (1981a). Analogue and digital filtering of auditory brainstem potentials. *Scandinavian Audiology, 10*, 81–89.

Doyle, D.J. and Hyde, M.L. (1981b). Digital inverse filtering of distorted auditory brainstem responses. *Scandinavian Audiology, 10*, 261–263.

Doyle, D.J. and Hyde, M.L. (1985). Wiener filtering of auditory brainstem responses. *Journal of Clinical Engineering, 10*, 331–337.

Elberling, C. and Don, M. (1984). Quality estimation of average auditory brainstem responses. *Scandinavian Audiology, 13*, 187–197.

Elberling, C. and Don, M. (1987). Detection functions for the human auditory brainstem response. *Scandinavian Audiology, 16*, 89–92.

Elberling, C. and Wahlgreen, O. (1985). Estimation of auditory brainstem response, ABR, by means of Bayesian inference. *Scandinavian Audiology, 14*, 89.

Eysholdt, V. and Schreiner, C. (1982). Maximum length sequences. A fast method for measuring brainstem-evoked responses. *Audiology, 21*, 242–250.

Gasser, T., Mocks, J., and Verleger, R. (1983). Selavco: a method to deal with trial-to-trial variability of evoked potentials. *Electroencephalography and Clinical Neurophysiology, 55*, 717–723.

Glaser, E.M. and Ruchkin, D.S. (1976). *Principles of neurobiological signal analysis*. New York: Academic Press.

Grandori, F., Comacchio, F., Martini, A., and Ravazzani, P. (1990). Field analysis of middle-latency auditory-evoked electric and magnetic responses. In F. Grandori, M. Hoke, and G.L. Romani (eds.), *Auditory evoked magnetic fields and electric potentials*, pp.119–140. *Advances in Audiology, V/6*. Basel: Karger.

Hamming, R.W. (1983). *Digital filters*. Englewood Cliffs, NJ: Prentice-Hall.

Hyde, M.L. (1976). Statistical inference in electric response audiometry. In S.D.G. Stephens (ed.), *Disorders of auditory function II*, pp.145–161. London: Academic Press.

Hyde, M.L. and Blair, R.L. (1981). The auditory brainstem response in neuro-otology: perspectives and problems. *Journal of Otolaryngology, 10*, 117–125.

Hyde, M.L. and Doyle, D.J. (1983). The polarity histogram in relation to the averaged evoked potential. *Electroencephalography and Clinical Neurophysiology, 55*, 357–360.

Jacobson, G.P. and Newman, C.W. (1990). The decomposition of middle latency auditory evoked potential (MLAEP) Pa component into superficial and deep source contributions. *Brain Topography, 2*, 229–236.

Jasper, H.H. (1958). The ten-twenty electrode system of the international federation. *Electroencephalography and Clinical Neurophysiology, 10*, 371–375.

Jervis, B.W., Nichols, M.J., Johnson, T.E., Allen, E., and Hudson, N.R. (1983). A fundamental investigation of the composition of auditory evoked potentials. *IEEE Transactions on Biomedical Engineering, BME-30*, 43–49.

Jewett, D.L., Martin, W.H., Sininger, Y.S., and Gardi, J.N. (1987). The 3-channel Lissajous' trajectory of the auditory brainstem response. Introduction and overview. *Electroencephalography and Clinical Neurophysiology, 68*, 323–326.

Kavanagh, R.N., Darcey, T.M., Lehmann, D., and Fender, D.H. (1978). Evaluation of methods for three-dimensional localization of electric sources in the human brain. *IEEE Trans. Biomed. Eng. BME-25*, 421–429.

Kileny, P. (1983). Auditory middle latency responses: current issues. *Seminars in Hearing, 4*, 403–413.

Kraus, N. and McGee, T. (1988). Color imaging of the human middle latency response. *Ear and Hearing, 9*, 159–167.

Kraus, N. and McGee, T. (1990). Topographic mapping of the auditory middle-latency response. In F. Grandori, M. Hoke, and G.L. Romani (eds.), *Auditory evoked magnetic fields and electric potentials*, pp.141–164. *Advances in Audiology, V/6*. Basel: Karger.

Marsh, R.R. (1988). Digital filtering of auditory evoked potentials. *Ear and Hearing, 9*, 101–107.

Mason, S.M. (1984). On-line computer scoring of the auditory brainstem response for estimation of hearing threshold. *Audiology, 23*, 277–296.

Mason, S.M. and Barber, C. (1984). Machine detection of the averaged slow cortical auditory evoked potential. In R. Nodar and C. Barber (eds.), *Evoked Potentials II*. London: Butterworth.

McGillem, C.D., Aunon, J.I., and Yu, K.B. (1985). Signals and noise in evoked brain potentials. *IEEE Transactions on Biomedical Engineering, BME-32*, 1012–1016.

McGillem, C.D., Aunon, J., and Childers, D.G. (1981). Signal processing in evoked potential research: Applications of filtering and pattern recognition. *CRC Critical Reviews in Bioengineering*, pp.225–265. Boca Raton, FL: CRC Press.

Norman, G.R. and Streiner, D.L. (1986). *PDQ statistics*. Toronto: B.C. Decker

Nunez, P. (1981). *Electric fields of the brain: The neurophysics of EEG*. New York: Oxford University Press.

Oppenheim, A.V. and Schafer, R.W. (1975). *Digital signal processing.* Englewood Cliffs, NJ: Prentice-Hall.

Ozdamar, O. and Delgado, R.E. (1990). Fiber tract model of auditory brainstem response generation using traveling dipoles. In F. Grandori, M. Hoke, and G.L. Romani (eds.), *Auditory evoked magnetic fields and electric potentials*, pp.141–164. *Advances in Audiology, V/6.* Basel: Karger.

Ozdamar, O., Delgado, R.E., Eilers, R.E., and Widen, J.E. (1990). Computer methods for on-line hearing testing with auditory brain stem responses. *Ear and Hearing, 11*, 417–429.

Parker, D.J. (1981). Dependence of the auditory brain stem response on electrode location. *Archives of Otolaryngology, 107*, 367–371.

Picton, T.W., Hillyard, S.A., Krausz, H.I., and Galambos, R. (1974). Human auditory evoked potentials. I. Evaluation of components. *Electroencephalography and Clinical Neurophysiology, 36*, 179–190.

Picton, T.W., Hink, R.F., Perez-Abalo, M., Linden, R.D., and Wiens, R.S. (1984). Evoked potentials: how now? *Journal of Electrophysiological Technology, 10*, 177–221.

Picton, T.W., Linden, R.D., Hamel, G., and Maru, J. (1983). Aspects of averaging. *Seminars in Hearing, 4*, 327–341.

Picton, T.W., Vajsar, J., Rodriguez, R., and Campbell, K. (1987). Reliability estimates for steady-state evoked potentials. *Electroencephalography and Clinical Neurophysiology, 68*, 119–131.

Pratt, H., Martin, W.H., Kaminer-Hazon, M., and Bleich, N. (1990). Three-channel Lissajous' trajectories of auditory brainstem evoked potentials. In F. Grandori, M. Hoke, and G.L. Romani (eds.), *Auditory evoked magnetic fields and electric potentials*, pp.330–356. *Advances in Audiology, V/6.* Basel: Karger.

Rabiner, L.R. and Gold, B. (1975). *Theory and application of digital signal processing.* Englewood Cliffs, NJ: Prentice-Hall.

Regan, D.M. (1989). *Human brain electrophysiology: Evoked potentials and evoked magnetic fields in science and medicine.* New York: Elsevier.

Ritter, W., Vaughan, H.G., and Costa, L.D. (1968). Orienting and habituation to auditory stimuli: A study of short-term changes in average evoked responses. *Electroencephalography and Clinical Neurophysiology, 25*, 550–556.

Salomon, G. (1974). Electric response audiometry (ERA) based on rank correlation. *Audiology, 13*, 181–194.

Sayers, B.McA., and Beagley, H.A. (1976). Identification of averaged auditory evoked potentials in man. *Nature, 260*, 461–462.

Sayers, B.McA., Beagley, H.A., and Henshall, W.R. (1974).

The mechanism of auditory evoked EEG responses. *Nature, 247*, 481–483.

Sayers, B.McA., Beagley, H.A., and Ross, A.J. (1979). Auditory evoked potentials of cortical origin. In H.A. Beagley (ed.), *Auditory investigation: The scientific and technological basis*, pp.489–506. Oxford: Clarendon Press.

Sayers, B.McA., Ruggiero, C., and Feuerlicht, J. (1981). Statistical variability of biomedical data: part 2. The influence of serial correlation on power estimates, and on comparative testing of samples. *Medical Informatics, 6*, 207–220.

Scherg, M. (1990). Fundamentals of dipole source potential analysis. In F. Grandori, M. Hoke, and G.L. Romani (eds.), *Auditory evoked magnetic fields and electric potentials*, pp.40–69. *Advances in Audiology, V/6.* Basel: Karger.

Scherg, M. and von Cramon, D. (1985). Two bilateral sources of the late AEP as identified by a spatio-temporal dipole model. *Electroencephalography and Clinical Neurophysiology, 62*, 32–44.

Scherg, M. and von Cramon, D. (1990). Dipole source potentials of the auditory cortex in normal subjects and in patients with temporal lobe lesions. In F. Grandori, M. Hoke, and G.L. Romani (eds.), *Auditory evoked magnetic fields and electric potentials*, pp.165–193. *Advances in Audiology, V/6.* Basel: Karger.

Scherg, M., Vajsar, J., and Picton, T.W., (1989). A source analysis of the late human auditory evoked potentials. *Journal of Cognitive Neuroscience, 1, 4*, 336–355.

Schimmel, H. (1967). The (±) reference: accuracy of estimated mean components in average response studies. *Science, 157*, 92–94.

Schimmel, H., Rapin, I., and Cohen, M. (1974). Improving evoked response audiometry with special reference to the use of machine scoring. *Audiology, 13*, 33–65.

Shi, Y. (in press). Nonlinear system identification by m-pulse sequences: application to brainstem auditory evoked responses. *IEEE Transactions on Biomedical Engineering.*

Sininger, Y.S., Gardi, J.N., Morris, J.H., Martin, W.H., and Jewett, D.L. The 3-channel Lissajous' trajectory of the auditory brain-stem response. VII. Planar segments in humans. *Electroencephalography and Clinical Neurophysiology, 68*, 368–379.

Snedecor, G.W., and Cochran, W. (1980). *Statistical methods.* Ames, IA: Iowa State University Press.

Spehlmann, R. (1985). *Evoked potentials primer.* Stoneham: Butterworth.

Stapells, D.R. and Picton, T.W., Technical aspects of brainstem evoked potential audiometry using tones. *Ear and Hearing, 2*, 20–29.

Stapells, D.R., Makeig, S., and Galambos, R. (1987). Auditory steady-state responses: Threshold prediction using phase coherence. *Electroencephalography and Clinical Neurophysiology, 67*, 260–270.

Steeger, G.H., Herrman, O., and Spreng, M. (1983). Some improvements in the measurement of variable latency acoustically evoked potentials in human EEG. *IEEE Transactions on Biomedical Engineering, BME-30*, 295–303.

Suzuki, T. and Horiuchi, K. (1977). Effects of high-pass filtering on auditory brainstem responses to tone pips. *Scandinavian Audiology, 6*, 123–126.

Sutter, E.E. (1987). A practical nonstochastic approach to nonlinear time-domain analysis. In V.Z. Marmarelis (ed.), *Advanced methods of physiologic system modelling*. Los Angeles: University of Southern California.

Swets, J. (1988). Measuring the accuracy of diagnostic systems. *Science, 140*, 1285–1293.

Valdes-Sosa, M.J., Bobes, M.A., Perez-Abalo, M.C., Perera, M., Carballo, J.A., and Valdes-Sosa, P. (1987). Comparison of auditory-evoked potential detection methods using signal detection theory. *Audiology, 26*, 166–178.

Vaughan, H.G., Jr. (1969). The relationship of brain activity to scalp recording of event-related potentials. In E. Donchin and D.B. Lindsley (eds.), *Averaged evoked potentials: Methods, results, and evaluations*, pp.45–94. NASA SP-191, Washington, DC: Government Printing Office.

Vaughan, H.G., Jr. and Ritter, W. (1970). The sources of auditory evoked responses recorded from the human head. *Electroencephalography and Clinical Neurophysiology, 28*, 360–367.

Wastell, D.G. (1977). Statistical description of individual evoked responses: an evaluation of Woody's adaptive filter. *Electroencephalography and Clinical Neurophysiology, 42*, 835–839.

Wastell, D.G. (1981). When Wiener filtering is less than optimal: an illustrative application to the brainstem evoked potential. *Electroencephalography and Clinical Neurophysiology, 51*, 678–682.

Weber, B.A. and Fletcher, G.L. (1980). A computerized scoring procedure for auditory brainstem response audiometry. *Ear and Hearing, 1*, 233–236.

Williston, J.S., Jewett, D.L., and Martin, W.H. (1981). Planar curve analysis of three-channel auditory brainstem response: a preliminary report. *Brain Research, 223*, 181–184.

Wong, P.K. and Bickford, R.G. (1980). Brain stem auditory evoked potentials: the use of noise estimate. *Electroencephalography and Clinical Neurophysiology, 50*, 25–34.

Woody, C.D. (1967). Characterization of an adaptive filter for the analysis of variable latency neuroelectric signals. *Medical and Biological Engineering, 5*, 539–553.

CHAPTER 4

STIMULUS CALIBRATION IN AUDITORY EVOKED POTENTIAL MEASUREMENTS

MICHAEL P. GORGA
STEPHEN T. NEELY

INTRODUCTION

In this chapter, we describe some procedures for calibrating stimuli used to elicit auditory evoked potentials. Some of these procedures are repeated from the first edition of this book because their applications remain appropriate. Additional topics include tests of attenuator accuracy and cross talk, and calibration of bone conducted stimuli. As in the first edition, it is assumed that the reader has a basic understanding of the physics of sound.

Standards exist that provide specific guidelines for describing the characteristics of many of the stimuli used in routine behavioral audiometry. However, this is not the case for instruments that are used to elicit physiologic responses from humans. Standards are currently evolving for stimuli produced by auditory evoked potential (AEP) systems. An effort has been made to recommend calibration procedures which will be compatible with these forthcoming standards.

STIMULUS LEVEL

The calibration of stimulus level is the process of specifying the amplitude of a test stimulus relative to some standard reference. The calibration procedure will depend, to a certain extent, on the *temporal characteristics* of the stimulus. For example, root-mean-square (RMS) sound pressure is an appropriate amplitude description

of continuous sinusoids and other long-duration stimuli such as broadband noise. The amplitude of short-duration stimuli, such as clicks or tone bursts, are better described by their peak (or peak-to-peak) sound pressure.

In addition to well defined sound pressure references such as RMS, peak, and peak-to-peak, we will also consider the use of the "just audible stimulus" as a reference, including such references as dB Hearing Level (HL), dB Sensation Level (SL), and dB Hearing Level for Normal Subjects (HL_n). Of these biologically based references, it should be remembered that dB HL is well established and is specified by measuring the RMS SPL of a stimulus (e.g., ANSI, 1989). A more detailed description of the issues associated with choosing an intensity reference are provided elsewhere (Gorga and Thornton, 1989). We will, however, describe procedures for calibrating the amplitude of many typical stimuli used in AEP evaluations.

dB SPL

Any decibel measurement represents the ratio of two values. Table 4.1 lists the pressure references for RMS sound pressure level (SPL), peak equivalent SPL (peSPL), peak pressure (pSPL), peak-to-peak equivalent SPL (ppeSPL), and peak-to-peak pressure (ppSPL). The most common amplitude reference for long-duration stimuli is 20 micropascal (μPa) RMS. This refer-

This work was supported in part by NIH. We thank Steve Barlow, Glenn Farley, and Beth Prieve for their comments on an earlier version of this manuscript.

ence has been standardized nationally (ANSI S1.8-1969) and is reasonably close to the average threshold of hearing for a continuous 1000 Hz tone presented in a free field for normal-hearing young adult listeners. A pascal is the standard measurement unit of pressure, with $1 \text{ Pa} = 1 \text{ N/m}^2 = 10 \text{ dyne/cm}^2$. The level of a stimulus (L_s) can be specified by determining the ratio of its RMS pressure (P_s) to the SPL of the reference ($P_r = 20 \text{ }\mu\text{Pa}$), and expressing this ratio in decibels, L_s (dB SPL) $= 20 \log 10 \text{ } P_s/P_r$.

Although the SPL reference roughly coincides with normal threshold of audibility only at 1000 Hz, this reference is frequency independent and the same 20 μPa reference is used at all frequencies. As such, it differs from many other references like dB Hearing Level (HL) and dB Hearing Level$_{normal}$ (HL$_n$) , which vary with frequency.

To measure transducer output in dB SPL, the transducer typically is attached to a calibrated microphone by means of a standard coupler (e.g., 9 NBS 6 cm^3 coupler for circumaural or supraaural earphones; 2 cm^3 coupler for insert earphones). The output of the microphone is a voltage which is proportional to sound pressure and thus can be read in units of pressure by a sound level meter (SLM) or in voltage with an RMS voltmeter. The entire measurement system, including the microphone, any voltage amplifiers, and the voltmeter (or SLM), are themselves calibrated against a known source, such as that provided by a pistonphone or other standard acoustic calibrator. Once the system is calibrated, the level of any long-duration stimulus can be determined by comparing the RMS output of

TABLE 4.1. Pressure references for various calibration methods.

dB	Reference Pressure	Measurement Method
SPL	20.00 μPa	RMS
peSPL	28.28 μPa	peak
pSPL	20.00 μPa	peak
ppeSPL	56.57 μPa	peak-to-peak
ppSPL	20.00 μPa	peak-to-peak

the microphone for the unknown stimulus with that obtained for the calibrated source.

dB Peak Equivalent SPL

Many of the stimuli used in AEP evaluations are transients that cannot be measured accurately by devices whose response time constants are long in relation to the duration of the stimulus. Peak equivalent SPL (dB peSPL) has been used to circumvent this problem. Measurements of peSPL are made using similar procedures to those used to obtain measures of RMS amplitude, with the following modification. A SLM is used to measure the RMS amplitude of a continuous sinusoid. At the same time, the AC output from the SLM is routed to an oscilloscope which is used to measure its peak voltage. This peak voltage is proportional to the peak (instantaneous) pressure of the tone being measured by the SLM. The conversion factor that relates voltage to pressure is referred to as the sensitivity of the SLM, and should be the same for peak or RMS measurements, regardless of how it is determined.

To illustrate the relation between voltage and pressure, consider a continuous, 1000 Hz sinusoid of 100 dB SPL that also has a peak voltage of 100 mV when the AC output of the SLM is measured with an oscilloscope. The oscillographic tracing of this sinusoid is shown in Figure 4.1. Since 0 dB SPL equals 20 μPa, and since peak pressure is 1.414 times greater than RMS pressure for sinusoids, peak pressure is 3 dB greater than RMS pressure. This ratio of peak to RMS pressure (with the DC component removed) is known as the crest factor. Since 100 dB SPL represents an RMS pressure of 2 Pa ($100 \text{ dB SPL} = 20 \log_{10} P_s/P_r$, where $P_s = 2 \text{ Pa}$ and $P_r = 20 \text{ }\mu\text{Pa}$), and since peak pressure is 1.414 times greater than RMS pressure, 100 mV represents a peak pressure of 2.828 Pa, or 103 dB relative to 20 μPa. This implies that the peak voltage/peak pressure sensitivity of our SLM is about 35 mV/Pa (100 mV/2.828 Pa). If a peak voltage of 200 mV is measured for a second continuous sinusoid, then peak pressure is 109 dB relative to 20 μPa. We know this because a peak voltage of 200 mV represents a peak pressure of 5.71 Pa ($200 \text{ mV}/\frac{35 \text{mV}}{\text{Pa}}$). Knowing the sensi-

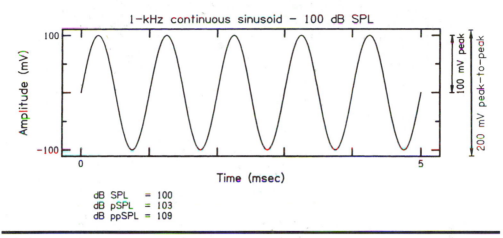

FIGURE 4.1.   Waveform of a 1000 Hz continuous sinusoid whose amplitude, when measured with a sound level meter, equals 100 dB SPL. Peak and peak-to-peak amplitude measures (in mV) are also shown.

tivity of the SLM enables us to measure the peak pressure of signals that differ from the reference by any factor, including factors of 2 or 10.

In order to extend this procedure to short duration sinusoids (or tone bursts) it is necessary to choose a reference signal for which both RMS and peak amplitude can be measured, such as the 1000 Hz continuous sinusoid, described above. The peak voltage of the tone burst can be measured on an oscilloscope in exactly the same manner described above for continuous sinusoids. This peak voltage is then compared to the peak voltage obtained for the 1000 Hz reference tone. We refer to the ratio of these two voltages (expressed in decibels) as peak equivalent sound pressure level (peSPL). When the duration of a tone burst becomes sufficiently long that it is indistinguishable from a continuous tone, then our measurements of SPL and peSPL are equivalent.

An example might make this procedure more clear. A 1000 Hz continuous sinusoid produces an SLM reading of 100 dB SPL (implying a peak pressure of 103 dB) and a peak voltage of 100 mV when the AC output of the SLM is measured with an oscilloscope. We are interested in measuring the level of a 2000 Hz tone burst, having a total duration of 4 ms (2 ms rise/

fall times with no plateau). The reference waveform (1000 Hz continuous sinusoid) and the tone burst (2000 Hz) are shown in Figure 4.2. Using an oscilloscope, we measure a peak voltage of 50 mV for the 2000 Hz tone burst. Thus, its peak voltage is one half the peak voltage of the 1000 Hz reference tone. We can infer that the peak pressure of the tone burst also is half the peak pressure of the reference tone, if we assume that the sensitivity of the SLM is the same at 1000 and 2000 Hz. (This assumption is valid with most of the equipment used to calibrate audiometers and AEP systems). Since the 1000 Hz reference signal has an SPL of 100 dB, the 2000 Hz tone burst has a peSPL of 94 dB. By this we mean that if the duration of the 2000 Hz sinewave were increased such that we would consider it continuous, then its level would be 94 dB SPL.

We could also have used our knowledge of the sensitivity of the SLM to accomplish this calibration. A peak voltage of 50 mV is equivalent to a peak pressure of 1.43 Pa (remember that we previously determined that 35 mV is equivalent to 1 Pa for our hypothetical example). Recall from Table 4.1 that the appropriate reference pressure for peSPL is 28 μPa. Therefore, the peak equivalent SPL of the 2000 Hz tone burst, expressed in dB, is 94 dB ($20 \log_{10} 1.43$ Pa/0.000028 Pa).

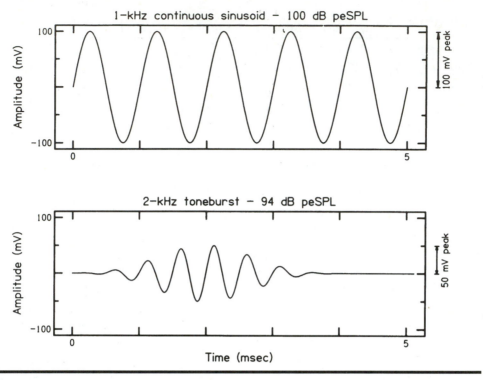

FIGURE 4.2. Waveforms of a 1000 Hz continuous sinusoid (reference) and a 2000 Hz tone burst, having 2 ms rise/fall times and no plateau. The reference stimulus, when measured with a sound level meter, has an amplitude of 100 dB SPL. The tone burst has a peak equivalent amplitude of 94 dB SPL.

Since RMS pressure is 3 dB less than peak pressure for sinusoids, the 2000 Hz tone has a pSPL of 97 dB.

In a similar manner, we can define the measurement of peak-to-peak equivalent sound pressure level (ppeSPL) by saying that a tone burst has a level of 100 dB ppeSPL when its peak-to-peak voltage measured on an oscilloscope is the same as the peak-to-peak voltage measured for a reference signal, such as a 1000 Hz continuous tone of 100 dB SPL. Often, the peak-to-peak voltage is easier to measure on an oscilloscope than the peak voltage.

Peak Sound Pressure

Some investigators use peak equivalent SPL to describe the amplitude of impulsive stimuli such as clicks. While it is appropriate to use the same measurement procedures, it may be inappropriate to maintain equivalency between the impulsive stimulus and the reference tone. Whereas sinusoids are symmetrical around zero amplitude, clicks typically are not. For these stimuli, it is imperative to know the sensitivity of the SLM. We determined SLM sensitivity using a 1000 Hz continuous sinusoid because this stimulus is commonly used to determine microphone sensitivity. We could have used many other stimuli, such a square waves or even broadband noise. However, the relation between RMS and peak pressure (i.e., the crest factor) is different for these types of stimuli in comparison to sinusoids. For example, the crest factor is 3 dB for a sinusoid, 0 dB for a square wave, and approximately 12 dB for gaussian noise. Yet SLMs typically only provide estimates of

RMS pressure (expressed in dB SPL). We need to know the relation between RMS and peak pressure for the reference signal in order to convert measurements of peak voltage into peak pressure. Thus, crest factor is important only when we are determining the relation between peak (instantaneous) pressure and peak voltage. Once this relation is known, the peak pressure of any stimulus can be calibrated.

For example, consider the waveforms shown in Figure 4.3. If a 1000 Hz continuous tone produces a 100 dB SPL signal, and a peak voltage of 100 mV when the AC output of the SLM is measured with an oscilloscope, then 100 mV represents a peak sound pressure of 103 dB. If a click now produces a peak voltage of 25 mV, its peak sound pressure is 12 dB less than the peak

sound pressure of the reference signal. We know this because its peak voltage is $\frac{1}{4}$ that of the reference peak voltage. Thus, it has a peak sound pressure of 91 dB. We also could calculate the peak pressure using our estimate of the SLM's sensitivity. We know that 25 mV represents a peak pressure of 0.714 Pa (25 mV/35 $\frac{mV}{Pa}$ = 0.714 Pa). We can convert this pressure into dB, using the equation, 20 $\log_{10}$ 0.714 Pa/0.00002 Pa. It is often the case that describing the amplitude of impulsive stimuli in RMS units is neither necessary or meaningful.

Likewise, we can define peak-to-peak sound pressure level (ppSPL) using an imaginary reference signal with the same pressure waveform, but with a peak-to-peak pressure of exactly 20 µPa. Estimates of peak-to-peak voltage are often easier than estimates of peak

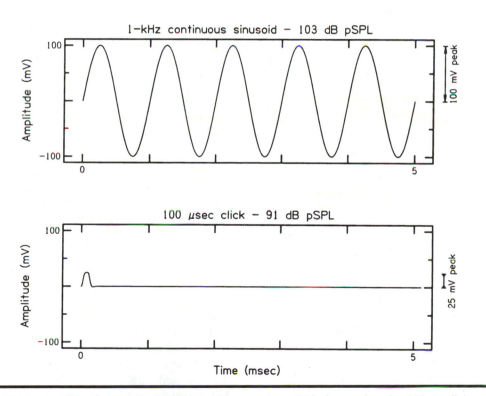

FIGURE 4.3. Waveforms of a 1000 Hz continuous sinusoid (reference) and a 100 µs click. The amplitude of the reference stimulus is 100 dB SPL when measured with a sound level meter. It has a peak voltage of 100 mV which is equivalent to a peak pressure of 103 dB re 20 µPa. The click has a peak voltage of 25 mV, which is equivalent to a peak pressure of 91 dB re: 20 µPa.

amplitude because there is no need to estimate a baseline. However, some individuals prefer to measure the amplitude of the largest peak of a click waveform (which is typically asymmetrical around zero). It should be recognized that the largest difference that is possible between peak and peak-to-peak amplitude estimates is 6 dB and this occurs only in the case when the impulsive stimulus is completely unidirectional. This occurs rarely with most clinical transducers.

dB HL

The threshold of audibility depends on frequency, due in large part to the middle ear, which transmits energy more efficiently for mid-frequencies (i.e., 1000 Hz to 2000 Hz) as compared to either low (250 Hz) or high (8000 Hz) frequencies. For example, the fact that, when TDH39 earphones are used, threshold at 250 Hz is 26 dB SPL whereas it is 9 dB SPL at 1000 Hz reflects the fact that there is less energy loss through the middle ear at 1000 Hz than at 250 Hz. Referencing stimulus level to dB HL (ANSI S3.6—1989), which is a common reference in clinical behavioral audiometry, takes into account this frequency dependence. It has the added advantage of providing a convenient normative reference (0 dB HL) to which clinical data from individual patients can be compared.

The procedures for calibrating stimuli in dB HL are identical to those used for SPL measurements. A calibrated microphone and a SLM (or a voltmeter) are required to measure RMS voltage. In this case, however, the measured RMS pressures are adjusted by the appropriate reference equivalent thresholds as a function of frequency. For example, the reference equivalent threshold at 1000 Hz for a TDH39 earphone is 9 dB SPL. Therefore, a measurement of 79 dB SPL at 1000 Hz is equivalent to 70 dB HL, the difference representing the reference equivalent threshold (in dB SPL) for this frequency.

dB HL$_n$

Pure-tone reference equivalent threshold levels have been established for a number of different earphones. See Wilber, Kruger, and Killion (1988) for a review

that includes data for the Etymotic ER-3A insert earphone as well as supraaural earphones such as the TDH39, TDH49, and the TDH50. These values were established from threshold measurements on large numbers of normal-hearing young adult subjects. Thus, these values have as their basis biological or behavioral threshold reference measures. By compensating for the transfer function of the external and, to a larger extent, middle ears, they provide values that produce uniform audibility across frequency.

A similar situation does not as yet exist for many of the stimuli used in EP evaluations. In the absence of standard reference equivalent thresholds, many clinics have used behavioral threshold measurements on small groups of normal-hearing subjects to establish intensity references for 0 dB. These values typically are referred to as dB HL$_n$ or $_n$HL. To obtain these values, behavioral thresholds are measured in normal-hearing subjects for the specific stimuli and the specific transducer that will be used in EP evaluations. The mean threshold for the group is assigned the value of 0 dB HL$_n$. It is important to recognize that behavioral thresholds will not only depend on the type of transducer (consider the differences between air-conducted thresholds using TDH49 earphones versus an ER-3A insert earphone [Wilber et al., 1988]) but also on transducer placement. For example, clinically we assume that interaural attenuation is 0 dB for bone conduction; however, reference equivalent force levels differ for bone conduction thresholds when the vibrator is placed at the forehead as compared to the mastoid (ANSI S3.26-1981). These differences are not uniform across frequency, ranging from 6.5 dB (4000 Hz) to 15 dB (500 Hz). Therefore, the value for 0 dB HL$_n$ should be determined not only for all possible transducer placements, but also for all stimuli that are used clinically.

Bone conduction requires special discussion because there are apparently many disagreements regarding the use of bone conduction in AEP evaluations (e.g., Mauldin and Jerger, 1979; Weber, 1984; Schwartz, Larson, and DeChicchis, 1985). When measured in units of force, the output of typical bone vibrators is greater for lower frequencies than it is for higher frequencies. However, thresholds by bone conduction are significantly lower for high frequencies than they are for low frequencies (Dirks and Kamm, 1975; ANSI, 1981). Bone-vibrator output limitations as a function of frequency provide clinical evidence of this differential sensitivity. Audiometrically, it is not uncommon for the maximum bone-conduction level at 250 Hz to be 40 dB HL whereas, at 2000 Hz, the limit is more typically 70 dB HL. Obviously, bone conducted sound is transmitted more efficiently at higher frequencies. Bone vibrators are low-frequency emphasis transducers only when their outputs are viewed in units of force. In terms of effective stimulation to the cochlea, they should be viewed either as high-frequency emphasis or broad-response transducers.

It also is essential that reference thresholds, such as dB HL_n, be developed in sound-isolated environments, even if clinically the test procedure will be used in a non-standard acoustical background. Otherwise, the peak pressure for 0 dB HL_n may be elevated, resulting in an underestimation of threshold for all hearing-impaired patients. For example, in normal-hearing subjects, the noise would have the effect of elevating their behavioral thresholds due to masking. Whereas 0 dB HL_n might require 35 dB peak sound pressure in a sound treated environment, 60 dB peak sound pressure might be needed in the noisy setting. In contrast, a patient with mild-to-moderate hearing loss might not experience any masking in the same noisy environment because the noise would be below threshold. This patient might have a click evoked ABR threshold of 80 dB peak sound pressure. If the reference condition was obtained in a sound-treated environment, threshold would be considered elevated by 45 dB relative to normal. In contrast, if we used a reference obtained in the noisy setting (i.e., 60 dB), threshold would be elevated by only 20 dB relative to normal. Thus, hearing loss would be underestimated by 25 dB. Clearly, the reference condition should be obtained under sound-isolated, controlled conditions for all applications, but especially when AEP measurements are to be used to estimate hearing sensitivity.

Finally, these references should be viewed as less rigorous than those obtained from published standards because there is no uniformity in terms of the number of normal subjects, the definition of a normal subject, the psychophysical technique used to measure threshold, or the precision with which these threshold measurements are made. Indeed, it is even difficult to recommend the number of normal subjects on which these measurements should be based. On the other hand, there is good consistency across laboratories and clinics, with 0 dB HL_n for 100 μs clicks, presented through supraaural, circumaural, or insert earphones, typically occurring at peak pressures ranging from 30 to 38 dB. Obviously, this range of values is due, at least in part, to differences in the responses of these transducers. Further validation of the consistency of these less formal threshold references is provided by the fact that ABR thresholds and latencies from different laboratories are remarkably similar for stimuli calibrated in dB HL_n. Whenever stimulus levels are expressed in terms of dB HL_n, we recommend that the relation to dB SPL also be provided in order to simplify comparisons across laboratories and clinics.

TEMPORAL CHARACTERISTICS

It is unlikely that the actual temporal characteristics of stimuli will differ significantly from nominal dial settings on typical AEP systems. On the other hand, these stimulus features are easy to measure with an oscilloscope and should be considered a part of routine calibration.

Stimulus Duration

For the purposes of this discussion, we will define duration as the entire stimulus envelope, including rise/fall times as well as any plateau. For clicks, the rise/fall time (when measured electrically) is essentially instantaneous so that pulse duration only includes the plateau. It also is more difficult to describe the duration of a click from the acoustic waveform because the frequency response of the transducer will alter the click's time waveform. As a consequence, it may be easier to make these measurements on the electrical signal prior to the shaping imposed by the earphone, and to rely on spectral analyses to provide more detailed descriptions of the transducer's response (see below). The electrical signal should be routed to an oscilloscope, which is triggered by the same pulse that starts averaging. Averaging should be started 1 or 2 ms prior to stimulus onset so that the complete stimulus waveform can be viewed. The duration can be measured directly from the oscillographic sweep as long as the oscilloscope's time base is calibrated. This procedure will work equally well for clicks and tone bursts.

Rise/Fall Time

Gated sinusoids are used in many clinical AEP evaluations. For example, short-duration tone bursts have been used to provide an estimate of the evoked potential equivalent of the pure-tone audiogram. The characteristics of gated sinusoids have been described elsewhere (Harris, 1978; Nuttall, 1981; below, in this chapter), as have some considerations for choosing temporal characteristics for the tone bursts used in EP evaluations (Gorga and Thornton, 1989). As a result, we will restrict our discussion only to the procedures that can be used to describe these temporal features. These procedures are identical to those used to measure stimulus duration, except that now the measurements are restricted to the portions of the waveform going from zero to maximum (rise) and from maximum to zero (fall) amplitude. It sometimes is difficult to measure rise/fall times from oscillographic recordings when a low-frequency stimulus is being gated because its sinusoidal oscillations may be slow in relation to the rise time. These measurements are made easier if a high-frequency sinewave is used because oscillations in these waveforms are likely to occur more rapidly than the changes in the waveform's envelope.

Stimulus Rate

Stimulus rate can be measured by following the procedures described above for duration and rise/fall time. The interval between identical points on successive stimuli can be measured from the oscillographic display. The reciprocal of this interval equals stimulus rate. For example, stimulus rate would be 25/s if the interval between successive stimuli was 40 ms (1/0.04 = 25). Devices known as counters/timers can be used to measure the interval between two events and thus could provide measures that could be used to estimate stimulus rate. However, these

devices may not be routinely available, whereas oscilloscopes typically are part of the AEP system.

POLARITY

Stimulus polarity may affect some AEP responses, although general agreement does not exist on whether polarity alters response latencies or the direction of these polarity effects, if they occur. It appears likely that polarity effects will be observed under those circumstances when short-latency responses (such as the ABR) are dominated by low-frequency energy in the signal. See Gorga and Thornton (1989) for a review of this hypothesis. This may occur when low frequency stimuli are used to elicit responses (Gorga et al., 1988) or when the configuration of hearing loss is such that the low-frequency components in a broadband stimulus dominate the response (Coats and Martin, 1977). Thus, it would appear that knowledge of stimulus polarity or phase has some clinical utility.

Cann and Knott (1979) described a procedure to measure stimulus polarity in which the earphone is disassembled in order to get access to the diaphragm. The earphone is firmly mounted and its diaphragm is brought into contact with a piston which is attached to a micrometer. The diaphragm of the earphone is placed into motion by applying a known DC voltage, such as that produced by a battery, and the direction of motion is measured with the micrometer. The positive and negative terminals on the earphone can be identified from the direction of the motion in relation to the way the earphone is attached to the battery terminals. One variation on this technique is to use a microscope and visually observe diaphragm motion when a voltage of known polarity is applied to the eaphone's terminals.

The above techniques require some specialized instrumentation which may not be readily available. An alternate and simpler approach uses equipment which is used routinely during the calibration of audiometers and thus should be available in all clinics. Place the earphone atop a standard coupler, the opposite end of which is fit with a microphone. The DC output from a SLM is routed to an oscilloscope, where it appears as a straight line. Gently press down on the earphone, creating a positive or condensation pressure in front of the microphone and note the direction of movement of the oscillographic trace. In this way, the entire measurement system is calibrated for polarity.

Next, connect the AC output from the sound level meter to the oscilloscope while a "rarefaction" or "condensation" click is presented by the earphone. Note the direction of the largest voltage peak of this waveform. If the motion is the same as that noted when the earphone was pressed, then this is a condensation click. If the voltage waveform goes in the opposite direction, then it is a rarefaction click. If the EP system produces a click of opposite polarity to its nominal setting, the wires connecting to the earphone typically can be reversed.

Tonal stimuli are typically symmetrical around zero voltage, having both rarefaction and condensation portions within each sinewave cycle. Thus, describing stimulus onset phase may be less relevant. Tonal stimuli also have durations which are longer than those used for clicks, and response waveforms are more likely to include both stimulus artifact and cochlear microphonic (CM), potentially making waveform component identification more difficult. As a result, alternating stimulus phase for such stimuli might be considered in order to cancel both stimulus artifact and CM. Under these circumstances, measurements of stimulus onset phase is of less interest, and it is only sufficient to know that phase reverses when stimuli of alternating polarity are presented. This can be accomplished by viewing waveforms on the oscilloscope, as described above, or by averaging the stimulus waveform. If phase reverses on each trial, the average waveform should be a straight line at zero voltage.

On the other hand, there may be reasons to present tone-burst stimuli with a fixed onset polarity. We know that hair cells are excited when their stereocilia are deflected in only one direction (Kiang et al., 1965; Goblick and Pfeiffer, 1969; Hudspeth and Corey, 1977). The temporal spacing between positive and negative half cycles of sinewaves depends on frequency, thus alternating stimulus phase would result in shifting the time at which excitatory events occur by one-half cycle. For high frequencies, such as 4000 Hz where the period is 250 μs, alternating polarity results in a maxi-

mal shift in excitatory events of only 125 μs, which may be too small to affect response morphology or latency. On the other hand, alternating polarity at 500 Hz results in a maximal shift of excitatory events by 1 ms. If, for example, wave V latencies were shifted by this amount, the portions of the response that share the same polarity might not align, and this temporal jitter might be sufficient to result in some response "cancellation" (Gorga et al., 1991). For these reasons, it might be useful to consider using fixed phase tone-burst stimuli, especially for low-frequency sinusoids. If tone-burst phase is important, then the procedures described above for measurement of click phase can also be used here.

AMPLITUDE SPECTRA

In addition to knowing the overall amplitude of a stimulus, it is useful to know how that energy is distributed across frequency. Such information is particularly important when one attempts to describe response properties for specific frequency (cochlear) regions. Plots of amplitude as a function of frequency are referred to as amplitude or power spectra, and there is an exact correspondence between the amplitude (and phase) spectrum of a stimulus and its time waveform, which are plots of amplitude as a function of time. Detailed descriptions of the issues related to choosing among time waveforms (and therefore, amplitude spectra) are described elsewhere (Gorga and Thornton, 1989). We will, however, review the effects of duration and rise/fall time on amplitude spectra for common AEP stimuli.

Clicks

The reciprocal of stimulus duration will determine the frequencies at which the amplitude is reduced. Thus, a 100 μs click will have spectral zeros at 10,000 Hz intervals. The rise/fall time will determine the relative amplitude of the side lobes in relation to the energy in the main energy lobe. See Harris (1978) and Nuttall (1981) for detailed descriptions of the effects of the windowing function on amplitude spectra. For example, a square-gated signal, such as a click, will have regions of reduced amplitude or spectral zeros at frequencies equal to one divided by click duration, the amplitude of the first side lobe will be 13 dB lower than the main energy lobe, and side-lobe energy will roll off or decrease at a rate of 6 dB/octave.

Gated Sinusoids

An identical pattern will occur for square-gated sinusoids, although these stimuli typically are not turned on and off with square functions. Instead, gated sinusoids usually are gated with windows that approach and descend from maximum amplitude more gradually. The effects of duration are the same but side-lobe energy will be 27 dB down from the main energy lobe for a linear (Bartlett) window and energy will continue to decrease at a rate of 12 dB/octave. For sinusoids gated with cosine-squared functions (Hanning windows), the first side lobe is 32 dB down and energy continues to roll off at a rate of 18 dB/octave. Stimuli that are becoming increasingly available on AEP systems are sinusoids gated with Blackman windows. For these windows, energy in the first side lobe is 58 dB below the energy in the main lobe and continues to roll off at a rate of 18 dB/octave. This reduction in side-lobe amplitude is gained at the expense of width in the main energy lobe, which is wider for a Blackman window than it is for Bartlett (linear or triangular) or Hanning windows of equivalent duration. Examples of the time waveforms and associated spectral representations for sinusoids gated with these windows are shown in Figure 4.4 (from Gorga and Thornton, 1989).

It is important to recognize that the rules governing these windows hold only when there is *no plateau* portion to the stimulus. Once a plateau is added, the amplitude spectra tend to be more complex. This fact is of little concern for short-latency responses, such as the ABR, because these AEPs are elicited by the onset portion of the stimulus; the contributions to the response from any steady-state or plateau portion of the stimulus are probably negligible. As a consequence, the temporal characteristics of stimuli probably should be chosen without steady-state portions. At the very least, it can be misleading to view stimuli with rapid onsets and

long plateaus as spectrally more narrow than the same stimulus without a plateau, especially for short-latency responses. Since these are onset responses, the spectrum during the earliest portions of the stimulus is important, but spectral characteristics due to the plateau are clearly less relevant.

There are many other windows that can be used to turn sinusoids on and off, each having slightly different characteristics. The three windows reviewed above were selected because they are commonly used in EP evaluations; however, it is important to recognize that this list

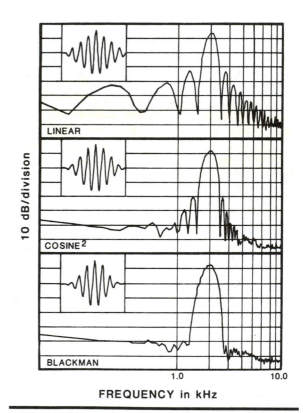

FIGURE 4.4. Time waveforms (inset) and amplitude spectra for 2000 Hz tone bursts having 2 ms rise/fall times and no plateaus. Top panel: Bartlett or linear window; middle panel: Hanning or cosine-squared window; bottom panel: Blackman window. Reproduced with permission, Gorga, M.P. and Thornton, A.R., The choice of stimuli for ABR measurements, *Ear and Hearing, 10, 4,* 217–230, © by Williams & Wilkins, 1989.

is not exhaustive and that other windows may prove to be superior to these for certain AEP applications.

Having reviewed the effects of stimulus duration and rise/fall time, we need to describe a way to measure the amplitude spectrum. There is a precise relation between the time waveform and the amplitude and phase spectra of any stimulus. If the time waveform is known, then the amplitude spectrum also is known. The method by which we transform a stimulus from its time-domain representation to its frequency- and phase-domain representations (or vice versa) is called Fourier analysis. Devices now exist that are capable of capturing time waveforms and performing Fourier transforms in order to derive the amplitude (and/or phase) spectra. These devices are referred to as spectrum analyzers. We can perform a spectral analysis of any stimulus on either its electrical waveform or its acoustical waveform (i.e., after transduction by an earphone). In the former, the input to the spectrum analyzer is taken prior to the earphone, while in the latter case, the AC output of a SLM is routed to the spectrum analyzer.

ATTENUATOR ACCURACY

We would like to know that attenuator settings controlling stimulus amplitude are accurate over their entire range. Attenuator accuracy is important in any clinical evaluation when there is a relation between characteristics of the response and stimulus intensity, such as latency-intensity functions or threshold. Each time we change an attenuator setting by 5 or 10 dB, the amplitude of the stimulus should change by the same amount. If stimulus intensity is calibrated at a high level, such as 80 dB HL_n, adding 70 dB of attenuation should result in a stimulus whose amplitude is equivalent to 10 dB HL_n.

Attenuator accuracy can be evaluated by measuring the amplitude of the stimulus over the range of values produced by the system. This can be accomplished by measuring the stimulus either electrically (i.e., at the input to the transducer) or accoustically (after transduction by the earphone). Either approach will work as long as the earphone remains connected to the system. Furthermore, either RMS, peak, or peak-to-peak amplitude measurements can be used to assess system linearity.

For high level conditions, the amplitude of the stimulus is typically above the noise floor of the measuring device or any ambient room noise. Thus, no signal treatment is necessary, and any suitable device, such as a voltmeter, a SLM, or an oscilloscope, could be used to directly measure stimulus amplitude. However, problems will occur once the amplitude of the stimulus is small in relation to the background electrical or acoustical noise. Under these conditions, it is not possible to measure amplitude accurately without some treatment of the signal. One way to improve the signal-to-noise ratio is signal averaging. Signal amplitude will remain unchanged but the amplitude of the noise will be reduced in relation to the number of samples included in the average. (Signal averaging is treated in greater detail by Hyde in Chapter 3).

It should be possible to accomplish these measurements using any clinical AEP system. The signal can be led to the averager in exactly the same way brain electrical activity is averaged when performing an AEP evaluation clinically. Stimuli can be presented at fairly high rates (e.g., 100/s) so that averaged waveforms consisting of many stimulus samples can be collected rapidly. The gain of the "response amplifier" will have to be adjusted, depending on stimulus amplitude, so that the input to the averager remains within the dynamic range of the analog-to-digital converter (ADC). As a consequence, measured amplitudes will need to be adjusted to account for any differences in "response" amplification. It also is useful to delay stimulus onset by about 2 ms relative to the onset of averaging in order to obtain a complete view of the stimulus. This very simple and rapid procedure can be used to improve stimulus-to-noise ratios, making it possible to measure stimulus amplitude over the entire range of values produced by a clinical AEP system.

CROSS TALK

It is not uncommon for a portion of the stimulus delivered on one channel to cross over to the opposite channel. This problem is referred to as cross talk. Typically, the level of the signal crossing over is very low and of little concern clinically as long as it is less than the minimum amount of interaural attenuation. Thus, we would be concerned about transcranial signal transmission before we would be concerned about cross talk. Consider a case with unilateral flat 50 dB sensorineural hearing loss, who is being evaluated with an AEP system which uses a TDH39 earphone housed in a standard cushion (such as an MX 41/AR) and whose cross-over signal is reduced by 60 dB. We might present masking noise to the non-test normal ear if we assumed (conservatively) that interaural attenuation was 40 dB. Because the cross talk is less than the signal that has crossed transcranially (i.e., –60 dB versus –40 dB), it too would be masked by the noise. If an appropriate masker was selected to eliminate the response from the non-test ear to the transcranially transmitted signal, it would also mask the response to that portion of the signal arriving at the non-test ear via cross talk.

However, insert earphones, which are used in many clinical situations, provide interaural attenuation that may be as great as 80 dB at some frequencies (Killion, 1984). With these earphones, the level of the signal due to cross talk (that was reduced by 60 dB from the signal delivered to the test ear) could be greater than the transcranially transmitted signal, thus obviating one advantage of using insert earphones. Under these circmustances, there would be some clinical utility in knowing the amount of cross talk produced by an EP system.

The simplest and most direct way to measure cross talk uses a procedure that is comparable to the one used to assess attenuator accuracy. Physically separate the two earphones so that they are accoustically isolated from each other. Place the earphone that is receiving the signal on a coupler attached to a SLM. Direct the AC output of the SLM to the averager as if it were an evoked potential. Present a stimulus at the maximum level possible while averaging the output. Measure the amplitude of this "test" signal. Next, place the "non-test" earphone on the coupler and repeat the above procedure. It may be necessary to adjust the gain on the "response amplifier" in order to remain within the dynamic range of the ADC because it is likely that the input signals will be very different in amplitude for these two conditions. Average this signal in order to improve signal-to-noise ratio and, thus, provide an accurate estimate of its amplitude. Compare the amplitude of the "test" signal to that for the "non-test" signal, making sure that differences in response amplification were taken into account. This amplitude ratio can be converted into dB in order to provide a measure of the separation (i.e., cross talk) between test and nontest ears.

SUMMARY

We have tried to provide a brief summary of some procedures which could be used when calibrating auditory stimuli used to elicit electrophysiological responses from humans. We have tended to weight our discussion towards the kinds of stimuli that are used in ABR evaluations because short-latency responses, such as the ABR, the whole-nerve action potential, and the summating potential, are the most common EPs measured in humans. A better understanding of calibration procedures can only lead to a more complete description of the stimuli we use to elicit these responses. This in turn should lead to more comparability of findings from different laboratories and clinics.

REFERENCES

American National Standards Institute (1969). *Preferred reference quantities for acoustical levels* (ANSI S1.8-1969), New York, NY.

American National Standards Institute (1989). *Specifications for audiometers* (ANSI S3.6-1969, R1973), New York, NY.

American National Standards Institute (1981). *Reference equivalent threshold force levels for audiometric bone vibrators* (ANSI S3.26-1981), New York, NY.

Cann, J. and Knott, J. (1979). Polarity of acoustic click stimuli for eliciting brainstem auditory evoked responses: A proposed standard, *American Journal of EEG Techechnology, 19*, 125–132.

Coats, A.C. and Martin, J.L. (1977). Human auditory nerve action potentials and brain stem evoked responses, *Archives of Otolaryngology, 103*, 605–622.

Dirks, D.D. and Kamm, C. (1975). Bone-vibrator measurements: Physical characteristics and behavioral thresholds, *Journal of Speech and Hearing Research, 18*, 242–260.

Goblick, T.J. and Pfeiffer, R.R. (1969). Time-domain measurements of cochlear nonlinearities using combination click stimuli, *Journal of Acoustical Society of America, 4*, 924–938.

Gorga, M.P. and Thornton, A.R. (1989). The choice of stimuli for ABR measurements, *Ear and Hearing, 10*, 217–230.

Gorga, M.P., Beauchaine, K.A., and Kaminski, J.K. (1991). The effects of stimulus phase on the latency of the auditory brainstem response, *Journal of the American Academy of Audiology, 2*, 1–6.

Harris, F.J. (1978). On the use of windows for harmonic analysis with the discrete Fourier transform, *IEEE Transactions of Acoustical Speech Signal Processing, 66*, 51–83.

Hudspeth, A.J. and Corey, D. (1977). Sensitivity, polarity, and conductance change in the response of vertebrate hair cells to controlled mechanical stimuli, *Proceeding of the National Academy of Science, 74*, 2407–2411.

Kiang, N.Y.S., Watanabe, T., Thomas, E.C., and Clark, L.F. (1965). Discharge patterns of single fibers in the cat's audi-

tory nerve, *Research Monographs, 35*, MIT Press, Cambridge, MA.

Killion, M.C. (1984). A new insert earphone for audiometry, *Hearing Instruments, 35*, 28–46.

Mauldin, L. and Jerger, J. (1979). Auditory brain stem responses to bone-conducted signals, *Archives of Otolaryngology, 105*, 656–661.

Nuttall, A.H. (1981). Some windows with very good sidelobe behavior, *IEEE Transactions of Acoustical Speech Signal Processing, 29*, 84–91.

Schwartz, D.M., Larson, V.D., and DeChicchis, A.R. (1985). Spectral characteristics of air and bone conduction transducers used to record the auditory brain stem response, *Ear and Hearing, 6*, 274–277.

Weber, B.A. (1983). Masking and bone conduction testing in brainstem response audiometry, *Seminars of Hearing, 4*, 343–352.

Wilber, L.A., Kruger, B., and Killion, M.C. (1988). Reference thresholds for the ER-3A insert earphone, *Journal of the Acoustical Society of America, 83*, 669–676.

PART TWO

AUDITORY ASPECTS

CHAPTER 5

ELECTROCOCHLEOGRAPHY

JOHN A. FERRARO
ROGER A. RUTH

INTRODUCTION

In the family of auditory evoked potentials (AEPs), the term electrocochleography (ECochG) refers to the general technique of recording the stimulus-related responses of the inner ear and auditory nerve (i.e., the "earliest" of the early- or short-latency AEPs). The specific components comprising the electrocochleogram (ECochGm) are shown in Figure 5.1. These may be recorded independently or in various combinations, and include the cochlear microphonic (CM) and summating potential(s) (SP) of the Organ of Corti, and the whole-nerve or compound action potential (AP) of the auditory nerve.

Attempts to record CM from humans date back almost to the time of its discovery by Wever and Bray in 1930 (Fromm, Bylen, and Zotterman, 1935; Andreev, Aropova, and Gersuni, 1939; Perlman and Case, 1941; Lempert, Wever, and Lawrence, 1947; Lempert, Meltzer, Wever, et al., 1950), whereas the first recording of the human auditory nerve AP was performed by Ruben and his co-workers in 1960. Comparatively speaking, the SP, first reported by Davis, Fernandez, and McAuliffe (1950), and von Bekesy (1950), has received little attention in humans until recently.

Although ECochG has long been available to the scientist/clinician, its application for clinical purposes was overshadowed following the discovery of the auditory brainstem response (ABR). This was primarily due to the audiometric advantages ABR offered in comparison to ECochG. Recently, however, there has been renewed interest in the clinical applications of ECochG. Several reasons can account for this. Certainly high among these is the widespread application and acceptance of AEP testing in general, and the ABR in particular. In addition, expanded and improved technology has made the very early components that constitute the ECochG waveform easier to extract using noninvasive, recording electrodes located peripheral to the tympanic cavity (extratympanic). Prior to this, the conventional method of performing ECochG involved penetrating the tympanic membrane to place the primary recording electrode on the round window or cochlear promontory (transtympanic).

Although there are still differences of opinion in the literature and among clinical investigators regarding the use of extratympanic versus transtympanic ECochG, the latter method has not been well accepted in North America primarily because of its invasiveness. Using extratympanic techniques, the ECochG examination can be performed by non-physicians without medical supervision using the same equipment and similar methodology to those employed for conventional ABR testing.

Certainly the most important factor in the acceptance and application of any clinical tool is the value of that tool in providing relevant and reliable clinical information. Several studies have now shown that ECochG can contribute significantly to the identification, assessment, and monitoring of certain audiologic, otologic, and neurologic disorders. More specifically, the currently most common clinical applications of ECochG include:

1. the objective identification and monitoring of Meniere's disease and endolymphatic hydrops;
2. the enhancement of wave I and the identification of the I-V Interwave Interval (IWI) of the ABR in the presence of hearing loss or less than optimal recording conditions; and

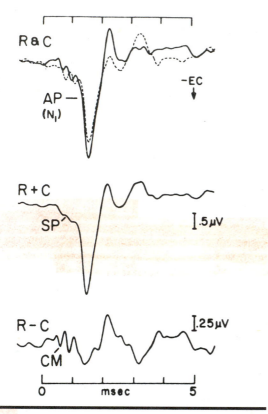

R & C

AP —
(N₁)

-EC

R + C

SP

].5 μV

R - C

].25 μV

CM

0   msec   5

FIGURE 5.1. Component potentials of the human electrocochleogram recorded using rarefaction (R) and condensation (C) click stimuli. Adding separate R and C responses enhances the Summating Potential (SP) and the Action Potential (AP). Subtracting R and C responses enhances the Cochlear Microphonic (CM). (from ASHA, 1988, pg. 9, based on data from Coats, 1981)

3. the monitoring of cochlear and auditory nerve function during surgical procedures that place the ear at risk for permanent damage (Ruth, Lambert, and Ferraro, 1988).

This chapter will provide an overview of the current theory, techniques and applications of clinical ECochG. The material has been organized to include descriptions of: the salient features of the CM, SP and AP; the various techniques and parameters employed to record these responses; normal and abnormal response char-

acteristics; and the various applications of ECochG in the clinical setting.

STIMULUS-RELATED POTENTIALS OF THE COCHLEA AND AUDITORY NERVE

There are considerable bodies of literature pertaining to each of the stimulus-related potentials utilized in clinical ECochG. The reader is referred to these for an indepth discussion of the specific features and functions of the CM, SP, and AP. Indeed, a thorough understanding and appreciation of the various electrical events associated with the transduction process in the cochlea and the transmission of neural impulses via the auditory nerve are essential for the recording and interpretation of ECochG. Given the scope and purpose of this chapter, the following section will confine the discussion of the CM, SP, and AP to their salient electrical features and respective applications in clinical ECochG.

Cochlear Microphonic

The CM, at least in animals, has been the most thoroughly investigated potential of the inner ear. The considerable magnitude of the response and the relative ease with which it can be recorded in the laboratory have certainly contributed to the CM's historical popularity. Whether the CM has an actual role in transduction at the hair cell level or is merely an epiphenomenon of the process is still a disputed issue. Nonetheless, the CM appears as an alternating current (AC) voltage that literally "mirrors" the waveform of the acoustic stimulus at low to moderate stimulus levels. Because of this characteristic, it is often difficult to differentiate between CM and stimulus artifact in clinical, non-invasive recordings. This presents certain technical problems to the examiner which, in turn, have discouraged the clinical utility of the CM.

The CM output stems primarily from the outer hair cells of the organ of Corti. When recorded from extracochlear sites such as the promontory, tympanic membrane, or ear canal, the primary generators are the outer hair cells of the basal turn of the cochlea (Dallos, 1973). The magnitude of the CM per se is reflective of hair cell output and a linear function of sound pressure over a fairly large range. The magnitude of the recorded response, however, also is dependent on the proximity of the recording electrodes to the hair cell generators. In general, as the distance between the electrode and generators increases, response magnitude decreases. This necessitates the application of signal averaging techniques when recording CM from extratympanic sites.

Despite its popularity in the laboratory, the CM has received far less attention than either the SP or the AP for clinical ECochG purposes. This is due in part to the variability observed in CM response patterns in both normal and abnormal ears and, as mentioned above, the technical difficulty of separating CM from stimulus artifact. In addition, the CM has not been shown to be consistently effective in the differential diagnosis of inner ear disorders. That is, changes in the CM waveform (reduction in amplitude and/or distortion) may indeed be reflective of cochlear and even middle ear pathology, but tend to be comparatively general and difficult to correlate with a specific disorder or pathologic agent. Elberling and Salomon (1973), for example, observed a reduction in response magnitude as the primary manifestation of cochlear pathology in CM recorded from the ear canal. Other investigators (Moriuchi and Kumagami, 1979; Morrison, Moffat, and O'Connor, 1980; Kumagami, Nishida, and Masaaki, 1982) have reported reduced CM magnitude and waveform distortion in Meniere's patients. Gibson and Beagley (1976), and Morrison, Moffat, and O'Connor (1980), described a "prolonged after ringing" of the CM in the early stages of endolymphatic hydrops, but this has been difficult to verify. More recently, Gerhardt, Wagner, and Werbs (1985), reported a reduced AP:CM amplitude ratio as a diagnostic criterion for acoustic neuromas.

Although the above studies show that CM response patterns may be useful in the identification of endolymphatic hydrops or acoustic tumors, abnormalities in other electrocochleographic and short-latency evoked potential components (i.e., SP, AP, ABR) appear to be more sensitive and reliable diagnostic indicators of these particular disorders. This is not to say, however, that we should abandon our efforts to utilize CM for clinical purposes. The current inadequacy of the CM as a clinical tool may indeed be attributable to an inadequate understanding of the mechanisms responsible for its production, its role in the transduction process, and cochlear mechanics in general. CM recordings from man may be very helpful in the study of these processes. Norton, Ferguson, and Mascher (1989), for example, observed both spectral and temporal similarities between CM recorded from the tympanic membrane and evoked otacoustic emissions (EAOEs) recorded from the ear canal. Their findings suggested that both CM and EAOEs may have a common, place-specific generator.

As our knowledge of transduction processes in the cochlea expands, and the techniques for recording the electrical events associated with these processes become more sensitive, the CM will most assuredly assume a more prominent role in clinical ECochG measurements.

Summating Potential

Since its identification over 40 years ago, the SP continues to be the least understood stimulus-related potential of the cochlea. This is certainly due in part to the complexity of the response, which comprises several components, and the effects on the recorded response attributable to an interaction between stimulus parameters and electrode location. As with the CM, the role of the SP in cochlear transduction is still a disputed issue. However, as a direct current (DC) response to an AC stimulus, at least some of the components of the SP are thought to be a reflection of nonlinear distortion in the transduction process (Tasaki, Davis, and Eldridge, 1954; Whitfield and Ross, 1965; Davis, 1968; Engebretson and Eldridge, 1968; Gulick, Gescheider, and Frisina, 1989).

The SP, like the CM, is stimulus-related and a product of hair cell generators. Unlike the CM, however, the SP is seen as a DC voltage that appears to be representative of the stimulus envelope rather than its waveform (Dallos, 1973). The polarity of the DC shift may be positive or negative depending on the frequency and intensity of the acoustic stimulus and the site of the recording electrode. When recorded extratympanically to click stimuli, the SP from a normal ear appears to be dominated by the negative differential (−DIF) component described by Dallos, Schoeny, and Cheatham (1972). This is characterized by a negative shift in the baseline of the recorded response which theoretically persists for the duration of the evoking stimulus. The term "theoretically" is used here because in conventional ECochG, click stimuli often are employed to evoke a complex waveform containing both the SP and AP. In such recordings, the SP to transient stimuli extends into the waveform of the AP making it difficult to study the parameters of each component independently, particularly the duration of the SP (Durrant and Ferraro, 1990).

Although the SP is historically the least studied ECochG component, recent, renewed interest in clinical ECochG is due in large part to changes reported in this particular response in suspected cases of endolymphatic hydrops (EH) or Meniere's disease. Several studies have now shown that the electrocochleograms of patients suspected of having EH are often characterized by an amplitude-enlarged SP, especially in comparison to the AP (Schmidt, Eggermont, and Odenthal, 1974; Gibson, Moffat, and Ramsden, 1977; Gibson, 1978; Moriuchi and Kumagami, 1979; Morrison, Moffat, and O'Connor, 1980; Coats, 1981, 1986; Kitahara, Takeda, and Yazama, 1981; Goin, Staller, and Ascher, 1982; Kumagami, Nishida, and Masaaki, 1982; Ferraro, Best, and Arenberg, 1983; Ferraro, Arenberg, and Hassanein, 1985; Staller, 1986; Ferraro, 1988a; Ruth, Lambert, and Ferraro, 1988). Unfortunately, the rationale for this finding remains unclear. Gibson, Moffat, and Ramsden (1977), for example, propose that an increase in endolymph volume may alter cochlear mechanics to result in an augmentation of the vibratory asymmetry of the basilar membrane. Since at least part of its components are thought be a reflection of this asymmetry, the SP would also be augmented or enlarged. Consistent with this hypothesis is the observation by Durrant and Dallos (1972, 1974) and Durrant and Gans (1977) that electrical biasing of the basilar membrane towards the scala tympani increases the amplitude of the SP. The latter studies, however, also lend support to an electrically as opposed to a mechanically induced alteration reflected in the SP.

Support for the above hypotheses are currently indirect at best. Given the relatively recent discovery and descriptions of active processes in the cochlea, it may be more reasonable to attribute an enlarged SP to micromechanical changes occurring at the level of the hair cells, rather than the basilar membrane. In addition,

biochemical and/or vascular changes that accompany or perhaps even cause EH cannot be ruled out as contributing factors (Goin, Staller, Ascher, et al., 1982; Staller, 1986). Further support for the notion that the enlargement of the SP is a physiological manifestation of endolymphatic hydrops may be found in clinical studies that have correlated changes in SP before and after glycerol dehydration (Moffat et al., 1978; Coats and Alford, 1981).

Regardless of specific pathophysiology, it is now well-documented that an enlarged SP may be pathognomonic of EH. This discovery, in turn, has been applied clinically to make ECochG one of the more powerful tools in the diagnostic test battery for Meniere's disease or EH.

Auditory Nerve Action Potential

Since its initial recording by Ruben, Sekula, and Bordley (1960) from patients undergoing ear surgery, the whole-nerve or compound AP of the auditory nerve has been the most widely studied component of the human ECochGm. In general, the AP represents the summed response of the synchronous firing of several thousand auditory nerve fibers. The response to click stimuli is often referred to as "whole-nerve" AP, implying that the stimulus has excited virtually the entire length of the basilar membrane in producing neural activity. When the evoking stimuli are tone-bursts, the term "compound" AP is used, which suggests that a more limited segment of basilar membrane contributes to the response (Gibson, 1978). In conventional ECochG, this terminology is misleading in that the synchronous activity essential for producing the AP occurs at the onset of the stimulus. This onset response, in turn, is dominated by neural contributions from the basal, high-frequency end of the normal cochlea (Kiang, 1965).

Similar to the CM, but unlike the SP, the AP appears as an AC voltage. The waveform of the AP is characterized by a short series of brief, predominantly negative deflections or sharp waves. The first and largest of these is referred to as N1. This component is virtually identical to wave I of the ABR, and arises from the distal portion of the auditory nerve (Møller and Janetta, 1983). Subsequent waves (i.e., N2) also are analogous to corresponding ABR components (wave II), but have received little, if any, clinical attention in

ECochG. The most relevant clinical features of the AP relate to its magnitude and latency. AP magnitude is a reflection of the number of fibers firing, whereas latency is generally defined as the time between stimulus onset and the peak of N1. A given latency value for N1 incorporates stimulus travel time, propagation time along the basilar membrane, and the time associated with the synchronization of neural impulses that produce the peak. In general, as stimulus intensity is decreased from suprathreshold levels, N1 magnitude decreases and latency increases, just as they do in ABR components.

As previously discussed, the ECochGms of patients suspected of having EH are often characterized by an enlarged SP component. The clinical consistency of this finding, however, improves when the SP amplitude is compared to the amplitude of the AP. In fact, an enlarged SP:AP amplitude ratio is currently considered to be the primary diagnostic indicator of EH in the ECochGm.

Several studies have now shown that the AP-N1 recorded with electrocochleographic techniques (i.e., from the ear canal or tympanic membrane) is larger and more sensitive than wave I of the conventionally recorded ABR (Ruth, Mills, and Ferraro 1988; Ferraro and Ferguson, 1989; Schwartz, Pratt, and Costello, 1989). This finding has provided another important application for ECochG. Namely, using a combined ECochG-ABR approach may improve the detectability of wave I of the ABR in the presence of hearing loss or less than optimal recording conditions, and thus facilitate the measurement of the I-V interwave latency under these circumstances.

Finally, when the integrity of the auditory nerve is at risk during surgical procedures, intraoperative recording of the AP has been shown to be an effective means of monitoring the status of the nerve (Ruth, Mills, and Jane, 1986; Ruth, Lambert, and Ferraro, 1988; Silverstein, Norrell, and Hyman, 1984; Silverstein, Wazen, Norrell et al., 1984).

RECORDING TECHNIQUES

Electrodes

Electrocochleography refers to the stimulus-related electrical potentials of the inner ear and auditory nerve. Thus, in the strictest sense, it would be appropriate to label conventionally recorded ABR as ECochG-ABR because responses from the auditory nerve (waves I and II) are components of the waveform. However, since the measurement of these components is more effective when the recording electrodes are closer to the response generators, the term ECochG currently tends to be used when at least one of the differential electrodes is located in the ear canal, on the tympanic membrane, or in the middle ear (promontory wall or round window). This necessitates the use of electrodes designed to provide optimal recordings from these sites. In general, these electrodes can be either invasive or non-invasive, depending on whether they penetrate the ear canal skin or tympanic membrane (TM), or merely rest on the surface of these structures (See Table 5.1).

Invasive Electrodes. The major advantage of using an invasive ECochG electrode is the acquisition of a clearer, more robust electrical response from the peripheral auditory system. This results simply from the fact that the recording electrode is usually very near the generators of the response. As such, the amplitude of the response is large in comparison to the background noise and thus presents a more favorable signal-to-

TABLE 5.1.   ECochG Recording Techniques

INVASIVE	NONINVASIVE
Transtympanic (TT-ECochG)	*Extratympanic* (ET-ECochG)
Needle electrode	Foam plug ear canal electrode
Round window ball electrode	Leaf electrode
	Tympanic Membrane (TM-ECochG)
	Flexible tubing with foam or cotton ball at end

noise ratio. An obvious disadvantage is the potential for some degree of discomfort to the patient. In addition, such an electrode must be placed by a physician which limits its use to medical settings.

The most frequently used invasive ECochG electrode is the transtympanic needle (Figure 5.2). The needle is generally insulated by a coating such as teflon except for a millimeter or two at its tip. Because of the relatively small surface area of contact, electrode impedance is generally high (ranging from 40 to 100+ kohms). It is usually placed, with the aid of an operating microscope, on the promontory wall of the middle ear near the round window niche by penetrating the tympanic membrane. Prior to placement of the transtympanic needle electrode, the tympanic membrane must be anesthetized. After placement the needle must be secured so as to prevent slippage due to minor head movements on the part of the patient.

ECochG recordings obtained with a transtympanic needle are often on the order of 20 to 40 microvolts in amplitude at high stimulus intensities (Ruth and Lambert, 1989). Given the relatively large amplitude of responses recorded in this fashion, fewer repetitions are required per average. For example, as few as 50 to 150 stimulus repetitions may be needed to resolve the response with this recording technique. This means that at a stimulus presentation rate of 10 per second a recording

can be obtained within 5 to 15 seconds, which is far less time than that required by most non-invasive procedures. More importantly, the AP response may be observed down to stimulus levels approximating hearing threshold. The transtympanic technique has become the standard of practice in many European countries.

Also shown in Figure 5.2 is a silver-ball electrode used for round window ECochG measurements. This type of electrode has been used for decades as a way of monitoring eighth nerve and cochlear potentials in animals. Its use in humans is more limited due to the fact that placement of the electrode requires that the ear drum be lifted so that the round window is visible to the surgeon. As such, this type of recording is generally reserved for those cases in which exposure of the middle ear is also needed for other purposes or for long term monitoring of the peripheral auditory system (i.e., intraoperative monitoring of the auditory nerve). In most cases round window ECochG recordings are similar to those obtained with the transtympanic needle electrode in terms of amplitude and response clarity.

Non-invasive Electrodes. The primary advantages of using non-invasive, extratympanic (ET) electrodes are that recordings can be achieved with no pain or discomfort to the patient, there is little if any risk of infection, and there is no need for sedation, anesthetics, or medical supervision. The major disadvantage is that the responses are considerably smaller than those recorded using invasive, transtympanic electrodes.

Although a variety of homemade devices have been reported in the literature, ET recording electrodes have been commercially available for several years. Figure 5.3 shows three of the more popular ones. The first of these to appear commercially was the so-called "eartrode" (middle) originally designed by Coats (1974). The eartrode consists of insulated silver wire with a ball tip glued to a strip of flexible plastic. The device is placed by pinching the leaves of the plastic strip together with fine forceps and inserting the unit tip-first into the ear canal. Releasing the forceps allows the leaves to spring open and serve as a wedge to hold the tip in place. Prior to insertion, the ear canal must be free of cerumen and cleansed in the anticipated vicinity of the gel-coated tip. Placement is generally in the posterior-inferior quadrant

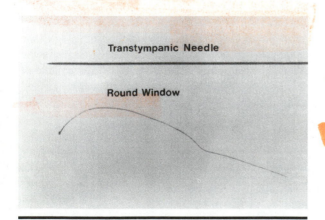

Transtympanic Needle

Round Window

FIGURE 5.2.   Transtympanic needle (top) and round window silver ball electrodes for use in ECochG testing.

of the canal at a depth that may range from shallow (mid-canal) to deep (base of the TM). The magnitude of the response will be larger for deeper insertions, however, positioning the eartrode near the TM usually creates some discomfort to the patient and increases the risk of traumatizing the membrane.

More recently, in the mid-1980's, a disposable foam earplug electrode (top, Figure 5.3) was introduced. The earplug consisted of front and rear nonporous rubber discs separated by a reticulated foam center saturated with electrode gel. A plastic tube running through the center of the earplug served as a sound channel. The earplug was connected to a special head-band unit that

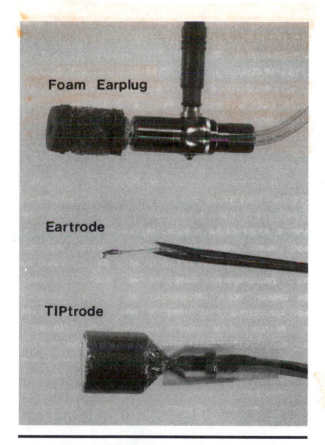

FIGURE 5.3. Commercially available ear canal electrodes. Foam earplug (top), Eartrode (middle), and TIPtrode (bottom). Reprinted by permission, Ruth et al. (1988), *The American Journal of Otology*, 9, 311.

coupled it to an electrode cable and stimulus transducer. The sound delivery tube of the transducer was continuous with the sound tube in the earplug.

The most recent version of the disposable ear plug electrode is shown in the bottom panel of Figure 5.3. This device is the "TIPtrode." The TIPtrode consists of compressible foam covered by a thin, pliable layer of gold foil. Like the foam earplugs, the TIPtrode can be coupled to an insert phone by flexible, silicon tubing.

Both of the earplug electrodes described above are designed to compress upon insertion into the ear canal, and expand to conform to the contour of the canal once in place. This allows for a large portion of the electrode surface to be in contact with the canal skin which helps to reduce electrical impedance. Depth of insertion, however, cannot extend beyond mid-canal.

Ferraro, Murphy, and Ruth (1986), compared ECochG recordings made with the eartrode (seated slightly beyond mid-canal), the foam earplug, and a gold-disc electrode on the mastoid process. Recordings from the ear canal using the eartrode and earplug were very similar and superior to those obtained from the mastoid process (that is, larger in amplitude, more sensitive and less distorted). The earplug, however, had considerably lower impedances, was easier and took less time to place, and was more stable after placement compared to the eartrode. Comparisons between the earplug and TIPtrode reveal similar performance between the two (Ruth, Lambert, and Ferraro, 1988; Bauch, 1988).

In attempts to optimize ET recordings, the TM has also been used as the primary recording site. In the early 1970's, Cullen, Ellis, Berlin, et al. (1972), utilized TM recordings to estimate hearing sensitivity in children. Their electrode consisted of silver wire attached to a saline-soaked wick, which rested on the unanesthetized TM. Although this provided good recordings, the discovery of the ABR at about this same time overshadowed subsequent development of TM-recorded ECochG for audiometric purposes. Several years later and as additional applications for ECochG have become apparent, using the TM as a recording site has received renewed attention.

Figure 5.4 displays an adaptation by Ferraro and Ferguson (1989) of a TM electrode described by

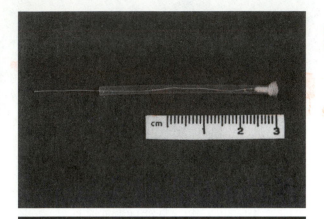

FIGURE 5.4. Adaptation of tympanic membrane electrode described by Stypulkowski and Staller (1987). (from Ferraro and Ferguson, 1989, pg.162)

Stypulkowski and Staller (1987). This device is constructed of small gauge silver wire attached to a small piece of soft, tightly packed foam sponge. The portion of the sponge attached to the wire and the wire itself are encased in flexible Silastic tubing. The portion of the sponge protruding from the tubing serves as the electrode tip. Prior to insertion, the tip is injected with gel using a small syringe. The electrode is inserted simply by running it along the ear canal until the tip rests against the tympanic membrane. Although this particular electrode was originally patented and designed for commercial distribution, it was unavailable in the marketplace at the time of this writing. The materials comprising the electrode, however, are relatively accessible and homemade adaptations of the device have been described (Ferraro, 1988b; Ferraro and Ferguson, 1989; Durrant and Ferraro, 1989; Ferraro and Durrant, 1989; Ruth et al., 1988; Ruth, 1990) as have other TM electrodes (Lily, Black, and Doucette, 1987).

Comparisons between TM and ear canal recordings reveal that TM responses are less distorted, more sensitive and much larger in amplitude than those measured from the canal (Stypulkowski and Staller, 1987; Ruth, Lambert, and Ferraro, 1988; Ferraro and Ferguson, 1989). Ruth and Lambert (1987) recorded simultaneously from the TM and cochlear promontory. Although the amplitudes of the TM responses were almost one magnitude

smaller than those from the promontory, overall waveform quality and identifiability of the waveform components were very similar (Ferraro et al.).

In a more recent study, Ferraro et al. (1991) obtained promontory and TM recordings to tone-bursts and clicks from a series of Meniere's patients. As expected, TM-recorded SPs were smaller in absolute amplitude than corresponding promontory SPs from the same patient, but the overall "pattern" of the responses leading to diagnostic interpretation was the same regardless of recording site.

Recording Parameters

Recording parameters for ECochG will vary according to which component or combination of components are to be measured. In general, these parameters are very similar to those employed for conventional ABR recording. As with the ABR, the most popular stimulus for noninvasive, clinical recordings has been the broad-band click, which produces the synchronization of neural firings necessary for a well-defined whole nerve AP. Unfortunately, the brevity of the click makes it considerably less than an ideal stimulus for studying the cochlear potentials whose durations are dependent on stimulus duration (i.e., the CM and SP). Nonetheless, the majority of recent literature regarding non-invasive ECochG reports the successful use of click stimuli for clinical purposes.

Separate ECochG responses to rarefaction (R) and condensation (C) clicks are displayed in Figure 5.1. The CM has a similar waveform and the same polarity as the stimulus whereas the polarities of the SP and AP are constant and independent of stimulus polarity. Thus, rarefaction clicks produce a CM 180 degrees out of phase with the CM produced by condensation clicks, while the SP and AP remain fixed. If these two waveforms are added together (R+C) the CM is canceled, leaving the SP and AP. If the waveforms are subtracted (R–C) the CM will be enhanced and the SP and AP canceled.

Cochlear Microphonic. As mentioned earlier, the CM has received considerably less attention than the SP and AP for clinical ECochG purposes. As can be

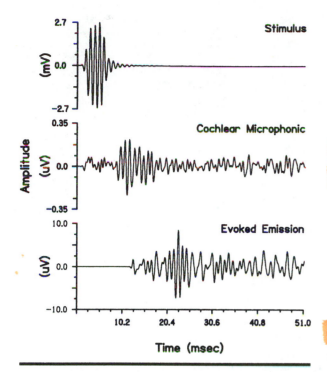

FIGURE 5.5. Data from Norton et al. (1989), displaying Cochlear Microphonic (CM) recorded from the tympanic membrane (middle) and an evoked otacoustic emission (EOAE) recorded from the ear canal (lower) to a 1000 Hz tone-pip stimulus (top). Onset of CM and EOAE delayed by using a long stimulus delivery tube.

seen in Figure 5.1, the CM to click stimuli is relatively small and can be especially difficult to differentiate in "noisy" recordings. When tone-bursts are used, it is often difficult to separate CM from stimulus artifact, since the two waveforms are almost identical. To help overcome this problem, one solution is to increase the stimulus travel time between the transducer and the ear, which will delay CM onset. This can be accomplished by using an insert-type transducer and a long stimulus delivery tube. Also, shielding the transducer with foil or other insulating material helps to reduce the amount of electromagnetic radiation picked up by the recording electrodes. Norton, Ferguson, and Mascher (1989), used a shielded insert phone coupled to a sound tube that introduced a 1 millisecond (ms)

delay between stimulus and CM onsets to record CM from the TM and acoustic emissions from the ear canal. Figure 5.5 displays an example of their responses. Both the CM and emission tracings represent signal-averaged waveforms to phase-locked tone-pips.

Summating Potential—Action Potential. The most popular clinical application of ECochG over the past decade has been in the diagnosis and assessment of Meniere's disease. Judgment of whether the ECochGm is positive or negative for this disorder is generally based on the relationship between the SP and AP. Thus, clinical recording parameters are selected to produce a complex waveform comprising both components. Table 5.2 illustrates the parameters suitable for doing this.

Electrode Array. As seen in Table 5.2, the primary (noninverted or voltage positive) recording site is the ear canal, TM or promontory. The reference or secondary site (inverted/voltage negative) can be the contralateral earlobe or mastoid or ear canal, with ground at the forehead or ipsilateral earlobe. When recorded with an ear canal/TM/promontory-positive configuration, the AP is displayed as a downward deflection. A vertex/forehead-to-ear canal/TM/promontory configuration could also be used, which is more analogous to conventional ABR recording. Using a vertex/forehead-positive array simply reverses the polarity of the AP to display it as an upward deflection.

An important aspect of recording ECochG with the eartrode or from the TM is that the impedance of the primary electrode generally is considerably higher than the impedances observed with conventional surface electrodes, or even the earplug electrodes described earlier. However, useful clinical recordings can be obtained in the face of very high impedances (i.e., greater than 20,000 ohms for extratympanic electrode locations and greater than 75,000 ohms for transtympanic electrode sites) (Ferraro, Best, and Arenberg, 1983; Ferraro, Murphy, and Ruth, 1986; Coats, 1986; Staller, 1986; Stypulkowski and Staller, 1987; Ruth and Lambert, 1989). The typical rules of thumb regarding impedance limits for suitable ABR recordings are generally not applicable when perform-

TABLE 5.2.   ECochG Recording Parameters

ELECTRODE ARRAY	
Primary	Ear Canal/ Tympanic Membrane/Promontory
Secondary	Contralateral Earlobe/Mastoid/Ear Canal
Ground	Forehead/Ipsilateral Earlobe
RESPONSE RECORDING	
Analysis Time	5–10 milliseconds
Amplification Factor	50,000X–100,000X (ET*)
	5,000X–25,000X (TT*)
Filter Bandpass	1 Hz–3,000 Hz
Repetitions	1,000–2,000 (ET)
	100–200 (TT)
STIMULI	
Type	Broad-band Clicks
Duration	100 Microsecond Electrical Pulse
Polarity	Alternating, Rarefaction and Condensation
Repetition Rate	5–11/second
Level	85–95 dB HL

*ET = Extratympanic; TT = Transtympanic

ing ECochG due to the more favorable signal to noise ratio associated with the latter.

Analysis Time.   ECochG components represent the first voltage changes to occur in the ear in response to sound. The analysis time or window for signal averaging must thus allow for a detailed visualization of physiological activity generated within 3–5 ms following stimulus onset. We generally extend our timebase to 10 ms, when we are interested in observing the ABR components.

Amplification Factor.   Preamplifier amplification factor for extratympanic recordings may be as high as 100,000X depending on the level of background electrical, myogenic, and electroencephalographic "noise". A factor of 50,000X is suitable under most conditions. The selection of the amplification factor also must take into account the sensitivity setting of the signal averager's analog-to-digital converter. Amplification/sensitivity settings will vary from laboratory to laboratory and even among different evoked potential units. The manipulation of this variable, however, is easily accomplished in most commercially available instruments, and the factors themselves are generally selected to provide for maximization of signal-to-noise ratio given the overall recording conditions. The amplification factor for transtympanic recordings is considerably less than that used for ET ECochG due to the proximity of the TT electrode to the response generators.

Filter Bandpass.   The bandpass of the preamplifier must be wide enough to allow for the amplification of a DC component (the SP) and AC component with a fundamental frequency of approximately 1000 Hz (the AP). This presents a technical problem in that the amplification systems generally employed to do this are primarily designed for AC signals. It should be recognized that the selection of a bandpass to allow for visualization of both the SP and AP together represents a compromise that introduces some degree of distortion to both components. That is, the DC component is actually frequency filtered, and the AC component may be distorted by the presence of low frequency noise in the extended bandpass. On the other hand, the SP to click stimuli is a transient response of very brief duration and should be tolerable of a certain degree of filtering. Durrant and Ferraro (1989), and Ferraro and Durrant (1989) examined the effects of high-pass filtering of the human ECochGm. Their results indicated that the low frequency cut-off could be raised as high as 30 Hz without producing significant alteration of the SP, AP, or the SP/AP amplitude ratio.

Number of Samples.   In general, the number of stimulus repetitions and summated responses needed to display a well-defined waveform will vary with recording conditions and the distance between the primary electrode and response generators. That is, it may be necessary to average more responses (2000) under noisy conditions, and, generally, fewer repetitions (100–1000) are needed as the recording site is moved medially from the ear canal to the promontory.

Stimuli.   As mentioned above, the broad-band click has been the most popular stimulus used for clinical ECochG. The duration of the electrical pulse from the stimulus generator is usually 100 microseconds (µs). It is important to recognize, however, that the stimulus transducer will modify the electrical input to produce an acoustical signal with a different waveform. Thus, the actual duration of the acoustic waveform is dependent on the characteristics of the transducer and is usually considerably longer than 100 µs. This aspect is very relevant to the recording of the SP since its duration is stimulus-dependent.

Stimulus polarity is an important factor for ECochG, just as it is for ABR. Delivering clicks in alternating polarity will help to inhibit the presence of stimulus artifact and CM in the resultant waveform. On the other hand, Margolis and Lily (1989) have presented evidence that separate responses to condensation (C) and rarefaction (R) clicks may provide useful clinical information. Separate R and C responses may also be added together "off-line" to reduce CM and stimulus artifact.

Stimulus repetition rate is generally selected to produce well-defined responses within a reasonable testing time. We have found click rates between 5–ll/s to be most suitable for this. Increasing repetition rate beyond 30/s may cause some adaptation of the AP. Rates on the order of 100/s will cause maximal depression of the AP, while leaving the SP relatively unaffected. Gibson, Moffat, and Ramsden (1977), and Coats (1981), have applied this feature clinically for better visualization of the SP. The success of doing this for improving the diagnostic power of ECochG has been mixed, in part because the AP contribution is not completely eliminated (Durrant, 1986; Harris and Dallos, 1989).

As shown in Table 5.2, we begin stimulus presentation at a level near or at the maximum output of the stimulus generator. The reason for this is that when the ECochG is performed to help diagnose Meniere's disease, the signal should be intense enough to evoke a well-defined SP-AP complex. When hearing loss in the higher frequencies (above 1000 Hz) is greater than 50 to 60 dB HL, it may not be possible to evoke well-defined components even at maximum levels of stimulation, particularly using ET recording techniques. This is especially true for the SP. However, it is important to remember that the primary generators of the recorded SP are the outer hair cells (OHCs) of the organ of Corti. The SP, in turn, may not be useful for diagnostic purposes if the degree and type of hearing loss suggest that the integrity of the OHCs is questionable.

Contralateral masking is unnecessary for ECochG because the magnitude of any response in the opposite ear to a reduced, bone-conducted signal will be too small to interfere with the response measured from the ear canal/TM/promontory of the stimulated side. It is also important to remember that the ECochG components are generated prior to cross-over of the auditory pathway.

Finally, as with other measures of auditory evoked potentials, we find it extremely useful to monitor background electrical "noise" simultaneously on a second oscilloscope during recording. This alerts us to potential problems associated with both procedural (e.g., electrode contact) and subjective (e.g., restless subject) variables.

CLINICAL APPLICATIONS

ECochG in Meniere's Disease/Endolymphatic Hydrops

Although much has been learned about Meniere's disease since its initial description in 1861, the true pathophysiology of the disorder continues to elude us. As a result, evaluation and treatment of Meniere's disease are often imprecise, lacking in specificity and efficacy. Patients presenting with the classic symptoms of unilateral sensorineural hearing loss, tinnitus and episodic vertigo usually do not present a diagnostic dilemma. However, a hallmark of Meniere's disease is its variable expression from one patient to the next or even within the same patient over time. The terms "Meniere's-like syndrome," "vestibular hydrops," and "cochlear hydrops" reflect this diagnostic uncertainty. As discussed earlier, several studies have shown that the ampitudes of the SP and AP recorded via ECochG may offer objective information to alleviate this uncertainty.

The absolute amplitudes of the SP and AP both show considerable variation across subjects. A more consistent amplitude feature within and across subjects is the SP-AP amplitude ratio (Eggermont, 1976). On the average an SP-AP ratio of 0.45 or greater is generally considered abnormal (i.e., SP amplitude $\geq 45\%$ of AP amplitude). However, Coats (1986) has noted that this ratio is not a simple linear relationship. In normal patients, for example, as the AP amplitude increases from 1 to 4 microvolts, the SP-to-AP ratio decreases from 0.4 to 0.25. Thus a single ratio differentiating normal from abnormal may be misleading. Using normative data, Coats (1986) has plotted SP amplitude against AP amplitude and derived a 95% confidence interval of normal values. He refers to this as the "AP-normalized SP amplitude plot," as shown in Figure 5.6.

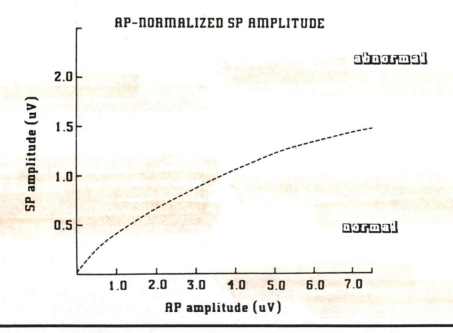

FIGURE 5.6.   Graph for plotting individual Summating Potential (SP) and Action Potential (AP) amplitudes (after Coats, 1986). Dashed line represents 95 percent confidence limit for normal SP-AP relationship.

The dashed line represents the 95% confidence interval for a normal SP-AP amplitude relationship. Therefore any values plotted above this line are considered to be abnormal (that is, the SP amplitude is larger than expected given the value of the AP amplitude).

Most investigators have found an abnormally enlarged SP-AP relationship in approximately two-thirds of the patients thought to have Meniere's disease (Gibson et al., 1977; Coats, 1981; Ferraro et al., 1983; Ferraro et al., 1985; Eggermont, 1986; Gibson and Prasher, 1983). The reason all such patients do not demonstrate this abnormality is unclear. It may relate to fluctuation in the extent of endolymphatic hydrops, to deterioration of outer hair cells in more advanced cases of Meniere's disease, to recording conditions or to other factors as yet unknown. It is apparent that the incidence of an abnormal SP-AP relationship is dependent on the extent of hearing loss and the presence of symptoms at the time of the recording. Patients with only a mild sensorineural hearing loss (less than 25 to 30 dB), for example, frequently have normal SP-AP relationships despite classic Meniere's symptoms. As degree of hearing loss increases (up to a moderate level), the incidence of recording an abnormal ECochG response is significantly greater. Ferraro et al. (1985) noted a very high correlation between an enlarged SP-to-AP ratio and the presence of symptoms at the time of the recording, especially aural fullness or pressure and some degree of hearing loss.

ECochG offers a valuable objective test for diagnosing Meniere's disease and endolymphatic hydrops, and this can be particularly helpful in atypical cases. There is indirect evidence that an enlarged SP reflects the pathologic condition of endolymphatic hydrops. The newer ear canal and tympanic membrane electrodes facilitate measurement of the ECochG response, permitting high quality recording with minimal professional time or patient discomfort. It is probable that the false-negative rate of the SP-to-AP ratio will be minimized if the recording is made while the patient is experiencing aural pressure or fullness and if the patient has at least a mild low frequency sensorineural hearing loss.

Using ECochG to evaluate the relationship of SP to AP in patients suspected of having Meniere's disease or endolymphatic hydrops requires a different set of pattern recognition skills from those we are accustomed to using in the evaluation of ABR recordings. With this application of ECochG, the primary measure is amplitude of the SP and the AP components of the response. Latency of these components has few, if any, diagnostic implications when applied to Meniere's patients. Figure 5.7 illustrates a normal and an abnormal SP-to-AP amplitude relationship. In this example, AP amplitude is measured from prestimulus baseline to the negative-most peak of the response. SP is measured from this same baseline to the "shoulder" preceding the onset of the AP. The SP is clearly seen in the normal response, but is less obvious in the abnormal recording. In the latter case, the SP may be distinguished from AP as a change in slope of the initial negative defection from baseline just prior to the peak of the AP.

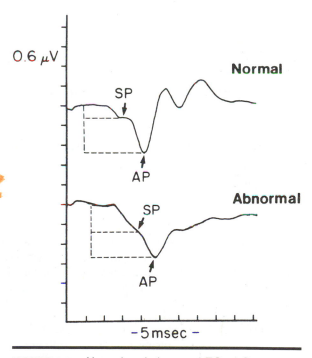

FIGURE 5.7.   Normal and abnormal ECochG waveforms obtained using a tympanic membrane electrode. SP, Summating Potential; AP, Action Potential.

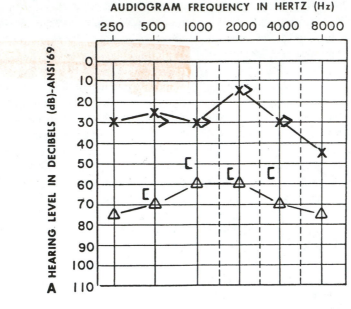

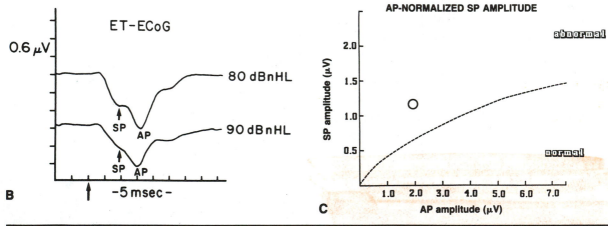

FIGURE 5.8. (A) Audiogram. (B) Click-evoked TM ECochG recordings. Solid arrow indicates stimulus onset. (C) Nonlinear SP-AP amplitude relationship. Circle represents the SP and AP amplitude values obtained from ECochGm.

The use of the ECochGm in the clinical evaluation of Meniere's disease is exemplified by the following case study:

A 51-year-old woman presented with a 12-year history of right-sided hearing loss, tinnitus, and dizziness. The dizziness was described by the patient as varying from an unsteadiness to a rare occasion of actual vertigo. She also described a "numbness" of her head that was present along with these other symptoms. During the last 6 months she experienced daily unsteadiness with no attacks of vertigo. The audiogram (Figure 5.8A) showed a mild sensorineural hearing loss in the left ear and a moderate to severe sensorineural hearing loss in the right ear. Because of facial paralysis and atypical vertigo an ABR and CT scan with contrast were accomplished. Neither test indicated retrocochlear involvement. The ECochG (Figure 5.8B) showed a clear abnormal SP-to-AP relationship which was consistent with a diagnosis of Meniere's disease. Medical therapy was unsuccessful and the patient eventually elected to undergo endolymphatic sac decompression. Post-operatively, her symptoms of dizziness and unsteadiness improved markedly.

Note that in this particular case the SP waveform was more clearly seen using an 80 dBnHL stimulus even though hearing thresholds in that ear were on the order of 60 to 70 dB HL for 1000–4000 Hz. We have observed this phenomenon in several patients. Thus, although we generally begin our testing at around 90 dB or higher, if responses are unclear at these higher levels, it is worthwhile to attempt an ECochG recording at levels 5 to 10 dB below.

Identification/Enhancement of wave I

Identification of waves I and V and the subsequent measurement of the I-V Interwave Interval (IWI) are essential to the use of the ABR for diagnostic purposes. However, when recorded from the scalp with surface electrodes, wave I is usually the first ABR component to disappear as stimulus intensity is lowered in normally hearing adults. In the presence of hearing loss, wave I may be immeasurable due to poor definition or total absence. Hyde and Blair (1981), for example, reported that only 42 per cent of 400 patients with sensory hearing loss had a reliable wave I. An even smaller percentage (38%) was found by Cashman and Rossman (1983), who also were unable to observe wave I in 86 percent of 35 patients with confirmed acoustic tumors. Thus, a key diagnostic feature of the ABR (i.e., the I-V IWI) may not be measurable in a large percentage of hearing-impaired patients.

Several studies have now shown that the use of ECochG in combination with conventional (i.e., scalp-recorded) ABR can improve the detectability and sensitivity of wave I (Coats, 1974, 1986; Durrant, 1977,

1986; Harder and Arlinger, 1981; Lang, Happonen, and Salmivalli, 1981; Walter and Blegvad, 1981; Yanz and Dodds, 1985; Ferraro, Murphy, and Ruth, 1986; Ruth, Mills, and Ferraro, 1988). Application of a combined ECochG-ABR technique is based on the assumption that the ECochG-N1 and wave I of the ABR are generated by the same neuronal population within the auditory nerve. This assumption is considered "safe" for clinical purposes even though slight differences between neural generators have been reported in the presence of low stimulus sensation levels (Coats and Martin, 1977; Coats, 1978).

Figure 5.9 illustrates the ABRs from a normally hearing subject recorded with forehead-ear canal (left panel) and forehead-mastoid (right panel) electrode configurations. The ear canal electrode used was the foam earplug device described previously in this chapter. As can be seen from this figure, wave I (or N1) is larger and observable at lower sensation levels for the

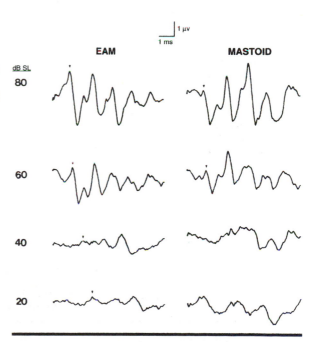

FIGURE 5.9. ABRs recorded using vertex-to-mastoid (left) and vertex-to-ear canal (i.e., combined ECochG-ABR) (right) configurations. (from Ruth et al., 1988, pg. 312)

forehead-ear canal configuration. In this same study, wave I was found to be approximately 65 percent larger when recorded from the ear canal versus the mastoid in a group of hearing impaired subjects. For comparative purposes, the abbreviation "N1" will subsequently be used with reference to the primary response recorded from the ear canal or TM, whereas the term "wave I" will refer to the initial component of the scalp-recorded ABR.

Ferraro and Ferguson (1989), combined TM-recorded ECochG with conventional ABR to compare the am-

plitudes and thresholds of N1, wave I and wave V in both normally and abnormally hearing subjects. For normal subjects, the amplitude of N1 from the TM was approximately one magnitude larger than either wave I or wave V amplitudes. In addition, there was no significant difference between N1 and wave V thresholds, whereas wave I threshold, by comparison, was elevated. In their hearing impaired group, N1 was always recordable from the TM when hearing reserve was sufficient to allow for a definable wave V in the ABR. Figure 5.10 from this study displays a representative

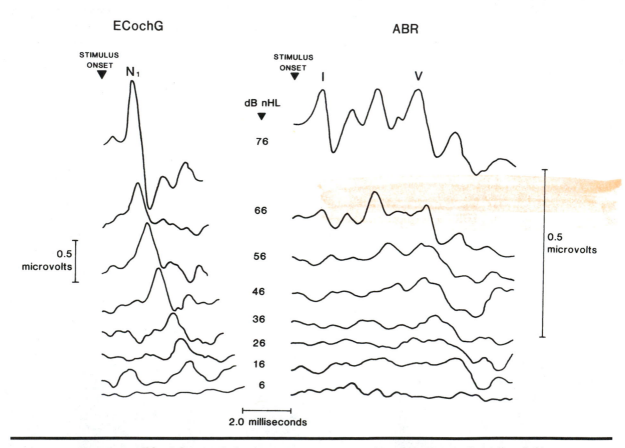

FIGURE 5.10.   ECochG recorded using a vertex-to-tympanic membrane configuration (left) and conventional vertex-to-mastoid ABRs (right) from a normally-hearing subject. Note the disparity between ECochG and ABR amplitude scales, showing how much larger the TM recordings were than their surface-recorded counterpart. Also, note that N1 and wave V have the same threshold, whereas wave I threshold (surface-recorded) is elevated by comparison (from Ferraro and Ferguson, 1989, pg. 163).

example of the tracings obtained from a normally hearing subject. The disparity between amplitude scales illustrates how much larger TM recordings were in comparison to scalp-recorded ABRs. In addition, N1 was identifiable at hearing levels below wave I threshold, and the thresholds of N1 and wave V were identical. Figure 5.11 compares the mean amplitudes of the TM-recorded N1 as a function of stimulus SL for their group of normally hearing subjects, with the amplitude-intensity functions for wave I observed by Ruth, Mills, and Ferraro (1988) using forehead-ear canal and forehead-mastoid electrode configurations. As shown in this figure, all three functions are virtually parallel with the largest values across all intensities observed for the TM recordings.

An important application of the above findings is that TM-recorded ECochG may be useful in the identification of N1 and the N1-V IWI in hearing-impaired subjects whose conventionally recorded ABRs do not contain an identifiable or reliable wave I. An example of this is seen in Figure 5.12. These data were obtained from a 56-year-old hearing-impaired patient whose pure-tone audiogram is illustrated on the righthand side of the figure. The audiogram revealed a mild, low-frequency hearing loss progressing to profound in the higher frequencies. Conventional, scalp-recorded ABR tracings to maximum stimulation (95 dB nHL) are shown in the upper left. Wave V was the only identifiable component observed using a vertex-earlobe electrode configuration. The lower tracings were recorded with a vertex-TM configuration using the TM electrode described previously in this chapter. The combined ECochG-ABR approach produced a waveform containing N1 and wave V, which allowed for measurement of the N1-V IWI.

INTRAOPERATIVE MONITORING

Several surgical operations within the posterior fossa place certain structures of the auditory system and their function at risk for permanent damage or impairment. The typical sources of injury include but are not limited to the following: 1) retraction of cerebellum, 2) compromise of blood supply to the auditory nerve and cochlea, and 3) excessive manipulation of the auditory nerve during tumor dissection. Intraoperative measurement of various electrophysiologic responses to sound has been increasingly utilized to assess the functional integrity of the peripheral and brainstem auditory pathway directly during the course of an operation so as to avert damage to such structures. The ABR, in particular has received widespread acceptance as a monitoring tool (see Chapter 18). Intraoperative measurements are also made using both ET and TT ECochG, as well as direct recording of the auditory nerve compound action potential.

A number of reports on intraoperative monitoring with auditory evoked potentials began appearing in the literature in the early to mid-1980s (Raudzens and Shetter, 1982; Grundy, Jannetta, Procopio, et al., 1982; Levine, Ojemann, Montgomery, et al., 1984; Møller and Jannetta, 1984; Silverstein, McDaniel, Wazen, et al., 1985; Ruth, Mills, and Jane, 1987). Since that time, the use of ABR, ECochG, and direct auditory nerve recordings has steadily increased. Virtually all major

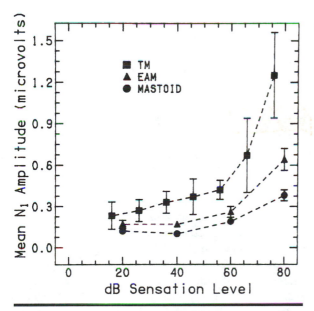

FIGURE 5.11. Normal N1 (wave I) amplitudes as a function of stimulus sensation level for vertex-to-TM (■), forehead-to-ear canal (▲), and forehead-to-mastoid (●) electrode configurations. Vertical lines represent +1 SE (from Ferraro and Ferguson, 1989, pg. 163).

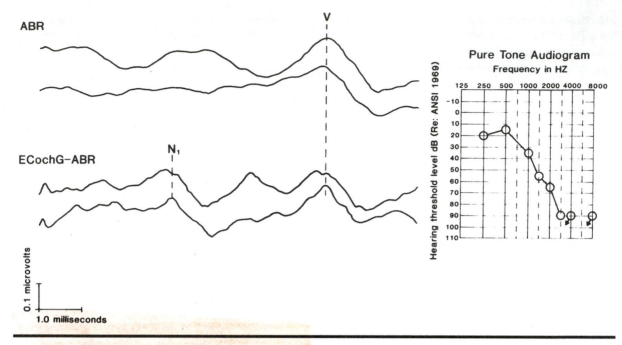

FIGURE 5.12.   ABR recorded conventionally using vertex-to-mastoid electrode configuration (top tracings) and ECochG-ABR tracings recorded using a vertex-to-tympanic membrane configuration (lower tracings) from a 56-year-old, hearing-impaired patient. Patient's pure-tone audiogram is shown to the right of the tracings. Wave I is absent in the conventional ABR, but N1 is observed in the ECochG-ABR tracings (from Ferraro and Ferguson, 1989, pg. 165).

medical centers in the country incorporate some form of intraoperative monitoring of auditory structures when preservation of residual hearing is considered both worthwhile and possible. As more experience with intraoperative monitoring has been gained, it has become apparent that a combination of recording techniques and responses sampled from various levels of the auditory system will optimize early detection of injury (Lambert and Ruth, 1988). For example, the ABR is known to reflect synchronous neural activity from the earliest potentials of the acoustic nerve through the brainstem auditory pathways. However, greater resolution of the earliest potentials can be achieved only with a more direct method of measurement, such as ECochG. ECochG naturally results in an improved signal-to-noise ratio (due to closer proximity to the generator of the response) and consequently a more optimal recording of the cochlear and auditory

nerve output. As a result of the improved signal-to-noise ratio, fewer averages are necessary to achieve a readable tracing, and thus more immediate feedback is available to the surgeon. A comparison of the time efficiency of the available AEP recording techniques is shown in Table 5.3. Note that whereas it may require as much as one to one-and-a-half minutes to adequately resolve a surface recorded ABR, it takes only a few seconds to measure a TT-ECochG recording.

It must be borne in mind that these various AEP measures reflect different aspects of the auditory system. For example, the ECochGm can provide rapid information on the status of the cochlea. However, it is not immediately sensitive to auditory nerve injury in the cerebellar pontine angle. Animal studies have shown that cessation of cochlear blood flow will alter the AP within 10 to 15 seconds and completely abolish the response within 30 to 45 seconds (Perlman, Kimura, and Fernandez, 1959).

TABLE 5.3.   Intraoperative Recording Options

	Amplitude (μV)	Number of Sweeps	Time (sec) @ (20/sec)
Surface Recorded ABR	0.1–0.5	500–1500	25–75
ET-ECochG	0.3–1.0	250–1200	12–60
TM-ECochG	2.0–6.0	100–500	5–25
TT-ECochG	10.0–20.0	40–100	2–5
Direct 8th nerve CAP	25.0–30.0	1	<1

Recovery of the AP is possible if vascular flow is re-established within eight minutes. Injury to the auditory nerve in the cerebellar pontine angle does not immediately change the ECochG response. Sectioning the auditory nerve, for example, does not abolish the AP until three or more days later, provided that the labyrinthine artery has been preserved (Ruben, Hudson, and Chiong, 1963). Thus, the use of the ECochGm alone during neuro-otologic surgery provides immediate information only on the direct or indirect (e.g., vascular compromise) labyrinthine injury and not on proximal auditory nerve integrity. Combination of ABR and ECochG allows for differentiation of neural from end organ damage and thus allows the surgeon to understand the actual source of injury better should it occur. Figure 5.13 shows a recording of the TT-ECochG (Figure 5.13A) and surface-derived ABR (Figure 5.13B) obtained from a patient undergoing removal of an acoustic tumor. Based on presurgical workup it was decided that this patient had sufficient residual hearing ability to warrant a hearing preservation procedure. The ABR exhibits a clear wave V but no apparent wave I, whereas in the case of the TT-ECochG the opposite is true. By simultaneous acquisition of both types of AEPs it is possible to continually observe changes to the peripheral and brainstem portions of the auditory pathway.

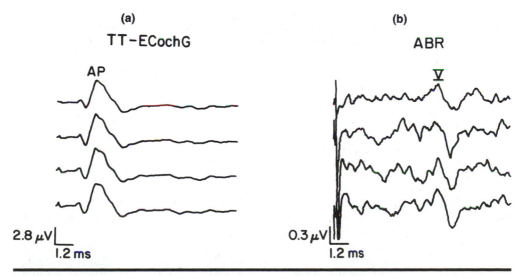

FIGURE 5.13.   (A) TT-ECochG and (B) surface-recorded ABR obtained during surgical removal of acoustic tumor.

REFERENCES

American Speech-Language-Hearing Association (1988). The short latency auditory evoked potentials: A tutorial paper by the Working Group on Auditory Evoked Potential Measurements of the Committee on Audiologic Evaluation.

Coats, A.C. (1981). The summating potential and Meniere's disease. *Archives of Otolaryngology, 107*, 199–208.

Coats, A.C. (1986). Electrocochleography: Recording technique and clinical applications. *Seminars in Hearing, 7*, 247–266.

Coats, A.C. and Martin, J.L. (1977). Human auditory nerve action potentials and brainstem evoked responses: Effects of audiogram shape and lesion location. *Archives of Otolaryngology, 103*, 605–622.

Cullen, J.K., Ellis, M.S., Berlin, C.I., and Lousteau, R.J. (1972). Human acoustic nerve action potential recordings from the tympanic membrane without anesthesia. *Acta Otolaryngologica, 74*, 15–22.

Dallos, P. (1973). *The auditory periphery: Biophysics and physiology.* New York: Academic Press.

Dallos, P., Schoeny, Z.G., Cheatham, M.A. (1972). Cochlear summating potentials: Descriptive aspects. *Acta Otolaryngologica, 301* (supplement), 1–46.

Davis, H., Fernandez, C., and McAuliffe, D.R. (1950). The excitatory process in the cochlea. *Proceedings of the National Academy of Science, 36*, 580–587.

Davis, H. (1968). Mechanisms of the inner ear. *Annals of Otology, Rhinology and Laryngology, 77*, 644–656.

Davis, H. (1968). Potentials and brainstem evoked responses: Latency-intensity functions in detection of cochlear and retrocochlear pathology. *Archives of Otolaryngology, 104*, 709–717.

Durrant, J.D. (1977). Study of a combined noninvasive ECochG and BSER recording technique. *Journal of the Acoustical Society of America, 62*, S87.

Durrant, J.D. (1986). Observations on combined noninvasive electrocochleography and auditory brainstem response recording. *Seminars in Hearing, 7*, 289–305.

Durrant, J.D. and Dallos, P. (1972). Influence of direct-current polarization of the cochlear partition on the summating potential. *Journal of the Acoustical Society of America, 52*, 542–552.

Durrant, J.D. and Dallos, P. (1974). Modification of DIF summating potential components by stimulus biasing. *Journal of the Acoustical Society of America, 56*, 562–568.

Durrant, J.D. and Ferraro, J.A. (1989). Analog model of human click-elicited SP and effects of high-pass filtering. *Program of the XI Biennial Symposium of the International Electric Response Audiometry Study Group, Tokyo, Japan, 68* (A).

Durrant, J.D. and Gans, D. (1977). Biasing of the summating potentials. *Acta Otolaryngologica, 80*, 13–18.

Elberling, C. and Salomon, G. (1973). Cochlear microphonics recorded from the ear canal in man. *Acta Otolaryngologica, 75*, 489–495.

Engebretson, A.M. and Eldridge, D.H. (1968). Model for the nonlinear characteristics of cochlear potentials. *Journal of the Acoustical Society of America, 44*, 548–554.

Ferraro, J.A. (1988). Electrocochleography. In Owen, J.H., and Donohoe, C.D. (eds.). *Clinical atlas of auditory evoked potentials.* Orlando, FL: Grune & Stratton.

Ferraro, J.A. (1988). Electrocochleographic recordings from the tympanic membrane: Technique and applications. *ASHA, 30*, 195 (A).

Ferraro, J.A., Arenberg, I.K., and Hassanein, R.S. (1985). Electrocochleography and symptoms of inner ear dysfunction. *Archives of Otolaryngology, 111*, 71–74.

Ferraro, J.A., Best, L.G., and Arenberg, I.K. (1983). The use of electrocochleography in the diagnosis, assessment and monitoring of endolymphatic hydrops. *Otolaryngologic Clinics of North America, 16*, 69–82.

Ferraro, J.A. and Durrant, J.D.(1989). Effects of high–pass filtering on the human electrocochleogram. *ASHA, 31*, 183 (A).

Ferraro, J.A. and Ferguson, R. (1989). Tympanic ECochG and conventional ABR: A combined approach for the identification of wave I and the I-V interwave interval. *Ear and Hearing, 10*, 161–166.

Ferraro, J.A., Murphy, G.B., and Ruth, R.A. (1986). A comparative study of primary electrodes used in extratympanic electrocochleography. *Seminars in Hearing, 7*, 279–287.

Ferraro, J.A., Thedinger, B., Mediavilla, S., and Blackwell, W. (1991). Human SP to tone-bursts: Comparison between tympanic membrane and promontory recordings. *IERASG meeting.*

Fromm, B., Bylen, C.O., and Zotterman, Y. (1935). Studies in the mechanisms of Wever and Bray effect. *Acta Otolaryngologica, 22*, 477–483.

Gerhardt, H. J., Wagner, H., and Werbs, M. (1985). Electrocochleography (ECochG) and brainstem evoked response recordings (BSER) in the diagnosis of acoustic neuromas. *Acta Otolaryngologica, 99*, 384–386.

Gibson, W.P.R. (1978). *Essentials of electric response audiometry.* New York: Churchill and Livingstone.

Gibson, W.P.R. and Beagley, M.A. (1976). Transtympanic electrocochleography in the investigation of retrocochlear disorders. *Revue Laryngology, 97 (suppl)*, 507–516.

Gibson, W.P.R., Moffat, D.A., and Ramsden, R.T. (1977). Clinical electrocochleography in the diagnosis and management of Meniere's disorder. *Audiology, 16*, 389–401.

Goin, D.W., Staller, S.J., Asher, D.L., and Mischke, R.E. (1982). Summating potential in Meniere's disease. *Laryngoscope, 92*, 1381–1389.

Grundy, B., Jannetta, P., Procopio, Lina, A., Boston, J. and Doyle (1982). Intraoperative monitoring of brainstem auditory evoked potentials. *Journal of Neurosurgery, 57*, 674–681.

Gulick, W.L., Gescheider, G.A., and Frisina, R.D. (1989). *Hearing: Physiological acoustics, neural coding, and psychoacoustics*. New York: Oxford University Press.

Harris, D.M. and Dallos, P. (1979). Forward masking of auditory nerve fiber responses. *Journal of Neurophysiology, 42*, 1083–1107.

Harder, H. and Arlinger, S. (1981). Ear canal compared to mastoid electrode placement in BRA. *Scandinavian Audiology, 13 (suppl)*, 55–57.

Hyde, M.L. and Blair, R.L. (1981). The auditory brainstem response in neuro-otology: Perspectives and problems. *Journal of Otolaryngology, 10*, 117–125.

Kiang, N.S. (1965). Discharge patterns of single nerve fibers in the cat's auditory nerve. *Research monograph 35*. Cambridge, MA: MIT Press.

Kitahara, M., Takeda, T., and Yazama, T. (1981). Electrocochleography in the diagnosis of Meniere's disease. In Volsteen, K.H. (Ed.). *Meniere's disease, pathogenesis, diagnosis and treatment*. New York: Thieme-Stratton.

Kumagami, H., Nishida, H., Masaaki, B. (1982). Electrocochleographic study of Meniere's disease. *Archives of Otology, 108*, 284–288.

Lambert, P. and Ruth, R. (1988). Simultaneous recording of noninvasive ECoG and ABR for use in intraoperative monitoring. *Otolaryngology—Head Neck Surgery, 98*, 575–580.

Levine, R., Ojemann, R., Montgomery, W., and McGaffigan, P. (1984). Monitoring of brainstem auditory evoked potentials during acoustic neuroma surgery: Insights into the mechanism of hearing loss. *Annals of Otology, Rhinology, and Laryngology, 93*, 116–123.

Lang, A., Happonen, J., and Salmivalli, A. (1981). An improved technique for the noninvasive recording of auditory brain-stem responses with a specially constructed meatal electrode. *Scandinavian Audiology, 13 (suppl)*, 59–62.

Lempert, J., Meltzer, P.E., Wever, E.G., and Lawrence, M. (1950). The cochleogram and its clinical applications: Concluding observations. *Archives of Otolaryngology, 51*, 307–311.

Lempert, J., Wever, E.G., and Lawrence, M. (1947). The cochleogram and its clinical applications: a preliminary report. *Archives of Otolaryngology, 45*, 61–67.

Lilly, D.J., Black, F.O., and Doucette, S.M. (1987). A comparison of three noninvasive systems for electrocochleography. *ASHA, 29*, 166(A).

Margolis, R.H. and Lilly, D.J.. (1989). Extratympanic electrocochleography: Stimulus considerations. *ASHA, 31*, 183(A).

Møller, A.R. and Jannetta, P.J. (1983). Monitoring auditory functions during cranial nerve microvascular decompression operations by direct monitoring from the eight nerve. *Journal of Neurosurgery, 59*, 493–499.

Møller, A. and Jannetta, P. (1984). Monitoring auditory nerve potentials during operations in the cerebellopontine angle. *Otolaryngology—Head and Neck Surgery, 92*, 434–439.

Moriuchi, H. and Kumagami, H. (1979). Changes of AP, SP and CM in experimental endolymphatic hydrops. *Audiology, 22*, 258–260.

Morrison, A.W., Moffat, D.A., and O'Connor, A.F. (1980). Clinical usefulness of electrocochleography in Meniere's disease: An analysis of dehydrating agents. *Otolaryngologic Clinics of North America, 11*, 703–721.

Norton, S.J., Ferguson, R., and Mascher, K. (1989). Evoked otacoustic emissions and extratympanic cochlear microphonics recorded from human ears. *Abstracts of the Twelfth Midwinter Research Meeting of the Association for Research in Otolaryngology, 227(A)*.

Perlman, M.B. and Case, T.J. (1941). Electrical phenomena of the cochlea in man. *Archives of Otolaryngology, 34*, 710–718.

Perlman, H., Kimura, R., and Fernandez, C. (1959). Experiments on temporary obstruction of the internal auditory artery. *Laryngoscope, 69*, 591–613.

Raudzens, P. and Shetter, A. (1982). Intraoperative monitoring of brainstem auditory evoked potentials. *Journal of Neurosurgery, 57*, 341–348.

Ruben, R., Hudson, W., and Chiong, A. (1963). Anatomical and physiological effects of chronic section of the eighth nerve in cat. *Acta Otolaryngologica, 55*, 473–484.

Ruben, R.J., Sekula, J., and Bordley, J.E. (1960) Human cochlear responses to sound stimuli. *Annals of Otorhinolaryngology, 69*, 459–476.

Ruth, R.A. (1990). Trends in electrocochleography. *Journal of the American Academy of Audiology, 1*, 134–137.

Ruth, R.A. and Lambert, P. (1989). Comparison of tympanic membrane to promontory electrode recordings of electrocochleographic responses in Meniere's disease. *Otolaryngology—Head and Neck Surgery, 100*, 546–552.

Ruth, R.A., Lambert P., and Ferraro, J.A. (1988). Electrocochleography: methods and clinical applications. *American Journal of Otology, 9*, 1–11.

Ruth, R.A. and Lambert, P. (1991). *Auditory evoked potentials*. Otolaryngology Clinics of North America, W.B. Saunders Company, Philadelphia.

Ruth, R.A., Mills, J., and Ferraro, J.A. (1988). Use of disposable ear canal electrodes in auditory brainstem response testing. *American Journal of Otology, 9*, 310–315.

Ruth, R.A., Mills, J., and Jane, J. (1986). Intraoperative monitoring of electrocochleographic and auditory brainstem responses. *Seminars in Hearing, 7*, 307–327.

Schmidt, P., Eggermont, J., and Odenthal, D. (1974). Study of Meniere's disease by electrocochleography. *Acta Otolaryngologica, 316 (suppl)*, 75–84.

Schwartz, D.M., Pratt, R.E., and Costello, J.A. (1989). Auditory brainstem responses in pre-term infants: Evidence of peripheral maturity. *Ear and Hearing, 10*, 14–22.

Silverstein, H., McDaniel, A., Wazen, J., and Norrell, H. (1984). Retrolabyrinthine vestibular neurectomy with simultaneous monitoring of eighth nerve and brain stem auditory evoked potentials. *Otolaryngology—Head and Neck Surgery, 93*, 736–742.

Silverstein, H., Norrell, H., and Hyman, S.M. (1984). Simultaneous use of CO_2 laser with continuous monitoring of eighth cranial nerve action potentials during acoustic neuroma surgery. *Otolaryngology—Head and Neck Surgery, 92*, 80–84.

Silverstein, H., Wazen, J., Norrell, H., and Hyman, S. (1984). Retrolabrynthine vestibular neurectomy with simultaneous monitoring of eighth nerve action potentials and electrocochleography. *American Journal of Otology, 5*, 552–555.

Staller, S. (1986). Electrocochleography in the diagnosis and management of Meniere's disease. *Seminars in Hearing, 7*, 267–277.

Stypulkowski, P.H. and Staller, S.J. (1987). Clinical evaluation of a new ECoG recording electrode. *Ear and Hearing, 8*, 304–310.

Tasaki, I., Davis, H., and Eldredge, D.H. (1954). Exploration of cochlear potentials in guinea pig with a microelectrode. *Journal of the Acoustical Society of America, 26*, 765–773.

Walter, B. and Blevgad, B. (1981). Identification of wave I by means of an atraumatic ear canal electrode. *Scandinavian Audiology, 13 (suppl)*, 63–64.

Wever, E.G. and Bray, C. (1930). Action currents in the auditory nerve in response to acoustic stimulation. *Proceedings of the National Academy of Science, 16*, 344–350.

Whitfield, I.C. and Ross, H.F. (1965). Cochlear microphonic and summating potentials and the outputs of individual hair cell generators. *Journal of the Acoustical Society of America, 38*, 126–131.

Yanz, J.L. and Dodds, H. (1985). An ear-canal electrode for the measurement of the human auditory brainstem response. *Ear and Hearing, 6*, 98–104.

CHAPTER 6

THE NORMAL AUDITORY BRAINSTEM RESPONSE AND ITS VARIANTS

DANIEL M. SCHWARTZ
MICHELE D. MORRIS
JOHN T. JACOBSON

Two decades have now passed since the seminal paper by Jewett, Romano, and Williston (1970) describing the characteristics and possible neural generators of the auditory brainstem response (ABR). During this time, the expansion of information on the clinical utility of the ABR has progressed at a rate that would challenge even the most ardent student of contemporary neurophysiology. Following publication of *The Auditory Brainstem Response* (Jacobson, 1985), we have come to appreciate better not only the pathologic correlates of the ABR, but also the normative aspects and statistical properties that underlie this neuroelectric response. The plethora of published data, as well as the increased neurodiagnostic and audiologic demand for this test, has enabled us to estimate the distribution of ABR peak latency and amplitude more precisely, both in normal and abnormal neurologic and otologic patients. Indeed, much that we have learned has reshaped our thinking about the establishment of individual laboratory data, defining the upper limits of normal and the influence of discrete parameters (e.g., age, gender, polarity, etc.).

This chapter on the normative aspects of the ABR reflects a modified philosophy relative to that which was underscored in *The Auditory Brainstem Response* (Schwartz and Berry, 1985). The development of computerized databases has enabled us to manage discrete parameters more efficiently, thus promoting more definitive statistical and/or clinical comparisons of various ABR measures between groups (e.g., male-female, young-old, normal-abnormal). While portions of this chapter may not differ significantly from its earlier counterpart, the majority of it is refocused toward these new perspectives.

CHARACTERISTICS OF THE NORMAL ABR

The exemplar ABR recorded from a normal neurologic and oto-audiologic adult is illustrated in Figure 6.1. The response consists of a sequential series of five to seven peaks occurring within approximately 7.0 milliseconds (ms) (depending on transducer type) following stimulus onset, when elicited by moderately-high intensity (110 dB peak sound pressure level, pSPL) clicks presented at a relatively slow repetition rate (e.g., <20/s). In clinical practice, the focus is on peaks I–V in general and I, III, and V in particular.

Waveform nomenclature is most commonly derived by labeling each peak with a Roman numeral (e.g., I–V) as advocated originally by Jewett et al. (1970); however, some Europeans continue to use sequential Arabic numerals (1–5) preceded by a polarity designate (N=negative; P=positive) as introduced by Sohmer and Feinmesser (1967). In neurophysiology (e.g., electroencephalography and electromyography) the convention is to plot negativity *up* relative to the neural activation recorded under the *active* electrode. Unfortunately, there is no such unified standard in evoked potential work, particularly in reporting ABR waveforms. (Although not universal, the general trend is to plot negativity *up* both for somatosensory and visual cortical evoked responses). Part of the problem

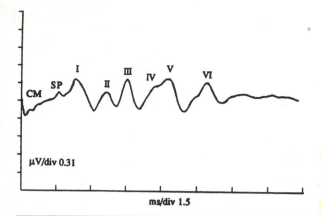

FIGURE 6.1. Auditory brainstem response from a neurotologic normal adult. Vertex-positive is *up* in this and all following figures. CM=cochlear microphonic, SP=summating potential.

with recording sensory evoked potentials is that both electrodes actually are *active*, but at different times. In other words, the ipsilateral ear electrode (A_i) that often is designated an *indifferent reference* when recording the ABR is not, in reality, unaffected by the underlying neural tissue. The contribution from each electrode depends primarily on the distance from and orientation to the neural generator. Hence, it is necessary to decide *a priori* which electrode is to be *active* and whether the deflection will be either in the negative or positive direction relative to how the electrodes are connected to the inputs of the differential amplifier. (See Hyde, Chapter 3, for a more detailed discussion on differential amplification). In North America, the prevailing polarity convention is to plot vertex-positivity (C_z+) relative to the A_i electrode as an upward deflection. Unlike differential amplifiers used in EEG instruments, there is not a unified standard for evoked potential systems. Many Canadians and most Europeans, however, prefer to maintain the neurophysiology standard as C_z+ down. This quagmire of nomenclature continues to hamper the simple exchange of clinical and research information and can be rather frustrating even to the most experienced clinical neurophysiologist. When faced with an ABR waveform of opposite

polarity from that which the reader is accustomed to, simply turn the printout upside down and backward while holding it up to a light source. This has the same effect as reversing the two inputs at the differential amplifier. Throughout this chapter, we shall adhere to the vertex-positive *up* convention.

ABR MEASUREMENT PARAMETERS

Diagnostic inferences from the ABR typically are derived by comparing wave latencies (conduction time) and amplitudes (voltage) calculated from an individual patient's ABR to those of laboratory and instrumentation specific average normal reference values having a known variance. An additional parameter that can be used in neurodiagnostics is wave shape, dispersion, or morphology. Unlike latency and amplitude measures which lend themselves to quantitative analysis, interpretation of the ABR based on response clarity is entirely subjective and at best, a qualitative descriptor.

Peak Latency

The amount of time elapsed in ms between the onset of the acoustic stimulus and the peak (positive or negative) of the averaged waveform defines the absolute latency of that peak and is illustrated in Figure 6.2. At present, no standard exists as to where exactly on the waveform latency should be measured. Some clinicians favor the apex of the waveform while others prefer a point representing the beginning of the downslope.

Our clinical bias is to calculate peak latency identification from the apex for several reasons. First, it is more consistent with that used in evoked potential recordings from other sensory systems (i.e., somatosensory and visual). In both of the latter cases, latency is calculated from the absolute peak of the primary waveform. Previous experience estimating wave latency from the downslope led us to the conclusion that this technique was much less consistent both within and between patients. Small differences in wave shape between ears, for example, resulted in much greater intra-subject variability with the downslope versus the apex procedure. Review of common variants to normal ABR morphology illustrates that identifying a *stan-*

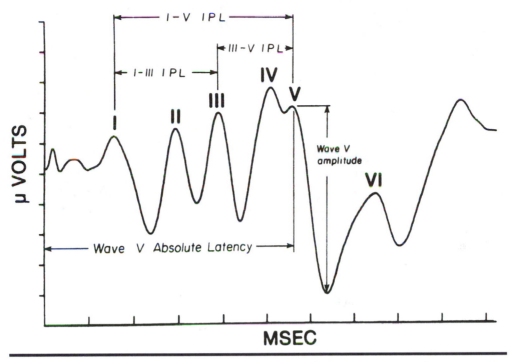

FIGURE 6.2. Method for labeling (Roman numerals) and calculating absolute and interpeak latency and peak-to-trough amplitude.

dard point on the downslope is much more difficult and less consistent than identifying the same at the apex. Alterations in signal-to-noise ratio (SNR) between recording trials can result in spurious peaks on the descending limb of the waveform that may be selected inadvertently as the point of downslope. At times a given peak, usually waves I and III, can be characterized by multiple components; that is, its shape is bifid as depicted in Figure 6.3. In such cases, we estimate latency of wave I from the second, typically more stable component, whereas that for wave III is determined by forming an isosceles triangle with the two equal sides emanating from each of the two peaks of the waveform, respectively. A vertical line is then drawn to intersect the midpoint. If latency is calculated from the downslope of this bifid waveform, it is possible to create temporal prolongation and thus, a Type I (false-positive) error since the point of estimation is on the descending flank of the second peak.

In clinical diagnostics, measurement of interpeak latency (IPL) is preferred to that of absolute latency because it is much less variable and more independent of subject, stimulus, and recording parameters; therefore, IPL is better able to distinguish peripheral from central pathology. Interpeak latency represents the time difference (Δ_t) between individual peaks of a given waveform as schematized in Figure 6.2, and reflects the conduction time between neural structures. In ABR practice, the I–III IPL depicts conduction time from the intracanalicular segment of the acoustic nerve across the subarachnoid space, through the ventral cochlear nucleus to the caudal pontine tegmentum (lateral pons). The III–V IPL, on the other hand, reflects conduction between the upper pons and low midbrain. The I–V IPL defines total conduction time between the acoustic nerve and low midbrain and is considered the ABR bench mark in neurodiagnostics (Nuwer, 1986; Chiappa, 1990; Schwartz and Morris 1991).

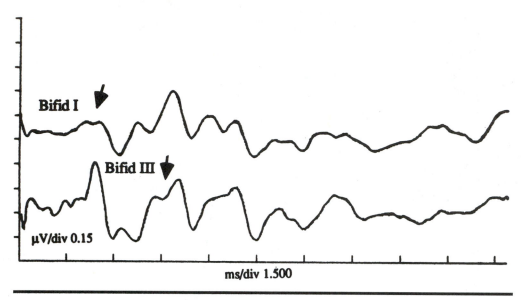

FIGURE 6.3. Illustrative example of auditory brainstem response showing bifid waves I (top) and III (bottom).

Peak Amplitude

The amplitude of an evoked potential can be measured in microvolts (μV) by four methods: 1) peak amplitude, 2) peak-to-peak amplitude, 3) amplitude ratio, and 4) amplitude difference. The first two can be considered absolute measures, whereas the others are more relative.

Peak amplitude represents the voltage difference, in μV, between a stable reference baseline level (0 μV) and the peak of the wave. The shortcoming of this approach to voltage computation is that all too often, a stable, zero voltage baseline is unavailable due to variations in background electrical activity (*noise*).

Peak-to-peak amplitude (Figure 6.2, wave V) does not depend on a zero voltage baseline and is thus the commonly preferred method for amplitude measurement. Voltage is calculated between the peak of one polarity and the immediately adjacent peak of the opposite polarity. For a C_z+ *up* deflection, amplitude would be measured from the peak of the waveform to the following trough. The problem with peak-to-peak amplitude is that successive peaks may vary independently of each other or a low amplitude peak may precede or follow one of equal or greater amplitude having the same polarity without returning to baseline as exemplified by a bifid wave shape.

The major limitation of either absolute amplitude measure is the inherent variability seen within and between normal neurologic and oto-audiologic patients. Most of the intrapatient variability is attributed to alterations in SNR between test runs. While the same holds true for interpatient amplitude variability, discrete factors such as click polarity and age have also been shown to influence peak voltage (Schwartz et al., 1989; Schwartz et al., 1990). Because the ability to detect neuropathology decreases with increasing dispersion among normal neurologic patients, neither baseline-to-peak nor peak-to-peak voltage is considered as useful in neurodiagnostics as measures of peak latency.

To circumvent the non-Gaussian (bell-shaped) distribution of normal absolute amplitude values, most clinicians compute relative amplitude expressed either as a ratio of the absolute amplitudes of any two peaks in the ipsilateral waveform or as the percent interside (e.g., interaural) amplitude difference (ΔμV) of like waves. In the former case, the derived value is compared to a normal reference whereas in the latter, the patient serves as his/her own control since the comparison is between like measures on opposites sides. By far the most popular yardstick of relative amplitude in ABR work is the V/I ratio which is calculated by dividing the absolute amplitude of wave V by that of wave I.

Wave Morphology

Wave morphology or dispersion refers to the clarity, resolution, and definition of the ABR either in part or overall. It is influenced by factors such as the SNR, stimulus intensity, recording montage, stimulus polarity, normal anatomical variants, high frequency sensory hearing loss, and neuropathology. Figure 6.4 shows a series of morphologic variations that are commonly observed in the classical normal ABR when the response is recorded from a single recording channel $(C_z + - A_i^-)$ using a narrow filter bandpass (e.g., 100–1500 Hz), relatively slow click rate (<17.1/s) and high signal intensity (>100 dB pSPL).

Wave I is seen as a vertex-negative peak (re: input to the differential amplifier) followed by a somewhat sharp down-going peak often labeled as NI'. In normal listeners, it will usually follow the two cochlear receptor potentials (cochlear microphonic [CM] and summating potential [SP]) when the stimulus is delivered through an insert transducer. In contrast to the CM, however, wave I does not reverse polarity with change in click phase (i.e., rarefaction to condensation). Among the more common morphologic aberrations is a bifid wave I (Figure 6.4A), especially when the ABR is recorded at very high stimulus intensities (>115 dB pSPL). In general, the first peak component has a greater amplitude than the second and appears more sensitive to intensity reduction and polarity reversal; therefore, decreasing stimulus intensity or reversing phase may resolve the morphologic dilemma.

In neurodiagnostics, the presence of a bifid wave I in one ear can lead to interpretive confusion relative to which component should be used for peak latency calculation. It is not good practice to compare the earlier peak of a bifid wave on one side with that of its later counterpart on the other; therefore, latency measure-

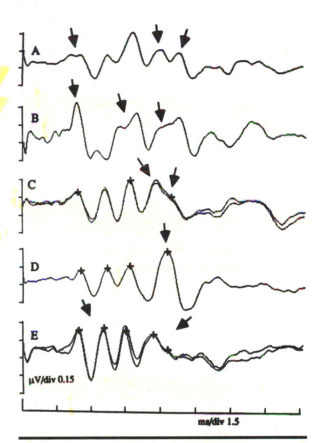

FIGURE 6.4.   Examples of normal auditory brainstem response morphologic variations. (A) Bifid wave I; the classic IV/V complex. (B) Hypervoltage of wave I; bifid wave III; wave IV is riding on the up-shoulder of wave V. (C) Wave V is riding on the downside shoulder of wave IV. (D) Fused IV/V complex. (E) Waves I and II amplitude is larger than the IV/V complex; wave V amplitude is greatly reduced on the downward slope of wave IV.

ments are best made from the second more stable component. Of course, the best approach to solving this anomalous morphology is to modify the recording strategy to resolve the problem. This is best achieved by decreasing stimulus intensity, reversing click polarity, decreasing stimulus rate, recording from a different electrode montage (e.g., horizontal or noncephalic reference), or by placing the ipsilateral ear recording electrode directly into the ear canal or onto the tympanic membrane. For a detailed description of strategies for optimizing the ABR waveform see Schwartz and Morris (1991).

On rare occasions, a normal patient may present with an unusually large (≥ 1 μV) wave I amplitude (Figure 6.4B) having a rather steep descending downstroke. In such instances, diagnostic interpretation can be confounded if wave V voltage is such that the V/I amplitude ratio appears abnormal, unless of course the same morphology is observed on both sides. When faced with this wave I *hypervoltage*, it is best to be careful to compare interaural interpeak latencies and wave V amplitude prior to developing the working diagnostic impression.

Wave II of the normal ABR usually is characterized by a much smaller voltage than wave I (Figure 6.4A and B). At times, it is difficult to define particularly in the presence of a noisy baseline. In other instances, wave II can ride on or merge with either the downward slope of wave I or the upward slope of wave III (Figure 6.4A) giving the illusion of a multiple component waveform. Recording from the contralateral ear (A_c) often is helpful in clarifying wave II since its amplitude tends to be larger than that in the ipsilateral response (A_i). Because of its variable amplitude among normal neurotologic patients, wave II is not considered to play a dominant role in ABR diagnostic interpretation.

Wave III is the central most vertex-positive peak of the I, III, V ABR triad. It is a rather prominent peak that is usually clearly defined by the amount of excursion on both sides. Like wave I, its most common morphologic irregularity is bifidity (Figure 6.4B). In contrast to wave I, however, estimation of peak latency is best made at the midpoint by forming an isosceles triangle from each of the two peaks of the waveform, respectively. Here again, however, response resolution can be improved greatly by altering the recording strategy as was described earlier for wave I.

Wave IV consists of the first component of the ubiquitous IV/V complex. In some cases waves IV and V are clearly separate forming the classical two peak configuration (Figure 6.4A). In others, it is seen as a small amplitude peak riding on the upgoing slope of wave V (Figure 6.4B) or it can actually appear to be the more prominent component of the complex where

wave V appears to be riding on the descending slope of the wave (Figure 6.4C). All too often, wave IV is partially or completely fused with wave V (Figure 6.4D). Partial fusion may appear as a trapezoidal formation wherein the apex of the complex is almost as wide as the base (Figure 6.4B). When totally fused, waves IV and V form a single large pyramid with a base that spans more than 1.5 ms across.

When faced with these normal variants, it is important to distinguish wave V for correct latency notation. As a rule, wave V usually begins above the baseline with its peak followed by a deep terminal downstroke (Figure 6.4A,B,D) that is maximal below the baseline. Schwartz and Morris (1991) have outlined various clinical strategies that can be used to isolate wave V. These include recording from the contralateral ear or from a noncephalic reference site, reducing stimulus intensity, increasing stimulus rate, reversing stimulus polarity, and/or reducing the high-pass filter setting. At lower signal intensities and increased click rates, wave V will typically emerge as the most robust and prominent peak.

FACTORS THAT INFLUENCE THE ABR

Over the past 15 years, there has been a long litany of reports that addressed the influences of so-called nonpathologic factors (e.g., age, gender, click polarity, signal intensity, filter bandwidth, electrode montage, etc.) on ABR wave latency, amplitude, and morphology. Nevertheless, controversy still remains whether to have separate normative data for male, female, young, and old patients and what recording parameters might be *optimal* both for neurodiagnostic and audiologic purposes. To be sure, there has been no consensus on how best to approach each of these issues and whether the reported influences are, in fact, clinically significant.

In evaluating the relevance of the myriad of reports on factors that influence the ABR, one must appreciate the difference between statistical and clinical significance. In routine clinical electrophysiology, group mean data can be quite misleading since it is rather sensitive to extreme measurements and has a tendency to obscure individual differences and to mask the degree of overlap within a given distribution. An excellent example of the difference between statistical and clinical significance is found from the studies on gender as discussed below. Although group mean data support earlier wave V latency for females versus males (Beagley and Sheldrake 1978; Jerger and Hall, 1980; Rosenhamer et al., 1980; Allison et al., 1983; Chu, 1985; Rosenhall et al., 1985; Jerger and Johnson, 1988), scatterplots of peak latency and amplitude demonstrate considerable overlap toward the middle of the distribution. What might represent statistical significance, therefore, may have little bearing on clinical interpretation.

Stimulus Considerations

Stimulus Intensity.   As with all sensory evoked responses, both amplitude and latency of the ABR are influenced by changes in signal strength as illustrated in Figure 6.5. This concomitant decrease in response voltage and increase in absolute peak latency in proportion to intensity reduction forms the basis of the latency-intensity (L-I) series which is the hallmark of ABR auditory evaluation. The most striking characteristic of the L-I series is the tenacity of wave V. The threshold of detection tends to be much lower for wave V than that for the earlier components, although the slope of the functions are approximately equal across all waves. On the average, wave V latency increases from about 6.5 ms at 110 dB pSPL to 9.1 ms at 40 dB pSPL in the normal ear, owing to the more apical spread of cochlear excitation and thus increased traveling wave time as intensity decreases. Evaluation of deviations in the slope of the wave V L-I function from normal facilitates the definition of hearing loss type. The threshold of wave V correlates best to frequencies between 2000 and 4000 Hz (Gorga et al., 1985; van der Drift et al., 1987; Bauch and Olsen, 1988) and is recognizable down to as low as 5 dB depending on the SNR (Elberling and Don, 1987). Shifts in wave V threshold can be used to estimate the behavioral hearing level within this high-frequency region.

In neurodiagnostics it is best to use as high a stimulus intensity as is necessary to maximize synchronous neural discharge so that the ABR reflects optimal auditory system capability (Schwartz and Morris, 1991). Signal level may have to be raised in patients with

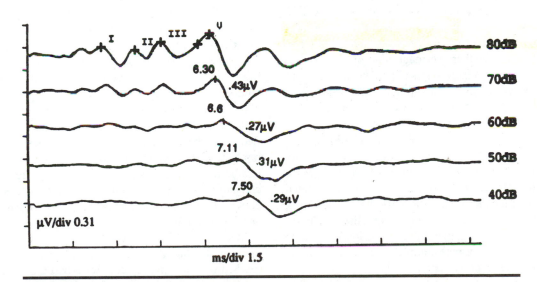

FIGURE 6.5.   Example of the relationship between stimulus intensity, wave latency, amplitude, and morphology. This paradigm is used to develop the latency-intensity series for threshold estimation. Intensity in dB normal hearing level (dB nHL).

cochlear hearing loss in order to insure that the ABR L-I series has approached or achieved asymptote as discussed in a subsequent section of this chapter.

In addition to its effect on amplitude and latency, stimulus intensity also influences ABR wave clarity. Thus, for example, a higher than normal intensity can help optimize wave I amplitude when unclear, whereas lowering intensity can assist in unbundling a bifid wave I or III or the often perplexing wave V double peak seen in patients with precipitous high-frequency cochlear hearing loss (Schwartz and Morris, 1991).

Signal Spectrum.   Although not without its shortcomings, the square wave click is the most common stimulus used in recording the ABR, whether it be for neuro-diagnostic or audiologic purposes. The temporal and spectral properties of abrupt onset, brief duration, and broad frequency composition promotes optimal neural synchrony from the aggregate of afferent auditory nerve fibers that mediate the response. Despite time-honored success with the click-evoked ABR, there are those who argue that its lack of frequency-specificity precludes accurate assessment of auditory threshold below 1000 Hz or in patients whose behavioral audiogram is characterized by a precipitous slope where the threshold at 1500 Hz is markedly better than that at and above 2000 Hz (Stapells, 1989). Stapells maintains that there is a tendency to underestimate degree of sensitivity loss with a click. Whether the magnitude of this error is consistent across a large series of patients with sensory hearing loss or will have any remarkable influence on patient management remains open.

There has been some call for frequency-specific stimuli in neurodiagnostics. Particularly problematic here is the patient whose ABR may have a wave V only due to precipitous high-frequency hearing loss above 1500 Hz. At least one clinical group has advocated supplementing the click with a 1000 Hz tone-pip in such cases. The latter appears to capitalize on the region of better hearing, thereby resulting in a recordable wave I for calculation of complete brainstem conduction time (Telian and Kileny, 1989).

Stimulus Phase.   The choice of click polarity (rarefaction, condensation, alternating) for recording the ABR in neurodiagnostics has long been the topic of debate (Terkildsen et al., 1973; Coats and Martin, 1977; Rosenhamer et al., 1978; Stockard et al., 1978; Hughes et al., 1981; Kevanishvili and Aphonchenko, 1981; Borg and Lofqvist, 1982; Emerson et al., 1982; Beattie and Boyd, 1984; Salt and Thornton, 1984; Tietze and Pantev, 1986; Coutin et al., 1987; Beattie 1988; Chan et al., 1988; Rawool and Zerlin, 1988; Schwartz et al., 1990).

Clinically, it appears that the majority of practitioners prefer either an alternating or rarefaction polarity. The original rationale for alternating onset phase was to reduce the magnitude of stimulus artifact imposed by magnetic radiation from an electrodynamic earphone that may obscure wave I. The underlying physiologic basis for rarefaction polarity emanates from the early single unit studies (Peake and Kiang, 1962; Kiang and Moxon, 1974; Zwislocki, 1975; Davis, 1976). They proposed that the afferent auditory nerve is excited only during the rarefaction phase of an acoustic click which results in basilar membrane movement towards the scala vestibuli and thus, excitatory hair cell activity. Polarity inversion to condensation causes the basilar membrane to reverse direction to the scala tympani thereby producing an inhibitory hair cell response.

From this one would presume, at least in principal, that such phase-dependent differences in basilar membrane movement should produce neural responses elicited by a condensation click that lags temporally behind those derived from rarefaction by one-half period of the stimulus waveform. Unfortunately, the quagmire of clinical investigation has failed to support either a one-half cycle assumption or the notion that excitatory deflection of the steriocilia occurs synchronously with the rarefaction phase of a stimulus. As a consequence, there had been no consensus as to whether there are, in fact, clinically salient polarity effects on the ABR, or what click phase is most advantageous to neurodiagnostic decision-making.

Because of this clinical ambiguity and because review of the literature indicated that the conclusions reached by most investigators were based on averaged data from normal listeners, Schwartz and coworkers (1990) sought to clarify the possible interaction between click phase and cochlear hearing loss in a large clinical series (N=340) of normal and hearing-impaired patients. Using two-dimensional plots of rarefaction minus condensation (R-C) differences as a function of average high-frequency hearing loss to probe for and express individual variation, they were able to demonstrate phase sensitivity as seen for waves I, III, and V in Figure 6.6. The zero line in each scatter plot represents no difference between polarity conditions. Data points falling below the zero line indicate longer latency to condensation stimuli while those above the zero cut-off denote the same for rarefaction. Although there is a clustering of data near the zero reference line for wave I, there is a clear trend toward longer peak latency to a condensation onset phase which has a definite propensity to increase as a function of high-frequency hearing loss. Similarly, the pattern of the data for wave V is reasonably clear for longer latencies to condensation clicks. In contrast to wave I, however, the structure of the data spread does not show any particular relationship to degree of hearing loss.

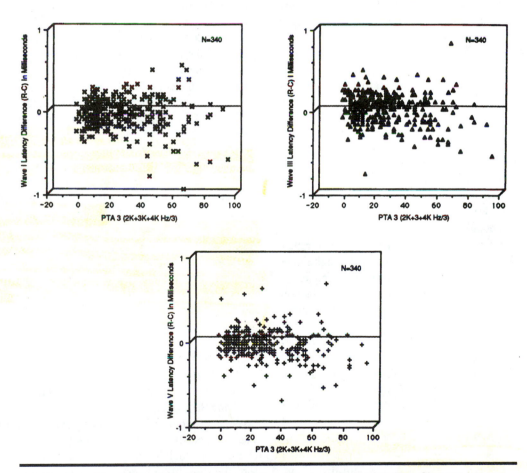

FIGURE 6.6.   Bivariate scatterplots of rarefaction minus condensation (R – C) wave latency differences as a function of average high frequency pure-tone hearing loss (PTA 3 = 2K Hz + 3K Hz + 4K Hz/3). Data points falling below zero reference represent longer latency to condensation clicks while those above zero reference represent longer latency to rarefaction events.

In addition to latency, Schwartz et al. (1990) also demonstrated a tendency toward larger amplitude with rarefaction clicks for all three ABR components (I, III, V). As high-frequency hearing loss increased, the magnitude of this R–C difference seemed to decrease for waves I and III. Wave V, on the other hand, continued to show larger amplitude to rarefaction versus condensation, regardless of high-frequency sensitivity loss.

Although the physiologic mechanism for this polarity effect remains unclear, one plausible explanation relates to the phase-locking properties of the afferent auditory receptors. Several studies have supported the premise that the direction in which basilar membrane displacement produces a neural response is governed by the characteristic frequency (CF) of a particular afferent fiber and that signal level, duration and spectrum have an interactive influence on the response (Zwislocki 1974; Antoli-Candela and Kiang, 1978; Salt and Thornton, 1984; Møller, 1986). Fibers with low CFs seem to respond best to rarefaction (i.e., basilar membrane displacement toward scala vestibuli) thus representing phase-locking. Conversely, auditory neurons having higher CFs tend to be phase-insensitive since they respond when the basilar membrane moves in either direction. Fibers with middle CFs are excited to condensation polarity.

As can be seen, the neural response to a click is rather complex. Functionally all of this means that at high signal levels as used in neurodiagnostics, the low-frequency, phase sensitive fibers which respond best to rarefaction take precedence, thus leading to an anticipated polarity effect. At low signal levels, however, as would be used in estimating auditory threshold, the high-frequency, phase-insensitive fibers are excited and the ABR should not be influenced by stimulus polarity. This latter point was supported by the recent findings of Sininger and Masuda (1990) who found that click polarity does not affect ABR threshold detection.

The clinical implications of the Schwartz et al. (1990) study are that rarefaction is preferable when using a monopolarity stimulus. There are occasions, however, where reversal to a condensation phase will help clarify an ambiguous rarefaction based ABR. When possible, the best strategy is to employ a dual polarity paradigm by recording the ABR individually

to rarefaction and condensation clicks. Alternating polarity can impose a latency and amplitude penalty by disrupting the phase-locking properties of the afferent auditory neurons. This is particularly true in patients with high-frequency hearing loss where the cochlea is better able to phase-lock to low frequencies. Alternating polarity can cancel the low-frequency phase-locked components while summing the input from fibers tuned to the high frequencies. This can yield responses that are out-of-phase, thus leading either to erroneously poor morphology or complete absence of the waveform.

Stimulus Delivery—Air Conduction.   During the past five years there has been an important change in the type of air conduction (AC) transducer used in routine ABR testing. No longer is the conventional electrodynamic audiometric earphone (i.e., TDH-39, -49) housed in either a circumaural or supraaural cushion the transducer of choice. Replacing it is the insert Tubephone™ (Etymotic ER3) which consists of a foam eartip (silicone for infants) attached to a small transducer assembly via a calculated length of polyvinyl tubing. The eartip is seated in the patient's ear canal, forming a reasonably tight, yet comfortable, acoustic seal. Because the tubing is separated from the actual transducer, a transmission delay based on the length of the tubing is imposed on the ABR waveform. This delay, which is usually around 0.9 ms, prevents the smearing of stimulus artifact on wave I as was commonly seen with the conventional earphone transducer. The Etymotic Tubephone also avoids the problems of ear canal collapse and SPL variability common to pediatric ABR evaluation (Schwartz et al., 1989; Schwartz and Schwartz, 1991).

An additional benefit of the Tubephone is the ability to record and visualize the cochlear receptor potentials (CM and SP) which typically were obscured by stimulus artifact when using an electrodynamic earphone. The foam ear-tip can also be modified by wrapping it in gold foil which is clipped to an electrode wire; therefore, the stimulus delivery system also becomes a non-invasive ear canal electrode for enhancing wave I amplitude as seen in Figure 6.7.

Whether one uses a Tubephone or the conventional audiometric earphone, frequency and temporal analy-

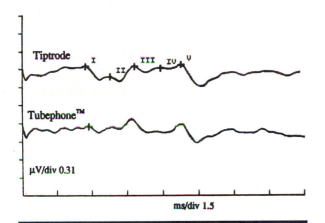

FIGURE 6.7. Comparison of wave I amplitudes for an auditory brainstem response recorded with a standard Tubephone (bottom trace) and Tiptrode (gold-foil wrapped ear-tip, top trace). Note the heightened wave I amplitude with the Tiptrode.

TABLE 6.1. Potential Problems in Bone-conducted ABRs

No existing calibration standard

Reduced undistorted output

Large electromechanical artifact

Crossover

Mastoid vs. forehead placement

Middle ear effects

---

sis should be part of routine calibration. Alterations in the acoustic spectra as a result of constant use or *misuse* can cause ABR latency prolongation reflecting the poor physical properties of the transducer and not neuropathology.

Stimulus Delivery—Bone Conduction. In pediatric testing, there are times when recording an ABR to AC stimuli simply is precluded or requires adjunctive auditory diagnostic information. For example, when attempting to estimate sensory reserve in a child with microtia, atresia, or congenital middle ear anomalies. In these select cases it may be necessary to substitute a bone-conduction (BC) oscillator for the Tubephone. While successful recording to BC stimuli certainly is possible, one should be acutely aware of the many inherent technical problems associated with the use of this transducer. Table 6.1 highlights some of the factors that must be considered when attempting to record the ABR to BC clicks or tone pips.

Among the most important of these factors is the narrow dynamic range or reduced undistorted output available with most commercial BC oscillators (Schwartz et al., 1985). The maximum output of a click

transduced through a Radioear B70 BC oscillator is equivalent only to about 35 dB HL (Schwartz et al., 1985), while those of its B71 or B72 counterparts are 15–20 dB less. Since the psychophysical threshold of a BC click through most commercial evoked response instruments is approximately 40 dB on the dial, one must assume that the BC ABR is probably limited only to those patients whose cochlear reserve does not exceed much more than 30 dB. In such cases one can dichotomize BC ABR results into normal or reduced sensory sensitivity as suggested by Stapells (1989). Attempts at driving the oscillator at high signal levels (e.g., 95 dB) can result in distorted waveforms which can confound test interpretation.

Masking the Non-test Ear. The application of masking in the non-test ear to eliminate crossover of the test stimulus is standard protocol in clinical audiometry. Certainly there would be good reason to believe that the same potential for crossover exists in ABR neurodiagnostic testing, particularly since the stimuli are presented monaurally at moderately high intensity levels. Yet, the question of whether masking is routinely needed has remained open to controversy for many years.

The need for masking was first questioned by Finitzo-Hieber et al. (1979) when two adults with unilateral congenital atresia failed to show repeatable ABRs when the impaired ear was stimulated at signal levels between 100–117 dB peak equivalent (pe)SPL. Opposite findings with adults were later reached by Chiappa, et al. (1979), Özdamar and Stein (1981) and Humes and

Ochs (1982), and more recently in infants by Hatanaka et al. (1990). In each case series, recognizable, albeit temporally delayed, ABRs were recorded initially without masking but were subsequently ablated with the introduction of masking to the normal ear of patients with unilateral deafness.

Interaural attenuation (IA) is influenced by factors such as the test stimulus and transducer type. For a click transduced either through a conventional earphone or ER-3 Tubephone, estimates of IA range from about 50–80 dB (Ozdamar and Stein, 1981; Humes and Ochs, 1982; Reid and Thornton, 1983; Van Campen et al., 1990) with the ER-3 offering no significant IA advantage over the circumaural earphone as it does with long duration pure tone stimuli (Van Campen et al., 1990).

From a conservative audiologic perspective, it would appear that the application of contralateral masking in ABR testing should follow the same principals as in behavioral audiometry using a minimum estimate of 50 dB IA; that is, you need to mask whenever the intensity of the stimulus exceeds sensory sensitivity in the non-test ear by more than about 50 dB (i.e., IA for a click).

An alternative method of determining *when to mask* is based on the interaural latency difference of corresponding peak components. The ABR produced by transcranial stimulation is significantly longer in latency and reduced in amplitude owing to the lower signal intensity reaching the contralateral cochlea. Such a crossover response would be so delayed relative to the better ear that the need for masking would be apparent. The advantage of this approach to determining *when to mask* is that it does not assume knowledge of cochlear sensitivity in the non-test ear.

Given the broad frequency response of a click and since the masking-noise intensity dial of evoked response instrumentation is not calibrated in effective levels, one might consider constructing an effective masking table as described originally by Sanders and Rintelmann (1964) and reviewed more recently by Sanders (1991). Unlike pure-tone audiometry where effective masking is computed for each pure tone center frequency, it need only be determined at the resonant frequency of the transducer for a click stimulus. This can be obtained from the spectral analysis during routine calibration. If this is not available, 3000 Hz

would serve as a good approximation. Although effective masking level can also be derived through direct measurement of ABR threshold in normal listeners, this method is inordinately time consuming.

In contrast to AC receivers, no study has evaluated IA for a click transduced through a BC oscillator. One would suppose that IA is probably no greater than 10 dB as in pure-tone audiometry, thereby necessitating the need for masking whenever a BC ABR is recorded. To circumvent the need for masking with infants and young children, Stapells (1989) recommends using the ipsilateral to contralateral latency and amplitude asymmetry seen with a two-channel ABR recording, where wave V is smaller in amplitude and prolonged in latency in the contralateral versus ipsilateral channel. According to Stapells (1989), at about 40 dB HL, the latency and amplitudes between the two channels are equivalent, suggesting probable crossover to the non-test ear. At lower signal levels, however, the ipsilateral (stimulated ear) shows the expected earlier wave V latency with larger voltage than its contralateral counterpart. The presumption here is that the ipsilateral response reflects no contribution from the opposite cochlea.

Stimulus Repetition Rate.   Since the ABR represents the summation of synchronous neural discharges along the afferent auditory pathway, waveform definition, latency, and amplitude all depend, to some extent, on the temporal characteristics of the stimulus. In general, the latency shift is greatest for wave V and least for wave I. In contrast, amplitude is most reduced for wave I and only minimally affected for wave V until the interstimulus interval becomes sufficiently short (e.g., 20 ms) to cause adaptation of the response.

In neurodiagnostic testing where waveform clarity of both the early and late components is essential, it is preferable to use relatively slow rates of stimulus presentation (<20/sec). It has been our experience that a rate of between 17.1–21.1/sec represents an excellent compromise between too slow for available testing time and too fast for optimal waveform clarity. When wave I is ambiguous, however, decreasing the rate below 10/sec (e.g., 3.1, 5.1, 7.1/sec) helps recruit the greatest aggregate of CN VIIIth nerve fibers and improves neural synchrony (Schwartz and Morris, 1991).

Because the amplitude of wave V is relatively stable even at high rates of stimulation (e.g., >65.1/sec), the latency shift between a slow (<20/sec) and rapid (>50/sec) rate is often used in neurodiagnostics to stress synaptic efficiency (Jacobson et al., 1987; Schwartz and Morris, 1991). On the average, increasing the rate from 17.1 to 65.1/sec prolongs wave V latency by 0.36 ms, in adults. Using a regression model, the adult wave V latency shift is estimated to be approximately 0.0075 ms per 10 Hz increase in repetition rate.

In the normal infant, increasing click rate between 17.1/sec and 57.1/sec creates an average wave V latency shift of 0.58 ms, representing a 0.28 ms greater prolongation than that seen in the adult. The estimated wave V latency shift in the newborn is approximately 0.145 ms per 10 Hz increase in click rate. This latency shift increase reflects the reduced neural encoding ability of the immature central auditory system, particularly when overloaded.

In addition to its value in neurodiagnostics, a high stimulus rate is also quite fruitful for ABR hearing screening or in recording a L-I series. Since, in each of these cases, the peak of interest is wave V, and since the amplitude of wave V is affected rather minimally at relatively high rates of presentation, one can purchase valuable testing time and permit a greater number of trials averaged thus improving the SNR (Schwartz and Schwartz, 1991).

Mode of Stimulus Presentation. The ABR amplitude to binaural stimulation is larger than that seen monaurally although its voltage is about 20–25 percent less than the linear sum of separate right and left monaural recordings (Dobie and Norton, 1980; Berlin et al. 1984). The difference between the sum of the two monaural responses from that of a binaural recording is known as the *binaural interaction component* (BIC). The major component (ß) is a small amplitude residual response occurring at a latency slightly longer than that of wave V (Dobie and Berlin, 1979; Dobie and Norton, 1980; Decker and Howe, 1981; Hosford-Dunn et al., 1981; Levine, 1981; Wrege and Starr, 1981; Berlin et al., 1984; Kelly-Ballweber and Dobie, 1984; Fowler and Leonards, 1985; Furst et al., 1985). ß is often preceded by an even smaller å component.

Although our neurophysiologic understanding of the BIC remains incomplete, it is thought to represent some form of binaural fusion via activation of auditory brainstem connections not excited by monaural stimulation. Whether the BIC is the result of transcranial stimulation (crossover) is open to discussion. Levine (1981), for example, found the BIC to be at signal levels below 50 dB HL where there is adequate interaural attenuation. Ainslie and Boston (1980), on the other hand, were unable to record a replicable response at low intensities. Moreover, when contralateral masking was introduced during monaural stimulation, the binaural difference waveform could not be seen.

At the present time, the clinical application of the BIC is limited by the difficulty in measuring such a small response and the observation that it is sometimes not even seen in normal neurologic and oto-audiologic listeners (Berlin et al., 1984; Wilson et al., 1985). In neuroelectrodiagnostics, therefore, it is unwise to stimulate binaurally since the response may mask a monaural brainstem abnormality. For audiologic purposes, however, a binaural stimulation approach will provide information about auditory sensitivity in the better ear when time does not permit monaural testing (Jerger et al., 1985; Schwartz and Schwartz, 1991).

Recording Considerations

The human body is replete with sources of bioelectric activity that can contaminate the ABR. Electrical activity from the brain (EEG), muscle (EMG), eye (ERG), and heart (ECG) have voltages many times greater than any component of the ABR and can pass through the recording electrodes. Non-biological sources of electrical interference also can enter the recording system and unite with the desired evoked response. Power cords from the evoked potential instrument itself as well as the 60 Hz power lines within the electrodiagnostic laboratory walls can broadcast 60 Hz electrical signals which can be *picked up* by the recording electrodes acting as a TV antenna. Together these *common-mode* sources of electrical *noise* can impose a harsh penalty on the resolution of the evoked response, particularly one with amplitudes less than 1 µV such as the ABR. Although total elimination of the *noise* from the *signal* is impossible, improvement in SNR can be achieved through: a) differential amplification, b) time-domain averaging, c) filtering, and d) artifact rejection. (See Hyde, Chapter 3, for a detailed discussion of differential amplification, signal averaging, and artifact rejection.) In addition to suppressing the background noise, response detectability can also be influenced by the location of the recording electrodes relative to the potential dipole field distributions that underlie the ABR.

Differential Amplification. Differential amplifiers are used in recording evoked potentials because of their ability to reject common-mode noise sources (e.g., EEG, EMG, 60 Hz). Equal or common voltages that are homophasic at the positive and negative inputs of the amplifier are rejected, whereas antiphasic signals of opposite polarity are amplified. In other words, the device amplifies only the difference in voltage between the two electrode inputs. In reality common-mode signals also get amplified to a small extent.

The degree to which an amplifier will reject a common-mode signal is known as the common-mode rejection ratio (CMRR) which can also be expressed in dB. The higher the dB value, the better the amplifier since the common-mode noise signals typically have much larger voltages than the desired evoked responses. For example, a CMRR of 100 dB (100,000:1) yields an amplifier gain some 10,000 times greater for antiphasic electrical potentials than for those that are homophasic. In clinical practice, the CMRR can also be optimized by maintaining the lowest impedance possible at each electrode site and by insuring that there is a close impedance balance between electrode pairs.

Time-Domain Averaging. The extent to which the ABR is embedded in background *noise* can be appreciated by comparing its voltages relative to normal EEG activity. Depending on the particular EEG wave, the patient's age and state of consciousness (e.g., awake, stage 2 sleep, etc.), EEG voltage can range from 5–150 μV, although neonates can have delta activity as much as 300 μV (Tyner et al., 1983). In comparison, the average amplitudes for waves I, III, and V of the ABR are 0.27, 0.25 and 0.43 μV, respectively (Schwartz et al., 1990). To be sure, clinical analysis of the ABR would

not be possible without some method of attenuating the background activity.

Time-domain averaging is the most common form of data reduction used to enhance the SNR. The assumptions underlying the theory of signal averaging are that: 1) the evoked potential activity, which is stationary over time, is buried in random, background noise, and 2) equivalent evoked responses are generated by repeated like stimuli; that is, electrical activity that is time-locked to the presentation of the stimulus. In clinical practice, of course, repeated like stimuli (i.e., clicks, tone-pips, etc.) do not necessarily generate identical ABR waveforms (Lauter and Loomis, 1988). In theory, however, averaging N samples of the two statistically independent waveforms (evoked potential + noise) should improve the SNR by the $\sqrt{N}$. With more averages, the amplitude of the signal ultimately exceeds that of the summed noise. Although it is often assumed that during the averaging process, the random noise will average to zero voltage, such is not the actual case. There is always some degree of noise component which varies across time thus adding further to violating the principal of identical stimuli generating identical ABR waveforms.

Since the purpose of signal averaging is to reduce random biologic and non-biologic electrical activity, the number of trials acquired should be based on waveform clarity and the estimated residual noise level rather than some fixed arbitrary number such as 2048. When a patient is myogenically quiet, a well-resolved ABR can be seen within 500–1000 averages. 500 trials will improve the SNR 22-fold ($\sqrt{500}$). With excessive movement, however, it may be necessary to average 4000 or more trials thereby gaining SNR improvement by a factor of 63. Consider, for example, an ABR peak component with an amplitude of 0.27 μV such as wave I. If embedded in an EEG signal of about 15 μV, the SNR is 0.018. Just to achieve a 1:1 SNR would require a 56-fold SNR enhancement which translates into 5500 averages.

While there are formal parametric methods available for estimating the level or statistical variance of the background noise during averaging, such as the $\pm$ reference (Schimmel, 1967) or Fsp calculation (Don et al., 1984; Elberling and Don, 1984), the most straightforward assessment of reliability is to see how well the response can be replicated via superimposition. If there is any deviation from overlap it is possible to calculate a *reproducibility index* (RI) to estimate relative residual noise in the response (Nuwer, 1986; Schwartz and Morris, 1991) as presented in Figure 6.8. The index represents the ratio between the amplitude (μV) of the largest peak in the evoked response and the difference amplitude ($\Delta\mu$V) at that portion of the two responses that is most incongruous. The smaller the index value, the more noise contaminated in the response. Schwartz and Morris (1991) suggest that a RI <3 is unacceptable for accurate neurodiagnostic or auditory threshold estimation purposes. It is often recommended that a *no stimulus input* serve as a baseline from which to judge the magnitude of noise in the stimulus evoked response. Such a recommendation assumes, however, that the physiologic background noise in the no-stimulus input recording will be the same as when the stimulus is introduced and will remain stable throughout the entire testing protocol. We know, of course, that this assumption is invalid and that the level of *noise* can be quite different between trials. A patient can be perfectly relaxed and myogenically quiet during the *control* run and excessively noisy upon testing.

There is no substitute for a well-defined, quiet ABR recording. If this cannot be accomplished within an appropriate period of testing time (<1.5 hours) because of excessive background interference, it is best to discontinue averaging and reschedule the patient to be tested under sedation. Continuing to average unacceptably high levels of residual noise serves no purpose since the relationship between the number of epochs averaged and the improvement in SNR is non-linear (Schwartz and Morris, 1991).

Automatic and Manual Artifact Rejection.   Commercial evoked response instruments customarily are designed to reject any incoming signal with an amplitude in excess of some preset voltage limit. Among the most villainous forms of contaminating artifact is myogenic activity. Unfortunately, merely engaging the automatic artifact reject does not guarantee a completely uncontaminated recording. Transient bursts of muscle activity often are below the rejection threshold and can interfere greatly with waveform definition.

Paramount to reducing the compromising influence of myogenic potentials is to ensure that the patient is comfortable and relaxed. Proper furniture—such as a well-padded reclining chair or bed allowing the patient to be placed in a supine or semi-supine position—as well as a darkened room in which the patient is left alone (the instrumentation and electrodiagnostician should not be in the same room as the patient) and instructed to keep eyes closed are among the best preventive measures. Rather than relying solely on the artifact reject capabilities of the system, it is better practice to view the input signal (EEG) as opposed to the averaged waveform, unless of course, the evoked potential system being used permits simultaneous displays. Whenever excessive or potentially contaminating artifact is seen in the *raw* EEG, the averaging should be manually interrupted until there is a return to a stable baseline.

Band-Pass Filtering.   The nonlinearity of signal-to-noise enhancement via time-domain averaging places a practical limit on the ability to resolve a noisy ABR waveform with averaging alone. Additional suppression of potentially contaminating noise is facilitated by filtering those portions of the incoming waveform that do not contain the evoked response of interest. Ideally,

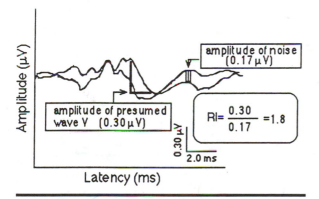

FIGURE 6.8.   Method for quantifying the reproducibility index (RI) of the evoked potential response. The noise is considered the irreproducible portion of the response.

the frequency response of the noise is different from that of the evoked response; however, there typically is some overlap in frequency content of signal and noise components.

To demonstrate the improvement in SNR with the addition of filtering, let us reconsider the ABR peak component with an amplitude of 0.27 µV illustrated in the previous discussion of signal averaging. Recall that to achieve a 1:1 ratio between the signal and noise would require 5500 averages. By filtering selected portions of the waveform that are not assumed to contain the ABR, it might be possible to reduce the noise component to ≤5 µV. Following the same method of computation, a 1:1 ratio would now be achieved by averaging across only 185 epochs. Averaging 2000 trails would make the signal almost 2.5 times larger than the noise component.

The choice of low-pass and high-pass filter settings should be predicated on the frequency content of various components of the response, in this case waves I–V of the ABR, and the contaminating noise sources. At high intensities (e.g., 115 pSPL) the frequency content of the ABR lies somewhere between 50 and 1000 Hz depending on the resolution of the instrument used for spectral analysis (Elberling, 1979; Kevanishvili and Aphonchenko, 1979; Boston and Ainslie, 1980; Laukli and Mair, 1981; Domico and Kavanagh, 1986; Kavanagh et al., 1988).

The digitally filtered ABR waveforms displayed in Figure 6.9 indicate composite energy of the fast components (i.e., waves I–III) between 500–1000 Hz with minimal additional energy above 1500 Hz; that is, when high-frequency cut-off is decreased from 1500 to 500 Hz, there is a significant amplitude suppression of the fast components. Low-pass filtering below 500 Hz virtually eliminates all waves with the possible exception of a low-frequency slow component that underlies wave V.

When filtering is used to suppress noise, it should be possible to preserve only portions of the ABR spectrum without compromising waveform definition. Since biologic and non-biologic noise often consist of considerable low frequency energy, it would seem rather safe to filter low frequency (<100 Hz) components of the response without compromising clarity of the salient peaks in the waveform as illustrated from the high-pass digitally filtered responses illustrated in Figure 6.10.

The problem is that analog filters used in commercial evoked potential systems introduce phase distortion that is a nonlinear function of frequency. Not only does this

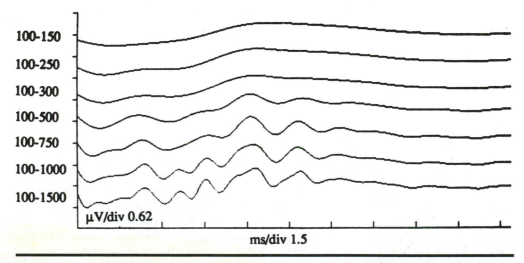

FIGURE 6.9.   Digitally filtered auditory brainstem responses demonstrating composite energy of the fast-components (waves I–III) between 500–1000 Hz with minimal energy above 1500 Hz.

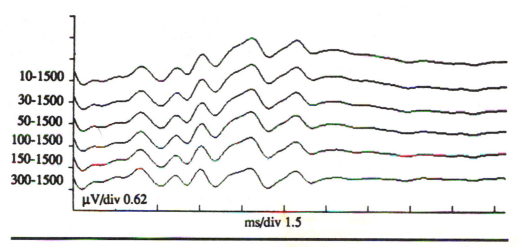

FIGURE 6.10. Digitally filtered auditory brainstem responses illustrating the frequency range of the slow component (wave V).

result in significant latency shifting across all ABR components, but the amount of shift in time for each specific peak is differentially governed by the frequency content of that component. Such nonlinearity prevents the use of a temporal correction factor to compensate for the latency shift. Moreover, analog filtering can also cause overall distortions of the waveform to include polarity inversion, introduction of non-standard peaks in the waveform, artifactual increases or decreases in peak-to-peak amplitude and general sharpening or broadening of the response (Dawson and Doddington, 1973; Ainslie and Boston, 1980; Boston and Ainslie, 1980; Doyle and Hyde, 1981; Møller, 1983; Domico and Kavanagh, 1986; Janssen et al., 1986). Most manufacturers of evoked potential instrumentation attempt to lessen the adverse effects of analog filtering by incorporating filter slopes of only 6 or 12 dB/octave, particularly for the high-pass filter stage. As filter slope increases to 24 or 36 dB/octave so does the adversity of the phase-distortion (Domico and Kavanagh, 1986).

In practice, the closest approximation to the true ABR is obtained for a bandpass between 30–1500 Hz. Although additional high-pass analog filtering can create artifactual alterations in the ABR waveform, one can actually turn this technical adversity into a clinical advantage. Increasing the high-pass cut-off frequency from 30 Hz to 100 or 150 Hz can result in an artificial voltage enhancement of waves I–III which can be most beneficial in neurodiagnostics (Schwartz and Morris, 1991). Alternatively, decreasing the high-pass filter setting to 30 Hz or 50 Hz can perpetrate up to a 20% spurious improvement in wave V amplitude. This is particularly beneficial in ABR threshold testing to estimate auditory sensitivity (Schwartz and Schwartz, 1991).

Most commercial evoked potential systems are equipped with a special purpose band-stop filter that is tuned to attenuate electrical activity within a narrow range of frequencies with 60 Hz at its center. The obvious importance of this *notch* filter is in the suppression of 60 Hz artifact that emanates from the main power lines supplying the wall outlets or other electronic instrumentation housed in the same room as the evoked potential system. While this feature might appear as a welcome addition in electrically noisy test environments, it actually has serious drawbacks. When the notch filter is engaged there is a summation of all electrical activity within its frequency band; that is, portions of the evoked response that may have spectral energy within that frequency region also will be affected. Moreover, since this too is an analog filter, it will introduce additional phase distortion that may compromise waveform clarity severely. Another undesirable feature of 60 Hz notch filters is their tendency to *ring* when excited by a transient. This so-called paradoxical artifact can actually give the false impression of a reproducible peak component where none actually exists. The clinical implication of such spurious peaks is intuitively obvious in neurodiagnostics, ABR threshold estimation, or intraoperative/acute care monitoring. Consequently, 60 Hz notch filters should not be used. Rather, the source of the interference should be identified and eliminated. (Suggestion: If the 60 Hz activity is not present in all channels, then it is possible that the source of the problem lies in the electrodes connected to those inputs. The first step toward the solution in this case is to insure low and matched impedances with reapplication or replacement if necessary.)

The Electrode Montage.   Perhaps with the exception of wave I, the peak components that define the ABR recorded from the surface of the scalp are the result of multiple discrete sources from deep neural substrates. What is recorded at the scalp represents electrical dipole vectors pointing outward from the center of a sphere (Scherg and von Cramon, 1985). Theoretically, the relative amplitude of specific peaks in the response should reflect how well the recording electrodes align with the direction of the electrical dipole.

The common practice for many clinicians is to record the ABR from a single pair of electrodes, one of which is affixed to the vertex (C_z) or high forehead (Fp_z) and the other either to the ipsilateral (stimulated ear) mastoid (M_i) or earlobe (A_i). In general, this electrode derivation assumes that ABR peaks represent maximum electrical source potential activity thereby permitting optimal visualization of all waveform components. Frequently, a second recording channel between C_z and the contralateral (non-stimulated) ear (A_c) is helpful in clarifying ambiguities such as a completely fused IV/V complex as illustrated in Figure 6.11. On the contralateral recording, peaks IV and V tend to separate owing to the rotational direction of the dipole vector loop of each peak relative to the stimulated ear. In normal neurologic patients, the direction of the wave V vector loop is toward the stimulated ear (Epstein, 1988) and reaches its maximum peak along the line from A_i to C_z earlier than it does from A_i to A_c. The vector loop for Wave IV, on the other hand, rotates in the opposite direction and thus achieves voltage maxima faster in the contralateral derivation. Table 6.2 summarizes additional characteristics of the contralateral ABR recording relative to its ipsilateral counterpart.

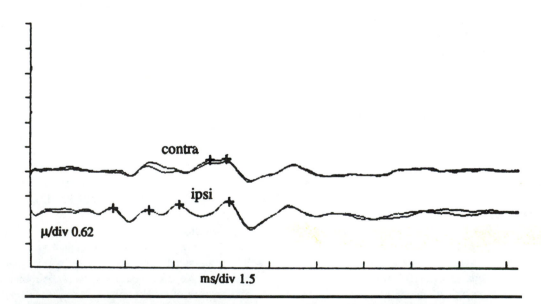

FIGURE 6.11.   Two-channel auditory brainstem response exemplifying the value of the second contralateral (A_c) recording channel for optimizing individual peak detection when there is fusion of the IV/V complex.

TABLE 6.2.   Latency and Amplitude
Characteristics of the Contralateral ABR

PEAK	CHARACTERISTIC
I	None
II	Larger
III	Smaller
IV	Earlier
V	Later

If we assume that the relative voltage of a given peak component is governed, in part, by how well the recording electrodes align with the direction of the electrical dipole responsible for that peak, then simultaneous recording from orthogonal electrode pairs should optimize waveform resolution for more accurate peak detection as demonstrated in the 4-channel recording in Figure 6.12.

Both inferential modeling of ABR generator sources from the scalp distribution in humans using spatio-temporal dipole modeling and planarity of the 3-channel Lissajous' trajectory (Starr and Squires, 1982; Pratt et al., 1985; Scherg and Von Cramon, 1985; Sininger et al., 1987) and extensive clinical experience in multiple channel montaging (Schwartz and Morris, 1991) have demonstrated that the equivalent dipole orientation for all peaks in the response lies either in the vertical or horizontal plane. The dipoles for waves I and III are oriented in the horizontal plane while those for waves II, IV, and V lie vertically. Optimization of wave I should thus be facilitated either by the conventional vertex-to-ipsilateral ear recording or to a horizontal (ear-to-ear) montage which lies along the general line of action potential propagation (Starr and Squires, 1982). In some patients, wave I amplitude is larger from vertex-to-ipsilateral earlobe than it is from ear-to-ear recordings, whereas in others, the opposite is true (Schwartz, 1991). Wave V is best recorded from vertex to the protuberance of a cervical spinous process (e.g., C7, C5, C2) which follows the axis of the brainstem as predicted both from inferential modeling (Scherg and von Cramon, 1985; Sininger et

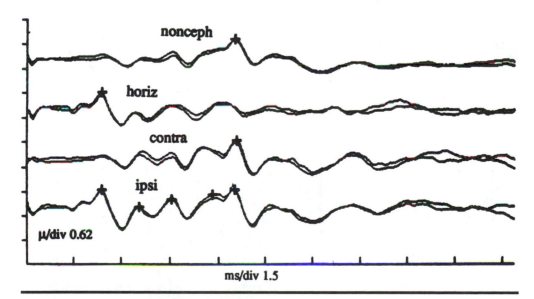

FIGURE 6.12.   Example of how a simultaneous four-channel auditory brainstem response can be used to highlight and clarify specific peaks of the response. (noncephalic, C_z-C2 spinous process of the second cervical vertebrae; horizontal, A_i-A_c; contralateral, C_z-A_c; ipsilateral, C_z-A_i).

al., 1987) and clinical measurement (Schwartz and Morris, 1991; Schwartz and Schwartz, 1991).

Patient Considerations

Influence of Gender and Age. On the basis of the difference in mean latency between males and females (Beagley and Sheldrake, 1978; Jerger and Hall, 1980; Rosenhamer et al., 1980; Allison et al., 1983; Chu, 1985; Rosenhall et al., 1985; Jerger and Johnson, 1988), it has been recommended that independent male and female ABR norms be generated for each clinical laboratory (Jerger and Hall, 1980; Schwartz and Berry, 1985; Jerger and Johnson, 1988). Recall, however, that the

foundation for this recommendation rested on measures of central tendency for wave V latency and amplitude.

Many investigators have suggested that wave V latency increases systematically with increasing age (Rowe, 1978; Jerger and Hall, 1980; Maurizi et al., 1982; Allison et al., 1983; Kelly-Ballweber and Dobie, 1984; Rosenhall et al., 1985; Debruyne, 1986; Jerger and Johnson, 1988; Lenzi et al., 1989) although there has been some conflicting opinion (Beagley and Sheldrake, 1978; Rosenhamer et al., 1980; Otto and McCandless, 1982; Chu, 1985). Here again, Jerger and Hall (1980), and Jerger and Johnson (1988), advocated independent normative data for young and aged (≥60 years).

It is apparent from the foregoing discussion that the

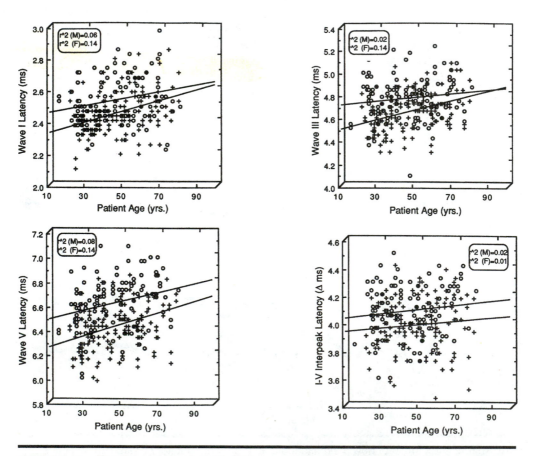

FIGURE 6.13. Bivariate scatterplots (N=240 normal listeners) of peak latencies as a function of age, gender, and cochlear hearing loss for waves I, III, V, and I–V IPL.

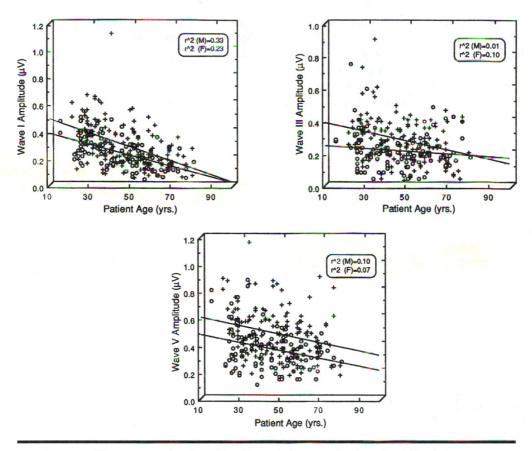

FIGURE 6.14.   Bivariate scatterplots (N=240 normal listeners) of peak amplitude as a function of age, gender, and cochlear hearing loss for waves I, III, and V.

discrete and continuous variables of gender and age have continued to perplex the auditory electrophysiologists for more than 10 years. Whether these two factors have a significant enough influence on ABR latency to warrant individual sets of normative data also remains controversial. In an extensive investigation on the clinical influences of age, gender and high-frequency cochlear hearing loss, we cast data from 240 normal listeners into bivariate scatter plots of ABR latency and amplitude for males and females as a function of age as shown in Figure 6.13 and 6.14 respectively.

Observe that the individual regression lines are consistently offset for males and females and there appears to be more males in the upper-half and more females in the lower-half of each latency distribution. When the data are examined more closely from the vantage point that 240 patients are represented in each plot, the relatively inconsequential number of males near the top and females near the bottom becomes rather apparent. What is most striking and more clinically meaningful is the high degree of overlap between the two gender groups toward the middle of the distribution.

Hence, what appears to be a statistically significant difference holds no clinical relevance. The implication here, of course, is that gender specific normative data are entirely unnecessary. The bivariate plots in Figure 6.13 are also self descriptive of a casual relationship, at best, between adult age and absolute latency, whereas age is shown unequivocally to have no influence on the I–V IPL. The overall scattering of the latency data and the individual simple regression lines for males and females indicated that only a small percentage of the variance was accounted for on the basis of age alone; that is, there was a very low correlation between adult age and peak latency.

In general, scatter plots of peak amplitude between males and females as a function of age revealed analogous findings to the latency counterparts as shown in Figure 6.14. That is, there was an overwhelming gender overlap at the center of the distribution, thus counteracting what might appear as a statistical mean difference due to the influence of extreme voltage values. Likewise, age contributes minimally to peak amplitude with the exception of wave I where voltage decreases slightly with increasing age. Whether this

finding represents the prologue of peripheral differentiation secondary to aging is entirely speculative. Once again, the more important clinical message from these data is that neither age nor gender specific normative data need be collected.

At the opposite end of the age continuum, data related to the latency and amplitude characteristics of the neonatal ABR seems to have enjoyed better agreement. It has generally been held that the newborn ABR is characterized as a series of three primary vertex positive peaks (I, III, V) all prolonged in latency compared to their adult counterparts (Salamy et al., 1975; Starr et al., 1977; Salamy et al., 1978; Goldstein et al., 1979; Jacobson et al., 1982; Starr and Squires, 1982; Weber, 1982; Stockard et al., 1983; Fria and Doyle, 1984; Jacobson, 1985; Morgan et al., 1987; Eggermont and Salamy, 1988). This prolongation has been attrib-

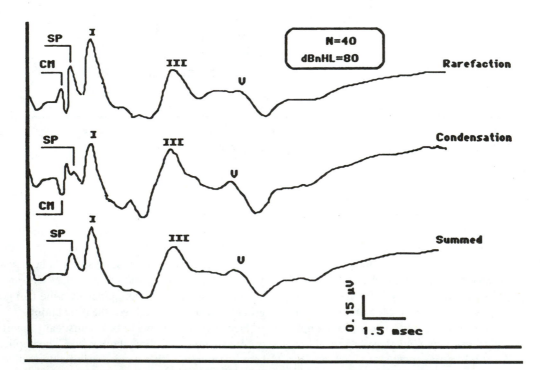

FIGURE 6.15.   Grand composite infant auditory brainstem response to rarefaction and condensation clicks and the computer summed response of the two monopolarities. CM=cochlear microphonic, SP=summating potential.

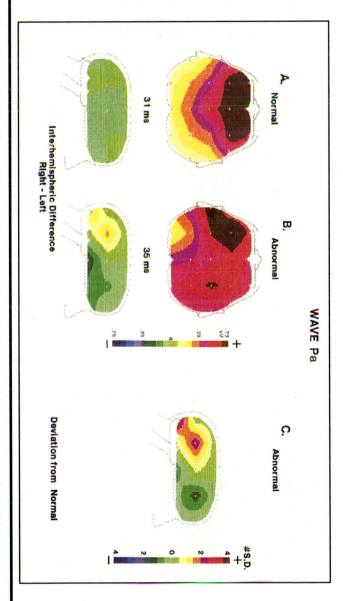

FIGURE 7.5. Top view of the scalp topography at the latency of wave Pa showing a normal (top left) and an abnormal response (top middle). When right hemispheric Pa values are subtracted from left hemispheric values, the resulting map is green, indicating little interhemispheric differences in normal subjects (bottom left). The interhemispheric Pa amplitude difference is illustrated for an abnormal-looking map (bottom right). When these differences are compared to the normal population using the Z statistic, this subject's data falls outside 2 standard deviations at several electrode locations (right). (Reprinted with permission, Kraus and McGee. (1988). *Ear and Hearing, 9,* 159-167.)

The editor would like to acknowledge Bio-logic System Corp. for its support in the publication of these color brain map illustrations.

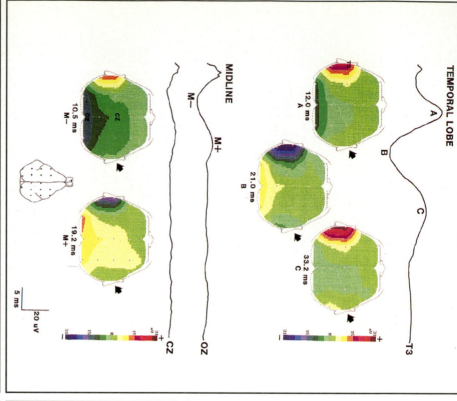

TEMPORAL LOBE

FIGURE 7.10. Top: Temporal response—The MLR obtained over the guinea pig temporal lobe contralateral to the stimulated ear consists of three components: A (12 ms), B (21 ms), and C (33 ms). The topographic maps illustrate the voltage measured at the latencies corresponding to each of these components. The electrode locations are shown on the schematic drawing of the guinea pig brain. Positive voltages are displayed with deeper hues of red; negative voltages with deeper hues of blue. Bottom: Midline response—The MLR obtained from the midline of the guinea pig consists of two components: M−, at 10 ms; and M+, at 19 ms. (Reprinted from Kraus, Smith, and McGee, 1988. *Electroencephalography and Clinical Neurophysiology*, 71, 541-558.)

Auditory Cortex Response: Lidocaine Effects

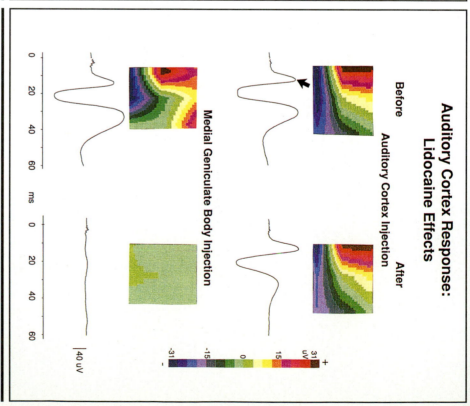

FIGURE 7.11. Lidocaine injection into auditory cortex affects auditory cortex activity differently from injections into the MGB. Responses from a 9-electrode recording device, positioned in the auditory cortex so as to record a polarity reversal of wave A, are shown in color. The polarity reversal at the latency of wave A is shown, where the positive wave (A) appears red and the waves showing reversed polarity at the latency appear blue. Representative waveforms recorded from the auditory cortex are shown before and after lidocaine injections. Top: Lidocaine injection into auditory cortex resulted in little change in auditory cortex response. Bottom: In contrast, auditory cortex activity was severely affected by lidocaine injection into the MGB. Inactivation of the MGB eliminated all activity measured from with the auditory cortex.

uted to external and middle ear effects (Morgan et al., 1987) as well as immaturity of the cochlear receptor and brainstem pathways (Starr et al., 1977; Salamy et al., 1978; Hecox and Burkhard, 1982; Eggermont, 1985).

In contrast, Schwartz and colleagues (1989) found that wave I latency and amplitude in the otherwise healthy preterm infant was no different than in the normal adult; that is, latency prolongation in the newborn is limited only to the *brainstem* components, waves III and V, owing to central auditory immaturity as displayed in Figure 6.15. Schwartz et al. (1989). This also provided indirect evidence for the consistent presence of cochlear receptor potentials in the preterm infant thereby providing additional support for peripheral auditory maturity. The principal difference between this study and its predecessors related to the stimulus intensity and transducer. Previous investigations with newborns delivered the click stimulus through a hand-held conventional electrodynamic earphone at a moderately high intensity around 90 dB pSPL. Conversely, Schwartz et al. (1989) employed a higher signal level (108 dB pSPL) that would optimize neural synchrony and neural transmission and delivered the click through an insert transducer that was taped securely into the infant's ear canal. They reasoned that use of an insert transducer circumvented the problems of collapsing ear canal and SPL reduction due to acoustic leakage from a hand-held earphone, both of which contribute to latency prolongation. On the basis of the Schwartz et al. (1989) data, as well as clinical findings in testing hundreds of term and preterm babies, it is now clear that the newborn ABR is characterized by a normal wave I latency followed by prolonged waves III and V secondary to reduced synaptic efficiency and incomplete overall neurodevelopment.

High-frequency Cochlear Hearing Loss. As in gender and age, the clinical influence of high-frequency cochlear hearing loss remains shrouded in opinion. The recurrent finding of prolonged wave V latency by previous investigators may be related primarily to insufficient signal intensity reaching the impaired cochlea (Møller and Blegvad, 1976; Coats and Martin, 1977; Selters and Brackmann, 1977; Jerger and

Mauldin, 1978; Stockard et al., 1978; Hyde and Blair, 1981; Rosenhamer et al., 1981; Prosser et al., 1983; Bauch and Olsen, 1986; Prosser and Arslan, 1987; van der Drift et al., 1987; Bauch and Olsen, 1988; Jerger and Johnson, 1988).

In the foregoing studies, there is a general failure to account for the differences in the slope of the latency-intensity (L-I) function between normal and cochlear impaired ears in the selection of click intensity. That is, wave V latency in the cochlear impaired ear may have not effectively achieved its asymptotic value at the stimulus intensities employed. Given that the slope of the L-I series is considerably steeper in patients with high-frequency hearing loss versus those with normal hearing, and accepting the increased traveling wave time needed to evoke a neural discharge in a more apical region of better hearing, it should not be too surprising that wave V latency tends to be delayed in these ears.

It is more prudent to optimize neural discharge by increasing stimulus intensity to maximum levels (110–130 pSPL) depending on degree of high-frequency hearing loss. In this way, wave V latency for most cochlear hearing losses will have achieved or come very close to asymptote, thus falling minimally within the upper limits of normal. To support this contention we scatter plotted latency and amplitude data from 385 ears as a function of high-frequency hearing status which was defined by the pure-tone threshold at 4000 Hz, the averaged hearing loss at 2000, 3000 and 4000 Hz (PTA_3) and the audiometric slope (4000–1000 Hz). Although the absence of a latency by high-frequency cochlear sensitivity loss effect was seen for individual waves I, III, and V, respectively, the most convincing evidence opposing the presumption of prolonged ABR latency as high-frequency hearing loss increases can be seen for the I–V IPL scatterplot (Figure 6.16). The broad scattering of data is self-evident of no relationship. The fact is that the complete brainstem transmission time never exceeded normal limits, regardless of severity of hearing loss at 4000 Hz. To this end, it appears that hearing loss in the high frequencies has negligible influence over peak latency as long as the level of stimulus presentation is compensatory. Consequently, additional justification is required to apply hearing loss correction factors as advocated by some investigators

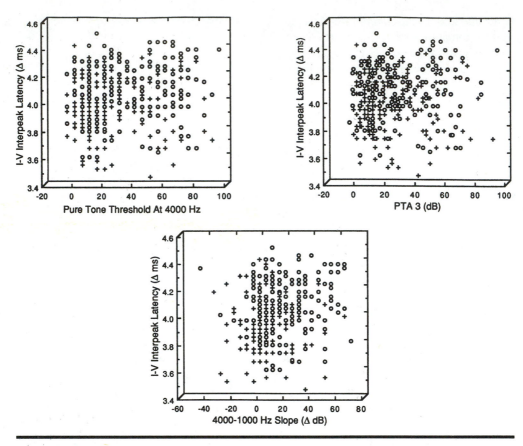

FIGURE 6.16.   Bivariate scatterplot latencies of the I–V IPL as a function of high-frequency hearing loss calculated by three different methods (4K Hz; 2K, 3K, and 4K average; and 4K–1K Hz slope). Data are from 385 neurologically normal ears with high-frequency sensory hearing loss.

(Selters and Brackmann, 1977; Jerger and Mauldin, 1978; Rossi et al., 1979; Hyde and Blair, 1981; Rosenhamer et al., 1981; Cashman and Rossman, 1983). (For additional discussion on the influence of peripheral hearing loss on the ABR see Fowler and Durrant, Chapter 10.)

DEFINING *NORMAL* LIMITS

In clinical practice, ABR interpretation is based on whether an individual patient's latency and/or amplitude values fall within or exceed a known distribution of such data established from normal neurologic patients.

Hence, it is necessary to define the distribution of these ABR measurement parameters in normal patients prior to clinical application with patients suspected of neurologic disease. A distribution is characterized by measures of central tendency (i.e., mean, median and mode) and dispersion (e.g., standard deviation, range, variance) and describes the probability of occurrence of all possible latency and amplitude values in the sample population under investigation; namely, the normal reference group. From these data one can calculate the Z statistic which represents the number of standard deviations (sd) away from the group mean that a specified latency or amplitude value lies.

Illustrated in Figure 6.17 is a cumulative frequency distribution of total central conduction time (I–V IPL) calculated for 296 normal neurologic patients. Observe that the I–V IPL is ≤4.5 ms in 100% of the cases. In most evoked clinical potential studies one is concerned primarily with the upper end of the frequency distribution since latency foreshortening is not considered an abnormal finding. When clinical decisions are made on the basis of amplitude, however, the salient region lies below the mean.

One way of defining the upper-limit of normal is simply to determine the boundary limit within which 100% of the reference population falls (e.g., 4.5 ms) for each measurement parameter and to consider any value found to exceed that limit for a given patient, an abnormal result. An alternative and more common method is to calculate the standard deviation as the measure of dispersion about the mean. The dashed

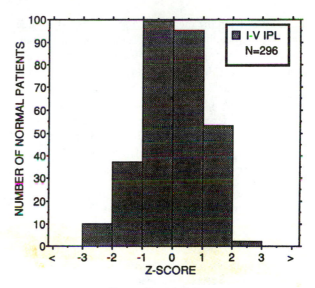

Range Restrictions

	Column Name:	Restriction:
AND	AVE 500-2K HZ	$-6 \le x \le 30$

FIGURE 6.18.   Z-distribution for determining how many standard deviations above the mean one should use to define the upper limits of normal. Note that the I–V IPL is well within 3 sd of the mean in all 296 normal patients.

lines in Figure 6.17 denote the mean (4.03 ms) +1 sd (sd = 0.2 ms). If the upper cut-off value was based on a 1 sd criterion, then approximately 20% of normal neurologic patients will be judged to have an abnormal I–V IPL (false-positives). The tradeoff for using this less stringent cut-off criterion, of course, is that it would essentially guarantee that all diseased patients, true-positives, will have an abnormal ABR, thus reducing the risk for a false-negative result. For detailed discussions on the principals of clinical-decision analysis see Hyde (1991), Schwartz (1987), and/or Turner (1991).

Although there is no rule as to how many standard deviations above the mean one should use to set the criterion level, the Z distribution can help in defining that boundary line as depicted in Figure 6.18. Recall that the Z-score denotes the number of standard devia-

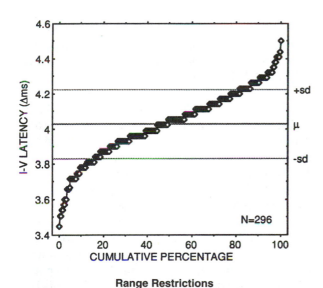

Range Restrictions

	Column Name:	Restriction:
AND	AVE 500-2K HZ	$-6 \le x \le 30$

FIGURE 6.17.   Cumulative frequency distribution of the I–V IPL from 296 normal neurotologic patients defining the upper limits of normal. The dashed lines denote the mean (4.03 ms +1 sd).

tions away from the mean that a given observed value lies. We can see that the I–V IPL is well within 3 standard deviations from the mean for all 296 normal neurologic subjects. In fact, the longest conduction time, 4.5 ms, is within 2.5 sd. In neurodiagnostic testing, the upper boundary of normal must include no less than 98% of the reference sample; therefore, either a 2.5 (98.8%) or 3.0 (99.7%) sd cut-off is appropriate. Anything less (e.g., 2.0 sd) is entirely unacceptable since it will increase the false-positive rate greatly.

Development of Laboratory Norms

In evoked potential study, it is commonly advised that each clinical facility establish its own normative database owing to the differences in instrumentation and recording parameters. The need for independent laboratory norms was underscored quite strongly in *The Auditory Brainstem Response* (Schwartz and Berry, 1985). Since that time, however, it has become readily apparent that it is entirely acceptable to base clinical decisions on normative data gathered by another facility, particularly one with a large practice. The ABR is so consistent that small differences in recording methods and sampling errors can easily be controlled by conservative cutoff limits for normalcy (e.g., 2.5–3.0 sd) if even detectable at all.

Figure 6.19 helps support this unconventional philosophy. Shown are mean I–V IPLs, +1 sd error bars and the upper limit of normal defined as +3 sd, extracted from four of the largest ABR databases published to date (Stockard and Rossiter 1977; Allison et al., 1983; Chu, 1985; Schwartz et al., 1990). Our purpose for choosing only the I–V IPL to illustrate the point was: 1) it would not be influenced by differences in transducer types, 2) interpeak latencies tend to have less intersubject variability than absolute latencies, and 3) the I–V IPL is the hallmark to ABR neurodiagnostics. It is clear that the data provide incontrovertible evidence as to the stability of the I–V IPL, despite marked differences in recording paradigms and techniques. Parenthetically, analogous results could have been shown for absolute latencies of peaks I, III and V.

Perhaps the best example to demonstrate how one could use published norms is to compare the two larg-

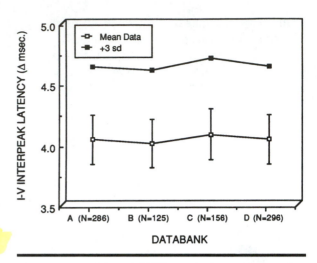

FIGURE 6.19. Mean I–V IPLs, +1 sd error bars and +3 sd upper boundary of normal from four studies. (Stockard and Rossiter, N=286; Allison et al., N=125; Chu, 156; Schwartz et al., 296.)

est databases, those from Allison et al. (1983) and Schwartz et al. (1990), whose normative sample sizes were 286 and 296 subjects respectively. In both cases the mean I–V IPL was 4.03 ms with a standard deviation of 0.20 ms. Note, however, that Allison et al. recorded the ABR to 75 dB SL alternating polarity clicks, transduced through an unconventional electrodynamic earphone (Clark 12507-G) and delivered at a rate of 10/sec. The bandpass filtering was broad from 30–3000 Hz. The stimulus in the Schwartz et al. study was a 110 dB pSPL (80 dB HL) rarefaction click, transduced through an insert tubephone (Nicolet Tip-10) and delivered at 17.1/s, and a narrower bandpass from 100–1500 Hz. Despite these important methodologic differences, the resulting group data were identical. Contrary to popular convention, therefore, the collection of independent laboratory and instrumentation specific normative data probably is not that critical. In fact, use of normative data from an active clinical practice which was based on a large number of unselected patients, including those with sensory hearing loss, would reduce the chance of diagnostic error compared to the use of normative data gathered on 10 young normal-hearing adults as is often the case. Contrary to conventional practice, the inclusion of normal neurologic patients with sensory hearing loss into the normative database will offset most of the minor differences in latency and amplitude manifested in the ABR. This should add further to reducing the possibility of a false-positive interpretation without influencing the false-negative rate.

AFTERWORD

Since the *Auditory Brainstem Response* (Jacobson, 1985), there have been significant advances in our understanding of the ABR. Not only has our knowledge on the influence of neuropathology increased substantially, but equally as important, our appreciation for what is normal has likewise improved.

When both stimulus and recording parameters are optimized in terms of signal intensity, SNR, electrode montage, etc., the likelihood of resolving all major components of the response in most normal neurologic patients is great, regardless of the patients' age, gender, or presence of cochlear hearing loss. While we recognize that there is greater reader excitement in seeing data from pathologic patients, it is our contention that errors in neurodiagnosis commonly derive from an inadequate understanding of what is normal and/or an unwillingness to spend the time necessary to optimize the clarity of the response. With the increased precision of imaging techniques for identifying neoplastic, vascular, and demyelinating diseases of the central nervous system, it is all the more critical that clinical impressions based on electrodiagnostic test results be accurate if they are to continue to serve as precursors and functional adjuncts to anatomic imaging studies. To achieve this we must begin with a clear understanding of what is *normal*.

REFERENCES

Ainslie, P. and Boston, J. (1980). Comparison of brainstem auditory evoked potentials for monaural and binaural stimuli. *Electroencephalography and Clinical Neurophysiology, 49*, 291–302.

Allison, T., Wood, C., et al. (1983). Brain stem auditory, pattern-reversal visual, and short latency somatosensory evoked potentials: Latencies in relation to age, sex, and brain and body size. *Electroencephalography and Clinical Neurophysiology, 55*, 619–636.

Antoli-Candela, F. J. and Kiang, N. (1978). *Unit activity underlying the N1 potential*. New York: Academic Press.

Bauch, C. and Olsen, W. (1988). Auditory brainstem responses as a function of average hearing sensitivity for 2000–4000 Hz. *Audiology, 27*, 156–163.

Bauch, C. and Olsen, W. (1986). The effect of 2000–4000 Hz hearing sensitivity on ABR results. *Ear and Hearing, 7*, 314–317.

Beagley, H. and Sheldrake, J. (1978). Differences in brainstem response latency with age and sex. *British Journal of Audiology, 12*, 69–77.

Beattie, R. (1988). Interaction of click polarity, stimulus level, and repetition rate on the auditory brainstem response. *Scandinavian Audiology, 17*, 99–109.

Beattie, R. and Boyd, R. (1984). Effects of click duration on the latency of the early evoked response. *Journal of Speech and Hearing Research, 27*, 70–76.

Berlin, C., Hood, L., et al. (eds.) (1984). Asymmetries in evoked potentials. *Hearing Science*. San Diego, CA: College-Hill Press.

Borg, E. and Lofqvist, L. (1982). Auditory brainstem response (ABR) to rarefaction and condensation clicks in normal and abnormal ears. *Scandinavian Audiology, 11*, 227–235.

Boston, J. and Ainslie, P. (1980). Effects of analog and digital filtering on brainstem auditory evoked potentials. *Electroencephalography and Clinical Neurophysiology, 48*, 361–364.

Cashman, M. and Rossman, R. (1983). Diagnostic features of the auditory brainstem response in identifying cerebellopontine angle tumours. *Scandinavian Audiology, 12*, 35–41.

Chan, Y., Woo, E., et al. (1988). The interaction between sex and click polarity in brain-stem auditory potentials evoked from control subjects of Oriental and Caucasian origin. *Electroencephalography and Clinical Neurophysiology, 71*, 77–80.

Chiappa, K. (1990). Brainstem auditory evoked potentials: Interpretation. *Evoked Potentials In Clinical Medicine*, Second ed., 223–305. New York: Raven Press.

Chiappa, K., Gladstone, K., et al. (1979). Brainstem auditory evoked responses: Studies of waveform variations in 50 normal human subjects. *Archives of Neurology, 36*, 81–87.

Chu, N. (1985). Age-related latency changes in the brain-stem auditory evoked potentials. *Electroencephalography and Clinical Neurophysiology, 62*, 431–436.

Coats, A. and Martin, J. (1977). Human auditory nerve action potentials and brain stem evoked responses. Effects of audiogram shape and lesion location. *Archives of Otolaryngology*, 103–622.

Coutin, P., Balmaseda, A., et al. (1987). Further differences between brain-stem auditory potentials evoked by rarefaction and condensation clicks as revealed by vector analysis. *Electroencephalography and Clinical Neurophysiology, 66*, 420–426.

Davis, H. (1976). Principles of electric response audiometry. *Annals of Otology and Laryngology, 85 (Suppl. 28)*.

Dawson, W. and Doddington, H. (1973). Phase distortion of biological signals: Extraction of signal from noise without phase error. *Electroencephalography and Clinical Neurophysiology, 34*, 207–211 .

Debruyne, F. (1986). Influence of age and hearing loss on the latency shifts of the auditory brainstem response as a result of increased stimulus rate. *Audiology, 25*, 101–106.

Decker, T. and Howe, S. (1981). Auditory tract asymmetry in brainstem electric responses during binaural stimulation. *Journal of the Acoustical Society of America, 69*, 1084–1090.

Dobie, R. and Berlin, C. (1979). Binaural interaction in brainstem-evoked responses. *Archives of Otolaryngology, 105*, 391–398.

Dobie, R. and Norton, S. (1980). Binaural interaction in human auditory evoked potentials. *Electroencephalography and Clinical Neurophysiology, 49*, 303–313.

Domico, W. and Kavanagh, K. (1986). Analog and zero-phase shift digital filtering of the auditory brain stem response waveform. *Ear and Hearing, 7*, 377–382.

Don, M., Elberling, C., et al. (1984). Objective detection of averaged auditory brainstem responses. *Scandinavian Audiology, 13*, 219–228.

Doyle, D. and Hyde, C. (1981). Analogue and digital filtering of auditory brainstem responses. *Scandinavian Audiology, 10*, 81–89.

Eggermont, J. (1985). Physiology of the developing auditory system. *Advances in the study of communication and affect: Auditory development in infancy*, 21–48. New York: Plenum Press.

Eggermont, J. and Salamy, A. (1988). Development of ABR parameters in a preterm and a term born population. *Ear and Hearing, 9(5)*, 283–289.

Elberling, C. (1979). Auditory electrophysiology: Spectral analysis of cochlear and brainstem evoked potentials. *Scandinavian Audiology, 8*, 57–64.

Elberling, C. and Don, M. (1984). Quality estimation of averaged auditory brainstem responses. *Scandinavian Audiology, 13*, 187–197.

Elberling, C. and Don, M. (1987). Threshold estimation of the human auditory brainstem response. *Acoustical Society of America, 81*, 115–121.

Emerson, R., Brooks, E., et al. (1982). Effects of click polarity on brainstem auditory evoked potentials in normal subjects and patients: Unexpected sensitivity of wave V. *Annals of the New York Academy of Science*, 710–719.

Epstein, C. (1988). The use of brain stem auditory evoked potentials in the evaluation of the central nervous system. *Evoked Potentials*, 771–790. Philadelphia, PA: W. B. Saunders Company.

Finitzo-Hieber, T., Hecox, K., et al. (1979). Brainstem auditory evoked potentials in patients with congenital atresia. *Laryngoscope, 89*, 1151–1158.

Fowler, C. and Leonards, J. (1985). Frequency dependence of the binaural interaction component of the auditory brainstem response. *Audiology, 24*, 420–429.

Fria, T. J. and Doyle, W.J. (1984). Maturation of the auditory brainstem response (ABR); additional perspectives. *Ear and Hearing, 5*, 361–364.

Furst, M., Levine, R., et al. (1985). Click lateralization is related to the ß component of the dichotic brainstem auditory evoked potentials of human subjects. *Journal of the Acoustical Society of America, 78*, 1644–1651.

Goldstein, P., Krumholz, A., et al. (1979). Brain stem evoked responses in neonates. *American Journal of Obstetrics and Gynecology, 135*, 622–628.

Gorga, M., Worthington, D., et al. (1985). Some comparisons between auditory brainstem response thresholds, latencies, and the pure tone audiogram. *Ear and Hearing, 6*, 105–112.

Hatanaka, T., Yasuhara, A., et al. (1990). Auditory brain stem response in newborn infants masking effect on ipsi- and contralateral recording. *Ear and Hearing, 11(3)*, 223–236.

Hecox, K. and Burkhard, R., (1982). Developmental dependencies of the human brainstem auditory evoked response. *Annals of the New York Academy of Science, 388*, 538–556.

Hosford-Dunn, H., Mendelson, T., et al. (1981). Binaural interactions in the short-latency evoked potentials of neonates. *Audiology, 20*, 394–408.

Hughes, J., Fino, J., et al. (1981). The importance of phase of stimulus and the reference recording electrode in brain stem auditory evoked potentials. *Electroencephalography and Clinical Neurophysiology, 51*, 611.

Humes, L. and Ochs, M. (1982). Use of contralateral masking in the measurement of the auditory brainstem response. *Journal of Speech and Hearing Research, 25,* 528–535.

Hyde, M. and Blair, R. (1981). The auditory brainstem response in neuro-otology: Perspectives and problems. *Journal of Otolaryngology,* 117–125.

Hyde, M., Davidson, M., et al. (1991). Auditory test strategy. *Diagnostic Audiology,* 295–322. Austin, Texas: Pro-ed.

Jacobson, J., (ed.) (1985). *The auditory brainstem response.* San Diego, CA: College-Hill Press.

Jacobson, J. (1985). Normative aspects of the pediatric auditory brainstem response. *Journal of Otolaryngology, 14,* 5–6.

Jacobson, J., Morehouse, R., et al. (1982). Strategies for infant auditory brainstem response assessment. *Ear and Hearing, 3,* 263–270.

Jacobson, J., Murray, J., and Duppe, N. (1987). The effects of ABR rate presentation in multiple sclerosis. *Ear and Hearing, 8,* 115–120.

Janssen, R., Benignus, V., et al. (1986). Unrecognized errors due to analog filtering of brainstem auditory evoked responses. *Electroencephalography and Clinical Neurophysiology, 65,* 203–211.

Jerger, J. and Hall, J. (1980). Effects of age and sex on auditory brainstem response. *Archives of Otolaryngology, 106,* 387–391.

Jerger, J. and Johnson, K. (1988). Interactions of age, gender, and sensorineural hearing loss on ABR latency. *Ear and Hearing, 9,* 168–175.

Jerger, J. and Mauldin, L. (1978). Prediction of sensorineural hearing level from the brain stem evoked response. *Archives of Otolaryngology, 104,* 456–461.

Jerger, J., Oliver, T., et al. (eds.) (1985). Auditory brainstem response testing strategy. *The auditory brainstem response.* San Diego, CA: College-Hill Press.

Jewett, D., Romano, M., et al. (1970). Human auditory evoked potentials: Possible brainstem components detected on the scalp. *Science, 167,* 1517–1518.

Kavanagh, K., Domico, W., et al. (1988). Digital filtering and spectral analysis of the low intensity auditory brainstem response. *Ear and Hearing, 9,* 43–47.

Kelly-Ballweber, D. and Dobie, R.A. (1984). Binaural interaction measured behaviorally and electrophysiologically in young and old adults. *Audiology, 23,* 181–194.

Kevanishvili, Z. and Aphonchenko, V. (1981). Click polarity inversion effects upon the human brainstem auditory evoked potential. *Scandinavian Audiology, 10,* 141–147.

Kevanishvili, Z. and Aphonchenko, V. (1979). Frequency composition of brain stem auditory evoked potentials. *Scandinavian Audiology, 8,* 51–55.

Kiang, N. and Moxon, E. (1974). Tails of tuning curves of auditory nerve fibers. *Journal of the Acoustical Society of America, 55,* 620.

Laukli, E. and Mair, I. (1981). Early auditory-evoked responses: Filter effects. *Audiology, 20,* 300–312.

Lauter, J. and Loomis, R. (1988). Individual differences in auditory electric responses: Comparison of between-subject and within-subject variability. *Scandinavian Audiology, 17,* 8792.

Lenzi, A., Chiarelli, G., et al. (1989). Comparative study of middle-latency responses and auditory brainstem responses in elderly subjects. *Audiology, 28,* 144–151.

Levine, R. (1981). Binaural interaction of brainstem potentials of human subjects. *Annals of Neurology, 9,* 384–393.

Maurizi, M., Altissimi, G., et al. (1982). Auditory brainstem responses (ABR) in the aged. *Scandinavian Audiology, 11,* 213–221.

Møller, A. (1983). Improving brain stem auditory evoked potential recordings by digital filtering. *Ear and Hearing, 4,* 108–113.

Møller, A. (1986). Effect of click spectrum and polarity on round window Nl-N2 response in the rat. *Audiology, 25,* 29–43.

Møller, K. and Blegvad, B. (1976). Brain stem responses in patients with sensorineural losses. *Scandinavian Audiology, 5,* 115–127.

Morgan, D., Zimmerman, M., et al. (1987). Auditory brainstem response characteristics in the full-term newborn infants. *Annals of Otology, Rhinology, and Laryngology, 96,* 142–151.

Nuwer, M. (1986). Basic electrophysiology: Evoked potentials and signal processing. *Evoked potential monitoring in the operating room,* First ed., 5–48. New York: Raven Press.

Otto, W. and McCandless, G. (1982). Aging and the auditory brain stem response. *Audiology, 21,* 466–473.

Özdamar, Ö. and Stein, L. (1981). Auditory brainstem responses in unilateral hearing loss. *Laryngoscope, 91,* 565–574.

Peake, W. and Kiang, N. (1962). Cochlear responses to condensation and rarefaction clicks. *Biophysical Journal, 2,* 23.

Pratt, H., Bleich, N., et al. (1985). Three-channel Lissajous' trajectory of human auditory brainstem potentials I. Normative measures. *Electroencephalography and Clinical Neurophysiology, 61,* 530–538.

Prosser, S. and Arslan, E. (1987). Prediction of auditory brainstem response wave V latency as a diagnostic tool of sensorineural hearing loss. *Audiology, 26,* 179–187.

Prosser, S., Arslan, E., et al. (1983). Evaluation of the monaurally evoked brainstem response in the diagnosis of sensorineural hearing loss. *Scandinavian Audiology, 12*, 103–106.

Rawool, V. and Zerlin, S (1988). Phase-intensity effects on the ABR. *Scandinavian Audiology, 17*, 117–123.

Reid, A. and Thornton, A. (1983). The effects of contralateral masking upon brainstem electric responses. *British Journal of Audiology, 17*, 155–162.

Rosenhall, U., Bjorkman, G., et al. (1985). Brain-stem auditory evoked potentials in different age groups. *Electroencephalography and Clinical Neurophysiology, 62*, 426–430.

Rosenhamer, H., Lindstrom, B., et al. (1978). On the use of click-evoked electric brainstem responses in audiological diagnosis. *Scandinavian Audiology, 7*, 117–123.

Rosenhamer, H., Lindstrom, B., et al. (1980). On the use of click-evoked electric brainstem responses in audiological diagnosis. II. The influence of sex and age upon the normal response. *Scandinavian Audiology, 9*, 93–100.

Rosenhamer, H., Lindstrom, B., et al. (1981). On the use of click-evoked electric brainstem responses in audiological diagnosis. III. Latencies in cochlear hearing loss. *Scandinavian Audiology, 10*, 3.

Rossi, G., Solero, P., et al. (1979). Brain stem electric response audiometry. *Acta Otolaryngologica, 364*, 2–13.

Rowe, M. I. (1978). Normal variability of the brain-stem auditory evoked response in young and old adult subjects. *Electroencephalography and Clinical Neurophysiology, 44*, 459–470.

Salamy, A., McKean, C., et al. (1978). Auditory brainstem response recovery process from birth to adulthood. *Psychophysiology, 15*, 214–220.

Salamy, A., McKean, C., et al. (1975). Maturational changes in auditory transmission as reflected in human brain stem potentials. *Brain Research, 96*, 361–366.

Salt, A. and Thornton, A. (1984). The effects of stimulus rise-time and polarity on the auditory brainstem responses. *Scandinavian Audiology, 13*, 119–127.

Sanders, J., Ed. (1991). Clinical masking. *Hearing assessment*. Austin, TX: Pro-ed.

Sanders, J. and Rintelmann, W. (1964). Masking in audiometry. *Archives of Otolaryngology, 80*, 541–556.

Scherg, M. and von Cramon, D. (1985). A new interpretation of the generators of BAEP waves IV: Results of a spatiotemporal dipole model. *Electroencephalography and Clinical Neurophysiology, 62*, 290–299.

Schimmel, H. (1967). The (±) reference: Accuracy of estimated mean components in averaged response studies. *Science, 157*, 92–94.

Schwartz, D. (1987). Neurodiagnostic audiology: Contemporary perspectives. *Ear and Hearing, 8 (Suppl. 4)*, 43S–48S.

Schwartz, D. and Berry, G. (1985). Normative aspects of the ABR. *The auditory brainstem response*, First ed., 65–97. San Diego, CA: College-Hill Press.

Schwartz, D., Larson, V., et al. (1985). Spectral characteristics of air and bone conduction transducers used to record the auditory brainstem response. *Ear and Hearing, 6(5)*, 274–277.

Schwartz, D. and Morris, M. (1991). Strategies for optimizing the detection of neuropathology from the auditory brainstem response. *Diagnostic audiology*. Austin, TX: Pro-ed.

Schwartz, D., Morris, M., et al. (1990). Influence of click polarity on the auditory brainstem response (BAER) revisited. *Electroencephalography and Clinical Neurophysiology, 77*, 445–457.

Schwartz, D., Pratt, R., et al. (1989). Auditory brainstem responses in preterm infants: Evidence of peripheral maturity. *Ear and Hearing, 10*, 14–22.

Schwartz, D. and Schwartz, J. (1991). Auditory evoked potentials in clinical pediatrics. *Hearing assessment*. Austin, TX: Pro-ed.

Selters, W. and Brackmann, D. (1977). Acoustic tumor detection with brain stem electric response audiometry. *Archives of Otolaryngology, 103*, 181–187.

Sininger, Y., Gardi, J., et al. (1987). The 3-channel Lissajous' trajectory of the auditory brainstem response. VII. Planar segments in humans. *Electroencephalography and Clinical Neurophysiology, 68*, 368–379.

Sininger, Y. S. and Masuda, A. (1990). Effect of click polarity on ABR threshold. *Ear and Hearing, 11(3)*, 206–209.

Sohmer, H. and Feinmesser, M. (1967). Cochlear action potentials recorded from the external ear in man. *Annals of Otology, Rhinology, and Laryngology, 76*, 427–435.

Stapells, D. (1989). Auditory brainstem response assessment of infants and children. *Assessing auditory system integrity in high-risk infants and young children*. J. Gravel, 10, 229–251. New York: Thieme Medical Publishers, Inc.

Starr, A., Amlie, R., et al. (1977). Development of auditory function in newborn infants revealed by auditory brainstem potentials. *Pediatrics, 60*, 831–839.

Starr, A. and Squires, K. (1982). Distribution of auditory brain stem potentials over the scalp and nasopharynx in humans. *Annals of the New York Academy of Science, 388*, 427–442.

Stockard, J. and Rossiter, K. (1977). Clinical and pathologic correlates of brainstem auditory evoked response abnormality. *Neurology, 27*, 316–325.

Stockard, J., Stockard, J., et al. (1983). Auditory brain stem response variability in infants. *Ear and Hearing, 4*, 11–23.

Stockard, J., Stockard, J., et al. (1978). Nonpathologic factors influencing brainstem auditory evoked potentials. *American Journal of EEG Technology, 18,* 177.

Telian, S. and Kileny P. (1989). Usefulness of 1000 Hz toneburst evoked responses in the diagnosis of acoustic neuroma. *Otolaryngology—Head and Neck Surgery, 101,* 466–471.

Terkildsen, K., Osterhamel, P., et al. (1973). Electrocochleography with a far-field technique. *Scandinavian Audiology, 2,* 141.

Tietze, G. and Pantev, C. (1986). Comparison between auditory brainstem responses evoked by rarefaction and condensation step functions and clicks. *Audiology, 25,* 44.

Turner, R., (ed.) (1991). Making clinical decisions. *Hearing assessment.* Austin, TX: Pro-ed.

Tyner, F., Knott, J., et al. (1983). *Fundamentals of EEG technology: Basic concepts and methods.* New York: Raven Press.

Van Campen, L., Sammeth, C., et al. (1990). Interaural attenuation using Etymotic ER-3A insert earphones in auditory brain stem response testing. *Ear and Hearing, 11(1),* 66–69.

van der Drift, J., Brocaar, M., et al. (1987). The relation between the pure-tone audiogram and the click auditory brainstem response threshold in cochlear hearing loss. *Audiology, 26,* 1–10.

Weber, B. (1982). Comparison of auditory brain stem response latency norms for premature infants. *Ear and Hearing, 3,* 257–262.

Wilson, M., Kelly-Ballweber, D., et al. (1985). Binaural interaction in auditory brain stem responses: Parametric studies. *Ear and Hearing, 6,* 80–88.

Wrege, K. and Starr, A. (1981). Binaural interaction in human brainstem auditory evoked potentials. *Archives of Neurology, 38,* 572–580.

Zwislocki, J. (1974). A possible neuro-mechanical sound analysis in the cochlea. *Acoustica, 31,* 354–359.

Zwislocki, J. (1975). Phase opposition between inner and outer hair cells and auditory sound analysis. *Audiology, 14,* 443.

CHAPTER 7

THE AUDITORY MIDDLE LATENCY RESPONSE

CLINICAL USES, DEVELOPMENT, AND GENERATING SYSTEM

NINA KRAUS
THERESE McGEE
LASZLO STEIN

The middle latency response (MLR) consists of a series of auditory evoked potentials that occur between 10 and 80 ms following the onset of an acoustic stimulus. By definition, the MLR follows the ABR, precedes the late auditory evoked potentials, and is characterized by waves Na, Pa, and P1 (or Pb), occurring at latencies of 18, 30 and 50 ms, respectively (Figure 7.1). Using a non-cephalic reference, a positive component at about 45 ms (TP41) can be recorded over the temporal area (Cacace et al., 1990).

In this review, we will outline the clinical applications of the MLR as currently practiced, review the effects of maturation, discuss what is currently known about the generating system, and finally, project the future place of MLR in clinical and research activities.

CLINICAL USES OF THE MLR

The MLR is used clinically in the electrophysiologic determination of hearing thresholds in the lower frequency range, the assessment of cochlear implant function, the assessment of auditory pathway function, and the localization of auditory pathway lesions.

Assessment of Hearing Thresholds

For assessing higher frequency sensitivity in cases of peripheral hearing loss, the auditory brainstem response (ABR) is the test of choice when behavioral methods cannot be used. The ABR, however, is highly dependent on neural synchrony and is best elicited by stimuli, such as clicks, with a rapid onset. Lower frequency stimuli (500–1000 Hz) inherently have a slower onset and therefore elicit a poorly defined ABR. The response is small, particularly when there is sensorineural hearing loss, and may be undetectable in clinical situations. Since the MLR is less dependent than the ABR on neural synchrony (Vivion, Hirsch, Frye-Osier, and Goldstein, 1980), it can be valuable in the assessment of low frequency sensitivity. Figure 7.2 illustrates the use of the MLR as a test of low frequency hearing sensitivity in a patient with a moderate-to-severe sloping hearing loss. No ABR was obtained to either click or 500 Hz stimuli. The MLR provided the only electrophysiologic indication that this patient had hearing in the lower frequencies.

It has been demonstrated in adults that the MLR will accurately reflect low frequency hearing thresholds (Zerlin and Naunton, 1974; Musiek and Geurnink, 1981; Scherg and Volk 1983). The MLR in children is of chief interest, however, since an accurate electrophysiologic measure of low frequency hearing thresholds is essential to the appropriate management of hearing loss in children too young to be tested by behavioral audiometric methods. The information obtained is particularly important for children who have

The participation of Trent Nicol is gratefully acknowledged.
Supported by NIH grant #R01 DC 00264.

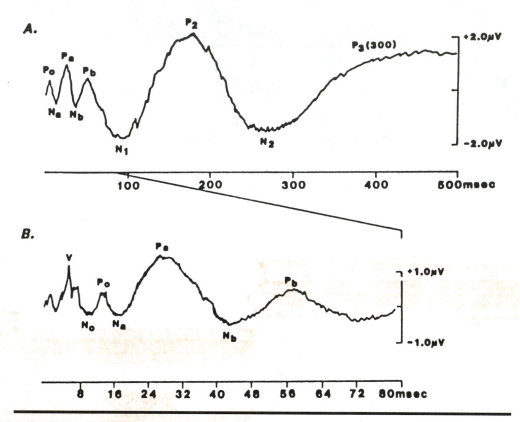

FIGURE 7.1.   Top: Representative evoked response showing the ABR, MLR and late potentials recorded from the vertex. Bottom: The post-stimulus epoch in which MLR waves are found is expanded for better visualization of MLR components.

residual hearing only in the low frequencies. For any hearing impaired child, knowledge of low frequency thresholds can be critical to the appropriate fitting of a hearing aid.

Since for practical reasons electrophysiologic testing is performed during sleep, the response must be reliable in sleeping children. Unfortunately, the MLR is only intermittently obtained in young children during certain stages of sleep. When the MLR is present, it provides information about low frequency hearing sensitivity. But the variability of the response even in normal children is such that the absence of a response cannot be interpreted as an indication of hearing loss if sleep stage is not monitored. Indeed, as will be discussed further in the development section of this chap-

ter, this inconsistency has been, although need not continue to be, a major factor limiting the clinical use of the MLR with children.

Clinical Procedure for Threshold Evaluation.   Our protocol for the evaluation of hearing sensitivity involves both the ABR and MLR (Kraus and McGee 1990a). Because many of our patients potentially have neurologic problems, the click-evoked ABR is used to assess the function of the brainstem. The click-evoked ABR is also used to assess hearing for the higher frequencies. Then we obtain both the ABR and the MLR in response to 500 Hz tone bursts as a measure of hearing sensitivity for the lower frequencies. The ABR and MLR are recorded simultaneously, either on separate

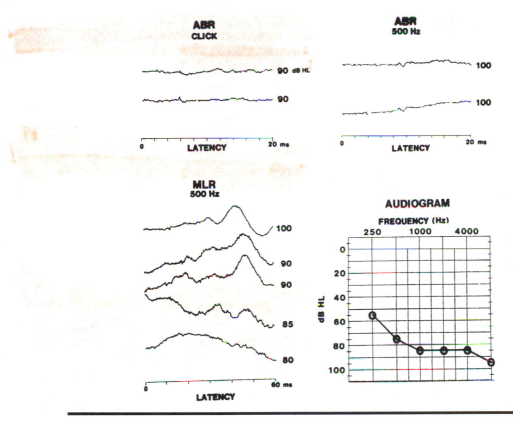

FIGURE 7.2.   ABR and MLR recordings from a patient with a moderate-to-severe sloping hearing loss. No ABR was obtained for either click or 500 Hz stimuli. The MLR threshold of 85 dB HL reflects this patient's hearing for the lower frequencies.

channels, or using a single channel, with a recording system having a fast sampling rate (<20 μsec/pt), and the capability to expand the initial portion of the 60–100 ms recording epoch. The primary differences between an MLR protocol and a typical ABR protocol are the wider filter settings and longer time base required for the MLR. The equipment settings for recording the MLR are summarized in Table 7.1.

Clinical experience over the past 10 years has indicated this procedure to be effective in predicting degree and configuration of hearing loss. We expect that a theoretical approach involving mathematical models (McGee, Kraus, and Wolters, 1988) will allow further refinement of the clinical protocol and more precise prediction of hearing thresholds.

Measuring Threshold when Neural Synchrony is Impaired.   Since the ABR is highly dependent on neural synchrony within the brainstem auditory pathway, damage can result in an abnormal or absent response. This occurs even when the peripheral hearing mechanism is functional, for example in infants sustaining diffuse neurologic damage as a consequence of perinatal asphyxia, hyperbilirubinemia or head trauma (Worthington and Peters, 1980; Kraus, Özdamar, Stein, and Reed, 1985). Nevertheless, the MLR can often be recorded in these patients. An example is illustrated in Figure 7.3. Although the ABR is absent, the click-evoked MLR reflects the patient's audiologic threshold of 30 dB HL. Kavanaugh, Gould, McCormick, and Franks (1989) obtained click-evoked MLRs in four

TABLE 7.1.   Stimulus and Recording Parameters
for Middle Latency Response

ELECTRODES

G1: Cz

G2: ipsi mastoid or earlobe

Ground: forehead

STIMULI

Monaural rarefaction clicks

Monaural tone bursts

        Envelope: 2–1–2 ms with linear ramp or
                     2–0–2 ms with Blackman ramp

RECORDING PARAMETERS

Time base: 60, 80 or 100 ms

Low filter:

    Adults: 3–15 Hz

    Children: 10–15 Hz

High filter: 2–3 kHz

Filter slope: 6 or 12 dB/octave or digital filtering

Rate: 11/sec

SIMULTANEOUS ABR AND MLR RECORDING

Computer capabilities to:

    1. record with a dual time base or
    2. record time window suitable for the MLR
        and expand initial segment to view ABR

---

hearing-impaired, multiply handicapped patients lacking ABRs. Although the peripheral hearing mechanism or the brainstem pathway may have been deficient in the synchrony necessary to produce an ABR, the MLR provided information about hearing sensitivity.

Assessment of Hearing in Patients with Cochlear Implants

Both ABR and MLR can be elicited by electric as well as acoustic stimuli. Termed the electrical auditory brainstem response (EABR) and the electrical middle latency response (EMLR), these electrically evoked potentials are proving useful with cochlear implant patients in the preoperative assessment of surviving neural elements of the central auditory system and as an objective measure of threshold and comfort level settings postoperatively.

The waveform morphology of the EABR and EMLR are similar to the acoustically elicited responses except that absolute latencies are shorter. Because an electrical artifact extends into the time-frame of the ABR thereby disrupting the ABR, the EMLR, which occurs after the artifact, has been suggested as the electrically evoked potential of choice for cochlear implant assessment (Gardi, 1985; Miyamoto, 1986; Kileny and Kemink, 1987).

MLR as Measure of Auditory Pathway Function

In the case discussed above (Figure 7.3), the presence of an MLR combined with the absence of an ABR implies dysfunction of the auditory brainstem pathways. Thus, a normal MLR rules out peripheral hearing loss as the cause of an abnormal ABR and thereby aids in the identification of auditory brainstem abnormalities.

The MLR is also useful in assessing damage to the higher auditory pathway. With unilateral auditory cortex lesions, the amplitude of wave Pa is diminished or absent over the lesioned hemisphere (Kraus et al., 1982; Scherg and von Cramon, 1986; Kileny et al., 1987). Testing requires the use of a coronal montage with electrodes at Cz and over each temporal lobe (halfway between Cz and the mastoid). An example of the response using a coronal electrode montage with a patient having left temporal lobe damage is shown in Figure 7.4.

The hemispheric asymmetry in these cases has sparked speculation that the scalp topography of the MLR holds clinical information. Fueling the speculation is the availability of brain mapping systems which allow recording and visualization of the scalp topography in a clinically practical manner (Kraus and McGee, 1988; Jacobson and Grayson, 1988; Pool et al., 1989; Kraus and McGee, 1990, review). For wave Pa, the analysis of interhemispheric symmetry can be used to assess abnormal response patterns. Figure 7.5 (see color plate) hows a top view of the scalp topography at the latency of Pa showing a normal (top, left) and an abnormal response (top, middle). When right hemispheric Pa values are subtracted from left hemispheric values, the resulting

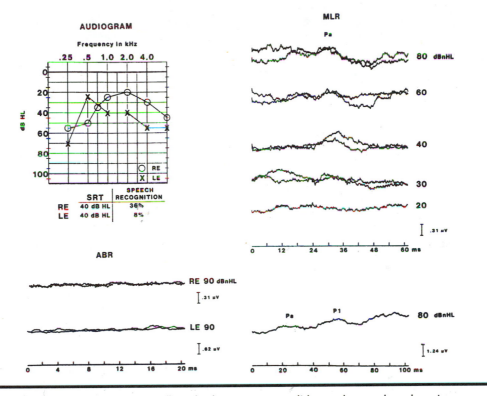

FIGURE 7.3.   Damage to the auditory brainstem can result in an abnormal or absent response, even when behavioral hearing thresholds show a mild or moderate hearing loss. The MLR often can still be recorded in these patients. In the example, although the ABR is absent, the click-evoked MLR reflects the patient's audiologic threshold of 30 dB HL. (Reprinted with permission from Kraus and McGee, 1990).

map is green, indicating little interhemispheric difference in normal subjects (bottom, left). The interhemispheric Pa amplitude difference is illustrated for an abnormal-looking map (bottom, middle). When these differences are compared to the normal population using the Z statistic, this subject's data falls outside 2 standard deviations at several electrode locations (right).

There are indications that alternative electrode configurations will yield additional human MLR components. Specifically, using a non-cephalic reference, a positive component at about 45 ms (TP41) can be recorded over the temporal area (Cacace et al., 1990).

Wave P1 (or Pb) has also been investigated an index of auditory pathway dysfunction. This wave is thought to reflect activity of the reticular activating system which modulates attention to sensory stimuli (Buchwald et al., 1981; Hinman and Buchwald, 1983; Erwin and Buchwald, 1986). Abnormalities of this MLR component have been associated with Alzheimer's disease (Buchwald et al., 1989), autism (Buchwald et al., 1988), schizophrenia (Erwin et al., 1988), and stuttering (Hood et al., 1987). P1 is also affected by handedness (Hood et al., 1989), which may suggest some modulatory influence from the cortex.

Summary of Clinical Uses

Clinical uses of the MLR include the electrophysiological determination of hearing thresholds for low frequencies, the assessment of hearing thresholds in patients

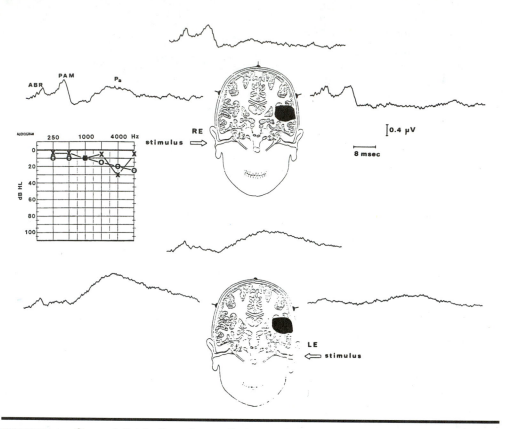

FIGURE 7.4.   Coronal distribution of wave Pa in a patient with a left temporo-parietal lesion and severe Wernicke's aphasia. Pa was largest over the intact hemisphere as compared to the vertex, and absent over the lesioned side, regardless of the ear stimulated. The patient's pure tone audiogram is shown on the left. "PAM" refers to posterior auricular muscle activity. (Reprinted with permission from Kraus, Özdamar, Hier, and Stein, *Electroencephalography and Clinical Neurophysiology, 54*, 275–287, 1982).

with abnormal ABRs due to neurological damage to the brainstem, and in the pre- and post-operative management of patients with cochlear implants. The MLR can be used in the localization of auditory pathway lesions and in the diagnosis of syndromes that compromise the MLR generating system.

However, two factors have limited the clinical use of the MLR:

1. As a hearing test for children, use of the MLR is hampered by the variability of the response in subjects younger than 12 years of age.

2. As a test of central brainstem function, interpretation of MLR results is limited by an incomplete understanding of the MLR generating system.

These facets of the MLR will be explored in the following sections. In the "Development" section we describe how the MLR changes with maturation, and the factors which influence MLRs in children. Data on the effects of sleep indicate that it may be possible to overcome the limitations which have faced the use of the MLR in pediatric populations. The "MLR Generating System" section is a review of both human and animal studies aimed at identifying the anatomic structures which contribute to the response.

DEVELOPMENT

Efforts to electrophysiologically assess low frequency thresholds are directed at very young, difficult to test patients. However, numerous studies have demonstrated that the MLR is obtained inconsistently in children (Engel, 1971; Skinner and Glattke, 1977; Okitsu, 1984; Hirabayashi, 1979; Suzuki et al., 1983a; Kraus et al., 1985; Stapells et al., 1988). Most of these studies have focused on wave Pa, which is reliable and robust in adults.

From birth to adolescence, the detectability of wave Pa increases monotonically, from 20% at birth to 90% at 12 years of age (Kraus, Smith, Reed, Stein, and Cartee, 1985). The response follows a systematic developmental course, and the trend of increased detectability with age exists regardless of whether the child is normally developing or has any of a wide range of neurologic, cognitive, or speech and language disorders. A trend of increased MLR detectability with age has also been observed in the more controlled context of an animal model (Kraus, Smith, McGee, Stein, and Cartee, 1987; Kraus, Smith, and McGee, 1987; Kraus, Smith, and McGee, 1988). Figure 7.6 shows the improved MLR detectability observed with age in humans and gerbils. Thus, both human and animal data suggest that a systematic developmental process underlies the detectability of MLR waves.

Factors that Influence MLRs in Children—Rate, Filtering, Sleep

Various factors have been considered in attempts to elicit the response more reliably in children. It appears that response filtering, stimulus repetition rate, and sleep stage all significantly influence the amplitude, latency and/or detectability of Pa in children.

Recording Filters

Ideally, filtering the neural activity will eliminate activity extraneous to the response, without distorting the response of interest. Differences in the adult and child EEG have led to the expectation that the testing of children requires special considerations in the choice of filtering parameters.

Low Filter Setting. Suzuki and colleagues (1983, 1984) reported that MLR variability in both children and adults can be reduced when EEG activity below 20 Hz is filtered out, although settings higher than 20 Hz caused unacceptable amplitude reductions in the child MLR. In a study of 217 children, Kraus et al. (1987a) examined MLR detectability, amplitude, and latency using two filtering conditions: 1) 3–2000 Hz with a 6 dB/octave slope and 2) 15–2000 Hz with a 12 dB/octave slope. In all age groups studied, the detectability of waves Na and Pa was better with highpass filter settings of 15 Hz than with lower settings. These results are consistent with the hypothesis that large amplitude, low frequency EEG activity obscures MLRs in children. That is, the MLR may be masked out by EEG activity in the 3–15 Hz range.

The amplitude of MLR waves increases as filter settings are lowered from 30 to 3 Hz, in human adults (McGee et al., 1987) and in developing experimental animals (Kraus, Smith, and McGee, 1987). In children, no trends are obvious.

Although a high-pass filter setting of 10–15 Hz can enhance MLR in children, it does not solve the problem of response liability. Even with optimum filter settings, response detectability varies with sleep, as will be discussed below.

High Filter Setting and Filter Slope. Two other technical issues arise with filtering. One concerns the high filter setting. The spectral energy for the MLR lies below 100 Hz, and no significant changes in the morphology or latency of Pa are seen with settings greater than 300 Hz (McGee, Kraus, and Manfredi, 1983). However, when the equipment is available, it is often desirable to open the filters to 2000–3000 Hz to allow simultaneous recording of the ABR (Suzuki et al., 1981; Özdamar and Kraus, 1983).

The second issue concerns the slope of the response filter. Izumi (1980), Scherg (1982), and Kraus, Smith, and McGee (1987) demonstrated that steep (24–48 dB/

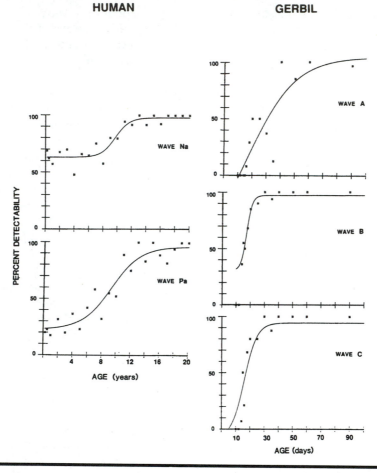

FIGURE 7.6. Percent detectability of MLR waves in humans (left) and gerbils (right) are shown as a function of age. Mean percent detectability was averaged across subjects in a given age group. A least squares nonlinear curve fitting procedure was used to obtain the curve of best fit (solid line). (Modified from Kraus, Smith, Reed, Stein, and Cartee, 1985. *Electroencephalography and Clinical Neurophysiology, 62*, 343–351; and Kraus, Smith, and McGee, 1987. *Hearing Research, 27*, 164–176).

octave) analog filtering causes distortion of the MLR and the emergence of non-physiologic peaks. That is, in patients with no MLR, the steep filters produce an MLR-like artifact. This artifact may be a distorted ABR and for this reason correlates with the presence of hearing. However, the ABR is better recorded with the filter settings usually recommended. In recording the

MLR, analog filtering of 6 or 12 dB/octave yields an undistorted waveform.

Stimulus Rate

The MLR is generally obtained at a rate of 10/sec (Picton et al., 1974), but there has been speculation that slowing down the stimulation rate may make the response more detectable in children. In adults there is a trend towards increasing amplitude with slower stimulation rates (McFarland et al., 1975; Picton et al., 1974). In experimental animals, some MLR waves also follow this trend (Buchwald et al., 1981; McGee, Özdamar, and Kraus, 1983; Knight et al., 1985), with a concurrent increase in detectability (Kraus, Smith, and McGee, 1987).

Jerger et al. (1987) describe a rate-dependent peak at about 50 ms in human infants which they suggest is a developmentally early version of Pa. It is observed at rates of 1–2/sec but seldom observed at rates above 4/sec. Also possible is that this peak may represent component P1 which is extremely rate sensitive even in adults (Erwin and Buchwald, 1986b). Our own experience is that slowing the rate enhances neither the detectability nor amplitude of wave Pa in children consistently. Nevertheless, we take the clinically conservative approach of reducing rate for cases in which the MLR is difficult to detect.

The issue of a clinically optimal rate remains controversial. Does the possibility of obtaining a larger response or increasing the likelihood of detection justify the additional time involved in obtaining the response at slower stimulation rates? As a practical matter, it is most efficient to begin with a fast stimulation rate. If no response is obtained, the rate may be reduced until a response is found.

The 40 Hz Response.   An exception to the general trend of decreasing amplitude with increasing stimulation rate occurs at a rate of 40/sec. This rate produces larger amplitude responses than are observed at slower rates (Galambos et al., 1981a; Suzuki et al., 1984; Stapells et al., 1984; Kileny and Shea, 1976).

This effect may be due to a superimposition of ABR and MLR waves, which are typically 21–25 ms apart in adults. Suzuki and Kobayashi (1984) found that in children, an amplitude maximum occurred at rates of 20–30/sec, corresponding with an average ABR-Pa latency difference of 31 ms observed in those children.

The 40 Hz response may be more than just a superimposition of waves, however. A 40 Hz response can also be elicited by visual and somatosensory stimuli (Galambos, 1981b). Possibly, the 40 Hz response is produced by generators different from those of the MLR and the ABR.

Sleep

Maturational changes in the EEG are known to occur during the first decade of life, when the MLR is variable (Feinberg and Carlson, 1968; Feinberg, 1974; Neidermeyer, 1982). The EEG and MLR frequency spectra overlap more in children than in adults. Consequently, the EEG may mask out the MLR in children, making it less detectable. However, the changes in the EEG and the MLR may be indicative of a more fundamental process involving the development of generators specific to both.

The EEG is the summation of widespread neural activity. As discussed below, the MLR, as well, is produced by multiple brain areas, some cortical and some subcortical. The MLR generating system includes auditory regions such as the thalamo-cortical pathway and other structures such as reticular formation, which modulate the general state of arousal and receptiveness to sensory input. If variations in the EEG, particularly during sleep, indicate changes in the activation of contributing centers, variations in the MLR during sleep may also indicate variations in the relative activation of components of the MLR generating system (reviewed in Kraus and McGee, 1993).

Since MLRs are obtained sometimes in infants, there must be certain periods during the recording session when the MLR generating system is active. Several investigators have suggested that sleep affects the detectability of MLR in children (Suzuki, Kobayashi, and Hirabayashi, 1983; Suzuki, Hirabayashi, and Kobayashi, 1983; Kileny, 1983; Kraus, Smith, Reed, Stein, and Cartee, 1985). This connection is important clinically, since recording could be concentrated at those times most likely to produce an MLR. This possibility motivated us to study the problem in a small cohort of children (Kraus, McGee, and Comperatore, 1989).

Simultaneous ABR, MLR, and EEG recordings were obtained in 6 children ranging in age from 4 to 9 years. The percent detectability (# present/# recordings) of wave Pa was calculated for each of the following arousal states: (a) wakefulness, (b) alpha and stage 1, (c) stages 2 and 3, (d) stage 4, and (e) REM sleep.

In this group of children, Pa was consistently detected during wakefulness, alpha, stage 1, and REM sleep. During stages 2 and 3, detectability was variable, while in stage 4, detectability was consistently poorer. Waveforms representative of the occurrence of wave Pa (during wakefulness, stage 1, or REM sleep) and of its absence (during stage 4) in the same subject, within the same recording session are shown in Figure 7.7.

Figure 7.8 shows the percent detectability of wave Pa for each child as a function of sleep state. Detectability was consistently high during wakefulness, alpha, stage 1, and REM sleep (81.8% to 100% detectability), poor during stage 4 (4.2% to 70%), and variable during stages 2 and 3. This is consistent with reports that Pa amplitude is largest during active (REM) sleep and smallest during quiet sleep (stages 3 and 4) (Osterhammel, Shallop, and Terkildsen, 1985; Collett et al., 1988). For the younger children (ages 4–6 years), the differences in detectability were dramatic, with Pa detectability being very low (<23.1%) during stage 4. The older children (ages 7–9 years) showed better Pa detectability in stage 4 (54.5%–70.0%). Thus, even in an unfavorable stage, there was a

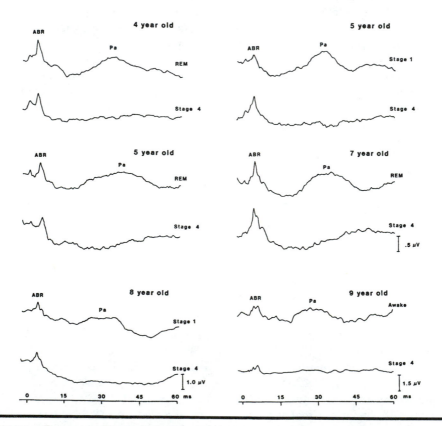

FIGURE 7.7. Representative waveforms showing presence of wave Pa during stages favorable for Pa, wakefulness, stage 1 and REM, and the absence of Pa during the stage unfavorable for Pa, stage 4. Representative waveforms are shown for each child. (Reprinted from Kraus, McGee, and Comperatore, *Ear and Hearing, 10*, 339–345. © Williams & Wilkins, 1989).

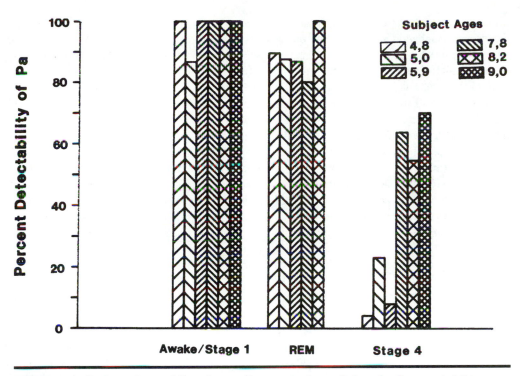

FIGURE 7.8. Percent detectability of wave Pa versus stage of sleep for 6 normal children. Each bar pattern denotes an individual child. Children's ages, in years and months, are shown. Detectability of wave Pa was high during wakefulness, stage 1, and REM sleep, and lower during stage 4. During stage 4, wave Pa was more likely to be present in the older children. (Reprinted from Kraus, McGee, and Comperatore, *Ear and Hearing, 10*, 339–345. © Williams & Wilkins, 1989).

trend toward increased Pa detectability with age (Kraus, Smith, Reed, Stein, and Cartee, 1985).

Clinical Implications of Sleep Data. It appears that the MLR is present only in certain sleep states. Very likely, effective clinical use will involve concentrating efforts to elicit the response during these optimal periods.

The most direct approach would involve signaling the clinician when the patient enters a sleep stage unfavorable for MLR recording, for example, signaling the presence of delta waves, a chief characteristic of stage 4 sleep (McGee et al., 1993; Kraus and McGee, 1993). Evoked potential recording equipment should incorporate a means to signal the clinician accordingly. Since

every auditory evoked potential protocol for the assessment of hearing requires recording of the ABR, the clinician could obtain the ABR when conditions were unfavorable for the MLR and concentrate MLR recording during optimal periods.

Mechanisms Underlying MLR Variability in Children

Maturational Sleep Effects. There is general agreement that sleep does not impede Pa detectability in adults, as it does in children. Some studies have reported the absence of any sleep effects on adult MLRs (Mendel and Goldstein, 1969; Mendel, 1974; Mendel and Kupperman, 1974; Picton et al., 1974; Mosko et al., 1984; Erwin and Buchwald, 1986a), while others have reported sleep-related amplitude and latency changes (Okitsu, 1984; Osterhammel, Shallop, and Terkildsen, 1985; Brown, 1982). Interestingly, Erwin and Buchwald (1986), who showed that Pa amplitude is virtually unaffected during stage 4 sleep in adults, obtained their data at slow stimulation rates, while the changes observed by Osterhammel et al. (1985) were observed with faster stimulation rates. In adults, 40 Hz responses are more affected by sleep than the ABR or MLR. This suggests that Pa in adults may consist of subcomponents that are differentially rate sensitive.

Developmental sleep stage studies by Feinberg and Carlson (1968) show a decrease in stage 4 sleep as well as an increase in wakefulness with age during the period of a night's sleep. These changes may account, in part, for the systematic increasing detectability of wave Pa with age. Still, even within stage 4, detectability improves with age. This improved detectability combined with decreased time in stage 4 sleep may account for the dramatic differences in Pa detectability seen between infants and adults.

Maturation of the Generating System—Early and Late Developing Components.   Below, we review the contribution of the auditory thalamo-cortical pathway and subcortical centers to the generation of the MLR. These results, combined with the data on MLR development, have led us to speculate that generators involving the primary auditory thalamo-cortical pathway are responsible for the robust MLR typically seen in adults and are always active (Kraus et al., 1988). Other inconsistently active generators such as the reticular formation and the non-primary auditory pathway also contribute to the response. Without the primary pathway contribution, the response comes and goes depending upon the patient's level of alertness.

We propose that in adults it is the primary thalamo-cortical pathway that imparts stability to the response, making it consistently detectable regardless of sleep stage. In children, this system is only partially developed, not reaching maturity until puberty. The observed MLR is then dominated by the other, more labile generators. There is evidence that myelinization of the human thalamo-cortical pathway and sensory

cortex continues until puberty (Yakovlev and Lecours 1967; Rabinowicz et al., 1977). The systematic development of MLR components observed in humans is consistent with such a maturational process (Kraus, Smith, and Reed, 1985). Therefore development of the temporal lobe and the auditory thalamo-cortical pathway may account for increases in detectability with age.

Data from gerbils support this division of generators into an early developing labile generating system and another later developing stable system. As will be described below, certain animal models allow the MLR to be broken down into component parts that represent contributions from distinct generating systems. In gerbils, one set of waveforms develops earlier than the other (Kraus, Smith, and McGee, 1987; Kraus, Smith, and McGee, 1988). One set of waves attains adult amplitude and becomes consistently detectable during the first postnatal month. A second set of components matures later, with amplitude reaching full adult values by 3 months, incidentally the same time when the gerbil is considered to be adult. The development of MLR components is shown in Figure 7.9. It is the later developing waves that have been linked closely to the primary auditory thalamo-cortical pathway. The early developing waves have been linked to the function of the reticular formation and the non-primary auditory system (McGee et al., 1991; Kraus et al., 1992).

Summary

Major clinical applications of the MLR are directed toward infants and children. Because the child MLR differs dramatically from the adult MLR, the maturation of the response is of considerable clinical interest. Wave Pa shows a systematic increase in detectability with age, and detectability correlates with sleep stage. Maturation of the generating system can be thought of as involving an early developing, variable response that is highly influenced by the reticular formation and a later developing, stable system dominated by the auditory thalamo-cortical pathway. Effective clinical use will involve concentrating efforts to elicit the MLR during optimal states of arousal. Evoked potential recording equipment should incorporate a means to sig-

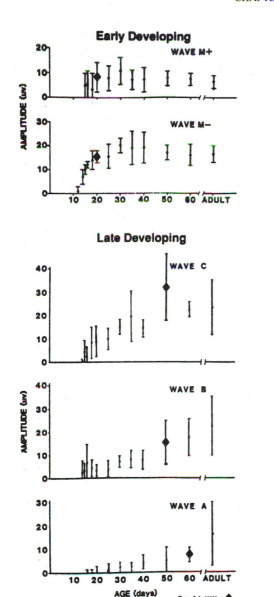

FIGURE 7.9. Amplitudes are shown for all MLR components in the gerbil as a function of age. The largest symbol in each graph represents the age at which amplitudes reached adult levels. Early developing waves (M−, M+) reached adult amplitude levels on day 20. Later developing wave A reached adult levels on day 60 while waves B and C reached adult levels on day 50. (Reprinted from Kraus, Smith, and McGee, 1988, *Electroencephalography and Clinical Neurophysiology, 71,* 541–558)

nal the clinician when conditions are favorable for MLR recording in children. The development of such a system is a research focus in our laboratory.

MLR GENERATING SYSTEM

Historically, each MLR wave has been studied as if it derived from a particular anatomic structure. However, it is likely that the MLR waves are the product of a complex system involving the interaction of many brain structures. The MLR generating system includes auditory specific structures central to and possibly including the inferior colliculus as well as structures outside the primary auditory pathway such as the reticular formation and multi-sensory divisions of the thalamus.

Human Research

Auditory Thalamo-Cortical Pathway. The temporal lobe has been postulated as one contributor to wave Na on the basis of electric source analysis of neuromagnetic and evoked potential data (Scherg et al., 1990) and from data from patients with auditory thalamo-cortical and cortical lesions (Scherg and von Cramon 1986; Scherg et al., 1989; Jacobson et al., 1990).

Hypotheses regarding a temporal lobe origin for wave Pa are derived from studies reporting a polarity reversal across the Sylvian fissure (Vaughan and Ritter, 1970; Cohen, 1982; Celesia, 1968; Wood and Wolpaw, 1982; Lee et al., 1984) and from others showing intracranial responses at the latency of Pa (Chatrian et al., 1960, Ruhm et al., 1967, Lee et al., 1984). Applying a model developed for the late (80–300 ms) potentials to the amplitude distribution of the MLR in the coronal plane, Vaughan and Ritter (1970) and Özdamar and Kraus (1983) proposed bilateral, vertically oriented dipole sources located in the temporal lobes as generators for Pa. The model predicts the greatest Pa amplitude at the midline, where the activity of the two hypothetical generators sum. This is further supported by the dipole modeling of Scherg and von Cramon (1986).

Case studies of patients with cortical lesions have largely supported a temporal lobe or thalamo-cortical origin for wave Pa. In patients with unilateral temporal lobe lesions, the most consistent finding has been a reduction in wave Pa amplitude over the lesioned temporal lobe in comparison to the intact hemisphere (Kraus, Özdamar, Hier, and Stein, 1982; Kileny et al., 1987; Scherg and von Cramon, 1986; Pool et al., 1989).

Wave Pa is usually disrupted but not necessarily absent when bilateral temporal lesions are present (Graham et al., 1980; Özdamar, Kraus, and Curry, 1983; Parving et al., 1980; Rosati et al., 1982; Woods et al., 1987). The persistence of wave Pa following some bilateral temporal lobe lesions suggests that the thalamus or the projections from thalamus may contribute substantially to the response. Woods (1987) has argued that only those temporal lobe lesions which have also damaged the thalamo-cortical pathway produce wave Pa abnormalities. Also feasible is that the intact Pa observed in some patients with bitemporal lobe lesions reflects the activity of an MLR generating system outside the auditory pathway.

For wave TP41, a radially oriented temporal lobe generator has been suggested based on dipole modeling (Scherg and von Cramon, 1986), data from patients with cortical lesions (Knight et al., 1988), and neuromagnetic studies (Hari et al., 1987).

For wave P1, neuromagnetic studies (Makela and Hari, 1987), correspondences between magnetic fields and electrical potentials (Scherg et al., 1990), and data from patients with auditory pathway lesions (Scherg and von Cramon, 1986; Scherg et al., 1989) point to a temporal lobe source for this wave, although as will become evident, this area is not the only contributing source.

Reticular Formation.   As reviewed above, wave Pa, especially in children, is affected by arousal state and by inference is tied to the reticular formation (Osterhammel, Shallop, and Terkildsen, 1985; Collett et al., 1988; Kraus, McGee, and Comperatore, 1989).

Buchwald and colleagues (1981; Hinman and Buchwald, 1983; Erwin and Buchwald, 1986*a*; 1986*b*) suggest that wave P1 is generated by thalamic nuclei that receive essential input from the midbrain reticular activating system. This wave is affected by stages of sleep (Erwin and Buchwald, 1986*a*). Interestingly, they have found that abnormalities in the P1 rate function correlate with disorders affecting arousal state such as Alzheimer's disease (Buchwald et al., 1989), autism (Buchwald et al., 1988), and schizophrenia

(Erwin et al., 1988). The 40 Hz response, consisting partially of MLR activity, has also been tied to the reticular formation and is affected by sleep (Galambos et al., 1981).

Midbrain.   Evidence exists for both cortical and subcortical contributions to wave Na, which is sometimes considered a slow component of the ABR (the SN10). Subcortical origins have been postulated on theoretical grounds (Dieber et al., 1988), its resistance to cortical lesions (Kileny et al., 1987), and the existence of a large negative wave at the latency of Na that is recorded at the level of the inferior colliculi (Hashimoto, 1982).

Animal Research

Animal research provides the strongest evidence for a generating system consisting of contributions and interactions from multiple sources. The topography of the surface response in some animal models offers a distinct advantage over the human response in the study of the MLR generating system. Human wave Pa is largest over the vertex and frontal lobes (Picton et al., 1974) and the scalp topography is such that both Na and Pa are obtained from widespread areas of the cortical surface (Kraus and McGee, 1990, 1988; Jacobson and Grayson, 1988). It appears that the multiple sources contributing to these waves are oriented such that they sum to produce one diffuse response, although there are indications that alternative electrode configurations will yield human MLR components with a more local topography (Cacace et al., 1990). However, Na and Pa show widespread activity.

In the cat, guinea pig, gerbil, chinchilla, and monkey, the MLR shows a complex distribution with components from different generating systems being well separated topographically (Kaga et al., 1980; Buchwald et al., 1981; Chen and Buchwald, 1986; Farley and Starr, 1983; Arezzo et al., 1975; Kraus, Smith, and McGee, 1988; Comperatore and Patterson, 1988).

An Animal Model.   In the guinea pig, two distinct MLR morphologies have been identified, one recorded over the temporal cortex and the other recorded over the posterior midline (McGee, Özdamar, and Kraus, 1983;

Kraus, Smith, and McGee, 1988). MLRs recorded from the surface of the temporal cortex exhibit a three component complex, beginning with a positive component at 12 ms (A), a negative component at 21 ms (B), and a positive component at 33 ms (C). MLRs recorded over the posterior midline are characterized by a negative component (M–), occurring at 10 ms followed by a positive component (M+), occurring at 20 ms.

The topography of these waves, referred to as "temporal" and "midline" components, is shown in Figure 7.10 (see color plate) where the MLR wave amplitude is expressed in color. Positive waves are shown in hues of red, negative responses in hues of blue, and voltages close to zero are expressed in green. The topographic maps illustrate the voltage measured at the latencies corresponding to each of these components. Areas of maximal MLR activity are the temporal lobe contralateral to the stimulated ear and the posterior midline.

The temporal and midline components differ in their response characteristics and appear to be mediated by distinct systems. The ABC complex is a large robust response, while the M–/M+ waveform is smaller in amplitude and more labile. Both the midline and temporal lobe responses can be affected by anesthetic agents, but often over different time courses. Rate functions are different for midline and temporal components; midline components do not change with stimulation rates of 1, 4, 10, 20, and 40/sec, whereas temporal component amplitudes decrease with increased stimulation rates (Kraus, Smith, and McGee, 1987). As reviewed above, in gerbils, maturation of the midline components precedes the temporal response. The differences in response and development indicate that the midline and temporal components reflect the activity of different generating systems, although the specific generators of these systems have yet to be identified. Additional experiments using this model are described below.

Auditory Thalamo-Cortical Pathway.   Ablation experiments in the cat have indicated that MLRs obtained over the temporal lobe are affected by lesions of the auditory cortex (Celesia, 1968, Kaga et al., 1980, Chen and Buchwald, 1986). Recent studies by Knight and Brailowsky (1990) identify a source in the auditory

thalamo-cortical pathway for one component and sources within primary auditory cortex for two other components that are best recorded over the temporal lobe. In the guinea pig, midline components persisted while temporal responses disappeared, both with unilateral and bilateral ablations of auditory cortex. In separate experiments, depth electrodes were used to make electrolytic lesions in auditory cortex at locations where polarity reversals occurred for wave A. The midline components persisted while the temporal components only were temporarily eliminated (Kraus, Smith, and McGee, 1988). This suggests both cortical and subcortical contributions for the MLR.

Thus, there are indications that the MLR generating system involves several brain areas. The questions then arise: Specifically what are the generators? What role does each play in producing the surface response? To investigate these questions, we utilized a technique in which lidocaine, a neural inactivating agent that functions by reducing membrane permeability to sodium, is injected into specific brain areas while simultaneous recordings of depth and surface activity are made. Local effects of intracranial microinjections are correlated with changes in the surface activity of the midline and temporal lobe components. The experiments described below have involved intracranial recording from the auditory cortex (AC), medial geniculate body of thalamus (MGB), the mesencephalic reticular formation (mRF), and the central nucleus of the inferior colliculus (IC) (McGee, Kraus, Comperatore, and Nicol, 1991; McGee et al., 1992; Kraus et al., 1992; Kraus and McGee, 1993, review).

Auditory Cortex.   Waveforms recorded from within auditory cortex are similar in latency and morphology to the surface temporal response. Representative waveforms are shown before and after the lidocaine injection in Figure 7.11 (see color plate), showing little effect of the injection. A 9-electrode device (Kraus, Jacobson, McGee, and Stark, 1988) was positioned in auditory cortex so as to record a polarity reversal of wave A as previously described (Smith and Kraus, 1988). Activity from the 9 electrodes at the latency of wave A is shown in Figure 7.11 (top). The polarity reversal can be visualized in color, where the positive wave (A) appears red and the waves showing reversed polarity at that latency appear blue. Lidocaine injection at this site resulted in no change in the responses measured by the 9 electrodes as illustrated by the color map (top). There were also no changes in surface potentials.

In general, pharmacologic inactivation of auditory cortex in the guinea pig did not disrupt waveform morphology although amplitude changes were observed with large volume injections (Kraus, Smith, and McGee, 1988). Since lidocaine injections interfered little with wave morphology but were associated with amplitude changes, one might speculate that the role of auditory cortex may be to modulate the MLR rather than to generate it. One could define modulation as an influence on response amplitude with no effect on response morphology. However, these findings do not rule out AC as a generator of MLR. An alternative interpretation is that the AC may be less sensitive to the effects of lidocaine than are other centers or the generators may be too large or too diffuse to be inactivated by discrete lidocaine injections.

Medial Geniculate Body.   Lidocaine injections into the ventral portion of the MGB disrupted the surface temporal response and eliminated MLR activity measured from auditory cortex. As shown in Figure 7.11 (bottom), inactivation of the MGB eliminated all activity measured from within auditory cortex. Also eliminated was the surface temporal response.

In Figure 7.12, the effects of a lidocaine injection into MGB are illustrated further. The amplitudes of surface and subcortical components were plotted over the course of the experiment. Lidocaine was injected into the ventral MGB after an initial baseline period, at time 0. Local amplitude reductions were seen in the MGB response following the injection. This was associated with the temporary disappearance of the three temporal components A, B, and C. The midline components were unchanged, as were the responses measured from the mesencephalic reticular formation and the inferior colliculus (McGee et al., 1991).

The relative contributions of the ventral (primary) and caudomedial (non-primary) subdivisions of the MGB were examined in another study (McGee et al.,

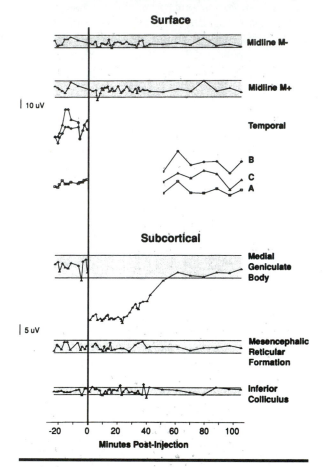

FIGURE 7.12.   Effects of lidocaine injection into the medial geniculate body on neural activity recorded simultaneously from multiple surface (midline, temporal) and subcortical (medial geniculate body, reticular formation, inferior colliculus) sites are shown. The amplitude of waveforms from these areas are plotted. Lidocaine was injected at point 0. Following the injection, wave amplitude reductions were seen in the MGB and the surface activity of the temporal components was disrupted (shown by the absence of data points). Midline surface components were unaffected, as were the responses from the mesencephalic reticular formation and the inferior colliculus. Shaded areas indicate the mean ± 2 sd of the baseline response amplitudes.

1992). The ventral MGB, a part of the primary auditory pathway, was found to contribute chiefly to the surface temporal response. The caudomedial MGB, which is linked to non-primary auditory pathways, contributed to both midline and temporal responses.

Thus it appears that the MGB or the thalamo-cortical pathway play an important role in the generation of the temporal response. Either the temporal component of the MLR is generated in the MGB, or the MGB provides critical input for cortical generation of the MLR.

Reticular Formation.   Several investigations in animal models have suggested that the mesencephalic reticular formation contributes to the generation of the MLR (Buchwald et al., 1981; Hinman and Buchwald, 1983; Molnár et al., 1988; Comperatore et al., 1989; Kraus et al., 1989). Based on ablation experiments and correlations between intracranial and surface recordings, the cat vertex component (22 ms) appears to be generated by ascending reticular formation in the midbrain and thalamus (Buchwald et al., 1981, Hinman and Buchwald, 1983). In humans, wave P1 has been shown to be affected by stages of sleep (Erwin and Buchwald, 1986*a*). The 40 Hz response, which consists partially of MLR activity, also has been linked to reticular formation activity and is affected by sleep even in adults (Galambos et al., 1981). In the reticular formation, decreases in neural activity have been reported during slow wave sleep with increases during REM sleep (Steriade et al., 1982). The surface recorded MLR components that are thought to reflect reticular formation activity in the cat have shown similar decreases in wave amplitude during slow wave sleep with increases during REM sleep (Chen and Buchwald 1986).

Lidocaine injections into the mRF of the guinea pig, affected both the midline and temporal responses (Kraus et al., 1992). The effects of lidocaine injections into the mesencephalic reticular formation are shown in Figure 7.13. The lidocaine injection simultaneously caused amplitude reductions in neural activity at the mRF and in both the midline and the temporal components. As with other injections associated with reductions in the temporal response, MGB activity was reduced. The IC response was unaffected.

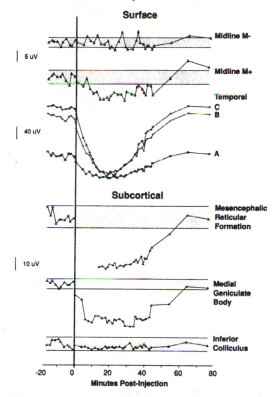

Lidocaine in Mesencephalic Reticular Formation

FIGURE 7.13.   Effects of lidocaine injections into the mesencephalic reticular formation on neural activity recorded simultaneously from multiple surface (midline, temporal) and subcortical (medial geniculate body, reticular formation, inferior colliculus) sites are shown. Following the injection, wave amplitude reductions were seen in the reticular formation and in the surface activity of both midline and temporal components. This injection also caused amplitude reductions in the medial geniculate body but left the inferior colliculus response unchanged. Shaded areas indicate the mean ± 2 sd of the baseline response amplitudes.

Midbrain.   The midbrain appears to be important to the generation of wave Na. Aspiration of the inferior colliculi in the guinea pig resulted in an amplitude reduction of the slow negative component following the ABR (Caird and Klinke, 1987).

Comparing effects over time (Figure 7.14), lidocaine injection into the inferior colliculus affected all of the waves both at surface and depth locations. Notice the widespread effects of the IC injection, including amplitude reductions over the temporal lobe, the MGB, and the mRF. The negative wave recorded from the IC electrode (at the same latency of surface wave M–), was most affected by the injection. The disruption of this wave correlated with the disruption of wave M–. We speculate that wave M– is the animal analogue of human wave Na.

Summarizing the lidocaine injection experiments in the guinea pig, the auditory primary thalamo-cortical pathway appears to play a critical role in the generation of temporal components A, B, and C. Still unclear are the relative roles of AC and MGB in the generation of the MLR. The mesencephalic reticular formation appears to influence both temporal and midline components, particularly the midline M+ response. The IC is likely to play a role in the generation of midline wave M–.

Summary

The multiple regions that contribute to the MLR include the auditory thalamo-cortical pathway, the mesencephalic reticular formation, and the inferior colliculus. In the guinea pig, two distinct MLR morphologies have been identified, one recorded over the temporal cortex and the other recorded over the posterior midline. These waves, referred to as "temporal" and "midline" components, appear to be mediated by distinct generating systems which differ both neuroanatomically and functionally. The midline components develop early, are rate resistant, variable over time, and sensitive to anesthetic agents. The midline response also persists following auditory cortex lesions. Temporal components develop later, are larger in amplitude, stable over time, rate sensitive, resistant to anesthetic agents, affected by auditory cortex lesions, and show significantly more binaural interaction than midline components. Pharmacologic inactivation of subdivisions of the medical geniculate body (ventral and caudomedial portions, MGv and MGcm, respectively) have revealed that the primary sensory pathway (MGv) selectively contributes to the

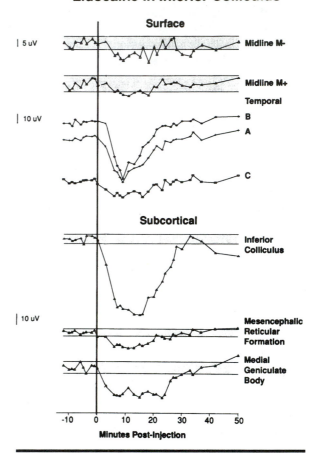

FIGURE 7.14.   Effects over time of lidocaine injection in IC on the amplitude of responses recorded simultaneously from multiple sites. The injection affected the amplitude of all surface and subcortical waves. Shaded areas denote the mean ± 2 sd of the baseline amplitudes.

temporal response while the non-primary afferent input (MGcm) contributes to both temporal and midline responses. The mesencephalic reticular formation appears to contribute to both components.

The inconsistency of the MLR in children when compared to adults also suggests that two components are involved in the human MLR. Scalp topography studies in normal adult subjects and patients with temporal lobe lesions support the concept of the involvement of the temporal lobes and/or thalamo-cortical pathway to the generation of wave Pa. Portions of the thalamo-cortical pathway that develop later in life appear to impart stability to the MLR. In children, Pa varies with sleep stage, possibly because at that age the MLR is dominated by the reticular formation and non-primary pathway activity.

These data are consistent with a model in which the MLR generating system receives contributions from both primary and non-primary auditory thalamo-cortical pathways, with reticular formation having a generalized activating effect on both systems. It is our speculation that primary and non-primary components are also present in the human MLR, and that the animal model has provided insights on how those components might be separated. The evaluation of primary and non-primary MLR components could have clinical implications. An assessment of the primary pathway may provide a neurophysiologic basis for evaluating specific aspects of central auditory processing. The non-primary pathway is likely to reflect different aspects of auditory processing. The non-primary pathway is likely to reflect different aspects of auditory processing as well as the modulation of attention and the integration of multi-modality information. A future challenge is to separate the contributions from these sources based on topography and response characteristics in humans so that dysfunction of components of the system can be identified clinically.

FUTURE DIRECTIONS

MLRs in Children

Since the MLR can be reliably obtained in children during certain arousal states, clinical use will become more practical if the clinician can be signaled when the patient is in a favorable state for obtaining the response. Research to develop this concept into its practical application and to validate it with clinical trials is necessary. At present, the MLR already provides information about low frequency hearing and auditory pathway function under appropriate conditions. In time it is likely to become more widely incorporated into the electrophysiologic battery.

Comprehensive Test Battery

As the ABR, MLR, and later cortical potentials have become more familiar to clinicians, there has been increasing speculation that it would be possible to develop a comprehensive electrophysiologic test of auditory pathway function. Although the technology for performing such a battery is available, more research is needed to ascertain the location of generators, and to correlate the evoked potential characteristics and patterns with the symptomatology and disorders they represent.

In addition to more information, there is a need for a more complex way of thinking about the clinical application of auditory evoked potentials. With the ABR, clinicians have worked hard to simplify the procedures and the concepts. Extraneous neural activity is filtered or averaged away. Abnormalities are expressed in narrowly-defined latency differences. Although the ABR is produced by multiple generators, for clinical interpretations, the generators are considered to be simple and sequential.

Very likely, the clinical use of MLR and the later potentials will not allow such simplifications. Even now, there is evidence that the MLR reflects functional damage to the thalamo-cortical pathway in adults and in children, but we must consider whether the patient is in an appropriate sleep/wakefulness state. Thus, contributions from the reticular formation must be considered, either by monitoring the EEG or by using a combination of electrodes that is sensitive to this contributing influence. Another evoked potential that reflects auditory thalamo-cortical activity, the mismatch negativity (Näätänen et al., 1978) is also likely to contribute to the clinical assessment of central auditory function (Kraus et al., 1993).

Almost every evoked potential wave represents activity from multiple contributing sources. These contributions tend to become more numerous and more complex the later the potentials occur in time. Lesion studies can be confusing because a lesion may interfere with a particular generator but the component may persist because it reflects activity from another contributing source which was not affected by the lesion. If a response persists even though the system is damaged, it is difficult to detect clinical abnormalities.

Probably compounding this difficulty is our tendency to record from a limited number of scalp locations. Typically, recordings are made only from the vertex. Likewise, reference sites are typically fixed at the mastoids. Yet the multiple components may have different optimal recording locations and reference sites.

If brain mapping allowed us to view the activity of the multiple aspects of the generating system simultaneously, then detailed analyses of scalp topography may allow a more sensitive detection of abnormalities. Mathematical analysis of topography, using techniques such as dipole source analysis (Scherg et al., 1989; Scherg and von Cramon, 1986), may allow better insight as to which generators are impaired.

This kind of thinking might also be helpful as a research tool in studying, for example, the contributions to the MLR generating system in children. This has been our approach using the animal model. This is also the approach we have taken in patients with cortical lesions in that rather than attend only to the MLR from the vertex, the relative amplitude of Pa at specific topographic locations is considered.

For such analysis, the placement of scalp electrodes need not conform to the conventional 10–20 montage, nor must the montage necessitate the use of a large number of electrodes. Clinically practical montages may include a few, well-placed electrodes. Much research may be required to determine which combinations of scalp electrodes will be important for deriving clinically meaningful information from individual auditory evoked components.

REFERENCES

Arezzo, J., Pickoff, A., and Vaughan, H.G. (1975). The sources and intracerebral distribution of auditory evoked potentials in the alert rhesus monkey. *Brain Research, 90,* 57–73.

Brown, D.D. (1971). The use of the middle latency response (MLR) for assessing low frequency auditory thresholds. *Journal of the Acoustical Society of America, 1,* 99.

Buchwald, J., Erwin, R., Schwafel, T., and Tanguay, P. (1988). Abnormal P1 potentials in autistic subjects. *Abstract, Neuroscience,* 771.

Buchwald, J.S., Erwin, R.J., Read, S., Van Lancker, D., and Cummings, J.L. (1989). Midlatency auditory evoked responses: Differential abnormality of P1 in Alzheimer's disease. *Electroencephalography and Clinical Neurophysiology, 74,* 378–384.

Buchwald, J.S., Hinman, C., Norman, R.S., Huang, C.M., and Brown, K.A. (1981). Middle- and long-latency auditory evoked potentials recorded from the vertex of normal and chronically lesioned cats. *Brain Research, 205,* 91–109.

Caird, D.M. and Klinke, R. (1987). The effect of inferior colliculus lesions on auditory evoked potentials. *Electroencephalography and Clinical Neurophysiology, 68,* 237–240.

Celesia, G.C. (1968). Auditory evoked response. *Archives of Neurology, 19,* 430–437.

Chatrian, G.E., Peterson, M.C., and Lazerte, J.A. (1960). Responses to clicks from the human brain: Some depth electrographic observations. *Electroencephalography and Clinical Neurophysiology, 12,* 479–489.

Chen, B.M. and Buchwald, J.S. (1986). Midlatency auditory evoked responses: Differential effects of sleep in the cat. *Electroencephalography and Clinical Neurophysiology, 65,* 373–382.

Cohen, M.M. (1982). Coronal topography of the middle latency auditory evoked potential in man. *Electroencephalography and Clinical Neurophysiology, 53,* 231–236.

Collett, L., Duelaux, R., Challand, M.J., and Revol, M. (1988). Effect of sleep on middle latency response (MLR) in infants. *Brain and Development, 10,* 169–173.

Comperatore, C.A. and Patterson, J.H. (1988). Mapping of cortical auditory middle latency responses in the chinchilla. *Association for Research in Otolaryngology, Abstract,* 75.

Dieber, M.P., Ibanez, V., Fischer, C., Perrin, F., and Manguiere, F. (1988). Sequential mapping favors the hypothesis of distinct generators for N1 and P1 middle auditory evoked potentials. *Electroencephalography and Clinical Neurophysiology, 71,* 187–197.

Engel, R. (1971). Early waves of the electroencephalic auditory response in neonates. *Neuropaediatrie , 3,* 147–154.

Erwin, R. and Buchwald, J.S. (1986a). Midlatency auditory evoked responses: Differential effects of sleep in the human. *Electroencephalography and Clinical Neurophysiology, 65,* 383–392.

Erwin, R. and Buchwald, J.S. (1986b). Midlatency auditory evoked responses: Differential recovery cycle characteristics. *Electroencephalography and Clinical Neurophysiology, 64,* 417–423.

Erwin, R., Mauhinney-Hec, M., and Gur, R.E. (1988). Midlatency auditory evoked responses in schizophrenics. *Abstract, Neuroscience, 14,* 339.

Farley, G.R. and Starr, A. (1983). Middle and long latency auditory evoked potentials in cat. II. Component distributions and dependence on stimulus factors. *Hearing Research, 10,* 139–152.

Feinberg, I. (1974). Changes in sleep cycle patterns with age. *Journal of Psychiatric Research, 10,* 283–306.

Feinberg, I. and Carlson, V.R. (1968). Sleep variables as a function of age in man. *Archives of General Psychiatry, 18,* 239–250.

Galambos, R., Makeig, S., and Talmachoff, P.J. (1981a). A 40 Hz auditory potential recorded from the human scalp. *Proceedings of the National Academy of Sciences, 78,* 2643–2647.

Galambos, R. (1981b). Tactile and auditory stimuli repeated at high rates (30–50 per sec) produce similar event-related potentials. *Annals of New York Academy of Science, 388,* 722–728.

Gardi, J.N. (1985). Human brain stem and middle latency responses to electrical stimulation: A preliminary observation. In: *Cochlear Implants,* pp 351–363. Schindler, R., Merzenich, M. (eds.) New York: Raven Press.

Graham, J., Greenwood, R., and Lecky, B. (1980). Cortical deafness: A case report and review of the literature. *Journal of Neurological Science, 48,* 35–49.

Graziani, L.J., Katz, L., Cracco, R.Q., Cracco, J.B., and Weitzman, E.D. (1974). The maturation and interrelationship of EEG patterns and auditory evoked response in premature infants. *Electroencephalography and Clinical Neurophysiology, 36,* 367–375.

Hari, R., Pelizzone, M., Makela, J.P., Hallstrom, J., Leinonen, L., and Lounesnaa, O.V. (1987). Neuromagnetic responses of the human auditory cortex to on- and offsets of noise bursts. *Audiology, 26,* 31–43.

Hinman, C.L. and Buchwald, J.S. (1983). Depth-evoked potential and single unit correlates of vertex midlatency auditory evoked responses. *Brain Research, 264,* 57–67.

Hirabayashi, M. (1979). The middle components of the auditory electric response. I. On their variation with age. *Journal of Otolaryngology (Japan), 82,* 449–456.

Jacobson, G.P. and Grayson, A.S. (1988). The normal scalp topography of the middle latency auditory evoked potential Pa component following monaural click stimulation. *Brain Topography, 1,* 29–36.

Jacobson, G.P., Privitera, M., Neils, J., Grayson, A., and Yeh, H. (1990). The effects of anterior temporal lobectomy (ATL) on the middle-latency auditory evoked potential (MLAEP). *Electroencephalography and Clinical Neurophysiology, 75,* 230–241.

Jerger, J., Chmiel, R., Glaze, D., and Frost, J.D. (1987). Rate and filter dependence of the middle latency responses in infants. *Audiology, 26,* 269–283.

Kaga, K., Hink, R., Shinoda, Y., and Suzuki, J. (1980). Evidence for a primary cortical origin of a middle latency auditory evoked potential in cats. *Electroencephalography and Clinical Neurophysiology, 50,* 254–266.

Kavanaugh, K.T., Gould, H., McCormick, G., and Franks, R. (1989). Comparison of the identifiability of the low intensity ABR and MLR in the mentally handicapped patient. *Ear and Hearing, 10,* 124–130.

Kileny, P. (1983). Auditory evoked middle latency responses: Current issues. *Seminars in Hearing, 4(4),* 403–412.

Kileny, P.R. and Kemink, J.L. (1987). Electrically evoked middle-latency auditory potentials in cochlear implant candidates. *Archives of Otolaryngology—Head and Neck Surgery, 113,* 1072–1077.

Kileny, P., Paccioretti, D., and Wilson, A.F. (1987). Effects of cortical lesions on middle-latency auditory evoked responses (MLR). *Electroencephalography and Clinical Neurophysiology, 66,* 108–120.

Kileny, P. and Shea, S. (1976). Middle-latency and 40 Hz auditory evoked responses in normal-hearing subjects: Click and 500-Hz thresholds. *Journal of Speech and Hearing Research, 19,* 20–28.

Knight, R. and Brailowsky, S. (1990). Auditory evoked potentials from the primary auditory cortex of the cat: Topographic and pharmacological studies. *Electroencephalography and Clinical Neurophysiology, 77,* 225–232.

Knight, R.T., Brailowsky, S., Scabini, D., and Simpson, G.V. (1985). Surface auditory evoked potentials in the unrestrained rat: Component definition. *Electroencephalography and Clinical Neurophysiology, 61,* 430–439.

Kraus, N., and McGee, T. (1990a). Clinical applications of the middle latency response. *Journal of the American Academy of Audiologists, 1,* 130-133.

Kraus, N. and McGee, T. (1993). Clinical implications of primary and non-primary components of the middle latency response. National Reserach Council, Committee of Hearing, Bioacoustics and Biomechanics (CHABA). *Ear and Hearing, 14*, 36-48.

Kraus, N. and McGee, T. (1988). Color imaging of the human middle latency response. *Ear and Hearing, 9*, 159–167.

Kraus, N. and McGee, T. (1990*b*). Topographic mapping of the auditory middle latency response. In: Auditory evoked magnetic fields and potentials. *Advanced Audiology, 6*, pp. 141–164. Basel: Karger.

Kraus, N., Jacobson, S., McGee, T., and Stark, C. (1988). Multichannel intracranial recording device using a color imaging brain mapping system. *Brain Topography, 1*, 61–64.

Kraus, N., McGee, T., and Comperatore, C. (1989). MLRs in children are consistently present during wakefulness, stage 1, and REM sleep. *Ear and Hearing, 10*, 339–345.

Kraus, N., McGee, T., Littman, T., and Nicol, T. (1992). Reticular formation influences on primary and non-primary auditory pathways as reflected by middle latency response. *Brain Research, 587*, 186–194.

Kraus, N., McGee, T., Micco, A., Carrell, T., Sharma, and Nicol, T. (1993). Mismatch negativity in school-age children to speech stimuli that are just perceptibly different. *Electroencephalography and Clinical Neurophysiology, 88*, 123-130.

Kraus, N., Özdamar, Ö., Hier, D., and Stein, L. (1982). Auditory middle latency responses in patients with cortical lesions. *Electroencephalography and Clinical Neurophysiology, 54*, 247–287.

Kraus, N., Özdamar, Ö., Stein, L., and Reed, N. (1984). Absent auditory brainstem response: Peripheral hearing loss or brainstem dysfunction? *Laryngoscope, 94*, 400–406.

Kraus, N., Reed, N.L., Smith, D.I., Stein, L., and Cartee, C. (1987). Highpass filtering effects the detectability of the auditory middle latency response in humans. *Electroencephalography and Clinical Neurophysiology, 68*, 234–236.

Kraus, N., Smith, D.I., and Grossmann, J. (1985). Cortical mapping of the auditory middle latency response in the unanesthetized guinea pig. *Electroencephalography and Clinical Neurophysiology, 62*, 219–226.

Kraus, N., Smith, D.I., and McGee, T. (1988). Midline and temporal lobe MLRs in the guinea pig originate from different generator systems: A conceptual framework for new and existing data. *Electroencephalography and Clinical Neurophysiology, 70*, 541–558.

Kraus, N., Smith, D.I., and McGee, T. (1987). Rate and filter effects on the developing auditory middle latency response. *Audiology, 26*, 257–268.

Kraus, N., Smith, D.I., McGee, T., Stein, L., and Cartee, C. (1987). Development of the middle latency response in an animal model and its relation to the human response. *Hearing Research, 27*, 165–176.

Kraus, N., Smith, D.I., Reed, N., Stein, L., and Cartee, C. (1985). Auditory middle latency responses in children: Effects of age and diagnostic category. *Electroencephalography and Clinical Neurophysiology, 62*, 343–351.

Lee, Y.S., Lueders, H., Dinner, D.S., Lesser, R.P., Hahn, J., and Klem, G. (1984). Recording of auditory evoked potentials in man using chronic subdural electrodes. *Brain Research, 107*, 115–131.

Makela, J.P. and Hari, R. (1987). Evidence for cortical origin of the 40 Hz auditory evoked response in man. *Electroencephalography and Clinical Neurophysiology, 66*, 539–546.

McGee, T., Kraus, N., Comperatore, C., and Nicol, T. (1991). Subcortical and cortical components of the MLR generating system. *Brain Research, 54*, 211–220.

McGee, T., Kraus, N., Killion, M., Rosenberg, R., and King, C. (1993). Improving the reliability of the auditory middle latency response. *Ear and Hearing, 14*, 76–84.

McGee, T., Kraus, N., Littman, T., and Nicol, T. (1992). Contributions of the subcomponents of the medial geniculate body of the MLR. *Hearing Research, 61*, 147-154.

McGee, T., Kraus, N., and Manfredi, C. (1987). Toward a strategy for analyzing the human MLR waveform. *Audiology, 27*, 119–130.

McGee, T., Kraus, N., and Wolters, C. (1988). Viewing the audiogram through a mathematical model. *Ear and Hearing, 9*, 153–156.

McGee, T., Özdamar, Ö., and Kraus, N. (1983). Auditory middle latency responses in the guinea pig. *American Journal of Otolaryngology, 4*, 116–122.

Mendel, M. and Goldstein, R. (1969). Stability of the early components of the averaged electroencephalic response. *Journal of Speech and Hearing Research, 12*, 351–361.

Mendel, M. (1974). Influence of stimulus level and sleep stage on the early components of the averaged electroencephalic response in clicks during all night sleep. *Journal of Speech and Hearing Research, 17*, 1–17.

Mendel, M.I. and Kupperman, G.L. (1974). Early components of the averaged electroencephalic response to constant-level clicks during rapid eye movement. *Audiology, 13*, 23–32.

Miyamoto, R.T. (1986). Electrically evoked potential in cochlear implant subjects. *Laryngoscope, 96*, 178–185.

Molnár, M., Karmos, G., Csépe, V., and Winkler, I. (1988). Intracortical auditory evoked potentials during classical aversive conditioning in cats. *Biological Psychology, 26,* 339–350.

Mosko, S.S., Knipher, K.F., Sassin, J.F., and Donnelly, J. (1984). Middle latency auditory evoked potentials in sleep apneics during waking and as a function of arterial oxygen saturation during apnea. *Sleep, 7(3),* 239–246.

Musiek, F.E. and Geurnink, N. (1981). Auditory brainstem and middle latency evoked response sensitivity near threshold. *Annals of Otology, 90,* 236–240.

Näätänen, R., Gaillard, A., and Mantysalo, S. (1978). Early selective attention effect on evoked potentials reinterpreted. *Acta Psychologica, 42,* 313–329.

Okitsu, T. (1984). Middle components of auditory evoked response in young children. *Scandinavian Audiology, 13,* 83–86.

Osterhammel, P.A., Shallop, J.K., and Terkildsen, K. (1985). The effect of sleep on the auditory brainstem response (ABR) and the middle latency response (MLR). *Scandinavian Audiology, 14,* 47–50.

Özdamar, Ö. and Kraus, N. (1983). Auditory middle latency responses in humans. *Audiology, 22,* 34–49.

Özdamar, Ö., Kraus, N., and Curry, F. (1983). Auditory brainstem and middle latency responses in a patient with cortical deafness. *Electroencephalography and Clinical Neurophysiology, 53,* 224–230.

Parving, A., Solomon, G., Elberling, C., Larsen, B., and Lassen, N.A. (1980). Middle components of the auditory evoked response in bilateral temporal lobe lesions. *Scandinavian Audiology, 9,* 161–167.

Picton, T.W., Hillyard, S.A., Krausz, H.I., and Galambos, R. (1974). Human auditory evoked potentials. I: Evaluation of components. *Electroencephalography and Clinical Neurophysiology, 36,* 179–190.

Pool, K., Finitzo, T., Chi-Tzong-Hong, Rogers, J., and Pickett, R.B. (1989). Infarction of the superior temporal gyrus: A description of auditory evoked potential latency and amplitude topology. *Ear and Hearing, 10,* 144–152.

Rosati, G., Bastiani, P.D., Paolino, E., Prosser, A., Arslan, E., and Artioli, M. (1982). Clinical and audiological findings in a case of auditory agnosia. *Journal of Neurology, 227,* 21–27.

Ruhm, H., Walker, E., and Flanigan, H. (1967). Acoustically-evoked potentials in man: Mediation of early components. *Laryngoscope, 77,* 806–822.

Scherg, M. (1982). Distortion of the middle latency auditory response produced by analogue filtering. *Scandinavian Audiology, 11,* 57–69.

Scherg, M., Hari, R., and Hamalainen, M. (in press). Frequency-specific sources of the auditory N19-P30-p50 response detected by a multiple source analysis of evoked magnetic fields and potentials, in: Williamson, S., ed., *Advances in biomagnetism.* New York: Plenum Publishing Corp.

Scherg, M., Vajsar, J., and Picton, T. (1989). A source analysis of the late human auditory evoked potentials. *Journal of Cognitive Neuroscience, 1,* 336–355.

Scherg, M. and Volk, S.A. (1983). Frequency specificity of simultaneously recorded early and middle latency auditory evoked potentials. *Electroencephalography and Clinical Neurophysiology, 56,* 443–452.

Scherg, M. and von Cramon, D. (1986). Evoked dipole source potentials of the human auditory cortex. *Electroencephalography and Clinical Neurophysiology, 65,* 344–360.

Skinner, P. and Glattke, T.J. (1977). Electrophysiologic responses and audiometry: State of the art. *Journal of Speech and Hearing Disorders, 42,* 179–198.

Smith, D.I., and Kraus, N. (1988). Intracranial and extracranial recordings of the auditory middle latency response. *Electroencephalography and Clinical Neurophysiology, 71,* 296–303.

Stapells, D., Galambos, R., Costello, J., and Makeig, S. (1988). Inconsistency of auditory middle latency and steady-state responses in infants. *Electroencephalography and Clinical Neurophysiology, 71,* 289–295.

Stapells, D.R., Linden, D., Suffield, J.B., Hamel, G., and Picton, T.W. (1984). Human auditory steady state potentials. *Ear and Hearing, 5,* 105–113.

Steriade, M., Oakson, G., and Ropert, N. (1982). Firing rates and patterns of midbrain reticular neurons during steady and transitional states of the sleep-waking cycle. *Experimental Brain Research, 46,* 37–51.

Suzuki, T., Hirabayashi, M., and Kobayashi, K. (1983). Auditory middle latency responses in young children. *British Journal of Audiology, 17,* 5–9.

Suzuki, T., Hirabayashi, M., and Kobayashi, K. (1984). Effects of analog and digital filtering on auditory middle latency responses in adults and young children. *Annals of Otology, 93,* 267–270.

Suzuki, T., Hirai, Y., and Horiuchi, K. (1981). Simultaneous recording of early and middle components of auditory electric response. *Ear and Hearing, 2,* 276.

Suzuki, T. and Kobayashi, K. (1984). An evaluation of 40-Hz event-related potentials in young children. *Audiology, 23,* 599–604.

Suzuki, T., Kobayashi, K., and Hirabayashi, M. (1983). Frequency composition of auditory middle responses. *British Journal of Audiology, 17*, 1–4.

Suzuki, T., Yamamota, K., Taguchi, K., and Sakabe, N. (1976). Reliability and variability of late vertex-evoked response audiometry. *Audiology, 15*, 357–369.

Vaughan, H. and Ritter, W. (1970). The sources of auditory evoked responses recorded from the human scalp. *Electroencephalography and Clinical Neurophysiology, 28*, 360–367.

Vivion, M.C., Hirsch, J.E., Frye-Osier, H., and Goldstein, R. (1980). Effects of stimulus rise-fall time and equivalent duration on middle components of AER. *Scandinavian Audiology, 9*, 223–232.

Wolpaw, J.R. and Wood, C.C. (1982). Scalp distribution of human auditory evoked potentials. I. Evaluation of reference electrode sites. *Electroencephalography and Clinical Neurophysiology, 54*, 15–24.

Woods, D.L., Clayworth, C.C., Knight, R.T., Simpson, G.V., and Naeser, M.A. (1987). Generators of middle- and long-latency auditory evoked potentials: Implications from studies of patients with bitemporal lesions. *Electroencephalography and Clinical Neurophysiology, 68*, 132–148.

Worthington, D.W. and Peters, J.F. (1980). Quantifiable hearing and no ABR: Paradox or error? *Ear and Hearing, 5*, 281–285.

Yakovlev, P.L. and Lecours, A.R. (1967). The myelogenetic cycles of the regional maturation of the brain. In *Regional Development of the Brain in Early Life*. Philadelphia, PA: Davis.

Zerlin, S. and Naunton, R. (1974). Early and late averaged electroencephalic responses at low sensation levels. *Audiology, 13*, 366–378.

CHAPTER 8

THE SLOW VERTEX POTENTIAL: PROPERTIES AND CLINICAL APPLICATIONS

MARTYN L. HYDE

INTRODUCTION

The auditory slow vertex potential (SVP) is generated in the cerebral cortex and typically consists of a vertex-negative peak at about 100 ms latency, followed by a positive peak at about 175 ms. It is a very useful clinical tool in subjects who are alert and will cooperate at least passively. Its main use is for estimating the pure-tone audiogram when a non-behavioral, frequency-specific and sensitive measure is needed, such as for many medico-legal and compensation assessments, and evaluations of suspected functional hearing loss. The SVP also has several other potential clinical applications, such as for non-behavioral measurement of frequency and temporal discrimination, localization, and speech perception.

The clinical value of the SVP is not widely appreciated, yet this potential has been used routinely and successfully for many years in several major clinics and laboratories worldwide. Such variations in perception and practice are certainly not in the interests of the hearing health care consumer. Thus, there is a need to reappraise the SVP, in relation to other auditory evoked potentials (AEPs) and also to audiologic assessment more generally.

The goals of this chapter are to inform audiologists about the SVP and its uses, and to provide practical information. After an outline of terminology and historical development, the properties of the SVP are reviewed. Clinical applications are discussed next and are followed by practical procedures for clinical measurements. The review of SVP properties contributes to the rationale for the clinical procedures recommended. Some of the material presented here is based on the author's experiences using and studying the SVP since 1968; the best test of the utility of that material will be the subsequent hands-on experience of the reader.

TERMINOLOGY AND NOMENCLATURE

There is little standardization of AEP classification and waveform nomenclature. The SVP, for example, is variously called the auditory (or not specified) slow (or long-latency, or late) vertex (or cortical) evoked potential (or response), and these combinations are not exhaustive. This is complicated further by distinction, or lack of it, between any AEP itself and the clinical technique based upon it. One approach is to add a response-specific prefix to a general term such as Electric Response Audiometry, yielding SVERA or BERA, for example, for the slow vertex and the brainstem potential techniques, respectively.

Part of this clutter is historic, part due to idiosyncracy, and part due to inherent complexity. The view adopted here is as follows: "auditory" is an optional

The author wishes to thank Krista Riko, Director of the Otologic Function Unit, Mount Sinai Hospital and The Toronto Hospital, for useful early discussions of this material. The underlying work was in part supported by the Ontario Ministry of Health, the Medical Research Council of Canada, and the Workers' Compensation Board of Ontario.

prefix; the latency classification into "first (cochlear)", "fast", "middle", "slow", and "late" potentials, (Davis, 1976; Davis and Owen, 1985) is empirically satisfactory, if applied consistently, so the SVP is "slow", not "late", which term is reserved here for longer-latency AEPs; "cortical" is redundant with "slow and also is unacceptably nonspecific, there being many AEPs of cortical origin; the term "vertex" specifies a potential with a particular topographic distribution over the head; lastly, "potential" is more informative than "response". With the advent of positron emission tomography, evoked electric currents, evoked magnetic fields and various kinds of source analysis, the word "response" is too imprecise. For these reasons, the term SVP has been adopted in this chapter.

Vaughan (1969) proposed the term "event-related potential" (ERP), defining "the general class of potentials that display stable time relationships to a definable reference event". This scheme included sensory evoked potentials and what are now known as late, endogenous, or cognitive potentials (see Chapter 9), as well as motor and extracranial potentials. Thus, AEPs are a subset of ERPs. There is a trend towards using the term ERP only for the endogenous potentials, but that is more narrow than Vaughan's definition. See Regan (1989, p.195), for another viewpoint.

Vaughan also suggested a concise response nomenclature, in which the general description of an ERP is typically of the form:

[Cz-A1: N(L1,A1)P(L2,A2) . . . . . . P(LN,AN)].

The placements of the noninverting and inverting electrodes are usually according to the "10–20 system" of the International EEG Federation (Jasper, 1958; Regan, 1989) and are followed by wave polarities, each with a latency and (optional) amplitude.

In this scheme, some particular SVP might be specified as:

[Cz-M2: N(96,–3.6)P(177,2.8)]

where the units are in milliseconds and microvolts, respectively. A simpler description of the "typical" SVP would be N100P175, referring to the features of the potential elicited by some typical or "standard" stimulus such as a 70 dB click. This type of nomenclature

was also proposed as a standard by Donchin, Callaway, Cooper, et al., (1977), but unfortunately, despite these efforts, wave labels that are arcane, outdated, and idiosyncratic are still in use for many AEPs (such as waves V, Pa, N1, etc.). Indeed, the SVP is often referred to as "N1-P2", which term is undesirable and can be confused with the "N1" potential from the cochlear nerve.

The SVP is a transient response, associated primarily with the onset of a stimulus such as a toneburst, as distinct from a sustained (DC) response to a lengthy stimulus or from a steady-state (overlapping) response to rapidly repeated stimuli. Also, the SVP is on the borderline between the exogenous response class governed by physical stimulus parameters, and the endogenous class governed by cognitive variables (John, 1967; Regan, 1989). The SVP is best classed as exogenous, but it is affected by arousal and attention.

HISTORY

The early history of AEPs was reviewed by Hallowell Davis (1976) in his monograph on Electric Response Audiometry (ERA). The earliest report of waking-state EEG changes evoked by sounds was due to Pauline Davis (Davis, 1939). Response description was extended by Gastaut (1953) and Bancaud, Bloch, and Paillard (1953), who suggested the term "V-potential" to emphasize the vertex-maximal scalp distribution. This was, in fact, the SVP.

The potential application to hearing assessment in very young children (Marcus, Gibbs, and Gibbs, 1949) spurred further study, but progress was hampered by the lack of a technology for response visualization. Using photographic superimposition of the post-stimulus EEG (Dawson, 1950), a triphasic, spatially diffuse response to clicks and 1 kHz tonebursts, with a latency of about 90 ms, was reported by Abe (1954). The click response was found by Calvet, Cathala, Contamin, Hirsch, and Scherrer (1956) to have "early" (about 50 ms) and "late" (about 150 ms) components. Following the development of on-line summing devices (Dawson, 1954, Goldstein, 1961), response properties were explored further by Geisler, Frishkopf, and Rosenblith (1958), Geisler (1960), Williams and Graham (1963), and by

Davis, Engebretson, Lowell, Mast, Satterfield, and Yoshie (1964). Geisler et al., (1958) had found what we now call the "middle-latency response" (MLR), but there are overlapping neurogenic and myogenic (post-auricular, inion) potentials in this latency region, and an ill-conceived debate about whether the "early" potentials were exclusively neurogenic or myogenic persisted for more than a decade, delaying the audiometric application of the MLR.

Davis (1964) reported a slow response with a latency of 160 ms to its largest positive peak. It was vertex-maximal, about 10 µV peak-to-peak with a 70 dB click, favored by low stimulus rates and detectable at 20 dB sensation level (SL) or lower. Use of this response to estimate hearing threshold was then examined by many investigators (Rapin, 1964; Barnet, 1965; Davis, 1965; Davis, 1966; Davis, Hirsh, Shelnutt, and Bowers, 1967; Beagley and Kellogg, 1968; Alberti, 1970), with generally favorable evaluations.

In the early 1970s, the initial enthusiasm for the SVP as an audiometric tool for very young or difficult-to-test children was tempered by the realization that for persons in natural or sedated sleep, the reliability of subjective SVP identification was poor, so the resulting audiometric threshold estimates were often inaccurate (Rapin, Schimmel, and Cohen, 1972; Osterhammel, Davis, Wier, and Hirsh, 1973). There were also reports indicating poor reliability even in cooperative adults (Rose, Keating, Hedgecock, Schreurs, and Miller, 1971).

Since the mid-1970s, there has been relatively little published research on SVP audiometry, partly due to widespread (but certainly not universal) lack of confidence in the technique and partly to an explosion of interest in the ABR. However, there have been several reports that SVP audiometry is accurate in passively cooperative, alert subjects (Davis, 1976; Alberti, 1981; Boniver, 1982; Davis and Owen, 1985; Coles and Mason, 1984; Hyde, Alberti, Matsumoto, and Li, 1986). As well, there is a growing awareness that for certain tasks, such as approximating the pure-tone audiogram, no single AEP is always the best tool. The various AEPs can have a complementary and synergistic role in clinical evaluation, and a multi-AEP testing strategy is often appropriate.

On a broader front, there is renewed and expanding interest in the use of the SVP to measure aspects of suprathreshold auditory performance (Durrant, 1987; McEvoy, Picton, Champagne, Kellett, and Kelly, 1990; Altman and Vaitulevich, 1990; Picton, 1991).

THE NATURE OF THE SVP

Early work on properties and applications of the SVP has been reviewed by Reneau and Hnatiow (1975), Davis (1976), Picton, Woods, Baribeau-Braun, and Healey (1977), and Gibson (1978). The SVP is a scalp potential evoked by any abrupt, perceptible change in the auditory environment. Usually, the evoking stimulus is a transient sound such as a click, toneburst or speech element, tonebursts being the most common stimuli for estimating the pure-tone audiogram. The SVP is best recorded with a vertex-mastoid electrode derivation, by averaging the response to about 20–50 tonebursts delivered at about one per two seconds. At moderate stimulus levels, the potential has a typical peak-to-peak amplitude of about 10–15 microvolts. Thus, it is more than ten times larger than wave V (P6) of the ABR.

The SVP is not a single, unitary phenomenon; the N100 and P175 components differ in basic characteristics and in their response to many physical and subject-related variables, and each probably has several overlapping sub-components. Some of the many discrepancies in reported properties of the SVP undoubtedly have resulted from this complexity of underlying structure.

Waveform

The morphology of waking-state slow AEPs in adults has been described extensively (Davis, 1965; Davis and Zerlin, 1966; Davis, Mast, Yoshie, and Zerlin, 1966; Onishi and Davis, 1968; Picton, Hillyard, Krausz, and Galambos, 1974). The typical full waveform can be notated as:

$$[Cz\text{-}M: P50N100P175N300].$$

Davis (1965) used the term "V-potential" for a triphasic portion of the response having latencies of about 60 to 200 ms. Goff, Matsumiya, Allison, and Goff (1969) reported similar morphology and topography for a diphasic negative-positive fluctuation start-ing at about 100 ms latency, with auditory, visual and somatosensory stimuli, calling this the "vertex poten-tial". As illustrated in Figure 8.1A, when recorded with wide bandwidth, the AEP is usually dominated by the components N100 and P175, which comprise the SVP proper. There is substantial variability of SVP ampli-tude, latency and waveform, both between and within subjects, with the individual components showing some independence. Latency measures have lower co-efficients of variation than amplitudes. Details of waveform are dependent upon many technical and sub-ject-related variables.

If the SVP is recorded with an amplifier bandwidth extending down to zero (DC) or near zero, the com-plete response waveform for a long (for example, 1s duration) toneburst includes a vertex-negative steady potential shift that lasts for as long as the stimulus (the "cortical DC potential"; Keidel, 1971), as well as a sec-ond, smaller SVP at the stimulus offset. Probably be-cause of poor signal to noise ratio (SNR) relative to very low frequency EEG energy, the DC potential has received little attention as an audiometric tool, and will not be discussed further.

Frequency Spectrum

The energy density spectrum of the SVP in an awake adult subject is illustrated in Figure 8.1B. Its appear-ance is quite predictable from the time-domain wave-form of Figure 8.1A, which is roughly sinusoidal, and its period would be twice the N-P interval, that is, about 160 ms. This corresponds to a frequency of about 6 Hz, which corresponds to the location of the spectral maximum in Figure 8.1B. At stimulus levels near threshold, the N-P interval expands and the spectral maximum reduces to about 4–5 Hz. There is negligible SVP energy below about 1 Hz and above about 12 Hz. In infants and young children, the distribution of energy shifts to lower frequencies, as also occurs during sleep.

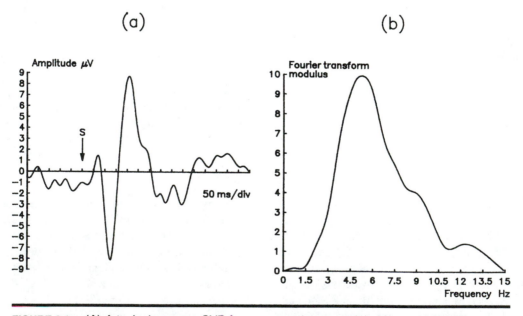

FIGURE 8.1.   (A) A typical average SVP from a normal young adult. Monaural 500 Hz tonebursts (10–40–10 ms) at 60 dB HL (TDH-39); 100 stimuli at 1/2s rate. Vertex-mastoid, vertex positive up. Recording bandwidth 0.1–20 Hz. Stimulus onset at 250 ms. (B) The frequency spectrum (Fourier transform modulus, 10-fold extension by zeroes, Hanning window) of the SVP in (A), showing typical SVP energy concentration at about 6 Hz.

Topographic Distribution

Early studies of the scalp topographic distribution of the N100 and P175 peaks showed a laterally symmetric, broad (diffuse) distribution over frontal and central regions, with an amplitude maximum over the vertex (Gastaut et al., 1967; Goff et al., 1969). Similar topographies were reported for seemingly analogous slow potentials evoked by visual and somatosensory stimuli. Recording with a "reference" (noninverting) electrode on the chin, Vaughan (1969) reported a diffuse, vertex-maximal topography with polarity reversal over the Sylvian fissure, the site of primary auditory cortex on the superior margin of the temporal lobe. In electroencephalography, polarity reversal (phase reversal) is often associated with location of the source of the potential beneath the point or contour of reversal. Kooi et al. (1971) found no such polarity reversal with a noncephalic reference electrode. See Regan (1989) and Nunez (1981) for discussion of problematic issues relating to electrode sites and source localization. Picton et al. (1974), using a chest reference, noted broad, vertex-maximal fronto-central distributions for both N100 and P175, with the latter being a little less broadly distributed; the mastoid was found to be isopotential (electrically equivalent) with the chest.

Generator Sources

The locations of the SVP sources are still not definitively established, but there have been significant advances recently. The lack of a good animal model has been a source of difficulty, and it is doubtful whether a genuine analog of the SVP exists in non-primates (Hardin and Castellucci, 1970). The issue has been whether the SVP is generated in the primary auditory cortex, and if so, whether the main contribution is contralateral to the stimulus, as might be expected from classical studies of the auditory pathway. The traditional alternative view was SVP generation via multiple pathways to widely distributed areas of cortex, not necessarily involving the primary auditory areas.

In the early years, nonspecific pathways outside the classical, lemniscal afferent auditory pathway were favored (Davis, 1976). Properties consistent with this

option were the breadth and lack of contralaterality of the scalp potential distribution, the positive correlation between changes in the SVP and the spontaneous EEG during sleep, the sensitivity of the SVP to barbiturates, its long time course, lability, and the slow response similarities across sensory modalities. Goff et al. (1969) noted that such a nonspecific generation pathway would allow SVP development even if the specific auditory afferent pathways were interrupted rostral to the brainstem, because of the collateral connections between the specific and nonspecific afferent systems at many levels in the brainstem. If so, this would pose a significant limitation on the audiometric validity of the SVP.

Vaughan (1969) considered that his topographic results were consistent with response generation in the primary auditory areas. Despite the arguments about effects of electrode position, this now appears to be a correct view. It is known that volume current flow in the head can create patterns of scalp potential with no obvious relationship to sources of potential (Vaughan, 1969; Nunez, 1981; Goff, 1978; Regan, 1989), so the broad topography of the SVP is not inconsistent with primary cortical origin. Furthermore, evidence has been accumulating that several concurrent sources contribute to scalp potentials in the latency region of the SVP (Wolpaw and Penry, 1975; Simson, Vaughan, and Ritter, 1976; Picton, Woods, Stuss, and Campbell, 1978; Wood and Wolpaw, 1982).

New insights into SVP source location have occurred in the last five years, because of advances in two areas. The first is dipole source analysis (Scherg and von Cramon, 1985; Scherg, 1990). This approach attempts to determine the location, strength and orientation of a small number of electrical "equivalent dipoles" that would cause the observed scalp potential distribution. (See Chapter 3, Signal Processing and Analysis, for a more detailed account.) The second advance is in the area of cortical auditory evoked magnetic fields (AEMFs; Hari, 1990). AEPs and AEMFs are complementary phenomena associated with current flow. AEMFs are associated primarily with lateral components of current flow, that is, with flow tangential to the surface of the skull; relative to AEPs, they have the advantage that the induced fields are spatially more restricted to scalp regions overlying the generator sites.

A detailed analysis of the sources of the slow and late AEPs was recently reported by Scherg, Vajsar, and Picton (1989); they used topographic and dipole analytic techniques. They concluded that N100 has bilateral, vertically oriented dipole sources located in the supratemporal plane, in or near the primary auditory koniocortex. These results are consistent with the properties of the N100 peak analog in the magnetic response (see reviews by Näätänen and Picton, 1987, and Hari, 1990). Scherg et al. (1989) also noted the variations in cortical anatomy between individuals, and that the sources of potential may alter with changes in stimulation parameters.

Despite these significant technical advances, the picture with respect to response generators is complex, incomplete, and not yet entirely clear. Current techniques of dipole source analysis require several constraining assumptions about the candidate dipoles and the electrical properties of the head, and the validity of these assumptions is an issue. Almost certainly, the definitive resolution of questions about slow auditory AEP generator sites will require integration of data from a wide variety of imaging modalities, in both normal and pathologic material and in both humans and other primates. It is fairly clear, however, that what at first sight might seem to be a single phenomenon (the SVP) is actually a composite of concurrent activity from several distinct anatomic sources, perhaps widely separated and perhaps having different functional properties and significance. This should be remembered when considering the further material presented about various properties of the SVP.

Whatever the source location, the exact electrophysiology of the neural elements that give rise to the SVP is also not established unequivocally. The prime candidates are postsynaptic potentials (PSPs) of radially oriented cortical pyramidal cells and their (superficial) apical dendrites (Creutzfeldt and Kuhnt, 1967).

Functional Correlates

An SVP is generated by any rapid change in any auditory percept. For example, SVPs are generated at both the onset and offset of a long toneburst, if they are sufficiently abrupt. The offset response amplitude increases with plateau duration asymptotically to half that of the onset response (Milner, 1969). Offset response latency is smaller than that of the onset response (Spreng, 1971). There is no evidence that SVPs occur during the stimulus plateau, but the lack of reference events for averaging would make them difficult to detect.

The SVP was implicated in the mechanism of arousal (Barnet and Goodwin, 1965), and Walter (1964) had noted that a neurologic mechanism functionally equivalent to mathematical differentiation (measuring the rate of change) of the perceptual environment would be useful for the establishment of conditional associations. Davis and Zerlin (1966) also suggested that the SVP reflects "a process or response related to a change of state rather than a channel for incoming sensory information". Clynes (1969) proposed that the SVP was associated with a dynamic control system of rate-sensitive units, allowing distinction between states of constancy and change in sensory variables (a "rest-motion" distinction). He found that the SVP is inhibited by low rates of change preceding the evoking event and that the system is not a simple differentiator, that is, not a simple rate-of-change detector.

The interpretation of the functional significance of the SVP is made even more difficult by the need to use a train of repeated stimuli to record it for averaging purposes. Especially when dealing with cortical responses, it is important to remember that the process of averaging tends to emphasize whatever part of the overall response to each stimulus is consistent over the set of stimuli; the relationship between the result of averaging and the actual AEPs evoked by the individual stimuli is obscure.

A distinction must be drawn between features of the SVP that relate to the parameters of a specific stimulus, for which the stimulus repetition is just an inconvenient requirement, versus features that depend on the existence of the entire set of repeated stimuli. For example, what may be an SVP is evoked by a missing stimulus in a periodic train (Keidel, 1971; Simson, Vaughan, and Ritter, 1976), and similar potentials are associated with recognition of any mismatch whatsoever between the expected and observed stimuli, even with respect to their timing (Näätänen, Pavilainen, Alho, Reinikainen, and Sams (1987). The topography and sources of this "mismatch negativity" (MMN) were examined in detail by Scherg, et al., 1989. It is a small step from here to the "oddball" paradigm for the elicitation of the P300 response (Sutton, Braren, Zubin, and John, 1965; Squires, Donchin, Herning, and McCarthy, 1977; see Chapter 9, in this text). However, the typical stimulus set used to estimate hearing sensitivity is one of periodic, identical stimuli, in which situation the MMN and P300 are of little concern.

Statistical Models

See the Chapter 3 in this text on Signal Processing and Analysis, as well as Regan (1989) for more detailed discussion of statistical models of AEP data. The usual model is an evoked potential "signal" that is identical for each stimulus repetition, additively superimposed on statistically independent electrical "noise". Sayers, Beagley, and Henshall (1974) concluded that this model is not valid for the SVP, because they could not detect the increase in overall energy that follows from the additive model. They proposed that the SVP arises by temporal reorganization of oscillatory energy that is already present in the ongoing EEG, by a kind of "phase-reordering" process. This is a radically different alternative model, and is still often quoted. However, using arguably more powerful statistical techniques, Jervis, Nichols, Johnson, Allen, and Hudson (1983) were able to detect an energy increment consistent with the additive model. Thus, at present, the additive model remains plausible. The significance of these models lies their potential implications both for neurologic mechanisms and for development of powerful and robust objective, computer-based response detection and classification systems.

Within the additive model, the assumption of constant AEP from stimulus to stimulus can be violated by both random or systematic changes. Of the random changes, latency jitter (random variation from trial to trial) has received the most attention (McGillem, Aunon, and Yu, 1985). Sayers, Beagley, and Ross (1979) described elegantly the waveform broadening, latency increase and amplitude reduction caused by

latency jitter, using simulated SVP data. However, as yet, there does not appear to have been a really convincing demonstration that significant latency jitter actually occurs for the auditory SVP. Systematic changes in the SVP from stimulus to stimulus are mentioned later, in the discussion of effect of the number of stimuli per average, and also in Chapter 3 on Signal Processing and Analysis in this text.

The additive model usually assumes that the electrical noise is statistically "stationary", that is, that it has constant average value, standard deviation, etc., over time. Under these conditions, the signal to noise ratio (SNR) in the average response to N stimuli is the square root of N times the SNR in a single sweep. In this respect, there are two main differences between SVP and, say, ABR data. First, the typical minimum number of sweeps acquired for an ABR is about 2000, whereas it is about 20 for the SVP. The stimulus repetition rates are such that the total acquisition time is similar, but because the SVP number is much smaller, changes in the EEG noise over time will cause larger variations in the final average records. Second, the recording bandwidth for the SVP is about 1–15 Hz, which covers the frequency range for several of the classical sinusoidal EEG "rhythms", such as alpha (8–13 Hz) and theta (4–8 Hz). These rhythms are nonrandom features of the EEG noise, and they violate the randomness assumption underlying the root-N law. These factors can conspire to increase the difficulty of evaluation of SVP records.

EFFECTS OF STIMULUS PARAMETERS

Caveat

There is often disagreement in the published reports regarding even basic properties of the SVP, and with some notable exceptions, many of the reports are of questionable value. Difficulties in this area include a lack of standardization of measurement conditions, methodologies, analyses and terminology. Better experimental designs and larger sample sizes are needed. Also, close attention must be paid to the many interactions between the effects of stimulus, recording and subject-related variables.

Type of Stimulus

The SVP can be evoked by a wide variety of transient sounds, such as clicks, tonebursts, noisebursts, syllables, and also by sudden changes in continuous sounds, such as in amplitude, frequency spectrum, or perceived point of origin (Jerger and Jerger, 1970; Arlinger, Jerlvall, Ahren, and Holmgren, 1976; Durrant, 1987; Maiste and Picton, 1989; McEvoy, Picton, Champagne, Kellett, and Kelly, 1990). It can also be evoked by "non-stimuli", such as by gaps in a tone or a noise, or omitted stimuli in a train (Keidel, 1971; Simson, Vaughan, and Ritter, 1976). By far the most common stimulus used for clinical assessment of hearing sensitivity is the toneburst. The stimulus can be delivered by headphone, insert receiver, bone conductor or loudspeaker.

Toneburst Level

SVP Amplitude. In subjects with normal hearing, SVP peak-to-peak amplitude generally increases with stimulus level, as shown in Figure 8.2. An early debate was whether amplitude increased linearly when plotted against stimulus level in dB (Antinoro, Skinner, and Jones, 1969), or whether it followed a power function, which would give a linear plot of log amplitude versus stimulus level in dB (Keidel and Spreng, 1965; Davis and Zerlin, 1966; Davis, Bowers, and Hirsh, 1968). Rothman (1970) showed that neither function fitted the data well. Literature review suggests that intersubject mean SVP amplitude increases approximately linearly with stimulus level, with a tendency to saturate at intermediate or high levels, and even to decrease at very high sensation levels (Beagley and Knight, 1967; Spoor, Timmer, and Odenthal, 1969; Picton, Goodman, and Bryce, 1970; Watts, 1976; Picton et al., 1977). The stimulus level at which saturation occurs tends to decrease at small values of ISI or at high stimulus frequencies (McCandless and Best, 1966; Nelson and Lassman, 1968; Moore and Rose, 1969; Picton et al., 1970; Rothman, 1970).

There are discrepant reports, some of which do not show saturation at high levels (Onishi and Davis, 1968; Kaskey, Salzman, Klorman, and Pass, 1980). There are several possible causes of these discrepancies. McCandless and Best (1966) noted that peak-to-peak measures may show complex properties due to differences in behavior of the component peaks; they also reported large intersubject variability in amplitude functions, probably reflecting effects of attention (Picton et al., 1977). Recently, Adler and Adler (1989) reported differences in the amplitude functions for N100 and P175.

SVP Latencies. In subjects with normal hearing, as stimulus level increases, the latencies of both N100 and P175 decrease rapidly just above the response threshold and then decline more gradually above about 20 dB SL (McCandless and Best, 1966; Rapin, Schimmel, Tourk, Krasnegor, and Pollak, 1966; Rose and Ruhm, 1966; Beagley and Knight, 1967; McCandless and Lentz, 1968; Onishi and Davis, 1968; Picton et al., 1977). See Figure 8.2. These relationships have been confirmed recently for both electric and magnetic responses (Pantev, Hoke, Lutkenhoner, Lehnertz, and Spittka, 1986). Adler and Adler (1989) found that at low levels the latency of P175 increases more than that of N100, so the SVP complex tends to expand.

Toneburst Frequency

Despite some reports of no effect, on balance it appears that the SVP diminishes with increasing toneburst frequency, at constant sensation level (Antinoro and Skinner, 1968; Evans and Deatherage, 1969). Antinoro, Skinner, and Jones (1969) showed that between 0.5 and 8 kHz this effect increases from zero at 20 dB SL to about 50% at 100 dB SL. Rothman (1969) showed the intersubject mean N100-P175 amplitude to be negatively correlated with frequency in the range 0.5 to 2 kHz, but the relationship was found to vary considerably between subjects. Grimes and Feldman (1971) reported no effect of frequency change from 500 Hz to 4 kHz on the difference between behavioral thresholds and SVP thresholds, in agreement with Beagley and Kellogg (1969). There are no apparent effects of stimulus frequency on SVP latency.

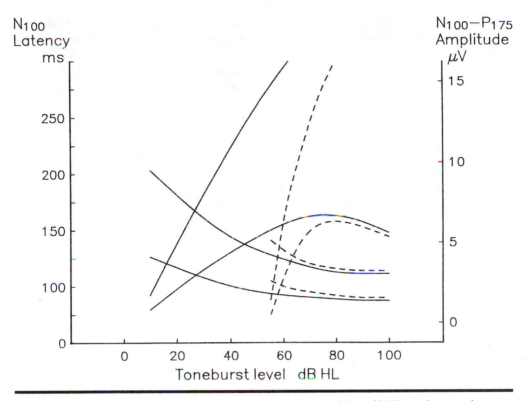

FIGURE 8.2.   Effects of toneburst level on N100 latency and N100–N175 peak-to-peak amplitude. The range of functions commonly observed is illustrated for persons with normal hearing (solid curves) and with moderate sensory hearing loss (dashed curves). Note the wide range of normal amplitude functions, some with rollover at high levels, and the tendency to more rapid, recruitment-like growth just above threshold in persons with hearing loss. Note marked latency shifts near threshold in normal persons, less marked with hearing loss.

Toneburst Waveform

Many toneburst envelopes have been explored, including ogival, exponential, and linear onset/offset profiles, usually combined with a plateau region. The rise and fall times are usually defined as the interval between the 10% and 90% points, the duration being the time between the 90% points.

Rise Time.   Onishi and Davis (1968) found that SVP amplitude remained constant until rise time increased beyond 50 ms, when it began to decline; this effect did not depend on toneburst level. N100 latency also increased with increasing rise time, the effect being most marked at low stimulus levels. Milner (1969) reported that response amplitude decreased monotonically with increasing rise time, the magnitude of the effect decreasing to zero at threshold, but she found the same latency effects.

Duration.   Onishi and Davis (1968) reported that amplitude was not affected by toneburst duration if the rise time was 30 ms, but for a 3 ms rise time the response amplitude increased linearly with duration up to 30 ms, and was constant beyond that. Hyde (1976) confirmed this, reporting a temporal integration time constant of about 15 ms, which effectively means that amplitude asymptotes at between 30 and 50 ms duration. Onishi and Davis (1968) also found that SVP latency decreased with increasing duration, especially at low stimulus levels and with small rise-times. They concluded that latency was governed by the rate of change of stimulus amplitude at the onset, regardless of the final stimulus amplitude. Cody, Klass, and Bickford (1969) confirmed that latency increased with rise time, more markedly at low sensation level.

In the small proportion of subjects who have prominent SVPs to toneburst offset, certain combinations of stimulus parameters, especially around durations of 75–100 ms, may cause interactions between the SVPs to tone onset and offset (Spreng, 1969; Keidel, 1976; Davis, 1976). The ensuing changes in the amplitude and latency of P175 can complicate studies of stimulus duration effects and can also make the SVP more difficult to recognize.

Interstimulus Interval

Several processes may mediate the effects of the number and timing of stimuli on averaged evoked potentials (Brazier, 1964; Sutton, 1969). Refractoriness is a general term describing any decrease in neuronal excitability mediated by a passive process, such as metabolic fatigue, whereas the term adaptation is often restricted to the sensory receptor or its immediate connections. Habituation usually implies active neuronal inhibition.

The usual stimulus set is N stimuli separated by (N-1) equal intervals. Cycle time (CT) is the time between some reference point on two successive stimuli, and interstimulus interval (ISI) is the time between the end of one stimulus and the start of the next. The two terms are often used interchangeably, which can cause confusion if the mark-space ratio, that is, the ratio of stimulus duration to ISI, is larger than about 0.1.

SVP amplitude increases markedly and monotonically with CT up to times of about 10 seconds (Davis, 1965; Keidel and Spreng, 1965; Davis and Zerlin, 1966; Davis et al., 1966), with little change in latency.

Nelson and Lassman (1968) found that peak and peak-to-peak amplitudes increased linearly with log CT, the regression slopes for the three measures being different; large intersubject variability of regression slope was observed. Milner (1969) proposed an exponential interstimulus recovery process with a time constant of about 4.5 seconds, consistent with the summarization presented by Picton et al. (1977). Recently, McEvoy et al. (1990) confirmed this model and time constant, in their study of the SVP for noise lateralization.

Number of Stimuli

The change in response with CT can be conceived as due to an interstimulus recovery process. The average response to a periodic set of stimuli will tend to reflect the asymptotic (adapted) state of the system. Of course, the response to the first stimulus will be different, and other processes, such as habituation, might cause the average response to change with the number of stimuli. These effects might themselves be a function of CT.

The dependence of SVP amplitude on both CT and the number of stimuli was studied by Fruhstorfer, Soveri, and Jarvilehto (1970). They proposed a post-stimulus inhibition that decays as a negative exponential function of time, and which cumulates for successive stimuli. Dishabituation was noted, and this is usually a necessary condition for a previous response decrement to be accepted as due to habituation (Groves and Thompson, 1970). Wastell (1980) suggested that, at least for CTs of 3s and greater, cumulation of inhibition throughout the stimulus train is related to the accuracy with which the arrival time of any stimulus can be predicted.

Henry and Teas (1968) showed that the mean amplitude of the first four responses in a train of 16 was generally greater than that of the last four. In an imaginative approach, Ritter, Vaughan, and Costa (1968) used a series of 24 blocks of 30 tonebursts, and averaged between blocks the responses at various intrablock positions. A rapid decrease in response was found over the first few stimuli of a block. The asymptotic amplitude was about 50% of its value for the first stimulus. It might be expected that this rapid habituation would be reduced by the use of non-periodic stimulation, such as by the addition of a random component to the interstimulus interval, but the literature is conflicting (Nelson, Lassman, and Hoel, 1969; Rothman, Davis, and Hay, 1970).

There is evidence for yet another process that causes response decrement but over a longer time course. Bogacz, Vanzulli, and Garcia-Austt (1962) reported a gradual decrease in AEP amplitude for successive blocks of 40 stimuli, and the decrement disappeared upon interference with photic stimuli. This was confirmed by several studies (Zerlin and Davis, 1967; Ritter, Vaughan, and Costa, 1968). Rothman et al. (1970) found no significant decrease in intersubject mean response amplitude throughout a test session of half an hour, but noted a marked decrease in one subject.

It is probable that intersubject variability, difficulties of controlling attention, and other differences in the measurement conditions have contributed to these inconsistencies. However, the consensus is that at least two changes in response amplitude occur over time: a large decrease over the first few stimuli, attributed to a cumulating, exponential recovery process, and a smaller, long-term decline over the course of many averages. There is at least case-report evidence that the true situation may be more complex than this (Hyde, 1976), in that systematic, slow variations of SVP amplitude sometimes appear to occur throughout the course of lengthy averages (see Chapter 3); some, but not all, of these variations are consistent with amplitude decline over time. Further research is required in this area, but there is evidently reason to conclude that the standard statistical model of constant elementary response may be invalid for the SVP.

Binaural Effects

In contrast to the binaural summation effects that occur for the ABR, the SVP for binaural stimulation is very similar, if not identical, to that for monaural stimulation (Davis, 1976). Pantev et al. (1986) reported the interesting finding that while there is no binaural summation for the SVP, there is summation for its magnetic analog. A review of binaural phenomena was provided by McEvoy et al. (1990). Their study of SVPs to shifts in noise image lateralization addresses the issue of direct AEP correlates of arguably the most important aspect of binaural function, but detailed discussion of such suprathreshold applications of the SVP is beyond the scope of the this chapter.

EFFECTS OF SUBJECT VARIABLES

Age

There appear to be no reports of gender differences for the SVP. The limited maturational data have been reviewed by Reneau and Hnatiow (1975) and by Musiek, Verkest, and Gollegly (1988). A comparative review of the maturation of various AEPs, in relation to development of the auditory system, was given by Eggermont (1989).

In neonates and infants, wave identification and maturational changes are complicated by response variability and changes with attention, state of arousal, and stimulation paradigms. Davis and Onishi (1969) reported that the development of response morphology was almost complete at about four months post-term, and the data of Barnet, Ohlrich, Weiss, and Shanks (1975) suggest that over the first three years, N100 latency decreases slightly, and P175 latency decreases markedly and linearly. Shucard and Shucard (1990) found an increase in amplitude though the first nine months, but no changes in latency. In contrast, Kurtzberg (1989), using speech stimuli, described a series of amplitude, latency, and waveform changes from term to two years. She stressed the need for norms specific both to age and to the type of stimulus used.

Callaway and Halliday (1973) and Callaway (1975) indicated that SVP peak-to-peak amplitude increases perhaps by as much as 50% from age 6 years to age 15 years. Their data also indicate a decrease in the latency of both N100 and P175, more marked for the latter. The data of Goodin, Squires, Henderson, and Starr (1978) showed that N100 latency is approximately constant from about 10 to 70 years of age, whereas P175 latency increases by about 25% over that age range. In adults, SVP amplitude decreased with age at a rate of about 1 microvolt every 5 years. These results match those of Brent, Smith, Michalewski, and Thompson (1976).

Attention

Psychological variables are apparently important, even for an "exogenous" response such as the SVP, when delivering to the subject a lengthy and monotonous set of stimuli. For example, Vaughan and Ritter (1970) noted that marked effects on response morphology can occur simply by changing from periodic to irregular stimulation sequences. Keating and Ruhm (1971) found that SVP variability was reduced with the subject reading, in comparison with counting the stimuli or merely sitting quietly. However, there are many discrepancies between studies in this area, some of which may have arisen from the methodological difficulties and subtleties inherent in attempts to measure or control attention (Hartley, 1970; Reneau and Hnatiow, 1975). An extensive review of attention and AEPs was provided by Picton, Hillyard, and Galambos (1976).

Most reports are of apparent increase in SVP amplitude with increased stimulus-oriented attention (Davis, 1964; Mast and Watson, 1968; Fruhstorfer, Soveri, and Jarvilehto, 1970; Picton and Hillyard, 1974). The amplitude changes are most marked at stimulus levels near threshold (Mast and Watson, 1968), and may differ between peaks. The exact mechanisms of these attentional affects are not clear, but changes in habituation are a prime candidate. Recently, it has also become clear that in studies that attempt to manipulate attention, very complex effects can arise because several distinct but concurrent slow evoked potentials that contribute to the overall scalp potential in the latency region of the SVP may be elicited. See Regan (1989, pp. 227–235) for a discussion. As yet, there is no clear consensus about the effects of attention on SVP peak latencies.

CLINICAL APPLICATIONS

Overview

In this chapter, the use of the SVP to estimate sensitivity thresholds for tonebursts, that is, to provide a non-behavioral analog of the pure-tone audiogram, is emphasized and considered in detail. However, the potential range of clinical applications of the SVP is much broader. One of the difficulties in developing clinically useful psychoacoustic measures of supra-

threshold function is the relative lack of sophistication and training of the subjects. Many of the more elaborate procedures are impracticable in the clinical context. Because the SVP is a correlate of any perceptible change in any aspect of the auditory environment, it can be used to explore the perceptibility of changes in the level, spectrum or source position of continuous sounds; it offers a non-behavioral approach to measurement of many psychoacoustical phenomena that have either proven or potential clinical relevance in diagnosis or in rehabilitation.

There are, of course, many other AEPs that can be used to estimate hearing sensitivity, and the question of comparative merit will be addressed in some detail shortly. However, AEPs from different levels within the auditory system can be used not only to cross-validate threshold estimates but also to suggest the site of lesions affecting the central pathways. Squires and Hecox (1983) reviewed such applications, including the use of the later "endogenous" potentials. Kileny (1985) examined the role of the middle-latency response and the SVP in the assessment of central auditory dysfunction, and it appears that SVP latencies may be increased in children with central auditory processing disorders (Jirsa and Clontz, 1990). Kurtzberg (1989) described an important role for slow potentials evoked by speech sounds in high-risk infants, and Gravel, Kurtzberg, Stapells, Vaughan, and Wallace (1989) as well as Stapells and Kurtzberg (in press) have described the role of multiple AEP procedures in an integrated approach to management of otoneurologic disorders in young children.

There have been several other reports showing possible direct (non-audiometric) neurologic use of SVP components in the detection and localization of lesions affecting cerebral cortex (Knight, Hillyard, Woods, and Neville, 1980; Goodin and Aminoff, 1986; Pool, Finitzo, Hong, Rogers, and Pickett, 1989). Most such applications often appear to require exploration of the scalp topography of the SVR. To date, one of the limiting factors has been uncertainly about the generator sites for the SVP. The recent clarification of those sites using dipole source analysis (Scherg et al., 1989) may explain some of the contradictory results to date in studies of cortical lesions. Source analysis seems to offer an approach to lesion detection and localization that is superior to direct topographical analyses (see Scherg and von Cramon, 1990).

Target Populations for SVP Audiometry

The target population for evoked potential audiometry aimed specifically at approximating the pure-tone audiogram is well-known: it includes any subject who is unable or unwilling to provide an acceptable behavioral pure-tone audiogram. This can embrace at-risk infants, difficult-to-test children, adults with certain mental or physical handicaps, and those with suspected functional hearing loss. It also includes persons for whom an "objective" measure of hearing is required, such as in medico-legal claims or compensation evaluations for occupational hearing loss.

The primary target population specifically for SVP audiometry is the subset of the above who are passively cooperative and alert. There are degrees of cooperation and of arousal, and the limits of feasibility of SVP audiometry depend on tester skill, the time available, and the audiometric accuracy required. If the subject will merely tolerate electrode application, then some finite amount of information about hearing can almost always be obtained, but the testing of very young children or of sleeping subjects with the SVP is far from straightforward and should only be done by experienced testers. Subjects who require sedation or anesthesia for AEP audiometry are best evaluated with some tool other than the SVP, such as with the ABR or by electrocochleography (ECochG).

A Conceptual Model of Audiogram Estimation

The word "estimation" is often used, here, reflecting two aspects of audiometry with the SVP, or with any other AEP. First, AEPs do not directly measure hearing, but provide a statistical correlate of it. Only behavior can unequivocally prove that a sound has been perceived, and it is wise to consider AEPs as epiphenomena, that is, as by-products of auditory processing. Second, the problem of interest is inherently statistical, involving the use of a sample measurement based on the SVP to derive the true value of an unknown quantity, the true perceptual

threshold. This estimation is conceptually more complicated than it first appears, and it will be useful to explore it briefly. Some elements of a proposed approach are shown in Figures 8.3A–D.

At low stimulus sensation levels, SVP amplitude increases steadily with stimulus level, and because of this, it is possible to define an SVP threshold. A statistical approach to threshold definition itself is necessary, because the recognition of SVPs in average records is intrinsically a signal-in-noise detection problem. The SVP threshold can be conceptualized in various ways, using a detection theory or statistical decision theory approach. For any particular stimulus level, imagine many averages obtained with that stimulus, and many more with no stimulus; let all the averages be sampled at random and judged for the presence of SVP, equating SVP presence with a suprathreshold stimulus, and SVP absence with a subthreshold stimulus. Whatever the method for evaluation of the averages, various outcome probabilities (hit or true positive, false alarm or false positive, miss or true negative, correct rejection or true negative) will ensue. Thus formulated, the problem of threshold definition relates closely to that of quantifying the accuracy of a yes-no diagnostic test, for which well-known techniques exist (Swets, 1988).

The obvious way of defining the SVP threshold is as that stimulus level that would lead to some particular true positive rate (say, 50% or 75%). The problem is that such a threshold will depend on the adopted false positive rate. Perhaps a better definition is as that stimulus level for which random pairs of stimulus and no-stimulus averages would be correctly discriminated in, say, 69% of cases, in a two-interval forced choice paradigm. For those familiar with the concept of the Relative Operating Characteristic (Swets, 1988), this is equivalent to adopting a d-prime of 1.0 as the threshold determinant (Macmillan and Creelman, 1991). There is nothing magical about the choice of 69% accuracy; other values between the random score of 50% and the perfect score of 100% could be used, and the threshold would shift accordingly. Note that the threshold so defined is not the level at which the SVP has zero amplitude, but is a level based on SVP detectability. It follows that both the intensity-amplitude input-output function and the residual electrical noise level in the

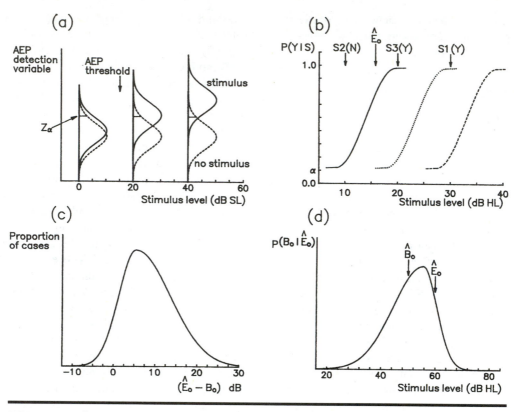

FIGURE 8.3.   A conceptual model of using AEPs to estimate behavioral pure-tone thresholds. (A) AEP detection in averages at various stimulus sensation levels is a signal-in-noise statistical decision problem based on an underlying family of hypothetical distributions of the decision variable; the distance between the "stimulus" and "no stimulus" distributions increases with level (below threshold they are identical). Given some value of the detection variable (Z) that defines a constant false-positive error rate (tail area alpha), the probability of correctly detecting AEP presence increases with level from alpha to almost unity. One such level is defined to be the true AEP threshold, based on its associated true positive rate. (B) When true behavioral and AEP thresholds are unknown, the first step is to estimate the latter. Any true AEP threshold has an associated ogive-like curve of correct detection probability; this is a conditional probability P ("yes", stimulus present) or P (Y/S). Curves for three AEP thresholds are shown. A stimulus and response sequence such as 30 dB (Y), 10 dB (N), 20 dB (Y) is used to estimate the AEP threshold crudely, that is to decide which all the possible ogives gave the observed decision pattern. The true AEP threshold is E_o, with estimation denoted by the hat ^. (C) For any true behavioral threshold B_o, there is a distribution of possible values of the E_o estimate. This is determined by large-sample normative studies, and usually has a mean 5–20 dB and positive skewness, depending on conditions. (D) The clinical problem is to estimate B_o, given an estimate of E_o. The normative distribution can be used in reverse to derive the best estimate of B_o, which is usually $\hat{E}_o$ minus the mean of the distribution in (c).

averages will affect the threshold. It follows in turn that many variables, such as the EEG noise level in the individual subject and average, and the number of stimuli used per average, will also affect the threshold.

In practice, the SVP threshold is never known exactly, but is estimated by making essentially yes-no SVP detection judgments on averages at a few stimulus levels, the overall approach being a bracketing process. Because SVP amplitude increases monotonically near threshold, the probability of judging any specific average as response-positive is also monotonic, increasing from the base false-positive rate through to almost unity at high stimulus sensation levels (Figure 8.3B). The efficiency of this procedure and the statistical properties of the ensuing threshold estimates can vary greatly, depending on the sequence of levels, the stopping rules and the AEP detection criteria (see later). Of course, with the very limited number of averages that it is feasible to collect in a clinical test, and with subjective evaluation of those averages, the threshold estimation process is usually quite crude. For example, if the response is judged definitely present at L dB HL, and definitely absent at, say, L-10, then the threshold estimate might be L-5. If the response is absent at L-10, questionable at L and definite at L+10, then L is the estimate. In many subjects, this causes little error, compared to the more quantitative threshold definitions, because the range of stimulus levels over which the response detectability goes from near-zero to near-unity is less than about 20 dB, and often 5 to 10 dB in the presence of substantial hearing losses.

Given an estimate of the SVP threshold, the clinical problem is to obtain a sufficiently accurate estimate of the true hearing threshold, and to determine the degree of accuracy expected. It cannot be assumed that the SVP and true perceptual thresholds are equal, but to the extent that they are correlated positively, over a hypothetical, large population of subjects, so the SVP threshold could be used to estimate an unknown perceptual threshold. In practice, the true SVP threshold is not available, so its estimate is used instead, but conceptually, there are two steps, one to derive the SVP threshold, and the other to infer the true perceptual threshold.

Overall, the statistical problem can be conceived simply as that of estimating the true mean of a distribu-

tion, given a single observation from it. The optimal distribution to use would be the (hypothetical) distribution of differences between all possible SVP threshold estimates and the true perceptual threshold, in the individual clinical subject, with the differences being attributed to random measurement error. Given that, it would be a simple matter to estimate the true threshold, given a single SVP threshold estimate. In practice, the distribution that must be used is that of the observed differences between the SVP threshold estimates and the behavioral thresholds, in a large, normative group that resembles the target clinical population (Figure 8.3C). The mean (expected value) difference is the statistical "bias" of the SVP threshold, positive bias meaning that the SVP threshold is larger numerically. Thus, the best point estimate of the perceptual threshold is the SVP threshold estimate minus the bias, and the bias is the mean estimation error (Figure 8.3D).

The accuracy of the estimated perceptual threshold can be expressed in terms of a confidence interval for it (Snedecor and Cochran, 1980). To derive this interval, information about the variability and shape of the error distribution must also come from the normative studies of differences between behavioral and SVP thresholds. The variance of the difference distribution governs the width of the confidence interval, and has a much greater impact on the clinical utility of the estimate than its mean (the bias), because the latter is simply subtracted out of the point estimate. The properties of the error distribution, including its shape, symmetry, width and mean value, will depend on many facets of the SVP test procedure, the characteristics and state of the subject, and especially the skill of the tester. Concomitantly, so will the bias and the interval estimate both depend on these many factors.

Accuracy of SVP Audiometry

Some case examples of near-threshold SVP waveforms in normal and impaired ears are shown in Figure 8.4, but the accuracy of SVP audiometry is more properly quantified in terms of the difference distributions for the SVP and behavioral thresholds. Most of the early studies (reviewed by Reneau and Hnatiow, 1975) found that SVP thresholds were within 10 dB of behav-

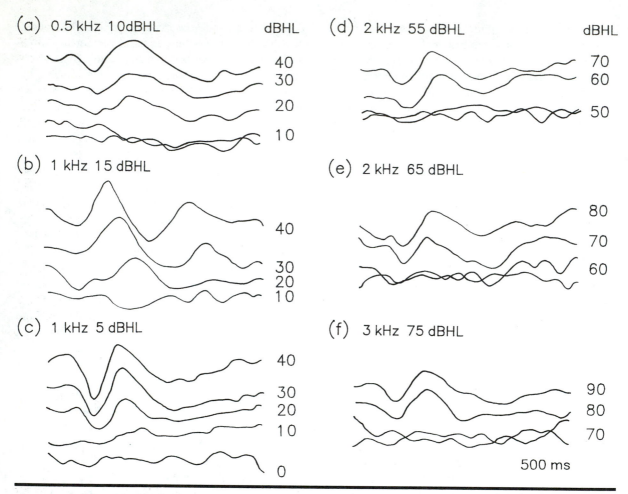

FIGURE 8.4.   Illustrative average SVP records near threshold, for several subjects, frequencies, and degrees of hearing loss (indicated). Note the tendency for large response and small latency shift at only 5–10 dB above the behavioral threshold, when there is moderate sensory hearing loss.

ioral thresholds in from 80% to 100% of cooperative adults with normal hearing (McCandless and Best, 1966; Price, Rosenblut, Goldstein, and Shepherd, 1966; Beagley and Kellogg, 1969). Alberti (1970) found that thresholds were within 10 dB in 90% or more of ears in both normal hearing and hearing impaired adults, for frequencies from 500 Hz to 4000 Hz; his SVP thresholds were obtained blind. Similarly, Beagley (1973) showed that in adults, thresholds were

within 15 dB over 95% of the time; for persons with hearing loss (over 20 dB), all the errors were within 0 to +15 dB, a positive error indicating a numerically larger SVP threshold. Jones, Harding, and Smith (1980) studied the threshold relationships in normal adults, and in adults and children aged 7–14 years with known hearing losses. All group mean errors were smaller than 5 dB. In the normal adults, the SVP threshold was within 10 dB of the behavioral threshold in all cases. In the hearing impaired adults and children, about 75% were within 10 dB, but there were occasional large discrepancies in both directions; they noted difficulties caused by high alpha rhythm. Several of these figures could be improved by adjusting the prediction using a correction factor (estimate of bias).

More recently, large-sample studies have found very good agreement between SVP and behavioral thresholds, in adult medico-legal cases and claimants of compensation for occupational hearing loss; Coles and Mason (1984) used a computer-assisted procedure for response detection, and Hyde et al. (1986) used blind subjective judgments. Some normative data from the latter study, in 254 compensation claimants, are shown in Figure 8.5, indicating 96.4% agreement within 10 dB, at 500 Hz. The scatterplot format is more informative than the overall histogram of differences

between SVP and behavioral thresholds, because of possible changes in the error distribution for various amounts of hearing loss. Indeed, Figure 8.5 suggests that both bias and variability are larger when the hearing is close to normal. SVP thresholds tend to be more sharply demarcated and easier to judge for moderate and severe hearing losses, especially if they are of cochlear origin; the cause of this is probably loudness recruitment and a positive correlation between SVP amplitude and stimulus loudness.

In contrast to these generally encouraging reports, Rose et al. (1971) had found that only 80% of cases fell within 20 dB, and frequently there were much larger errors. They cautioned about the difficulty of response judgments near threshold. Mendel, Hosick, Windman, Davis, Hirsh, and Dinges (1975) concurred, finding an SVP threshold range of 10–45 dB SL, using blind re-

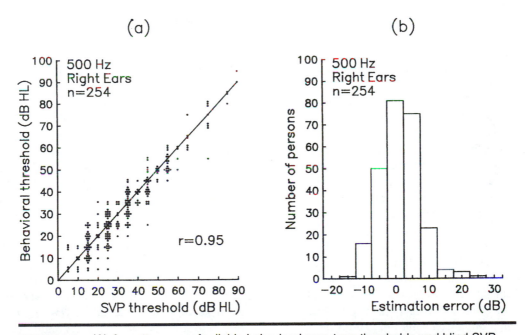

FIGURE 8.5. (A) A scattergram of reliable behavioral pure-tone thresholds and blind SVP threshold estimates in 254 adult claimants for occupational hearing loss compensation. Note the excellent correspondence, and the slight tendency for the SVP threshold to overestimate the perceptual threshold more at low levels. (B) The normative histogram of differences between the SVP threshold estimate and the behavioral threshold, collapsed (for simplicity) over the entire range of SVP thresholds.

sponse judgments. Russ and Simmons (1974) also reported difficulty and unreliability of subjective response detection judgments.

Clearly, there are significant discrepancies between reports about the accuracy of SVP techniques in cooperative adults. There are several sources of difficulty in such studies, in addition to the obvious sources of potential discrepancy such as random error and population differences. First, the behavioral audiometry against which the SVP is compared must be valid and accurate, and this was not always the case. Second, any study that does not involve blind or computer-based evaluation of SVP records is questionable because of possible bias in response detection judgments. Third, differences in many details of SVP technique, such as instructions to the subjects, recording bandwidth and data window, the number of stimuli averaged and the number of averages used, the selection strategy for stimulus levels, and response recognition criteria, can affect the accuracy of results strongly. The effect is one of a chain, only as strong as its weakest link, and the potential causes of poor results are legion. Many of these matters are covered further, later in this chapter.

A very important subject characteristic is the amount of EEG alpha rhythm. High levels of alpha activity increase greatly the difficulty of SVP detection judgments. These activity levels are randomly distributed throughout the population, so differences between groups can arise by chance. The impact of rhythmic EEG on the accuracy of SVP results depends very much on some of the details of technique, and some of the published reports describe techniques that are possibly ineffective.

All of these sources of discrepancy are compounded by frequent reporting of studies with insufficient sample sizes. It is very important to note that sample size requirements for research studies are strongly dependent upon the precise intent of the study. Most studies deal with group mean values of various measures, but in the area of SVP audiometric accuracy, it is the entire error distribution that is of interest, and this is much more demanding. When examining distribution features such as shape, variance, and the proportion of cases in the tails, sample sizes of at least several hundred cases are absolutely essential, or the results will be unstable and potentially misleading.

A very important option in SVP audiometry, and one that is frequently ignored in normative studies, is to abandon the SVP procedure if the EEG conditions are very poor, either as a result of movement artifacts or of high levels of alpha activity. This simple strategy will avoid most of the large errors. It follows that the rules that govern test abandonment will have a profound effect on the error distributions. The appearance of the background EEG and the clarity with which the first attempted SVP threshold is defined will provide the necessary clues as to the probable success of the SVP technique in the individual subject.

In one percent or less of persons, the SVP threshold is much higher than the behavioral threshold, for no obvious cause. This is reminiscent of the occasional subject with normal pure-tone thresholds who has no ABR (Worthington and Peters, 1980). In terms of predictive error in SVP audiometry, this means that there is a small probability (less than 0.01) that the true hearing level is as much as 50 dB better than the observed SVP threshold. Usually, that possibility is ruled out by other audiometric tests.

There is greater consensus regarding the audiometric accuracy of the SVP in very young children: it is relatively insensitive (large bias) and inaccurate (large variability), especially in infants or whenever there is a need to test in natural or sedated sleep (McCandless, 1967; Osterhammel, Davis, and Weir, 1973). The special causes of difficulty in that population include greater variability of response waveform, higher amplitude and more variable EEG, movement artifacts, and changes in attention or level of arousal (Gibson, 1978). However, it is generally agreed that in older, cooperative children, the accuracy of SVP audiometry is comparable to that in adults (Davis, 1966; Claus, Handrock, and Arentsschild, 1975; Jones, Scott, Binnie, and Roberts, 1975; Beagley and Fisch, 1981).

In summary, it appears that accurate threshold estimation by SVP audiometry is problematic in infants and more generally in any subject who is not both awake and passively cooperative. However, if those conditions are satisfied, it is possible to estimate the behavioral pure-tone threshold to within 10 dB in at least 90% of cases. To achieve this accuracy, appropriate instrumentation and testing protocols are essential. Adequate tester skill in response detection judgment is also crucial, unless an automatic procedure is available. Exclusion of subjects with obviously unfavorable EEGs will further improve the test accuracy.

Resource Requirements

The general instrumentation and test facilities required for the SVP are similar to those needed for measurement of other AEPs such as the ABR or MLR. However, an additional bandpass filter will usually be required, because most commercial EP units do not have appropriate filter options; also, some units do not permit external filtering and without it, SVP testing will be considerably more difficult. An audiometric soundroom with adjacent control area is preferred, but it need not be electrically shielded.

A single tester is usually sufficient, for the older child or adult. Adequate tester training and sufficient case load to maintain testing and interpretive skills are absolutely essential. An appropriate training program would include a sequence of observation and instruction, supervised testing, and a practice period of testing hearing impaired subjects whose behavioral thresholds are known; the tester should be blind to the true thresholds until after the interpretation of SVP records. To maintain skills, a clinical case load of at least one per week is desired, and again, these tests should be performed without detailed foreknowledge of any behavioral results. It will usually require a substantial group practice or health care center setting to sustain a successful SVP practice; sporadic SVP testing is simply not clinically viable, because of the skills issue.

Outline of Test Procedures

The SVP test is basically a set of SVP threshold estimations. Typically, it takes between five and ten minutes to estimate a single SVP threshold. Even in a co-operative adult, factors such as boredom, fatigue, or discomfort will limit the test length to about an hour.

Thus, it is rarely possible to obtain a full audiogram. In a single test session, there is a trading relationship between the accuracy of the threshold estimate and the number of stimulus frequencies and routes tested. The use of efficient stimulus selection strategies directed towards specific clinical questions is essential.

With respect to choice of stimulus frequency, route (AC, BC, soundfield), and contralateral masking requirements, SVP audiometry should be regarded simply as a time-consuming version of behavioral audiometry, substituting the detection of a response waveform in the average record for the conventional behavioral response.

Integration of SVP Results

Because AEPs are only correlates of hearing, the results of SVP audiometry should not be taken in isolation, but should be integrated into the overall audiologic picture. Medical or audiologic management should not be based exclusively on SVP results, unless it is absolutely necessary. For example, if the SVP thresholds are very much better than those volunteered behaviorally, a functional component is very likely. Armed with this information, a non-confrontational approach towards re-instruction of the subject is usually indicated, the goal being to obtain some degree of concordance between behavioral and AEP measures. In subjects with functional hearing loss, often the SVP results will be consistent with the clinical impression, or with the BC, SRT, or ART results, and this concordance lends validity to the overall assessment.

Comparison to Other AEP Techniques

The audiometric utility of several AEPs has been reviewed comparatively by Davis (1976), Gibson (1978), Davis (1981), Davis and Owen (1985), Hyde (1988), and Picton (1991), among others. Click stimuli are of little value for quantifying the pure-tone audiogram, except in conjunction with high-pass filtered ipsilateral masking noise, that is, using the relatively time-consuming derived-band technique. The present discussion is restricted to AEPs generated by tonepips or tonebursts (long pips). The most promising candidates are the cochlear nerve compound action potential (CAP) recorded by transtympanic electrocochleography (ECochG), the vertex positive-to-negative potentials starting with ABR wave V that is sometimes called the "wave V - SN10 complex", the MLR (both regular and 40 Hz varieties), and the SVP.

Important dimensions upon which these options can be compared are validity, accuracy, efficiency, and practicability, and these factors are highly interlinked.

Validity. With respect to validity, the question is whether the AEP is reflecting what it is intended to reflect. One obvious cause for a lack of validity would be the occurrence of a lesion at a place in the auditory pathway that is higher (more rostral) than the site of generation of the AEP. See Ozdamar, Kraus, and Curry (1982) for a good case example. The order of AEP preference in this matter is clearly SVP, MLR, ABR, and CAP, with the SVP having the advantage because it is mediated by primary auditory cortex.

The other major threat to validity is lack of frequency-specificity, the risk being that the hearing sensitivity at frequencies other that the frequency being tested at any particular point in time will contribute to, or confound, the measurements. The main ways this could happen are acoustic (Harris, 1978) and physiologic (Folsom, 1984) spectral spread of the effective stimulus energy. See Stapells, Picton, Perez-Abalo, Read, and Smith (1985) for a detailed discussion.

The order of AEP preference with respect to frequency-specificity is SVP, MLR, ABR, and CAP. It can be argued that the ABR and CAP should trade places, but regardless of this, for both of these peripheral phenomena the rapid stimulus onset needed to evoke the required neural synchrony and the brevity of the interval over which the response-determinant events occur are basically incompatible with a narrow effective stimulus frequency spectrum. See Gorga and Worthington (1983), Hyde (1985), and Picton (1991) for further discussion. In contrast, for the MLR and even more so for the SVP, both stimulus rise times and the duration of response-determining events (the integration time) increase. Thus, the problem of effective spectral spread diminishes.

The SVP is highly frequency-specific: there is no apparent clinically significant difference between the frequency specificity of SVP audiometry and that of behavioral pure-tone audiometry itself. Thus, high-slope and notched audiograms can be reproduced accurately. The author's impression is that frequency-specificity of the MLR is less than that of the SVP and better than that of the notch-masked ABR, but there has been insufficient definitive research in this area. The interrelated issues of accuracy and frequency specificity have been examine for certain, specific AEPs, such as by Stapells et al. (1990) for the ABR to notch-masked tonepips, but there appears to have been no definitive comparative study across AEPs in a common group of subjects. Such a study would be difficult, because the test protocol for each AEP technique would have to be near-optimal, the sample size statistically sufficient, and the subjects would have to cover several etiologies and have several specific and relatively uncommon pure-tone audiometric profiles, such as very steep, notched, and low-frequency losses. All in all, it is not yet clear whether the MLR and masked ABR techniques are sufficiently frequency specific for, say, medico-legal evaluation in a person with a possible high-slope audiogram.

An interesting point discussed by Picton (1991) is that some of the masking techniques that are used to increase the frequency specificity of the ABR or CAP, such as the derived-band or notch-masking techniques, actually force response to originate from a restricted place in the cochlea. Place does not always equate to frequency in a simple way. The pure-tone audiogram involves no such place constraint, so if there is damage to the low-frequency region of the cochlea, the behavioral response to a low-frequency stimulus can be mediated by relatively basal hair cells; that is why there is no such thing as a precipitous low-frequency hearing loss. It is possible, therefore, that AEP thresholds obtained using these masking methods will not be reflecting the same aspects of cochlear function as the pure-tone audiogram would. Which of the measures should be the gold standard is debatable, but if the explicit goal is to estimate the pure-tone audiogram, such a phenomenon may cause lack of validity of the AEP thresholds. This is not a concern with the SVP or MLR, for which ipsilateral masking is not necessary.

Accuracy.   The components of accuracy are bias (sensitivity) and variability. Bias is intimately related to the desired test frequency range, because whereas ECochG may actually have the least bias at middle frequencies, the need to evaluate 500 Hz causes difficulty with the more peripheral AEPs, and even with the MLR (Weber, 1987). At 500 Hz, there is no bias problem at all with the SVP. Again, there is a general lack of definitive reports, but it appears that the SVP has the most appropriate range of applicability; the only area of difficulty is at frequencies above 4 kHz, where the SVP thresholds tend to be less well demarcated.

With regard to variability, there are conflicting reports and some of the data for the SVP were reviewed earlier. It is difficult to believe that any AEP, with the possible exception of the CAP recorded transtympanically in subjects with low-slope audiometric profiles, could yield better results than the 90% confidence interval of 15 dB reported earlier for the SVP. The other key issue here is the applicability of the various techniques to the individual subject, which is governed mainly by EEG noise properties. Thus, the subject with a very strong alpha rhythm is not a good candidate for SVP measurement but may be fine for the MLR, whereas a subject with a high level of electromyogenic activity (about 25–250 Hz), associated either with tension in the head and neck musculature or with gross movement, will be unsuitable for MLR testing, and will probably just as difficult with the ABR, because with tonepip stimulation, especially at 500 Hz, the ABR recording bandwidth must be extended to below 100 Hz.

Efficiency.   Conceptually, this dimension addresses the time required to achieve a specific degree of threshold estimation accuracy, when the basic constraints of validity, acceptable bias and applicability to the individual are satisfied. Efficiency relates most strongly to variability, because it is perhaps best expressed in terms of the averaging time needed to achieve a target signal-to-noise ratio at near-threshold stimulus levels. It is assumed that optimal test protocols are used. There have been few, if any, explicit studies of this matter, and certainly not comparative studies. However, it is clear that ECochG will be by far the most efficient (see Eggermont, Odenthal, Schmidt, and Spoor, 1974, for a detailed exposition); the efficiencies of SVP, MLR and ABR testing are probably similar, but this is an area that requires further research.

Practicability.   Despite low complication rates, transtympanic ECochG is at a significant disadvantage relative to the other candidate AEPs, especially in litigious societies, because of its invasiveness and the accompanying transient discomfort. Also, there is the added requirement that the electrode placement be done by a physician. The SVP is at a slight disadvantage relative to the MLR and ABR, because of the common need for additional data filters in order to optimize the recording conditions. On the other hand, some modern AEP instruments cannot even provide ipsilateral masking, so that is a disadvantage for the ABR, given that unmasked tonepips are unlikely to provide sufficient frequency-specificity for the most demanding cases.

The SVP, regular MLR, and ABR require comparable skills from the tester, in terms of session management, and audiometry with any of these AEPs certainly requires a higher level of skill than does otoneurologic ABR measurement, for example. The 40 Hz MLR technique may enjoy a slight advantage because of the simple, oscillatory form of the target response waveform, which makes the response detection judgment a little easier. The ability to use completely standard audiometric judgments in matters of stimulus transducers and contralateral masking favors the SVP and MLR over the ABR, for which there are still some unresolved issues about the accuracy of bone-conduction measurements.

A significant drawback of the SVP is its dependency on the level of arousal. None of the AEP techniques works well in an active, tense, or uncooperative subject, but at least for ECochG and ABR measurement, the options then include natural or sedated sleep, or general anesthesia. Under these conditions, accurate audiometry with the SVP is difficult or impossible; the SVP waveform changes that occur during sleep make response detection judgments more difficult, and also they undermine the process of signal averaging, which is based upon the assumption of constant response waveform for each stimulus. It is possible to perform "SVP" testing during sleep, but the most prominent response component in the sleeping adult is a large negative wave at about 200–300 ms latency (Picton et al., 1974). This means that in the sleeping subject, it is not the regular N100-P175 complex that is providing the threshold estimate, so some additional uncertainty is introduced. Also, the SVP is altered or abolished by many sedative or anesthetic agents. Parving, Elberling, and Salomon (1981) concluded that in young, uncooperative children, ECochG or ABR audiometry are preferable to SVP testing.

Overall Comments.   Despite the probable experiential bias of the author, the SVP has several points in its favor. Perhaps the biggest fallacy, however, is the notion that there is one, best procedure. This is a simplistic view that is unlikely to lead to proper clinical assessment and management. The importance of all of the dimensions considered above will be governed by local circumstances and by the exigiencies of the individual subject. For example, in medico-legal assessments, and where financial compensation is involved, the accuracy needed is usually greater than for clinical assessment of, say, a

person suspected of a functional overlay of emotional origin. Furthermore, the characteristics of the individual subject can affect the viability and accuracy of the various AEP procedures profoundly and unpredictably, so the only proper approach is a multi-AEP decision protocol that takes the pertinent factors into account. See Figure 8.6 for an example of such a protocol.

PROCEDURES FOR CLINICAL SVP TESTING

This section offers more detailed practical information on SVP testing methods. The material is directed primarily at use of the SVP to estimate the pure-tone audiogram in an awake, passively cooperative subject aged about 7 years or more, although in several areas the material may be of broader relevance.

Subject Management

General Points.   Proper management of the subject so as to promote favorable EEG noise conditions is perhaps the most important factor in successful SVP

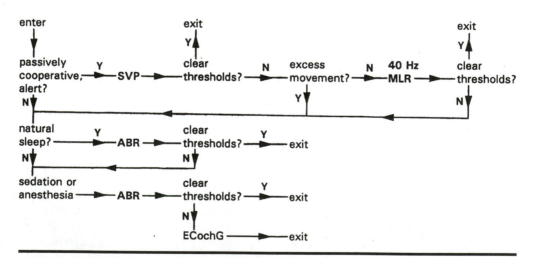

FIGURE 8.6.   A decision protocol for estimating the audiogram using several frequency-specific AEP procedures. The SVP is the tool of choice in the passively cooperative, alert subject. If it fails because of high movement artifact, there is little point in trying the MLR or ABR. If the SVP fails due to large alpha activity (8–13 Hz) in the EEG, the 40 Hz MLR has the best chance of success. Otherwise, testing is done asleep (ABR, but not SVP or MLR) or anesthetized (ABR, then ECochG, but not SVP or MLR). For ECochG and ABR tests, notch masking or high-pass masking noise may be required for adequate frequency-specificity.

audiometry, because it promotes accuracy of SVP detection in average records. Generally, it is unwise to rely solely on technologic maneuvers such as filtering and artifact rejection, to solve EEG noise problems.

The ideal subject is sufficiently cooperative not to move much during the test, because movements generate EEG artifacts that can complicate the evaluation of records (Figure 8.7). These artifacts are not the relatively high-frequency (50–200 Hz) myogenic potentials from head and neck musculature that confound in ABR and MLR measurements. Rather, they are slow (0.5–5 Hz) potential shifts caused mainly by movement of the electrode-skin interface, resulting in changes of the steady potentials that exist in the skin and at the electrode (polarization). For initial instruction, usually it is sufficient to explain the test, to emphasize that no response is required, and to indicate that the subject should read quietly, and not go to sleep. The subject should also be made fairly comfortable, because discomfort causes muscle tension, fidgeting, and movement artifacts. The ongoing EEG should be monitored for artifact, and the subject should be visible and audible to the tester. Earphones can become very uncomfortable after half an hour or so, and the subject should be told to indicate any discomfort, not to tolerate it. Sometimes it is beneficial to have a mid-session break. Any kind of anxiety can also lead to movement artifacts, so it is usually appropriate to keep in touch with the subject occasionally throughout the test. Sitting in a sound room for over an hour, with endless stimuli and no human contact can be quite disturbing, even if there is no physical discomfort, so an occasional reassuring remark can help in maintaining a low level of movement artifact. The best position for the adult subject is probably in a dentist-type adjustable examination chair, providing good head and neck support, but an ordinary, comfortable chair is usually satisfactory. Too much comfort promotes drowsiness.

The subject should remain alert, with eyes open, throughout the test. Eye closure and drowsiness are associated with high levels of alpha rhythm (8–13 Hz) in most subjects, and must be avoided. See Figures 8.7C and 8.8. Averaging is most effective, and the root-N law for SNR increase is valid, if the EEG noise process is random. The more energy there is in sinusoidal EEG components such as the alpha rhythm, the less

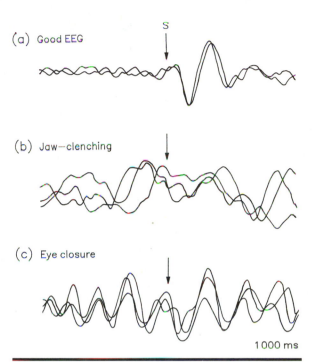

FIGURE 8.7. The adverse effects (despite artifact rejection) of jaw-clenching (B) and eye closure (C) on the ability to detect a clear SVP (A). 40 dB SL, 500 Hz toneburst, onset at 500 ms; bandwidth 1–15 Hz, 24 dB/octave (Butterworth). Note the apparent response cancellation by artifact in (B), and the response-like concordance by chance between records pre-stimulus in (C).

random the EEG becomes; in some persons it resembles the output of a sine wave generator more than a noise generator, even with the eyes open. When the level of alpha is high, it can summate to produce response-like waveforms at stimulus levels far below threshold, or alternatively, it can obscure even large, genuine responses (Figure 8.7). If possible, the subject should read light but interesting material, because it helps to maintain alertness and visual attention itself tends to suppress alpha activity. Flipping through reading material, on the other hand, causes movement artifacts. Lighting levels should be moderately high.

Functional Hearing Loss.   If there is a prior indication that there may be a functional component, acoustic

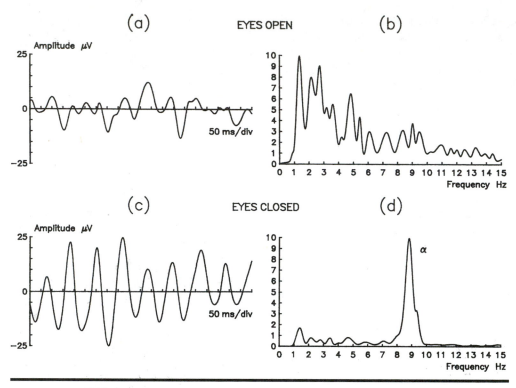

FIGURE 8.8.   EEG activity (sweep length 1s) and frequency spectra (from 100s records, full-scale linear magnitude, scaled to unit maximum), illustrating good SVP recording conditions (A and B), and a large increase in alpha activity associated with eye closure (C and D). Accurate SVP audiometry is difficult when such activity occurs.

reflex measurements and SVP audiometry are best positioned early on in the assessment protocol. The lack of need for behavioral response can be highly disconcerting, if there is deliberate exaggeration of hearing loss. If there is a high index of suspicion of exaggeration, it may be advisable to modify the initial instruction so as to avoid giving clues about how to defeat the SVP test, for example, by covert movement such as jaw-grinding, or by eye closure. In this situation, it is sometimes useful to explain to the subject that he/she should specifically not pay any attention to the stimuli "because it can mess up the test. Don't count them or anything like that." The exaggerator will promptly attend to the stimuli, which will usually increase the size of the SVP as well as reduce levels of alpha rhythm.

The occasional subject will even count out loud stimuli delivered at levels far below the admitted threshold.

Young Children.   The unresponsive but passively cooperative child is no more difficult to test with the SVP than a cooperative adult is. However, the handling of a difficult-to-test child is often as problematic for SVP testing as it is for behavioral testing. This should only be attempted by very experienced SVP testers. The three milestones are: toleration of electrodes, toleration of headphones, and achievement of quiet play. If the child will not tolerate the electrodes, the game is over before it began. If electrodes are tolerated but headphones are not, then soundfield SVP testing is an option, but has the same limitations as for behavioral testing. If both are tolerated, then a skillful SVP tester can almost always obtain useful clinical information. An assistant or a parent is usually needed in the test room, to play with the child; talking to the child causes no problem, as long as it is not continuous. When testing the difficult-to-test child, skill in artifact recognition and management of averaging, as well as efficient stimulation strategy, are absolutely essential.

Test Environment

The most important factors here are electrical interference, acoustics, and distraction. Low-frequency electromagnetic fields are a minor problem, the most common sources generating power-line frequencies (50 or 60 Hz). This problem can usually be dealt with by appropriate siting of power sources, shielding of power lines, and by low-pass filtering of the EEG. The test room acoustics are very important if free-field testing is envisaged, because of standing wave effects at the subject's head. Ambient noise is a concern only if it is distracting or continuous and loud enough to mask the test stimulus. The amount of distraction in the test environment is important for child testing, because distractions are not conducive to quiet play or to the establishment of rapport with the audiologist.

Electrodes

Type.   A detailed review of electrode issues was given by Regan (1989). Electrodes can be needle, cup, or disk. There is little justification for the use of needles. The author's preference is for silver/silver chloride cup or disk. There is a possibility that gold electrodes have higher noise levels at very low frequency than the electrochemically reversible Ag/AgCl electrodes. However, for the SVP recorded with appropriate high-pass filters (with cutoff at 1–2 Hz), the difference is small.

Number and Site.   As is usual for single-channel differential recording, three electrodes are required: one noninverting, one inverting, and one common. The sites are dictated mainly by the scalp topography of the SVP and its associated electrical noise. The noninverting electrode should be at the scalp vertex, or

near to it. The vertex (Cz) is in the midline (that is, equidistant from the left and right preauricular points) and halfway from the nasion (the indentation at the top of the nose, between the eyes) to the inion (the small, bony bump in the midline at the back of the head). The size of the SVP decreases most rapidly posterior to the vertex, to a lesser extent laterally, and even less anteriorly. Thus, placement error anterior to the vertex matters little, but it is important to be within about 1 cm of the midline and definitely not behind the vertex. Although the decrease in response amplitude anterior to the vertex is gradual, the forehead is too far forward for efficient SVP recording.

The site of the inverting electrode has been much debated, but there is some consensus that on or near the mastoid process is most appropriate. This derivation is approximately isopotential with the vertex, for corneoretinal potentials (Hillyard, 1974), and this is important for minimizing eye movement artifacts. Apparently, it matters little which mastoid forms the differential pair, but the author's preference is to use the ipsilateral mastoid, with the other mastoid as common. The mastoid is preferable to the earlobe, if earphone comfort is a consideration.

Preparation and Attachment.   Electrode problems are a very common cause of difficulty in SVP recording. The effect of a poorly attached electrode is to increase the susceptibility to low-frequency movement artifact and other electrical noise. As in other AEP procedures, the electrode sites should be cleaned and lightly abraded, and there are many ways of doing this. In the author's experience, a gauze prep pad soaked with alcohol is very satisfactory. The vertex requires more rubbing than the other sites. Bald persons usually need the most site preparation. However, it is never necessary to cause significant discomfort when preparing the electrode site.

If the vertex is hairy and the sticky disk electrodes are to be used, then the hair must be cut over an area about the size of a quarter. Alternatively, a water-soluble electrode paste that is both conductive and adhesive can be used; then there is rarely a need to cut hair, unless it is dense and wiry, but the area must be cleaned and a layer of paste applied to the scalp. Sufficient paste must also be applied to the electrode, which is then lightly pressed into the paste bed on the scalp, and the whole is covered with a small gauze square. Whatever the electrode, it is important to use sufficient paste or gel, and not to press down hard on the electrode when attaching it; doing so can cause a pocket free of conducting medium when pressure is removed.

Impedance.   With proper preparation of the skin, electrode impedances should be below about 5 kohm, and preferably, should not differ by more than 20%. Higher impedance increases the pickup of movement artifacts and unequal impedance reduces the common mode rejection ratio (CMRR) of the preamplifier. Most instrumentation has built-in impedance checking, but some clinicians prefer to use an independent impedance meter. Usually, the impedance will improve during the testing session, as the electrode/skin interface hydrates and equilibrates electrochemically.

If the clarity of SVP threshold is poor, or if there is a marked change in the EEG at some point during the test, with no obvious behavioral cause, the first step is to check the electrodes. A common problem is raising of the vertex electrode off the scalp, if the attachment procedure was inadequate. This is usually detectable by monitoring the impedance while pressing the electrode gently; if there is a marked reduction in impedance, the electrode must be removed and re-attached. Curiously, it appears that it is not always possible to detect a deficient electrode attachment by impedance checking; another approach is to monitor the ongoing EEG with the bandwidth opened up beyond 60 Hz, and touch the electrode. If the two electrodes (other than the common) are very different in terms of the amount of power line pickup, the one with the larger amount is suspect and should be replaced.

Care and Maintenance.   Reusable electrodes should be washed gently and thoroughly, preferably with a soft toothbrush under clean running water. If necessary, they can be soaked briefly in a non-corrosive disinfectant solution. This must be followed by thorough rinsing. Once cleaned, the electrode surface should not be touched. It should be stored carefully. Dirt particles, scratches or the slightest deposition of grease can in-

crease artifact and noise levels. The junction between the electrode and its lead is often a point of mechanical weakness and susceptibility to corrosion. The junction should not be subjected to stress, such as through pulling the electrode off the skin using the lead.

Preamplifiers/Filters

Standard preamplifiers are used to record the SVP. The typical gain is about 20,000. A suitable recording bandwidth for most cases has 3 dB points at 1–2 Hz (high pass) and 15 Hz (low pass). This is dictated mainly by the spectra of the SVP and the concurrent electrical noise (see Figures 8.1B and 8.8). Correct choice of filters is important. The filter characteristics, especially the low-frequency edge of the pass-band, can make the difference between a useful and a useless test by suppressing high-amplitude, low-frequency EEG energy that will otherwise obscure the SVP, especially when there is a significant amount of movement of the subject. In SVP audiometry, the signal-to-noise ratio is paramount and waveform distortion due to filtering is not usually a concern (see Chapter 3 for a more detailed discussion of filters and waveform distortion). Thus, stronger filters can be used than would be appropriate for situations in which the actual waveform of the AEP is of greater interest, such as in otoneurologic testing with the ABR. For SVP work, a 24 dB/octave Butterworth filter is adequate but 48 dB/octave is better, and the much more common 12 dB/octave is often not enough. Unfortunately, the filters that are supplied with many commercial EP units, whether analog or digital, are not steep enough and do not have enough choices of cut-off frequency for efficient SVP audiometry. Often, it is necessary to augment the instrumentation with a variable band-pass filter, and it must be verified that it is feasible to introduce such a filter into the signal processing channel. Filtering post-hoc, often available digitally, is not a total solution here because one of the problems is in the data acquisition process: insufficient filtering at frequencies below about 2 Hz can lead to unnecessarily high rates of sweep loss due to artifact rejection.

With a bandwidth of about 1–15 Hz, at 24 dB/octave, power line interference at 50 or 60 Hz is not usually a problem. The real issue is the alpha rhythm, which in some subjects can obscure the SVP even when the subject is alert and visually attending. If the alpha is a problem and is of relatively high frequency, perhaps in the 11–13 Hz range, it is sometimes possible to improve the records dramatically by setting the filter cutoff at, say, about 8–10 Hz. This works only if the filter has a steep rolloff, such as 48 dB/octave. However, if the alpha is of lower frequency, such as about 8 Hz, attempts to remove it by filtering end up removing too much of the energy in the SVP itself.

The cutoff slope should not be much greater than 48 dB/octave, nor should the bandwidth be much narrower than about 2–10 Hz. Both these factors tend to promote "ringing" when a high-frequency artifact such as a burst of myogenic activity hits the filter. Also, if the bandwidth is very narrow, there is a loss of response waveshape cues, because the filter output resembles a sine wave at the band center frequency, regardless of the input waveshape.

Window Parameters

To be sure to cover the latency of occurrence of any SVP, a post-stimulus epoch of 500 ms is ideal. However, some pre-stimulus analysis should also be included. In contrast to the situation for the ABR and MLR recorded at high stimulation rates, the bandwidth and interstimulus interval for SVP recording are such that the epoch just before the stimulus should be free of any significant SVP-like evoked potential, so it is a useful baseline against which to judge the post-stimulus epoch. Thus, the recording window should be at least 750 ms long, with a post-stimulus epoch of 500 ms and at least 250 ms of pre-stimulus analysis. Statistically, the preferred window is 1 s long with stimulus onset at 500 ms, because then the probabilities of response-like artifact occurring are equal pre- and post-stimulus. The usefulness of this pre-stimulus analysis as an aid in SVP detection judgments is often not appreciated. This approach is much better than the use of "no-stimulus" or "control" averages, because the EEG noise conditions actually occurring at the time of stimulation are examined. In the minute or two between a control run and a run with stimulation, the EEG conditions can change so

much that the value of any control average is dubious, except to explore nonphysiologic noise.

The main effect of the prestimulus epoch is in reducing false-positive response detection. Often, it can be seen that there is a pre-stimulus transient waveform at least as prominent as that which might be identified as an SVP in the post-stimulus epoch, or it may be seen that the putative response is just a continuation of rhythmic activity starting before the stimulus. To anyone who has used this approach, working without a pre-stimulus analysis is like working in the dark.

Sampling Rate and Number

The sampling theorem dictates use of a digitization rate of at least twice the highest frequency at which there is significant energy in the data, to avoid aliasing errors (Regan, 1989). Using real filters, with their gradual rolloff, a margin of at least 2.5 times the low-pass cutoff frequency is commonly used. For direct visualization of the digitized average AEP, without interpolation to recover the full waveform, in practice the digitization rate should be at least ten times the highest frequency of interest in the AEP, to avoid significant amplitude loss and latency errors. For the SVP, the highest frequency of interest is not more than 15 Hz, so a sampling rate of about 150/s is sufficient. Usually, there will be 256 or more samples in a data window of length 1 s.

Averaging

For a description of the basic theory of averaging, see Chapter 3, which also outlines some more advanced averaging methods. For a detailed exposition of several aspects of averaging and artifact management, see Sayers et al. (1979), Picton et al. (1983), and Regan (1989).

There is no fixed number of accepted sweeps that should be used. Ideally, the number used per average should covary with the EEG energy, so as to promote constant variance in the averaged record, but this is difficult to achieve without computer control. The danger with too few sweeps is that the resulting averages are very variable; if the urge to halt the acquisition arises from on-line monitoring of the accumulating sum or average, a response-like waveform seen initially may well be merely summed noise that would become insignificant after further averaging. The problem with using very many sweeps is that it is potentially inefficient, in the sense that a response might be clearly visible after 20 sweeps, so why continue for 50 sweeps? Also, the return in terms of increase in SNR per unit test time decreases steadily as averaging proceeds, governed usually by the root-N law. Thus, to double the SNR after 10 sweeps takes another 30 sweeps, for a total of 40, whereas to double the SNR after 40 sweeps takes another 120 sweeps, to total 160. If a putative response is unclear at 10 sweeps, going on to 40 sweeps will double the SNR and take perhaps another minute or so. If the same uncertain situation pertains after 40 sweeps, at that point it would cost over four minutes to double the SNR.

The practice recommended here is to use between 10 and 40 accepted sweeps per average, and to replicate a lot. The view is that a single average is worth very little, on its own, no matter how clear the response in it appears to be. With this approach, two averages of 10 sweeps each are the absolute minimum needed for any single stimulus condition; two records of 20 sweeps would usually be sufficient if the stimulus were at a moderate sensation level or higher, and would always be more informative than a single average of 40 sweeps (taking the same test time), because of the importance of showing reproducibility in independent averages. In the case of putative response but substantial discrepancy between two averages of, say, 20 sweeps, it is necessary at least to run another average of 20 sweeps and apply "2 out of 3" scoring. Near to threshold, the use of larger averages and three replicates will increase. To score a near-threshold condition as response-negative requires at least two "negative" averages of 20 sweeps.

The general size of the averages and the number of replicates per stimulus condition will also depend on the EEG characteristics of the individual subject. For example, a subject with high alpha rhythm (despite attempts to reduce it) will tend to need more averaging than someone with a low-amplitude, desynchronized EEG pattern. Also, some subjects have well-behaved EEGs but small SVPs, which tends to result in a lack of clarity of the SVP threshold; under these circumstances, too, the size and number of averages should be

increased. Because the goal is usually to estimate the SVP threshold with a particular, consistent amount of accuracy, it seems reasonable to try and compensate in this way for between-person differences in SVP and EEG noise characteristics.

Artifact Rejection

The simplest approach, available in almost all commercial AEP instruments, is to reject a sweep if its amplitude exceeds some critical value, often corresponding to a full-scale deflection on a display of the ongoing activity. The practical problem is where to set the artifact rejection limits, and whether to change them during the session. In statistical terms, this is akin to the problem of deciding on a rejection criterion for outliers in a one-sample location test (Snedecor and Cochran, 1980). The most common error is to set the limit too high, so that very few sweeps are rejected. There is no fixed value of the rejection limit that will be appropriate for all subjects and conditions. A useful approach that is also applicable to ABR and MLR measurement is to set the limit so that about ten percent of sweeps are rejected even when the EEG is "quiet", i.e., relatively free from movement artifacts and high-amplitude sinusoidal rhythm. This approach trades a small (about 5%) loss of efficiency when the EEG is good for a large gain when it is bad. It also is a sufficiently liberal rejection policy that there is no need to interrupt the averaging if the subject shows a burst of bad EEG: the limit will take care of it and none of the sweeps will be accepted.

It is a significant problem (for all AEP measurements, not just the SVP) that many commercial instruments do not allow sufficiently fine control of the rejection limits. If, for example, the limits are simply at full scale, and the only change possible is by changing the gain, then if the gain control steps are large, such as from 10k to 25k to 50k, the rejection control resolution is inadequate. The tendency is to have too little rejection or too much; within reason, it is better to err on the side of liberal rejection (see Chapter 3).

When someone's EEG "goes bad" in the middle of a session, the best thing to do is try and find out what the problem is and then fix it. It may be discomfort, anxiety, or drowsiness, or it may be a deterioration in an electrode attachment. It is far better to correct the cause of a poor EEG than to rely upon filtering and artifact rejection to cope with the problem.

Sometimes the EEG conditions start off unacceptable and never improve, or become unacceptable and remain so for no obvious reason. The urge to increase the artifact rejection limits so as too allow more sweeps to be averaged should be resisted. If the limits are increased, the reliability of the results will decrease. A deterioration to even a 50% rejection rate is probably best tolerated. If it becomes necessary to raise the limits, then the ensuing records should be treated with caution; there should be an increase in N to 50, and more replication. Essentially, there is no way to get something for nothing: if the EEG deteriorates, then it will take longer to achieve the accuracy targets. The main thing to avoid is pretending that the EEG has not deteriorated, and just changing the artifact rejection limit without any other change in strategy or without recording the deterioration somehow. A useful general practice is to document the rejection limits and the accepted and rejected sweep count for each average.

At some point, the EEG noise levels may have to be considered unacceptable, and the SVP test must be abandoned. What constitutes "unacceptable" is a matter of judgment, and will depend on the precision of measurement required, the skill of the tester, and the state of the subject. Generally, if the EEG is highly rhythmic, testing will be difficult and the emphasis must be upon larger averages, more replications and fewer stimulus conditions. It is better to get one answer that can be believed, albeit at only one frequency in one ear, rather than a more complete audiogram that is wholly unreliable.

Stimuli

Type. The stimuli can be delivered monaurally by headphone, insert earphones, bone conductor, or loudspeaker. Contralateral masking noise is required in accordance with normal pure-tone audiometric criteria. Click stimuli could be used to evoke the SVP, but usually it makes little sense to use such a wide-band stimulus. In contrast to the situation with more caudal AEPs, the click offers no advantage in terms of response clarity, with the SVP. Audiometrically, the click is not usu-

ally an appropriate stimulus, unless only a rough correlate of the best threshold in the 500 Hz to 4 kHz range is required. Click stimulation is certainly not appropriate in medico-legal or compensation assessments, because many, very different audiograms can give exactly the same click results.

To estimate the pure-tone audiogram with the SVP, the most suitable stimuli are shaped tonebursts, with rise and fall times in the range 10–20 ms and a plateau of 20–40 ms. With these rise and fall times the frequency-specificity of the stimulus (and of the elicited SVP) is sufficient for estimating any pure-tone audiogram, regardless of whether the rise/fall envelope is linear or one of the nonlinear forms that restrict spectral energy spread and are preferable for use with more caudal AEPs, such as the ABR.

Repetition Rate. There are several factors underlying the choice of stimulus repetition rate. The higher the rate, the smaller the response evoked by each stimulus, but the more averaging can be done per unit test time. One approach is to optimize the ratio of response amplitude divided by the standard deviation of the averaged noise (Hyde, 1973; Picton et al., 1983). If there is a negative exponential SVP recovery process with a time constant of 4.5 s, as noted earlier, the optimal rate would be about one per six seconds, but the efficiency of one per three seconds is only slightly lower. To get the most total response amplitude per test, a rate of one per second is more efficient, and another problem with very low rates is that the number of stimuli per average tends to be small, which increases the variation in averaged noise from average to average. The optimal rate varies between subjects, but overall, the most suitable rate for clinical testing is one every two to three seconds. The author's preference is for a two-second base CT, with a random increment of up to one second, but this will usually require custom instrumentation.

Stimulus Frequency Tactics

For toneburst nominal frequencies below 500 Hz, at the highest stimulus levels there may be a problem with elicitation of a vibrotactile SVP that is indistinguishable from the auditory SVP. Above 4 kHz, the test difficulty may increase because of the flattening of the amplitude input-output function for stimulus level. Given those constraints, the main point is to select the test frequencies in a "top down" fashion, that is, to ensure that the most important information is gained first. Even when testing a cooperative adult, it is a good idea to behave as if the test session could be terminated at any time. When testing a child, that may well be a very realistic position.

The question to ask, of course, is "If I can test only one frequency, which is it to be?" The process of thinking about the audiometric information in that way can often be quite revealing, in terms of relating the audiometric measurements to the actual critical features in clinical management.

Stimulus Level Tactics

At any frequency, the tactics for selecting the sequence of stimulus levels strongly influence the quality of results and should reflect several principles, some of which are illustrated in Figure 8.9. The key issues are goal-directedness and efficiency. The tactics must be matched to the goals of testing in the individual subject, and those goals should reflect crucial decisions in clinical assessment or management. There is no point in wasting valuable and strictly limited testing time taking measurements that are either clinically irrelevant or which constitute overkill.

The approach reflected in Figure 8.9 is that there are three basic types of measurement goal: threshold classification, in which a fairly crude categorization of hearing sensitivity is sufficient for management, and there is no credible prior information about the true hearing status; second, threshold estimation, in which there is also no good prior information, and a numeric estimate of the threshold is desired, say, within about 10–15 dB; third, there is threshold verification, in which there is a fair degree of prior belief in some particular hearing threshold, and validation of it is required. The estimation problem generally requires the most averages; classification is less demanding because the required measurement precision is less, and verification is less demanding because some use can be made of the prior information, to shorten the test se-

quence. In the case of verification, care must be taken to minimize subjective bias in evaluation of SVP records. In general, especially with limited experience, it is preferable to be blind at least to the precise details of prior audiometry, when performing and interpreting SVP tests.

A general principle is that no endpoint of the stimulus level sequence can be reached without at least two replicated averages at the endpoint level. For the classification problem, the test time is spent obtaining replicated averages at very few levels that are widely separated; ascent or descent is governed by SVP absence or presence, respectively, erring on the side of ascent in case of doubt. For the 30 dB step size shown in Figure 8.9, a total of four averages at two levels is required to reach an endpoint. By then, it is possible to infer the degree of hearing loss with a resolution of about 30 dB. A skilled interpreter, by using clues in the size, latency and clarity of the SVPs, could usually achieve better resolution than that, by interpolation or extrapolation.

For the threshold estimation problem, common mistakes are the use of sequences of levels that are too close together, that start too high or too low, or that are not sufficiently adaptive. In Figure 8.9, the estimation sequence starts in a similar way as for classification, but progresses rapidly to finer resolution of stimulus levels. The guiding principle for the early part of the sequence is the choice of levels that roughly bisect the current range of uncertainty about the threshold (this approach is also reflected in the classification sequence). Note that after only three averages, the domain of possible hearing level from below 15 dB to over 110 dB has been sampled with a resolution of 15 dB or less. This helps to ensure that even if the test session terminates unexpectedly, perhaps due to radical deterioration of EEG conditions caused by drowsiness, anxiety or intolerance, at least classificatory information will have been obtained.

The other important feature of the estimation sequence is that any endpoint that is not at the limits of the hearing loss scale involves at least two pairs of replicate averages, separated by at most 15 dB and usually 10 dB, with the SVP judged present in one pair and absent in the other. When an average is equivocal, a third replicate may resolve the issue, with increase in level if it does

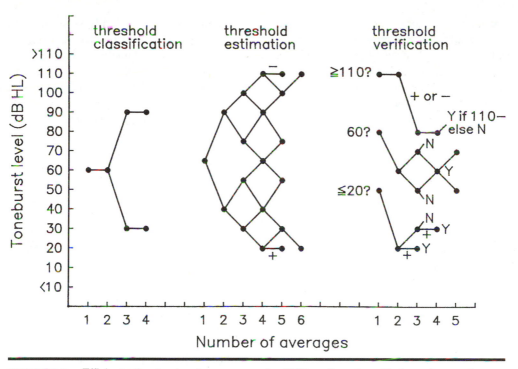

FIGURE 8.9.   Efficient stimulus level sequences for SVP audiometry with three types of clinical goal: a rough classification of hearing, a more precise estimate of the actual threshold, and verification of a particular threshold (three values indicated). Each dot represents an averaging run at the stimulus level indicated. Apart from repeat averages at a given level, generally, if an average is judged positive for SVP, then the level is decreased, otherwise it is increased; exceptions are indicated by + or − signs.

not. It is important to try and obtain an unequivocally positive pair of averages as soon as possible in the sequence of levels, to provide a rough template against which the other records may be compared. Especially if the EEG conditions are unfavorable, failure to do this often results in a very inefficient series, with much time wasted hunting around for threshold in a region that is actually far below the true threshold. The converse of failing to identify a clearly positive level is failing to identify a clearly negative level; here, it is important that proper opportunity for response development was provided, so it is a good idea to require at least two averages of 40 sweeps at any near-threshold level that is considered to be probably negative.

The final result at one frequency can be taken into

account when selecting the initial level for the next test frequency in the same ear. For example, in a noise-exposed adult, if the first frequency tested was 500 Hz and the behavioral threshold estimate was 90 dB, it seems obtuse to start a higher-frequency sequence at 65 dB. The problem is one of possible subjective bias in the interpretation of records; especially when inexperienced, SVP testers are biased to obtain the results they expect. Provided that the general principles of getting an unequivocally positive record quickly, bisecting the range of current uncertainty, and replicating liberally near threshold, are followed, the risk of serious bias or inefficiency is reduced.

The problem of threshold verification, also exemplified in Figure 8.9, could be regarded as a kind of limiting case with strong prior information about the probable hearing level. The tactical principles remain unchanged. In addition, when verifying profound hearing loss it is desirable to check for response presence at a much lower stimulus level, because of the possibility of intensity-amplitude function inversion at high sensation levels, noted earlier. When verifying normal hearing, the relatively high starting level and the subsequent sequence reflect the fact that the true threshold shows a greater tendency to be better than the SVP threshold when hearing is near normal.

Response Detection Judgments

In the absence of computer-based or computer-assisted evaluation of records, the reliance is upon the human observer's judgment of response presence or absence. These judgments are complex, and contain much that is hard to express quantitatively. This is an area in which the interpretive skill resembles an art. The skill is trainable to a point, but there are large differences in aptitude and ultimate performance, even between trained testers. It is desirable to monitor that performance with blind trials, and unless SVP testing is done at a rate of at least one per week, it is doubtful that skills will be maintained, let alone improved. It follows that a large or highly selective referral base is required if high-quality SVP testing is to be offered.

Several factors contribute to accurate subjective detection judgments. The importance of obtaining an unequivocal response at a high sensation level, as early as possible in the test session, has been noted. Such a response can serve as a rough template for subsequent waveform judgments. Perhaps the strongest criterion for a putative SVP waveform to be accepted as genuine is its reproducibility across two or two out of three independent averages. Another criterion relates to the pre-stimulus/post-stimulus contrast, that is, there must not be a similar and equally prominent waveform in the pre-stimulus epoch, nor must there be a coherent oscillatory wavetrain that starts before the stimulus onset. A third criterion is that the putative SVP should exhibit appropriate latency, allowing for a plausible fluctuation of no more than about 25 ms from average to average same stimulus level, and taking account of

the high-level template and the usual increase in latency to be expected just above threshold.

Another useful adjunctive aid is the "+− reference" method (Schimmel, 1967; Picton, Linden, Hamel, and Maru, 1983), in which the regular average is compared against the average of the same data, but with the polarity of half of the sweeps reversed. The reference average retains many of the noise features of the regular average, but should contain no SVP, which will have canceled out. Thus any putative response in the regular average must be absent in the reference average.

The application of judicious SVP detection criteria cannot transmute lead into gold: detection judgment accuracy is strongly affected by many of the technical factors discussed earlier, such as electrode technique, recording bandwidth and artifact rejection. Correct technical procedures and good subject management, as well as interpretive skill, are necessary to achieve accurate results.

Recently, much research has been directed towards the development of computer-based AEP detection methods, most of these being statistically based and oriented towards the ABR or MLR; see Chapter 3 for a more detailed discussion. The early work in this area was applied to the SVP (Rapin, Schimmel, and Cohen, 1974; Salomon, 1974; Hyde, 1976; Sayers and Beagley, 1976; Mason and Barber, 1984). With computer-based statistical response detection methods, is easy to objectively outperform a naive judge, but it is difficult to match the most skilled judges, using Relative Operating Characteristic (ROC; Swets, 1988; Hyde, Davidson, and Alberti, 1991) evaluative methods and blind trials with low-level stimulus delivery or non-delivery as the gold standard. There are several promising approaches, but a method that is unequivocally best has not yet emerged, nor has the performance of the various methods been fully explored. A method that is good for one type of AEP may not be so good for another; the SVP is a relatively demanding problem, because of the small number of sweeps per average, and the degree of violation of assumptions of the classical signal in noise model.

In the medico-legal or compensation assessment context, unless computer-based record scoring is to be used, it is especially important that the SVP tester should not know any of the behavioral results. Coding the averages and scrambling the levels for a given frequency and route of stimulation, followed by interpretation by a third party, is one approach, provided that the interpreter is skilled at SVP testing.

Reporting of Results

The point estimates of the true, perceptual pure-tone thresholds, whether obtained by soundfield, air conduction, or bone conduction, with masking as indicated conventionally, can be reported in a similar format to the behavioral pure-tone audiogram. The main concern is how to deal with the issues of validity and accuracy. Evoked potential audiometry of one kind or another can often be a decisive component of audiologic assessment, but it is important that those who will be making clinical management decisions keep in mind that AEPs are only statistical correlates of hearing, not causative elements. Also, even the most skilled SVP testers will not be able to achieve a level of audiometric accuracy that is equal to that of reliable, behavioral pure-tone audiometry, and it is desirable that the degree of uncertainty in the threshold estimates should be expressed somehow, in the SVP report, because it may affect management.

The usual scientific method would be to provide confidence intervals (90%, say) for the true threshold. The usual clinical method would be to classify the reliability of the result, for example, as good, fair or poor. The problem with such rating scales is that they are subjective and not anchored in any consistent standards. Moreover, unskilled testers tend to over-rate the accuracy of their results—a comment sometimes heard from novices is that they really do not understand the need for all the training and quality control—after all, SVP audiometry is actually quite easy.

The confidence interval approach is not without its problems, either. Clearly, the general performance of tester A cannot be equated with that of tester B, and neither can be equated with accuracy figures from the literature, so which confidence interval is the one to use? One approach is to try and assemble tester-specific accuracy data, but it may be more feasible to develop over-all local norms and rely on proper training and quality assurance to maintain reasonable accuracy and homogeneity between testers. So, the problem is how to express that accuracy on a report, and how to incorporate the genuine differences between subjects in the apparent accuracy of the test; such differences certainly can be recognized by properly trained testers.

The data of Figure 8.5, as well as review of the literature, suggest that it is difficult to do better than a 90% interval width of 15 dB; because there are more reasons why a behavioral threshold would be overestimated (greater hearing loss than there really is) rather than underestimated, the interval would not be symmetric about the estimated SVP threshold. For example, an SVP at 60 dB HL and no SVP at 50 dB would lead to an estimated SVP threshold of 55 dB. The associated approximate confidence interval for the perceptual threshold would be from 45 to 60 dB HL. If there is anything difficult about the SVP test, such as thresholds that are not sharply defined, the interval should be increased to, perhaps, a width of 25 dB. Clearly, this is a very approximate procedure; prehaps the most important feature of it is that by actually plotting a confidence interval on the audiogram, albeit a crude estimate, the clinician making use of the audiometry is reminded explicitly that there is a possibility of error.

CONCLUDING REMARKS

New techniques often undergo an evolution that includes as elements: validation, often in idealized circumstances; adoption, often overenthusiastic, such as in the bandwagon effect; rejection, partly justified, and partly over-reactive; finally, there may (or may not) be rational integration. A quarter-century after the start of this process, SVP audiometry may now be entering the integration phase (Durrant and Wolf, 1991). Part of the confusion about its clinical value was due to the need for careful attention to the many procedural variables that underlie accurate test results. Furthermore, there has been a tendency to over-generalize conclusions about SVP test accuracy, across subject populations, thereby discarding the baby with the bath water.

In recent years, it has become clear that the concept of a single, ideal AEP procedure that is applicable to all populations is intrinsically flawed. Rather, there is a set of procedures that must be matched logically and progressively to the clinical goals and idiosyncracies in the individual subject. The SVP belongs in any such protocol directed at estimation of the pure-tone audiogram.

As noted by Davis and Owen (1985), SVP audiometry is "ideal for a limited class of applications". Performed correctly, it is arguably the best AEP procedure for estimating the pure-tone audiogram in passively cooperative, alert subjects aged over about six years. This includes most medico-legal, DVA/compensation, and functional (non-organic) hearing loss evaluations. More broadly, this test should be considered whenever the patient is passively cooperative and alert and there is any question of audiometric unreliability or inconsistency.

Anticipated developments in automated test control and objective statistical detection of AEPs will accelerate the proper integration of the SVP into the audiologic armamentarium, not only as a tool for estimation of the pure-tone audiogram, but also as a method for objective and practicable testing of suprathreshold auditory performance.

APPENDIX

Synopsis of Clinical Protocol. See text for details.

Indications: Audiometric uncertainty or need for objectivity subject passively cooperative, aged over 6 years.

Subject State: Quiet, alert, sitting comfortably, eyes open, preferably reading.

Test Environment: Soundroom preferred. Electrical shielding unnecessary.

Electrodes: Disk or cup, AgCl preferred, vertex to either mastoid, forehead unsuitable.

Instrumentation: Standard systems, but with added filter.

Preamplifier/Filter: Gain about 20,000, filter 1–2 Hz to 10–15 Hz, Butterworth, Chebychev, or Elliptic modulus, at least four poles (24 dB/octave), phase function irrelevant.

Analysis Window: 500 ms post-stimulus, 250–500 ms pre-stimulus.

Artifact Rejection: Set for 10% rejection during quiet EEG, or as close as possible within equipment limitations.

Stimuli: Monaural via standard AC or BC transducers, conventional contralateral masking. Tonebursts, 10–20 ms rise and fall 20–40 ms plateau, detailed shaping and onset phase irrelevant. Repetition rate about one per 2 s.

Frequencies: 500 Hz to 4 kHz, more difficult at 8 kHz. 6–12 combinations of ear/route/frequency feasible per session.

Stimulus Levels: 10 to 110 dB HL (ANSI, 1989). Efficient, adaptive strategy essential. Obtain response-positive record early. Replicate averages at levels bracketing SVP threshold.

Threshold Estimation: Test blind to any detailed behavioral results. Use high-intensity SVP template, consistency between averages, pre/post stimulus comparison and (+−) reference, where possible, to aid subjective SVP detection judgment.

Reporting: As conventional pure-tone audiogram, but including approximate confidence intervals for perceptual threshold.

REFERENCES

Abe, M. (1954). Electrical responses of the human brain to acoustic stimulus. *Tohoku Journal of Experimental Medicine, 60,* 47–58.

Adler, G. and Adler, J. (1989). Influence of stimulus intensity on AEP components in the 80- to 200-millisecond latency range. *Audiology, 28, 6,* 316–324.

Alberti, P.W. (1970). New tools for old tricks. *Annals of Otology, Rhinology and Laryngology, 79, 4,* 800–807.

Alberti, P.W. (1981). Non-organic hearing loss in adults. In H.A. Beagley (ed.), *Audiology and audiological medicine,* V/2, pp. 910–931. Oxford: Oxford University Press.

Altman, J.A. and Vaitulevich, S.F. (1990). Auditory image movement in evoked potentials. *Electroencephalography and Clinical Neurophysiology, 75,* 323–333.

Antinoro, F. and Skinner, P. (1968). The effects of frequency on the auditory evoked response. *Journal of Auditory Research, 8,* 119–123.

Antinoro, F., Skinner, P., and Jones, J. (1969). Relation between sound intensity and amplitude of the auditory evoked response at different stimulus frequencies. *Journal of the Acoustical Society of America, 46,* 1433–1436.

Arlinger, S., Jerlvall, L.B., Ahren, T., and Holmgren, E.

(1976). Slow evoked cortical responses to linear frequency ramps of a continuous pure tone. *Acta Physiologica Scandinavia, 98*, 412–424.

Bancaud, J., Bloch, V., and Paillard, J. (1953). Contribution EEG à l'étude des potentiels évoques chez l'homme au niveau du vertex. *Revue de Neurologie, 89*, 382–399.

Barnet, A.B. (1964). Averaged evoked electroencephalographic responses to clicks in the infant. *Acta Otolaryngologica, Suppl. 206*, 134–146.

Barnet, A. and Goodwin, R. (1965). Averaged evoked electroencephalographic responses to clicks in the newborn. *Electroencephalography and Clinical Neurophysiology, 18*, 441–450.

Barnet, A., Ohlrich, E., Weiss, I., and Shanks, B. (1975). Auditory evoked potentials during sleep in children from ten days to three years of age. *Electroencephalography and Clinical Neurophysiology, 39*, 29–41.

Beagley, H.A. (1973). The role of electrophysiological tests in diagnosis of non-organic hearing loss. *Audiology, 12*, 470–480.

Beagley, H.A. and Fisch, L. (1981). Bio-electric potentials available for electric response audiometry: Indications and contra-indications. In H.A. Beagley (ed.), *Audiology and audiological medicine*, V/2, pp. 755–768. Oxford: Oxford University Press.

Beagley, H.A. and Kellogg, S.E. (1969). A comparison of evoked response and subjective auditory thresholds. *International Audiology, 8*, 345–353.

Beagley, H.A. and Kellogg, S.E. (1970). A survey of hearing by evoked response audiometry in a group of normally hearing school children. *Journal of Laryngology and Otology, 84*, 5, 481–493.

Beagley, H.A. and Knight, J.J. (1967). Changes in auditory evoked response with intensity. *Journal of Laryngology and Otology, 81*, 861–873.

Bogacz, J., Vanzulli, A., and Garcia-Austt, E. (1962). Evoked responses in man. IV. Effects of habituation and conditioning upon auditory evoked responses. *Acta Neurologica Latinamericana, 8*, 244–252.

Boniver, R. (1982). Interet de l'etude des potentiels evoques corticaux en expertise. *Acta Oto-rhino-laryngologica Belgica, 36*, 377–381.

Brazier (1964). Evoked responses recorded from the depths of the human brain. In R. Katzman (ed.), Sensory evoked response in man, pp. 33–59. *Annals of the New York Academy of Sciences, 112*.

Brent, G.A., Smith, D., Michalewski, H., and Thompson, L. (1976). Differences in the evoked potential in young and old subjects during habituation and dishabituation procedures. *Psychophysiology, 14*, 96–97.

Callaway, E. (1975). *Brain electrical potentials and individual psychological differences*, p. 34. New York: Grune & Stratton.

Callaway, E. and Halliday, R.A. (1973). Effects of age, amplitude and methods of measurement. *Electroencephalography and Clinical Neurophysiology, 34*, 125–133.

Calvet, J., Cathala, H.P., Contamin, F., Hirsch, J., and Scherrer, J. (1956). Potentiels evoques corticaux chez l'homme: étude analytique. *Revue de Neurologie, 95, 6*, 445–454.

Claus, H., Handrock, M., and Arentsschild, O. (1975). Comparison between conventional audiometry and ERA for deaf children in a serial test. *Revue de Laryngologie, 96*, 133–137.

Clynes, M. (1969). Dynamics of the vertex evoked potentials: The R-M brain function. In E. Donchin and D.B. Lindsley (eds.), *Averaged evoked potentials: Methods, results and evaluations*, pp. 363–375. *NASA SP-191*, Washington, DC: Government Printing Office.

Cody, D.T.R. and Klass, D.W. (1968). Cortical audiometry: Potential pitfalls in testing. *Archives of Otolaryngology, 88*, 396–406.

Coles, R.R.A. and Mason, S. (1984). The results of cortical electric response audiometry in medico-legal investigations. *British Journal of Audiology, 18*, 71–78.

Creutzfeldt, O.D. and Kuhnt, U. (1967). The visual evoked potential: Physiological, developmental and clinical aspects. In W. Cobb and C. Morocutti (eds.), *The evoked potentials*, pp. 29–41. *Electroencephalography and Clinical Neurophysiology, Suppl. 26*.

Davis, H. (1965). Slow cortical responses evoked by acoustic stimuli. *Acta Oto-laryngologica, 59*, 179–185.

Davis, H. (1966). Validation of evoked response audiometry (ERA) in deaf children. *International Audiology, 5,2*, 77–81.

Davis, H. (1976). Principles of electric response audiometry. *Annals of Otology, Rhinology and Laryngology, 85, 3, Suppl. 28*.

Davis, H. (1981). Electric response audiometry: past, present and future. *Ear and Hearing, 2*, 5–8.

Davis, H., Bowers, C, and Hirsh, S.K. (1968). Relations of the human vertex potential to acoustic input: Loudness and masking. *Journal of Acoustical Society of America, 43, 3*, 431–438.

Davis, H., Engebretson, M., Lowell, E.L., Mast, T., Satterfield, J., and Yoshie, N. (1964). Evoked responses to clicks recorded from the human scalp. In R. Katzman (ed.), *Sensory evoked response in man*, pp. 224–225. *Annals of the New York Academy of Sciences, 112.*

Davis, H., Hirsh, S.K., Shelnutt, J., and Bowers, C. (1967). Further validation of evoked response audiometry (ERA). *Journal of Speech and Hearing Research, 10, 4*, 717–732.

Davis, H., Mast, T., Yoshie, N., and Zerlin, S. (1966). The slow response of the human cortex to auditory stimuli: Recovery process. *Electroencephalography and Clinical Neurophysiology, 21*, 105–113.

Davis, H. and Onishi, S. (1969). Maturation of auditory evoked potentials. *International Audiology, 8*, 24–33.

Davis, H. and Owen, J. (1985). Brainstem auditory evoked responses. In J.Owen and H.Davis (eds.), *Evoked potential testing*. Clinical applications, pp. 55–108. Orlando, FL: Grune & Stratton.

Davis, H. and Zerlin, S. (1966). Acoustic relations of the human vertex potential. *Journal of the Acoustical Society of America, 39*, 109–116.

Davis, P.A. (1939). Effects of acoustic stimuli on the waking human brain. *Journal of Neurophysiology, 2*, 494–499.

Dawson, G.D. (1950). Cerebral responses to nerve stimulation in man. *British Medical Bulletin, 6*, 326–329.

Dawson, G.D. (1954). A summation technique for the detection of small evoked potentials. *Electroencephalography and Clinical Neurophysiology, 6*, 65–84.

Donchin, E., Callaway, E., Cooper, R., Desmedt, J., Goff, W., Hillyard, S., and Sutton, S. (1977). Publication criteria for studies of evoked potentials (EP) in man. Report of a committee. *Progress in Clinical Neurophysiology, 1*, 1–11.

Durrant, J.D. (1987). Auditory-evoked potential to pattern-reversal stimulation. *Audiology, 26*, 123–132.

Durrant, J.D. and Wolf, K.E. (1991). Auditory evoked potentials: Basic aspects. In W. F. Rintelmann (ed.), *Hearing Assessment*, 2nd edition, pp. 321–382. Austin, TX: Pro-Ed.

Eggermont, J.J. (1989). The onset and development of auditory function: contributions of evoked potential studies. *Journal of Speech-Language Pathology and Audiology, 13, 1*, 5–27.

Eggermont, J.J., Odenthal, D.W., Schmidt, P.H., and Spoor, A. (1974). Electrocochleography: Basic principles and clinical application. *Acta Oto-Laryngologica, Supplement 316.*

Evans, T.R. and Deatherage, B.H. (1969). The effect of frequency on the auditory evoked response. *Psychonomic Science, 15*, 95–96.

Folsom, R.C. (1984). Frequency specificity of human auditory brainstem responses as revealed by pure-tone mask-ing profiles. *Journal of the Acoustical Society of America, 66*, 919–924.

Fruhstorfer, H., Soveri, P., and Jarvilehto, T. (1970). Short term habituation of the auditory evoked response in man. *Electroencephalography and Clinical Neurophysiology, 28*, 153–161.

Gastaut, Y. (1953). Les points negatives evoquées sur le vertex. Leur signification psycho-physiologique et pathologique. *Revue de Neurologie, 89*, 382–399.

Gastaut, H., Regis, H., Lyagoubi, S., Mano, T., and Simon, L. (1967). Comparison of the potentials recorded from the occiput, temporal and central regions of the human scalp, evoked by visual, auditory and somato-sensory stimuli. In W.Cobb and C. Morocutti (eds.), *The evoked potentials*, pp.19–28. *Electroencephalography and Clinical Neurophysiology, Suppl. 26.*

Geisler, C.D. (1960). *Average responses to clicks in man recorded by scalp electrodes.* Technical report, no. 380. Research Laboratory of Electronics, Massachusetts Institute of Technology. Cambridge, MA: MIT Press.

Geisler, C.D., Frishkopf, L.S., and Rosenblith, W.A. (1958). Extracranial responses to acoustic clicks in man. *Science, 128*, 1210–1211.

Gibson, W. P. (1978). *Essentials of clinical electric response audiometry.* Edinburgh: Churchill Livingstone.

Goff, W.R. (1978). The scalp distribution of auditory evoked potentials. In R.F. Naunton and C. Fernandez (eds.), *Evoked electrical activity in the auditory nervous system*, pp. 505–524. New York: Academic Press

Goff, W.R., Matsumiya, Y., Allison, T., and Goff, G.D. (1969). Cross-modality comparisons of averaged evoked potentials. In E. Donchin and D.B. Lindsley (eds.), *Averaged evoked potentials: Methods, results and evaluations*, pp. 95–141. *NASA SP-191*, Washington, DC: Government Printing Office.

Goldstein, M.H., Jr. (1961). Averaging techniques applied to evoked responses. In M.A.B. Brazier (ed.), *Computer techniques in EEG analysis*, pp. 59–63. *Electroencephalography and Clinical Neurophysiology, Suppl. 20.*

Goodin, D. and Aminoff, M. (1986). Electrophysiological differences between sub-types of dementia. *Brain, 109*, 1103–1113.

Goodin, D., Squires, K., Henderson, B., and Starr, A. (1978). Age-related variations in evoked potentials to auditory stimuli in normal human subjects. *Electroencephalography and Clinical Neurophysiology, 44*, 447–458.

Gorga, M.P. and Worthington, D.W. (1983) Some issues relevant to the measurement of frequency-specific auditory brainstem responses. *Seminars in Hearing, 4, 4*, 353–362.

Gravel, J., Kurtzberg, D., Stapells, D., Vaughan, H., and Wallace, I. (1989). Case studies. In J.S. Gravel (ed.), *Assessing auditory system integrity in high-risk infants and young children. Seminars in Hearing, 10, 3, 272–287.*

Grimes, C.T. and Feldman, A. (1971). Evoked response thresholds for long and short duration tones. *Audiology, 10, 358–363.*

Groves, P.M. and Thompson, R. (1970). Habituation: A dual-process theory. *Psychological Review, 77, 419–450.*

Hardin, W.B. and Castellucci, V. (1970). Analysis of somatosensory, auditory and visual averaged transcortical and scalp responses in the monkey. *Electroencephalography and Clinical Neurophysiology, 28, 488–498.*

Hari, R. (1990). The neuromagnetic method in the study of the human auditory cortex. In F. Grandori, M. Hoke and G. Romani (eds.), *Auditory evoked magnetic fields and electric potentials*, pp. 222–282. *Advances in Audiology*, Vol. 6. Basel: Karger.

Harris, F.J. (1978). On the use of windows for harmonious analysis with the discrete Fourier transform. *Proceedings of the IEEE, 66, 51–83.*

Hartley, L.R. (1970). The effect of stimulus relevance on the cortical evoked potentials. *Quarterly Journal of Experimental Psychology, 22, 531–546.*

Henry, G.B. and Teas, D.C. (1968). Averaged evoked responses and loudness: Analysis of response estimates. *Journal of Speech and Hearing Research, 11, 2, 334–342.*

Hillyard, S.A. (1974). Methodological issues in CNV research. In R.F. Thompson and M.M. Patterson (eds.), *Bioelectric recording techniques*, pp. 282–304. New York: Academic Press.

Hyde, M.L. (1973). *Properties of the auditory slow vertex response in man.* Ph.D. thesis, Institute of Sound and Vibration Research, University of Southampton, U.K.

Hyde, M.L. (1976). Statistical inference in electric response audiometry. In S.D.G. Stephens (ed.), *Disorders of auditory function II*, pp. 145–161. London: Academic Press.

Hyde, M.L. (1985). Frequency-specific BERA in infants. *Journal of Otolaryngology, 14, Suppl. 14, 19–27.*

Hyde, M.L., Davidson, M.J., and Alberti, P.W. (1991). Auditory test strategy. In J.T. Jacobson and J.L. Northern (eds.), *Diagnostic Audiology*, pp. 295–322. Austin, TX: Pro-ed.

Hyde, M.L., Alberti, P.W., Matsumoto, N., and Li, Y. (1986). Auditory evoked potentials in audiometric assessment of compensation and medicolegal patients. *Annals of Otology, Rhinology and Laryngology, 95, 514–519.*

Jasper, H.H. (1958). The ten-twenty electrode system of the international federation. *Electroencephalography and Clinical Neurophysiology, 10, 371–375.*

Jerger, J. and Jerger, S. (1970). Evoked response to intensity and frequency change. *Archives of Otolaryngology, 91, 433–436.*

Jirsa, R.E. and Clontz, K.B. (1990). Long latency auditory event-related potentials from children with auditory procesing disorders. *Ear and Hearing, 11, 222–232.*

John, E.R. (1967). *Mechanisms of memory.* New York: Academic Press.

Jones, B.N., Scott, S., Binnie, C., and Roberts, J. (1975). Clinical and evoked response audiometry in late infancy. *Developmental Medicine and Child Neurology, 17, 726–731.*

Jones, L., Harding, G., and Smith, P. (1980). Comparison of auditory cortical EPs, brainstem EPs and post-auricular myogenic potentials in normals and patients with known auditory defects. In C. Barber, (ed.), *Evoked potentials*, pp. 337–344. Baltimore, MD: University Park Press.

Kaskey, G.B., Salzman, L., Klorman, R., and Pass, H. (1980). Relationships between stimulus intensity and amplitude of visual and auditory event-related potentials. *Biological Psychology, 10, 115–125.*

Keating, L.W. and Ruhm, H. (1971). Within average variability of the acoustically evoked response. *Journal of Speech and Hearing Research, 14, 1, 179–188.*

Keidel, W.D. (1971). DC potentials in the auditory evoked response in man. *Acta Oto-laryngologica, 71, 242–248.*

Keidel, W.D. (1976). The physiological background of the electric response audiometry. In W.D. Neff and W.D. Keidel (eds.), *Handbook of Sensory Physiology*, V/3, pp. 105–231. Berlin/New York: Springer Verlag.

Keidel, W.D. and Spreng, M. (1965). Neurophysiological evidence for the Stevens Power function in man. *Journal of the Acoustical Society of America, 38, 191–195.*

Kileny, P. (1985). Middle latency (MLR) and late vertex auditory evoked responses (LVAER) in central auditory dysfunction. In M.L.Pinheiro and F.E. Musiek (eds.), *Assessment of central auditory dysfunction: Foundations and clinical correlates*, pp. 87–102. Baltimore, MD: Williams & Wilkins.

Knight, R.T., Hillyard, S., Woods, D., and Neville, H. (1980). The effects of frontal and temporal-parietal lesions on the auditory evoked potential in man. *Electroencephalography and Clinical Neurophysiology, 50, 112–124.*

Knight, R.T., Scabini, D., Woods, D.L., and Clayworth, C. (1988). The effects of lesions of superior temporal gyrus and inferior parietal lobe on temporal and vertex components of the human AEP. *Electroencephalography and Clinical Neurophysiology, 70*, 499–509.

Kooi, K.A., Tipton, A.C., and Marshall, R.E. (1971). Polarities and field configurations of the vertex components of the human evoked response: A reinterpretation. *Electroencephalography and Clinical Neurophysiology, 31, 2,* 166–169.

Kurtzberg, D. (1989). Cortical event-related potential assessment of auditory system function. In J.S. Gravel (ed.), *Assessing auditory system integrity in high-risk infants and young children. Seminars in Hearing, 10, 3,* 252–261.

Macmillan, N.A. and Creelman, C.D. (1991). Detection theory: A user's guide. New York: Cambridge University Press.

Maiste, A.C. and Picton, T.W. (1987). Auditory evoked potentials during selective attention. In C. Barber and T. Blum (eds.), *Evoked Potentials III.* London: Butterworth.

Marcus, R.E., Gibbs, E.L., and Gibbs, F.A. (1949). Electroencephalography in the diagnosis of hearing loss in the very young child. *Disorders of the Nervous System, 10,* 170–173.

Mason, S.M. and Barber, C. (1984). Machine detection of the averaged slow cortical auditory evoked potential. In R. Nodar and C. Barber (eds.), *Evoked Potentials II.* London: Butterworth.

Mast, T.E. and Watson, C. (1968). Attention and auditory evoked responses to low detectability signals. *Perception and Psychophysics, 4,* 237–240.

McCandless, G.A. (1967). Clinical application of evoked response audiometry. *Journal of Speech and Hearing Research, 10,* 468–478.

McCandless, G.A. and Best, L. (1966). Summed evoked responses using pure tone stimuli. *Journal of Speech and Hearing Research, 9,* 266–272.

McCandless, G.A. and Lentz, W.E. (1968). Evoked response (EEG) audiometry in non-organic hearing loss. *Archives of Otolaryngology, 87,* 123–128.

McEvoy, L., Picton, T., Champagne, S., Kellett, A., and Kelly, A. (1990). Human evoked potentials to shifts in the lateralization of a noise. *Audiology, 29,* 163–180.

McGillem, C.D., Aunon, J.I., and Yu, K. (1985). Signals and noise in evoked brain potentials. *IEEE Transactions on Biomedical Engineering, BME-32, 12,* 1012–1016.

Mendel, M.I., Hosick, E.C., Windman, T.R., Davis, H., Hirsh, S.K., and Dinges, D.F. (1975). Audiometric comparison of the middle and late components of the adult auditory evoked potentials awake and asleep. *Electroencephalography and Clinical Neurophysiology, 38,* 27–33.

Milner, B.A. (1969). Evaluation of auditory function by computer techniques. *International Audiology, 8,* 361–370.

Moore, E.J. and Rose, D.E. (1969). Variability of latency and amplitude of acoustically evoked responses to pure tones of moderate to high intensity. *International Audiology, 8,* 172–181.

Musiek, F.E. and Baran, J.A. (1987). Central auditory assessment: thirty years of challenge and change. *Ear and Hearing, 8, 4 (Suppl.),* 22S–35S.

Musiek, F.E., Verkest, S., and Gollegly, K. (1988). Effects of neuromaturation on auditory-evoked potentials. In D.W. Worthington (ed.), *Seminars in hearing, 9, 1,* 1–13.

Näätänen, R. and Picton, T.W. (1987). The N1 wave of the human electric and magnetic response to sound: A review and an analysis of the component structure. *Psychophysiology, 24,* 375–425.

Näätänen, R., Pavilainen, P., Alho, K., Reinikainen, K., and Sams, M. (1987). Interstimulus interval and the mismatch negativity. In C.Barber and T. Blum (eds.), *Evoked potentials III,* pp. 392–397. Boston: Butterworth.

Nelson, D.A. and Lassman, F.M. (1968). Effect of intersignal interval on the human auditory evoked response. *Journal of the Acoustical Society of America, 44,* 1529–1532.

Nelson, D.A., Lassman, F., and Hoel, R.L. (1969). The effects of variable-interval and fixed-interval signal presentation schedules on the auditory evoked response. *Journal of Speech and Hearing Research, 12,* 199–209.

Nunez, P. (1981). *Electric fields of the brain: The neurophysics of EEG.* New York: Oxford University Press.

Onishi, S. and Davis, H. (1968). Effects of duration and rise time of tone bursts on evoked potentials. *Journal of the Acoustical Society of America, 44,* 582–591.

Osterhammel, P.A., Davis, H., Wier, C., and Hirsh, S. (1973). Adult auditory evoked vertex potentials in sleep. *Audiology, 12,* 116–128.

Pantev, C., Hoke, M., Lutkenhoner, B., Lehnertz, K., and Spittka, J. (1986). Causes of differences in the input-output characteristics of simultaneously recorded auditory evoked magnetic fields and potentials. *Audiology, 25, 4–5,* 263–276.

Parving, A., Elberling, C., and Salomon, G. (1981). Slow cortical responses and the diagnosis of central hearing loss in infants and young children. *Audiology, 20, 6,* 465–479.

Picton, T.W. (1991). Clinical usefulness of auditory evoked potentials: a critical evaluation. *Journal of Speech-Language Pathology and Audiology,* in press.

Picton, T.W., Woods, D., Stuss, D., and Campbell, K. (1978). Methodology and meaning of human evoked potential scalp distribution studies. In D.A. Otto (ed.), *Multidisciplinary perspectives in event-related brain po-*

tential research, pp.515–522. Washington, DC: U.S. Environmental Protection Agency.

Picton, T.W., Goodman, W.S., and Bryce, D.P. (1970). Amplitude of evoked responses to tones of high intensity. *Acta Oto-laryngologica, 70*, 77–82.

Picton, T.W. and Hillyard, S. (1974). Human auditory evoked potentials. Part II: Effects of attention.

Picton, T.W., Hillyard, S., and Galambos, R. (1976). Habituation and attention in the auditory system. In W.D. Keidel and W.D. Neff (eds.), V/3. *Auditory system. Clinical and special topics*, pp. 343–389. Berlin/New York: Springer-Verlag.

Picton, T.W., Hillyard, S.A., Krausz, H.I., and Galambos, R. (1974). Human auditory evoked potentials. I. Evaluation of components. *Electroencephalography and Clinical Neurophysiology, 36*, 179–190.

Picton, T.W., Linden, R.D., Hamel, G., and Maru, J. (1983). Aspects of averaging. *Seminars in Hearing, 4, 4*, 327–341.

Picton, T.W., Woods, D.L., Baribeau-Braun, J., and Healey, T.M. (1977). Evoked potential audiometry. *Journal of Otolaryngology, 6, 2*, 90–119.

Pool, K.D., Finitzo, T., Hong, C.-T., Rogers, J., and Pickett, R.B. (1989). Infarction of the superior temporal gyrus: A description of auditory evoked potential latency and amplitude topology.

Price, L.L., Rosenblut, B., Goldstein, R., and Shepherd, D.C. (1966). The averaged evoked response to auditory stimulation. *Journal of Speech and Hearing Research, 9*, 361–370.

Rapin, I. (1964). Practical considerations in using the evoked potential technique for audiometry. *Acta Oto-laryngologica, Suppl. 206*, 117–122.

Rapin, I., Schimmel, H., and Cohen, M. (1972). Reliability in detecting the auditory evoked response (AER) for audiometry in sleeping subjects. *Electroencephalography and Clinical Neurophysiology, 32*, 734–738.

Rapin, I., Schimmel, H., Tourk, L.M., Krasnegor, N.A., and Pollak, C. (1966). Evoked responses to clicks and tones of varying intensity in waking adults. *Electroencephalography and Clinical Neurophysiology, 21*, 335–344.

Regan, D.M. (1989). *Human brain electrophysiology: Evoked potentials and evoked magnetic fields in science and medicine*. New York: Elsevier.

Reneau, J. and Hnatiow, G.Z. (1975). *Evoked response audiometry: A topical and historical review*. Baltimore: University Park Press.

Ritter, W., Vaughan, H., and Costa, L. (1968). Orienting and habituation to auditory stimuli: A study of short term changes in average evoked responses. *Electroencephalography and Clinical Neurophysiology, 25*, 550–556.

Rose, D.E., Keating, L.W., Hedgecock, L.D., Schreurs, K.K., and Miller, K.E. (1971). Aspects of acoustically evoked responses—interjudge and intrajudge reliability. *Archives of Otolaryngology, 94, 4*, 347–351.

Rose, D.E. and Ruhm, H.B. (1966). Some characteristics of the peak latency and amplitude of the acoustically evoked response. *Journal of Speech and Hearing Research, 9*, 412–422.

Rothman, H.H. (1970). Effects of high frequencies and intersubject variability on the auditory evoked cortical response. *Journal of the Acoustical Society of America, 47*, 569–573.

Rothman, H., Davis, H., and Hay, I. (1970) Slow evoked cortical potentials and temporal features of stimulation. *Electroencephalography and Clinical Neurophysiology, 29*, 225–232.

Russ, F.M. and Simmons, F. (1974). Five years of experience with electric response audiometry. *Journal of Speech and Hearing Research, 17*, 184–193.

Salomon, G. (1974). Electric response audiometry (ERA) based on rank correlation. *Audiology, 13*, 181–194.

Sayers, B.McA. and Beagley, H.A. (1976). Identification of averaged auditory evoked potentials in man. *Nature, 260*, 461–462.

Sayers, B.McA., Beagley, H.A., and Ross, A.J. (1979). Auditory evoked potentials of cortical origin. In H.A. Beagley (ed.), *Auditory investigation: The scientific and technological basis*, pp. 489–506. Oxford: Clarendon Press.

Sayers, B.McA., Beagley, H.A., and Henshall, W.R. (1974). The mechanism of auditory evoked EEG responses. *Nature, 247*, 481–483.

Scherg, M. (1990). Fundamentals of dipole source potential analysis. In F. Grandori, M. Hoke, and G. Romani (eds.), *Auditory evoked magnetic fields and electric potentials*, pp. 40–69. Advances in Audiology, Vol. 6. Basel: Karger.

Scherg, M. and von Cramon, D. (1985). Two bilateral sources of the late AEP as identified by a spatio-temporal dipole model. *Electroencephalography and Clinical Neurophysiology, 62*, 32–44.

Scherg, M. and von Cramon, D. (1990). Dipole source potentials of the auditory cortex in normal subjects and in patients with temporal lobe lesions. In F. Grandori, M. Hoke, and G. Romani (eds.), *Auditory evoked magnetic fields and electric potentials*, pp. 165–193. *Advances in Audiology, Vol. 6*. Basel: Karger.

Scherg, M., Vajsar, J., and Picton, T.W., (1989). A source analysis of the late human auditory evoked potentials. *Journal of Cognitive Neuroscience, 1, 4*, 336–355.

Schimmel, H. (1967). The (+−) reference: Accuracy of estimated mean components in average response studies. *Science, 157,* 92–94.

Shucard, J.L. and Shucard, D. (1990). *Maturational changes in the AEP: A longitudinal study of alert infants.* Presented at the Fourth International Evoked Potentials Symposium, Toronto, Canada.

Simson, R., Vaughan H., Jr., and Ritter, W. (1976). The scalp topography of potentials associated with missing visual or auditory stimuli. *Electroencephalography and Clinical Neurophysiology, 40,* 33–42.

Snedecor, G.W. and Cochran, W.G. (1980). *Statistical methods.* Ames, IA: The Iowa State University Press.

Spoor, A., Timmer, F., and Odenthal, D.W. (1969). The evoked auditory response (EAR) to intensity modulated and frequency modulated tones and tone bursts. *International Audiology, 8,* 410–415.

Spreng, M. (1969). Problems in objective cerebral audiometry using short sound stimulation. *International Audiology, 8,* 424–429.

Squires, K.C., Donchin, E., Herning, R., and McCarthy, G. (1977). On the influence of task relevance and stimulus probability on event-related potential components. *Electroencephalography and Clinical Neurophysiology, 42,* 1–14.

Squires, K.C. and Hecox, K.E. (1983). Electrophysiological evaluation of higher level auditory processing. *Seminars in Hearing, 4, 4,* 415–432.

Stapells, D. (1983). *Studies in evoked potential audiometry.* Doctoral dissertation, University of Ottawa, Ottawa, Canada.

Stapells, D.R. and Kurtzberg, D. (in press). Evoked potential assessment of auditory system integrity in infants. *Clinics in Perinatology.*

Stapells, D.R., Picton, T., Durieux-Smith, A., Edwards, C., and Moran, L. (1990). Thresholds for short-latency auditory evoked potentials to tones in notched noise in normal-hearing and hearing-impaired subjects. *Audiology, 29,* 262–274.

Stapells, D.R., Picton, T., Perez-Abalo, M., Read, D., and Smith, A. (1985). Frequency specificity in evoked potential audiometry. In J.T. Jacobson (ed.), *The auditory brainstem response,* pp. 147–177. San Diego, CA: College-Hill.

Swets, J.A. (1988). Measuring the accuracy of diagnostic systems. *Science, 240,* 1285–1293.

Sutton, S. (1969). The specification of psychological variables in an average evoked potential experiment. In E. Donchin and D.B. Lindsley (eds.), *Averaged evoked potentials: Methods, results and evaluations,* pp. 237–297.

NASA SP-191, Washington, DC: Government Printing Office.

Sutton, S., Braren, M., Zubin, J., and John, E.R. (1965). Evoked potential correlates of stimulus uncertainty. *Science, 150,* 1187–1188.

Vaughan, H.G., Jr. (1969). The relationship of brain activity to scalp recording of event-related potentials. In E. Donchin and D.B. Lindsley (eds.), *Averaged evoked potentials: Methods, results and evaluations,* pp. 45–94. *NASA SP-191,* Washington, DC: Government Printing Office.

Vaughan, H.G., Jr., and Ritter, W. (1970). The sources of auditory evoked responses recorded from the human head. *Electroencephalography and Clinical Neurophysiology, 28,* 360–367.

Walter, W.G. (1964). The convergence and interaction of visual, auditory and tactile responses in human nonspecific cortex. In R. Katzman (ed.), *Sensory evoked response in man,* pp. 320–361. Annals of the New York Academy of Sciences, 112.

Wastell, D.G. (1980). Temporal uncertainty and the recovery function of the auditory EP. In C. Barber, (ed.), *Evoked potentials,* pp. 491–495. Baltimore, MD: University Park Press.

Watts, D. (1976). *Input/output functions for the auditory evoked slow vertex response in man.* M.Sc. thesis, Institute of Sound and Vibration Research, University of Southampton, U.K.

Weber, B.A. (1987). Assessing low-frequency hearing using auditory evoked potentials. *Ear and Hearing, 8, 4 (Suppl.),* 49S–54S.

Williams, W.G. and Graham, J.T. (1963). EEG responses to auditory stimuli in waking children. *Journal of Speech and Hearing Research, 6,* 57–62.

Wolpaw, J.R. and Penry, J.K. (1975). A temporal component of the auditory evoked response. *Electroencephalography and Clinical Neurophysiology, 39,* 609–620.

Wood, C.C. and Wolpaw, J.R. (1982). Scalp distribution of human auditory evoked potentials. I. Evidence for overlapping sources and involvement of auditory cortex. *Electroencephalography and Clinical Neurophysiology, 54,* 25–38.

Worthington, D.M. and Peters, J. 1980. Quantifiable hearing and no ABR: Paradox or error? *Ear and Hearing, 1,* 281–285.

Zerlin, S. and Davis, H. (1967). The variability of single evoked vertex potentials in man. *Electroencephalography and Clinical Neurophysiology, 23,* 468–472.

CHAPTER 9

COGNITIVE AUDITORY RESPONSES

JAYNEE BUTCHER

INTRODUCTION

Classification of AEPs

Auditory evoked potentials (AEPs) consist of a series of bioelectric events generated at various levels of the auditory system. Although there is no formally accepted classification system, AEPs have been described by their common name, physiologic description, anatomical source, latency epoch, latency range, response type, and the response's temporal relationship with the eliciting stimulus. The reader is referred to Chapter 1 for a detailed description of AEP classification.

An alternative method of describing AEPs is to specify whether the electrical potential is elicited directly by an external stimulus (exogenous response), or whether it is of a nonobligatory nature (endogenous response). For example, the earlier and most common cortical AEP components are considered to be exogenous responses and are always elicited by external (environmental) stimuli. Exogenous responses are, therefore, dependent on the physical parameters of the eliciting stimuli (Donchin, Ritter, and McCallum, 1978). These various AEPs have been used to aid in the diagnosis of auditory nervous system disorders, and in the determination of auditory sensitivity in difficult to test patients.

The long latency auditory evoked potentials consist of both exogenous and endogenous components. Specifically, the exogenous components include the N1, P2, and N2 responses that are thought to arise from the temporal and temporal-parietal region of the brain (Celesia and Puletti, 1969; Wood and Wolpaw, 1982). While clinical interest in the long-latency potentials preceded interest in the short-latency responses, the

acceptance of their utility has vacillated over time (Squires and Hecox, 1983). One of the reasons for their waning popularity is undoubtedly that they are more affected by changes in patient state than are the earlier auditory potentials. Exogenous AEPs are reviewed extensively throughout this book.

In contrast, endogenous (event related) responses occur in proximity to the stimuli, but are relatively invariant to changes in the physical parameters of the eliciting stimulus (Desmedt and Debecker, 1979a; Donchin et al., 1978). Endogenous responses (internally generated) are dependent on the contexts within which the stimuli are presented as well as the psychologic status of the individual (Squires and Hecox, 1983).

An example of an endogenous response is the P300. The response is so named because it is a vertex positive wave component occurring from 250–600 ms poststimulus. It is thought to result from cognitive processes related to relevant stimuli. As such, the same stimulus may or may not result in a P300 waveform in an individual, depending on the relevance of the stimulus to the individual. In addition, the P300 may be elicited by the absence of a stimulus if that absence is task relevant (Donchin et al., 1978).

Support for the differences between exogenous and endogenous potentials in terms of the processing required for each can be found in the data related to recovery rates. Specifically, the refractory cycles for the exogenous components typically increase as a function of component latency (Allison, 1962), whereas the P300 component recovers more quickly than do the earlier N1-P2 exogenous components (Woods, Hillyard, Courchesne, and Galambos, 1980). Therefore, while the recovery period for the exogenous components appears to exceed the time required for an individual to evaluate stimuli, the P300 response recovery is apparently more directly related to processing rates (Woods et al., 1980).

It is noteworthy to mention that the endogenous components, as a group, can be generated in various stimulus modalities. For example, a P300 component can be seen in response to auditory, visual, and/or somatosensory stimuli. While various researchers have reported that the scalp distribution and amplitude of the P300 response are independent of stimulus modality (Squires, Duncan-Johnson, Squires, and Donchin, 1977), there is conflicting evidence regarding whether the P300 is a unitary phenomenon (Johnson, 1989*a,b*).

Long-Latency Component Overview

The endogenous long-latency potentials are thought to reflect higher level processing than are the exogenous potentials. While this group of potentials has not received much attention in terms of its application to clinical audiology until recently, it has been studied fairly extensively by scientists interested in studying central processing. The group consists of both negative and positive components that seem to reflect some type of information processing. Figure 9.1, taken from Squires and Hecox (1983), is a schematic representation of the various endogenous evoked potential components that have been described in the literature. The characteristics of the responses in the long latency group differ dramatically from the earlier responses in that they are highly variable and appear to be subject dependent manifestations of perceptual and cognitive activity (Polich and Starr, 1983). It is this potential group which is the subject of the remainder of this chapter. Since the P300 has probably been the most studied of the long-latency endogenous potentials, and because it appears to have the most immediate relevance to clinical audiology, the bulk of the chapter will be focused on the P300 response.

P300 Recording Procedures. The event-related potentials, particularly the P300 response, are most commonly recorded using an "oddball" paradigm (see Figure 9.2). The oddball paradigm involves the presentation of a random sequence of two or more different

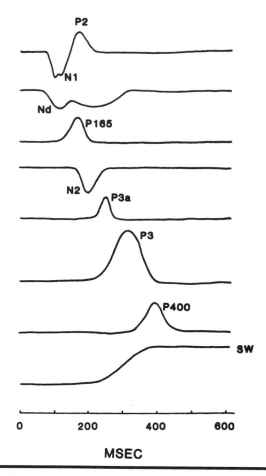

ENDOGENOUS EVOKED POTENTIAL COMPONENTS

FIGURE 9.1. Schematic representation of the long latency endogenous evoked potential components. Copied with permission from Squires and Hecox, 1983.

stimuli, one of which occurs less frequently than the other(s). For auditory testing, the use of tonal stimuli has been most frequently reported, and the tones usually differ in terms of frequency. The subject is instructed to acknowledge the presence of the rare stimuli (Donchin et al., 1978). Investigators have reported the use of active discrimination or signal detection paradigms, in which subjects are required to make

ODDBALL PROCEDURE

Two stimuli, S1 and S2

Train with fixed intervals

Probabilities of S1 and S2 unequal

S1 and S2 mixed randomly

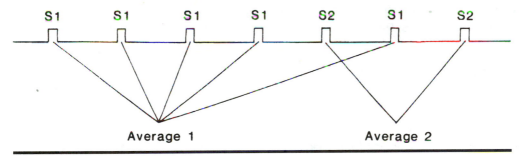

FIGURE 9.2. Schematic representation of an oddball procedure. Copied with permission from Squires and Hecox, 1983.

an active response behaviorally when the targets are heard, and passive paradigms, in which no active behavioral responses are required. While the response mode has been shown to affect the response characteristics, presence of the response does not require active participation on the part of the subject.

When the oddball procedure is employed, the averaged evoked potentials are computed separately for the various stimulus types. Therefore, instrumentation requirements include the capability of presenting at least two kinds of stimuli at variable presentation ratios, as well as the ability to average and store the resulting bioelectrical activity separately. Table 9.1 is a sample protocol for the elicitation of the P300 response. Depending on the purpose of the test, modifications of the stimulus parameters are possible. Using this method, a large P300 response is expected to occur for the target (rare) stimuli only, whereas the earlier ERPs are anticipated in response to all stimulus types. Finally, the response is normally maximal in the temporal-parietal regions of the head (Picton and Hillyard, 1974).

Audiologists have recently become interested in the P300 response because of its potential application in

evaluating patients having suspected problems affecting the central processing of complex auditory stimuli. Inasmuch as the response typically results from an active discrimination, and because the examiner has considerable flexibility regarding the nature of the stimulus employed, the potential exists for examining high level processing skills using a physiologic response. The review which follows will describe the characteristics of and variables related to the P300 response. Subsequently, the clinical application of P300 will be discussed.

CHARACTERISTICS OF AND VARIABLES RELATED TO P300

The P300 vertex positive response has been considered to be an endogenous event-related potential (Donchin, 1979; Snyder, Hillyard, and Galambos, 1980). As such, task relevance is a factor that directly affects the P300 response. Generally, when subjects are asked to attend to a target stimulus, there is typically a larger P300 wave amplitude following the target, regardless of the physical cue involved (Hillyard and Picton, 1979). Whether a

TABLE 9.1. Sample P300 Recording Parameters Using Tonal Stimuli and an Oddball Paradigm.

RECORDING PARAMETERS

Stimulus Parameters:

Stimulus Type	500–4000 Hz Tone Bursts
Rise-Fall	9.9 ms
Plateau Time	30 ms
Delivery Rate	.999 per second
Rare/Frequent Ratio	1/5, Randomized

Other Parameters:

Electrode Montage	Cz and/or Pz to Az
Electronic Impedance	< 3000 Ohms
Filter Bandpass	1–100 Hz
Latency Epoch	800 ms
Patient Response	Count the Rare Tones

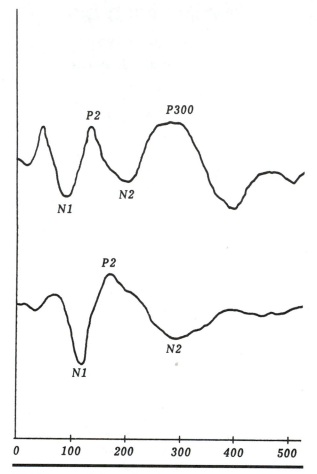

FIGURE 9.3. Schematic representation of responses to target (top trace) and nontarget (bottom trace) tonal stimuli presented using an oddball procedure.

given stimulus serves as a task relevant signal or as a nonsignal is a function of the instructions given to the subject (Pritchard, 1981). More specifically, if the subject is presented with two types of tonal stimuli, both of which are clearly audible, and is told to count silently one stimulus type and to ignore the other type, the counted stimuli will result in a P300 waveform whereas the uncounted stimuli will not. Figure 9.3 illustrates a normal P300 response elicited using tonal stimuli. In normal listeners, the audible target stimulus results in a clearly identifiable P300 response (see top trace), while the nontarget stimulus does not (see bottom trace).The stimulus must in some way be task relevant to elicit a response (Donchin et al., 1978).

Signal Detection and P300

Several investigators have utilized a signal detection paradigm to examine variables affecting the P300 response (Desmedt and Debecker, 1979*a,b*; Hillyard, Squires, Bauer, and Lindsay, 1971; Ruchkin, Sutton, Kietzman, and Silver, 1980; Squires, Squires, and Hillyard, 1975). Stimuli are delivered following a

warning signal at an intensity level that has been determined to allow for a certain percentage correct detection. Subjects are asked to make a decision about whether a target stimulus was presented during each trial. Subjects may or may not be asked to make an overt response.

Various authors have described the relationship between P300 responses and signal detectability. Specifically, Hillyard et al. (1971) found that when AEPs were averaged separately for hits, misses, false alarms, and correct rejections using a signal detection paradigm, a large P300 was evident only for hit trials. They also found that the P300 response increased monotonically as a function of the percentage of correct detections as performance grew from chance to 90% correct. Similarly, Ruchkin et al. (1980) found an increase in P300 amplitude with increasing accuracy. They also found that P300 latency tended to increase as signal detection accuracy decreased.

A signal detection paradigm has also been implemented to examine the relationship between P300 and decision confidence. Squires et al. (1975) utilized an eight-point confidence rating scale, averaging waveforms separately for each decision category. A P300 component was evident for both hit and false alarm trials of the highest confidence rating. As ratings became less confident, there was a systematic decrease in the size of the P300 component for both hits and false alarms, as well as an increase in mean peak latency.

Other investigators have also concluded that the P300 seems to be sensitive to manipulations of confidence (Hillyard et al., 1971; Pritchard, 1981). The lower the subjects' confidence in their perceptions, the lower the P300 amplitude (Pritchard, 1981) and the longer the P300 latency (Snyder et al., 1980). Paul and Sutton (1972) proposed that the increase in P300 amplitude with increased sensitivity or increased detection performance might reflect the degree of confidence felt by the subjects in their decisions with respect to the signals. As intensity is increased, the subjects become increasingly confident in the accuracy of their decisions that the signal was presented.

Stimulus Probability and P300

Another variable that has been demonstrated to affect the P300 waveform is stimulus probability (Donchin et al., 1978). The relationship between a priori probability and subjective probability is complex and somewhat vague. Although the a priori probability has been shown to have an effect on the P300 waveform, the effect is only as great as the relationship between the physical stimulus probability and the subjective probability. In terms of the relationship between the subjective probability and P300 amplitude, there seems to be a inverse linear relationship between subjective prob-

ability of the stimulus and P300 amplitude (Johnson and Donchin, 1980). The more improbable the event, the larger the amplitude of the P300 that results (Donchin, 1979; Polich, 1987b). Furthermore, a reduction in P300 amplitude with increased task probability has been reported in children as well (Ladish and Polich, 1989).

Various researchers have concluded that the subjective probabilities assigned to an event by a subject vary from trial to trial, depending on the specific sequence of stimuli preceding the event (Duncan-Johnson and Donchin, 1977; Johnson and Donchin, 1980; Squires, Petuchowski, Wickens, and Donchin, 1977; Squires, Wickens, Squires, and Donchin, 1976).The size of the P300 complex elicited by a given stimulus increases with the number of different stimuli preceding it. Conversely, the size of the P300 complex decreases as runs of like stimuli precede the target.

Squires et al. (1976) used the word "expectancy" to refer to the complex relationship between stimulus probability, stimulus sequence, and P300. These authors hypothesized that expectancy is determined in a linear fashion by three factors: 1) the memory for event frequency within the prior stimulus sequence; 2) the specific structure of the prior sequence; and 3) the global probability of the event. Given the complexity of the relationship of these factors with P300 and the data reported by various investigators, it seems as though the expectancy model is a reasonable way to describe the relationship between probability and P300.

Emitted versus Evoked P300

As was discussed earlier in this chapter, the data relative to P300 suggest that both task relevance and stimulus probability have an effect on the waveform of the P300 component. Various studies have reported that an absent stimulus will also result in a P300 when that absence is task relevant and relatively improbable (Desmedt and Debecker, 1979a; Ruchkin and Sutton, 1978a, b; Ruchkin, Sutton, and Tueting, 1975; Squires et al., 1975). Ruchkin and Sutton (1978a) differentiated between the two P300 components by using the terms "emitted" and "evoked." The emitted P300 occurs at the time of the expected but absent sensory stimulus, whereas the evoked P300 occurs in response to a present sensory stimulus. They reported, furthermore, that the emitted and evoked P300s differ in waveshape detail; emitted P300s have lower amplitudes and longer duration than their evoked counterparts.

Ruchkin and Sutton (1978a) conceded that the differences they found between evoked and emitted P300s may have been due to the lack of a precisely timed external stimulus for the emitted trials. They investigated that hypothesis by conducting a study that used latency compensated averages in addition to conventional averages to examine amplitude relationships. They found that the average emitted potential was smaller than the averaged evoked potential, and that the decrement from evoked to emitted was greater when the interstimulus interval was longer. Emitted potentials decreased in size with increased interstimulus intervals. They also found that emitted P300 latency was related to time estimation; those subjects who increased most in their time judgment variability as a function of increase in duration of the interval being judged were also subjects whose emitted P300 latency variability increased most.

Evidence suggests that the emitted and evoked P300s are manifestations of the same process. Both are similarly affected by stimulus probabilities (Ruchkin et al., 1975; Squires et al., 1975), and have similar scalp distributions (Squires et al., 1975). It seems clear, then, that like the evoked P300, the emitted P300 can be produced endogenously when the experimental conditions allow the subject to make a definite time-locked decision that an expected stimulus was absent (Desmedt and Debecker, 1979a).

P300 and Reaction Time

A large portion of the P300 literature has involved the examination of the relationship between P300 and reaction time (RT). The consensus of the studies was that, although P300 and RT are related, they are not indices of the same process (Ford, Roth, Mohs, Hopkins, and Kopell, 1979). P300 latency is affected by only some of the component processes that contribute to RT. McCarthy and Donchin (1981) indicated

that the processes concerned with the categorization of stimuli affect both P300 latency and reaction time, whereas processes of response selection and execution have no effect on P300 latency. Several investigators have also concluded that P300 latency is sensitive to the duration of stimulus evaluation processes and is relatively insensitive to response selection processes (Donchin, 1979; Kutas, McCarthy, and Donchin, 1977; Ritter, Simson, Vaughan, and Friedman, 1979). As Donchin et al. (1978) concluded, the latency of P300 depends on the time required by subjects to recognize a stimulus for what it is.

If the latency of the P300 waveform is sensitive to the duration of stimulus evaluation time, then variables affecting the latter should also affect the former. Difficult discriminations are known to lengthen reaction time. Donchin et al. (1978) reported that longer P300 latencies were also associated with more difficult discriminations between targets and non-targets. Similarly, Polich (1987b) reported that increased task difficulty yielded a decrease in P300 amplitude, and an increase in P300 latency.

Stimulus repetitions also affect stimulus evaluation time, and therefore the P300 response. Johnson and Donchin (1980) concluded that the reduction in P300 amplitude with stimulus repetitions indicated that subjects tend to expect a stimulus to repeat. Because of the subjects' expectations that a stimulus will repeat, when it does repeat, subjects take less time to respond. The RT is shorter for repeated trials, and the P300 latency and amplitude are reduced.

In summarizing the relationship between P300 and RT, Donchin (1979) commented that if P300 latency represents stimulus evaluation time, then its relation to reaction time should depend primarily on the extent to which the subjects' reaction time depends on stimulus evaluation. The data from reaction time studies have supported this notion.

VARIATIONS OF P300

To this point, the discussion has been concerned with the P300 as a unitary phenomenon. However, there is some controversy regarding whether that is in fact the case. Squires et al. (1975) made direct comparisons between late-positive waves evoked by shifts in ongoing trains of tones in conditions of active attention versus non-attention (reading). They found that two types of P300 waves could be identified; the two differed from one another in latency, scalp topography, and psychological correlates. The P300 component which was evident during the ignore condition in response to infrequent stimuli was referred to as "P3a"; the counted rare stimuli resulted in a complex called "P3b." Squires et al. reported that the mean latency of P3a was between 220 and 280 ms, whereas the P3b component had its major peak between 310 and 380 ms. In terms of scalp topography, P3a had the largest amplitude at Fz or Cz, whereas P3b was largest at Cz or Pz. The researchers concluded that the P3a and P3b waves are indices of different brain phenomena.

Polich (1989*a*) compared the event-related potentials obtained using a passive procedure with those obtained while patients completed active discriminations. Additionally, he examined responses from the passive ignoring condition with those obtained while the subject was actively involved in a task of another modality (puzzle-solving). In the first case, he found no differences in the P300 waveforms in terms of scalp distribution and peak latencies across conditions. In the second instance, he found a reduction in the amplitude of the P300 during the puzzle-solving task, but did not report a change in latency of the response.

Pritchard (1981) mentioned two additional types of P300 responses. He observed that attended, task-relevant, and intermittent stimuli that are easily encoded evoke a P300 that appears to be similar to the P3b of Squires et al. (1975). However, with repeated presentations, the component undergoes a decrease in amplitude. Also, Pritchard observed that the amplitude of this third type of P300 seems to be more a function of physical contrast with background stimuli than of stimulus probability. In those respects, the third type of P300 described by Pritchard appears to be a different phenomenon than the P3b described earlier.

The fourth type of P300 reported by Pritchard appears in response to "novel" stimuli. According to Pritchard, the response to novel stimuli initially has a frontal scalp distribution, however, with repetition it gradually shifts in location until it resembles a P3b in scalp topography. It also decreases in amplitude with repeated presentations.

It is not clear how many varieties of P300 truly exist, nor are the characteristics of each completely clear. There are some data that suggest that previous efforts to interpret the P300 in terms of a single mode of information processing have been complicated by evidence that there may be different varieties of the late positive P300 waves (Snyder et al., 1980). It is apparent that additional research is necessary before this controversy can be resolved.

SUMMARY OF P300

Although the research related to P300 has been highly variable in terms of its purposes, methods, and results, there are some common threads which run throughout. First, the process manifested by P300 appears to be related to the ongoing process by which the subject interacts with the environment rather than the specific response-selection mechanisms activated on a given trial (Duncan-Johnson and Donchin, 1977). Although a task-relevant event, whether it be the presence of a stimulus or the absence of one is typically involved in the elicitation of a P300, the simple stimulus-response relationship which is characteristic of the exogenous components is not characteristic of the P300 complex. The P300 is a robust component of the human event-related potentials which is apparently endogenous (Donchin et al., 1978).

Previous data have also supported the conclusion that the P300 is elicited independent of stimulus modality, although the degree to which it is truly a unitary phenomenon remains unclear. It has been suggested that the appearance of the P300 wave seems to reflect some special cognitive processes that are invoked by certain psychological operations, such as stimulus meaning, independent of the physical characteristics of the stimulus (Ford, Roth, Dirks, and Kopell, 1973; Hillyard and Picton, 1979). This cognitive process concept is supported by the fact that both latency and amplitude of the P300 can be modulated by variations in the psychologic context in which stimuli are presented (Donchin et al., 1978; Roth, Ford, and Kopell, 1978; Sutton, 1979).

Desmedt and Debecker (1979a) proposed that the P300 denotes the completion of a cognitive epoch and the clearance of the processing capabilities for the next upcoming items rather than the actual operation of any specific cerebral processor; P300 is a post-decision event. Picton and Hillyard (1974) concluded that the P300 complex indexes the perceptomotor sequelae of the decision that an event has occurred; the sequelae might involve the registration of pertinent sensory information in memory, the resetting of perceptual analyzers, or an appropriate behavioral response. Similarly, Klein, Coles, and Donchin (1984) reported that their data may be interpreted as supporting the notion that the P300 reflects processing activities related to the maintenance of representations of external events in "working memory." Furthermore, Squires et al. (1976) reported that the P300 seems to be associated with the evaluation of contextual hypotheses generated about the environment.

Clearly, there has been no general agreement upon how to best formulate the psychological correlates of P300 (Squires et al., 1975). It appears to be part of a decision complex, and undoubtedly overlaps with other late components having different scalp distributions (Snyder et al., 1980). Perhaps the best approach for now is to continue systematically investigating the characteristics of and variables relating to the P300 component. Eventually, continued careful study may lead to lawful answers for the questions related to the psychologic and physiologic origin of the P300.

AUDIOLOGIC APPLICATIONS OF P300

Audiologists have become increasingly more interested in the cognitive responses over the last several years because they form a class of responses which has potential in providing a means of evaluating higher level processing skills. Although there has been no absolute agreement about how to formulate the psychological correlates of P300, the data support the concept that a task relevant event is a necessary, if not sufficient, condition for eliciting a P300. Because it is, in that respect, a measure or index of stimulus processing, it appears to have potential value in the assessment

of hearing sensitivity and auditory processing abilities. In fact, Hillyard et al. (1971) reported that the P300 wave on hit trials was six to eight decibels more sensitive than any other component in the passive vertex AEP typically used in clinical audiology.

Another distinct advantage of the P300 response is that it is less dependent on the physical characteristics of the stimulus employed than are the exogenous potentials. As such, a complex stimulus can be employed to elicit the response. Additionally, although it does require attention to task relevant stimulus items, no active behavioral response is required from the subject. For those reasons, there is renewed interest in the use of this response in the evaluation of patients having suspected or confirmed diagnoses of disorders affecting cognitive function.

Before discussing the literature pertaining to P300 data obtained from various patient groups, consideration of the literature pertaining to the normal aspects of P300 is essential. Specifically, a review of stimulus effects, response mode effects, and the effects of subject characteristics (i.e., age, gender, and alertness) is critical.

Normal Aspects of P300

Stimulus Effects.   Numerous investigators have reported that P300 latency and amplitude vary as a function of psychological parameters rather than the physical characteristics of the stimulus. However, few studies have systematically examined the effects of changes in stimulus frequency or intensity on the P300. Butcher (1983) utilized an oddball paradigm to investigate the above-mentioned relationship with normal adult subjects. She found that changes in the intensity of the rare stimulus had a significant effect on the latency of the P300 response. Specifically, as the stimulus was increased in intensity from 10 dBSL to 50 dBSL, the average reduction in P300 latency was 29.3 ms. Changes in stimulus frequency had no significant effect on the P300 response.

Polich (1989b) examined the effects of changes in stimulus frequency, intensity, and duration on the auditory P300 response. He reported that both the latency and amplitude of the response were affected significantly by changes in frequency, and that P300 latency was affected by an interaction of stimulus intensity and duration. Similarly, Polich, Howard, and Starr (1985*a*) reported that increased target tone frequency yielded decreased P300 latency. Additionally, they reported that the use of masking resulted in an increase in P300 latency. No gender differences were noted in their data. Therefore, while the changes noted by these investigators are sometimes small, they are reliable.

Response Effects.   Another important consideration in the application of the P300 response to clinical audiology is the task assigned to the subject. Clearly, if the aim is to obtain optimal responses, selection of the appropriate task is important. Although researchers have commented regarding the effects of task complexity on P300, few studies have systematically compared the types of responses typically used to determine whether the response mode contributes to variability in the P300.

Butcher (1983) compared the P300 responses obtained using three response types. Specifically, subjects were instructed to: (i) mentally acknowledge, (ii) silently count, or (iii) silently count and press a button in response to rare stimulus presentations. The data indicated that changes in response mode had a significant impact on P300 amplitude. To be specific, whereas no differences were noted between the two counting conditions, a large amplitude reduction was present when the subjects were only mentally acknowledging the tones. No latency effects were present as a function of response mode.

Polich (1987*a*) also examined the response mode effects on the P300 across three conditions during a discrimination task. In comparing the responses obtained while subjects silently counted, tapped an index finger, or pressed a button in response to target stimuli, he reported that P300 amplitude was greater when subjects counted the targets than for the other two conditions. Furthermore, he reported an increase in P300 latency when subjects counted. Therefore, it is apparent that the auditory P300 response is sensitive to response mode for discrimination tasks, and should be taken into account during auditory evaluation.

A final issue to be considered regarding the normal aspects of the P300 response related to its application in clinical audiology is that of task difficulty. Specifi-

cally, if the response is to be utilized with patients having suspected cognitive or auditory processing deficits that may affect the perceived task difficulty, it is important to determine whether that variable has an impact on the responses obtained in the normal population. Polich (1987*b*) examined P300 responses obtained for "easy" and "hard" auditory discriminations, and concluded that processing difficulty does affect the latency and amplitude of P300 responses. Results also suggest that the effects are independent of stimulus probability unless differences in task requirements affect the encoding of the stimuli employed.

In summary, then, although the P300 response is considered to be an endogenous potential, and is therefore less sensitive to the physical attributes of the stimuli employed than the exogenous responses, it is clear from the literature that stimulus and response characteristics do have reliable effects on the P300 latency and amplitude of the P300 response. Therefore, in comparing the results from various studies, as well as the clinical findings across settings, stimulus and response parameters are important considerations.

Effects of Subject Characteristics.   The developmental aspects of the P300 response have been studied by various investigators. Martin, Barajas, Fernandez, and Torres (1988) examined event related potentials in normal children using an oddball paradigm. They grouped subjects in two ways according to age, and completed separate age versus P300 latency and amplitude regression analyses for a subgroup of subjects ages 6–14 years versus the entire subject age range of 6–23 years. They reported a significant negative correlation between age and P300 latency. Interestingly, the slope of the regression line was different for the two age groups, with the young subjects demonstrating a more steeply sloping function than did the older children. The authors concluded that P300 latency decreases with increasing age during childhood until it reaches an asymptote sometime during the second decade of life.

Similarly, Pearce, Crowell, Tokioka, and Pacheco (1989) examined age-related changes in P300 latency in children ranging in age from 5–13 years. These authors reported significant age trends in P300 latency which appeared to be linear in nature. The slope of the curve reported was approximately 20 ms, which is in good agreement with the 19 ms slope reported by Martin et al. (1988) for children aged 15 years and younger. Pearce et al. hypothesized that the neurodevelopmental processes, such as increased myelination and dendritic arborization, may underlie the changes in P300 latency seen in children.

At the other end of the age continuum, the effects of aging on the latency of the P300 response have been investigated in adult subjects. Age-related effects in the normal population are particularly important considerations in applying this response to elderly patients having cognitive impairments. Polich, Howard, and Starr (1985b) reported a significant increase in P300 latency with advancing age which was evident in both the P3a and P3b components. The average increase in latency seen between 20 and 70 years of age was 65 ms. These authors also reported increased variability of the P3 components with advanced age.

Diagnostic Applications of P300

The diagnostic application of P300 which has received the most attention in the literature is the use of the response in the evaluation of patients who are suspected of having disorders which affect their cognitive function. Specifically, Alzheimer's disease and other forms of dementia have been studied, as have patients having aphasia, head trauma, epilepsy, multiple sclerosis, autism and schizophrenia, and alcoholism. With these patient types, the theoretical function of the response appears to be the detection of a processing impairment in response abnormalities before the patient's behavior on traditional measures of cognitive function would be affected.

A second category for potential application of the P300 response is directly related to auditory perceptual skills. In particular, the evaluation of sensitivity and discrimination abilities could be evaluated using a physiologic response. Because the response appears to be present when a patient perceives something relevant about a stimulus, regardless of whether an active behavioral response is made, it may be used with some difficult-to-test patients for whom auditory processing abilities are questionable. Additionally, it could be used

to determine whether a patient is capable of perceiving a difference between two or more stimuli. For example, Kileny (1991) used the P300 response to monitor tonal discriminations in cochlear implant recipients.

The remainder of this section will consist of a discussion regarding the clinical utility of the P300 response with various patient populations, and some suggestions for future research in that regard.

Dementia. Several studies have compared P300 and other event-related potentials obtained for young adults and/or normal elderly versus elderly demented patients (Ball, Marsh, Schubarth, Brown, and Strandburg, 1989; Polich, Ehlers, Otis, Mandell, and Bloom, 1986; Slaets and Fortgens, 1984; Neshige, Barrett, and Shibasaki, 1988; Sara, Kraiuhin, Gordon, Landau, James, Howson, and Meares, 1988). Some investigators have reported significant response abnormalities in demented patients relative to normal controls (Neshige et al. 1988; Ball et al. 1989; Polich et al. 1986), while other investigators have failed to see significant differences across groups (Sara et al. 1988; Slaets and Fortgens, 1984).

Neshige et al. (1988) used an auditory oddball paradigm to compare the long latency event related potentials obtained from two groups of patients, one having known Alzheimer's disease, and the other having multi-infarct dementia. Abnormality was based on a 95% confidence level determined from a regression equation employed on data obtained from normal subjects. The investigators were interested in knowing whether P300 was a useful diagnostic test for dementia. They were also interested in clarifying whether there is a correlation between P300 and intelligence measurements in demented patients.

Neshige et al. (1988) reported that significant prolongation of both the N2 and P300 responses was evident for both groups of demented patients overall. However, in examining the data more closely, it was evident that abnormal responses were evident in less that half of the demented patients tested. Additionally, no significant amplitude changes were reported. In comparing the P300 response latencies to WAIS scores, a negative correlation was evident.

Ball et al. (1989) conducted a longitudinal study comparing latency changes in the auditory P300 response for probable Alzheimer's disease (pAD) patients and normal controls. At the beginning of the study, the pAD group had significantly prolonged P300 latencies relative to normal subjects. Additionally, over the course of the study, the rate of change in the pAD group was significantly greater than in the normals. The authors concluded that the increased rate in P300 latency shifts in the demented patients may be reflective of an accelerated aging process in that group.

Polich et al. (1986) evaluated the relationship between P300 latency and cognitive function in normal elderly and cognitively impaired elderly patients. They found that the response latency was significantly longer in patients diagnosed as having dementia and other cognitive impairment. Furthermore, neurologists' ratings of cognitive decline were positively correlated with P300 latency. However, it is of interest to note that no significant latency differences were evident between categories of dementia.

Slaets and Fortgens (1984) were interested in knowing whether P300 is of value in the differential diagnosis of dementia. They compared event-related potentials for demented elderly, nondemented elderly, and normal young adult subjects. Contrary to the results of the studies discussed previously, these authors did not report a significant difference in P300 latency between the two groups of elderly patients. They did report that P300 latency increased as a function of age by an average of 0.3 ms per year, but the response did not differentiate the demented from the nondemented elderly subjects. Additionally, they did not report any change in the N100 and P200 components as a function of age or dementia. Finally, the authors reported that the latency of the P300 responses obtained for elderly patients were highly variable overall.

Similarly, Sara et al. (1988) investigated the ability of the P300 latency measure to discriminate demented patients from normals. They hypothesized that, in part, the conflicting evidence in the literature regarding the utility of the P300 response as a diagnostic tool, stems from the fact that studies have varied in terms of the degree of dementia of the subjects studied, as well as the procedures employed. Specifically, some investigators have averaged responses from target stimuli without regard to the patient's attention to and percep-

tion of the targets. Because the response mode employed is known to have an impact on the P300 (Butcher, 1983), the variable of attention to task may be important to control. Finally, in some cases, the diagnostic criteria for determining severity of dementia have been unclear.

Interestingly, when the patients' ability to perform the required task was monitored and only clearly identified targets contributed to the averaged response, no significant difference was noted in the responses obtained for the demented subjects relative the their age-matched controls (Sara et al., 1988). Furthermore, several of the demented subjects were unable to perform the required button-press response task correctly. Finally, only two of 15 demented subjects fell outside the 95% confidence regression.

Rather than considering only P300 latency across patient groups, Patterson, Michalewski, and Starr (1988) examined response latency variability as well in their comparison of demented elderly, depressed elderly, normal elderly, and normal young subjects. They reported increased latency and increased variability of the P300 response relative to the normal controls and the depressed patients. Contrary to the findings of Slaets and Fortgens (1984), Patterson et al. (1988) did not find any change in latency variability as a function of increased age alone.

Despite the statistical significance of the differences in P300 latency and variability between groups, only 27% and 13% of the demented patients were correctly identified using P300 variability and latency, respectively (Patterson et al., 1988). Therefore, these authors concluded that, while event-related potentials were useful in describing group differences, they were not sufficiently sensitive to be used in differentially diagnosing demented patients on an individual basis.

In summary, depending on the criteria employed in subject selection and the determination of normalcy, the P300 response may or may not vary significantly from normal in patients diagnosed as having dementia. In terms of the clinical utility of the P300 response in sorting individual patients from age-matched normal controls, the data do not convincingly support the clinical use of this test. As Sara et al. (1988) pointed out, the insensitivity of the response in the early stages of dementia constitutes a limitation in the clinical utility of the test. Apparently, the diagnosis of dementia is most difficult in the early stages. Therefore, it is at that point that an objective measure of function would be most useful.

Other Neurologic Disorders.   One of the neurologic disorders that has been studied using event-related potentials is minor head injury. Specifically, Pratap-Chand, Sinniah, and Salem (1988) examined changes in the P300 responses over time for patients having concussion and normal controls. They found abnormal latency and amplitude values initially for the patients. However, the observed abnormalities seen resolved in time. Therefore, the authors suggested that the P300 response may be a useful measure of cerebral dysfunction in head trauma patients.

The P300 responses of patients having multiple sclerosis (MS) have also been studied. Newton, Barrett, Callanan, and Towell (1989) compared the ERPs of MS patients with age-matched controls. While all subjects had normal exogenous responses, approximately half of the patients had abnormal cognitive responses. It is noteworthy to mention that, of the patients with abnormal endogenous potentials, all but two had prolonged reaction time. Additionally, they all had more grossly abnormal MRI scans and a longer duration of illness with greater physical disability than did the patients having normal P300 responses.

Rodin, Khabbazeh, Twitty, and Schmaltz (1989) studied the P300 response characteristics of epilepsy patients, comparing their responses to those of age-matched control subjects. They found that 10% of the patients had response latencies beyond three standard deviations of the mean. They did not find any seizure type or medication effects on the responses.

Investigators have also examined the P300 characteristics in autistic and Down's syndrome patients. Niwa, Ohta, and Yamazaki (1983) compared P300 responses from four autistic subjects with four Down's syndrome patients and five normal controls using three response modes. Half of the autistic subjects were unable to participate in the active discrimination task, so comparisons for that response mode were not possible. In examining the data from a passive sequence, autistic subjects had decreased response amplitude relative the other subject groups. It is important to mention, however, that the number of subjects evaluated was very small. Therefore, the generality of the findings is questionable.

Dawson, Findley, Phillips, Galpert, and Lewy (1988) examined the relationship between response characteristics and language impairment and intelligence in autistic children. These investigators used a modified tonal stimulus and a consonant-vowel syllable (/da/) to elicit responses during a discrimination task. For this study, responses were recorded from three scalp locations in an effort to determine whether hemispheric differences exist. While no differences across subject groups were evident to the tonal stimulus, the autistic children exhibited decreased response amplitude at the vertex and left hemisphere sites, and increased amplitude at the right hemisphere site to the syllable stimulus. Furthermore, degree of language impairment was correlated with increased response amplitude for the right hemisphere. The authors concluded that there was differential hemispheric involvement in autistic children.

Another population for which hemispheric differences were found is aphasic subjects. Selinger, Prescott, and Shucard (1989) compared ERPs obtained using a verbal and a nonverbal paradigm from aphasic subjects with those of normal adults. They also compared the patient's endogenous responses to traditional aphasia tests. The results yielded hemispheric differences in the aphasic group during the verbal task which were not evident in the normal subjects.

As was the case with the literature pertaining the utility of the P300 response in the differential diagnosis of dementia, the evidence suggests that P300 responses obtained from patients having a variety of neurological disorders may be abnormal. In fact, in a statistical sense, each of the groups studied demonstrated response characteristics which differ from a normal population. In that regard, it is useful in discussing group differences relative to the normal population. However, when the standard is one of clinical sensitivity, the P300 response does not appear to be useful in differentiating individual patients, nor does it appear to be valuable in the differential diagnosis of various possible disease processes.

Auditory Perception.   To this point, the discussion of the clinical application of the P300 response has been centered on latency, amplitude, and variability measures, and a comparison of those characteristics in disordered populations relative to normal subjects. Inasmuch as P300 has been described as an index of cognitive function, the attempt has been to use it in that capacity to assess patients having suspected cognitive decline. As was mentioned earlier, the utility of the response in that regard appears to be limited.

Audiologists interested in obtaining information about auditory perceptual skills may prefer to use the presence or absence of the response to index cortical processing of auditory stimuli. As was discussed earlier in this chapter, in certain contexts, the P300 response occurs following various environmental events, apparently as a function of a subject's decision about or evaluation of those events (Picton and Hillyard, 1974; Squires et al., 1976). Specifically, in an oddball paradigm, a P300 component is expected to occur when a subject successfully attends to the rarely occurring stimulus. Additionally, either simple or complex discrimination paradigms can be used in its elicitation (Kileny, 1991). Therefore, the response appears to have potential in the evaluation of patients for whom the ability the discriminate and perceive stimuli is an issue. However, it is important to reiterate at this juncture that, in this application, the clinician or researcher would be concerned about the presence or absence of a response, rather than the response characteristics per se.

Recently, Kileny (1991) reported the use of cognitive ERPs in children who have been implanted with cochlear implants. In the P300 paradigm, the earlier ERPs (N1 and P2) are evoked by both the frequent and rare auditory stimuli, and indicate that the signals have been detected. Secondly, the presence of a P300 component indicates that the patient is able to discriminate the rare from the frequent stimuli. In a cochlear implant patient, then, the presence of the P300 response could be used to determine whether implant patients hear as different two stimuli that are known to be audible, and that should stimulate different pairs of an electrode array.

Kileny (1991) reported data obtained from four implanted children using both passive and active task paradigms. Prior to experimentation, it was determined that the patients were able to detect all of the stimuli employed in the study. His data demonstrated that some of the cochlear implant recipients were able to differentiate the frequent and rare stimuli, as evidenced by the presence of distinct, reproduceable P300 components in response to rare stimuli. Additionally, while other subjects were apparently unable to discriminate the two stimuli, the presence of robust N1-P2 components supported the audibility of both stimuli. Finally, the P300 component was present in both the active and passive conditions for subjects who were capable of discriminating between the frequent and the target (rare) stimuli. Figure 9.4 illustrates the responses to the two stimulus types from a twelve-year-old cochlear implant recipient. The top trace is the response to the frequent stimulus (500 Hz tone bursts), while the bottom trace is the response to the target or infrequent stimulus (2000 Hz tone bursts). This patient, reportedly, was an excellent responder who had no difficulty detecting or discriminating the two stimuli employed. As can be seen in the figure, this patient exhibited a prominent P300 component with a peak latency of 440 ms.

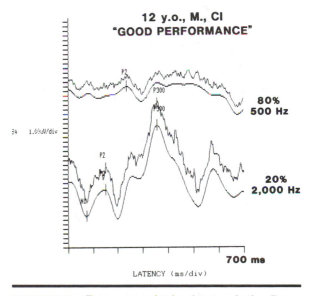

FIGURE 9.4.   Responses obtained to tonal stimuli from a 12-year-old cochlear implant recipient. Copied with permission from Kileny, 1991.

Based on his preliminary work with cochlear implant recipients, Kileny concluded that the cognitive ERPs may be useful in the ongoing monitoring of detection and discrimination abilities in cochlear implant recipients. Furthermore, he suggested that the use of this paradigm with phonetic or phonemic stimuli may facilitate additional monitoring of the progress in this young patient population.

In a similar fashion, the P300 paradigm could be used to evaluate discrimination abilities in patients who are unable or unwilling to cooperate with behavioral tests of discrimination. For example, patients for whom the peripheral function has been determined to be normal via behavioral or physiological tests (e.g. ABR testing), but who behave as if they are hearing-impaired, may be evaluated. Recently, one such patient was presented to the author for testing because he insisted that he could hear nothing, but previous audiological testing had suggested that he had normal or near normal hearing sensitivity. Because his educational placement was dependent on a determination of his auditory function, and because of the conflicting evidence present in the patient's records, the issues of cortical deafness and central auditory processing ability were raised.

While the patient refused to cooperate with an active discrimination task, he was physically quiet enough to enable the examiner to complete AEP testing. Specifically, ABR, MLR, and ERP components were evaluated. The earlier responses were indicative of normal peripheral auditory function. Additionally, reliable P300 components were present in response to the rare stimuli, thereby confirming the patient's ability to differentiate the frequent and rare tones.

It is interesting to note that most of the research completed in the area of auditory EPRs has involved the use of tonal stimuli, despite the fact that the paradigm can be adapted for the use of more complex stimulus items. Specifically, visual ERPs have been elicited using written words, and there is no reason why linguistic units could not be presented auditorially. While the instrumentation involved in the use of external stimuli for AEP testing is somewhat more complex than is required for using stimuli which are generated by the recording instrument itself, the possible benefits of having a physiological indicator of speech processing is worth the additional effort. Additionally, because the use of complex auditory stimuli has not been widely investigated, it would be important to compare behavioral discrimination data for comparison with P300 data for normal subjects before employing it with patients. Specifically, a categorical perception experiment is necessary in which test stimuli are used both to test patients' behavioral responses and their ERPs. If the P300 response is truly an indication of auditory speech discrimination abilities, the category boundaries obtained for the behaviorally obtained responses should correspond with the presence of P300 responses. Such an investigation has not yet been reported in the literature.

Audiologic Applications Summary

A review of the literature to date suggests that there is widespread interest in the P300 response, both on the part of audiologists and on the part of other professionals interested in cognitive and auditory processing abilities. The applications of the test fall into two categories: 1) the diagnosis of disorders affecting cognition; and 2) the evaluation of specific auditory perceptual skills. While both applications have been investigated and reported in the literature, differences exist between them in terms of the clinical utility of the response.

In one application type, the examiner is interested in comparing response characteristics (i.e., amplitude, latency, and variability) for waveforms obtained from patients against those obtained from normals. As was discussed earlier in the chapter, researchers have demonstrated that a number of patient populations exhibit response abnormalities as a group when compared to normal listeners. In a clinical environment an examiner is typically interested in evaluating the responses of a single patient in an effort to contribute to a diagnosis. Inasmuch as the sensitivity of the test appears to be relatively poor, the value of the response in the clinical assessment of patients having cognitive impairments seems limited.

Conversely, in the second type of application described, the examiner is interested in the presence or absence of a response, and the goal is to determine whether a patient is capable of discriminating between two or more stimuli presented. Specifically, examples outlined include the evaluation of cochlear implant patients and patients who are unable or unwilling to cooperate with behavioral auditory discrimination procedures. At the present time, the clinical utility in this regard is limited to the use of tonal stimuli. However, if experimentation using complex auditory stimuli with normal listeners demonstrates that the response is, in fact, a marker of specific auditory discrimination, its potential application in the evaluation of central auditory processing abilities in various patient populations is exciting. Certainly, the data to date suggest that the response has value, and the potential applications of the response warrant further study.

REFERENCES

Allison, T. (1962). Recovery functions of somatosensory evoked responses in man. *Electroencephalography and Clinical Neurophysiology, 14,* 331–343.

Ball, S., Marsh, J., Schubarth, G., Brown, W., and Strandburg, R. (1989). Longitudinal P300 latency changes in Alzeimers disease. *Journal of Gerontology, 44,* 195–200.

Butcher, J. (1983). P300 as a clinical diagnostic tool: The effects of changes in stimulus frequency and intensity and response mode on P300 (Doctoral dissertation, University of Kansas, 1983). *Dissertation Abstracts International.*

Celesia, G. and Puletti, F. (1969). Auditory cortical areas of man. *Neurology, 19,* 221–220.

Dawson, G., Findley, C., Phillips, S., Galpert, L., and Lewy, A. (1988). Reduced P3 amplitude of the event-related brain potential: Its relationship to language ability in autism. *Journal of Autism and Developmental Disorders, 18,* 493–504.

Desmedt, J.E. and Debecker, J. (1979a). Waveform and neural mechanism of the decision P350 elicited without prestimulus CNV or readiness potential in random sequences of near-threshold auditory clicks and finger stimuli. *Electroencephalography and Clinical Neurophysiology, 47,* 648–670.

Desmedt, J.E. and Debecker, J. (1979b). Slow potential shifts and decision P350 interactions in tasks with random sequences of near-threshold clicks and finger stimuli delivered at regular intervals. *Electroencephalography and Clinical Neurophysiology, 47,* 671–679.

Donchin, E. (1979). Event-related brain potentials: A tool in the study of human information processing. In H. Begleiter (ed.), *Evoked brain potentials and behavior.* New York: Plenum Press.

Donchin, E., Ritter, W., and McCallum, W.C. (1978). Cognitive psychophysiology: The endogenous components of the ERP. In E. Callway, P. Tueting, and S.H. Kolson (eds.), *Event-related brain potentials in man.* New York: Academic Press.

Duncan-Johnson, C.C. and Donchin, E. (1977). On quantifying surprise: The variation of event-related potentials with subjective probability. *Psychophysiology, 14,* 456–466.

Ford, J.M., Roth, W.T., Dirks, S.J., and Kopell, B.S. (1973). Evoked potential correlates of signal recognition between and within modalities. *Science, 181,* 456–466.

Ford, J.M., Roth, W.T., Mohs, R.C., Hopkins III, W.F., and Kopell, B.S. (1979). Event-related potentials recorded from young and old adults during a memory retrieval task. *Electroencephalography and Clinical Neurophysiology, 47,* 450–458.

Hillyard, S.A. and Picton, T.W. (1979). Event-related brain potentials and selective information processing in man. In J.E. Desmedt (ed.), *Cognitive components in cerebral event-related potentials and selective attention.* Basel, Switzerland: Karger.

Hillyard, S.A., Squires, K.C., Bauer, J.W., and Lindsay, P.H. (1971). Evoked potential correlates of auditory signal detection. *Science, 172,* 1357–1360.

Johnson, R. Jr. (1989a). Auditory and visual P300s in temporal lobectomy patients: Evidence for modality-dependent generators. *Psychophysiology, 26,* 633–650.

Johnson, R. Jr. (1989b). Developmental evidence for modality-dependent P300 generators: A normative study. *Psychophysiology, 26,* 651–667.

Johnson, R. Jr. and Donchin, E. (1980). P300 and stimulus categorization: Two plus one is not so different from one plus one. *Psychophysiology, 17,* 167–178.

Kileny, P.R. (1991). The use of electrophysiological measures in the management of children with cochlear implant: Brainstem, middle latency, and cognitive (P300) responses. *American Journal of Otology, Supplement, 12,* 37–47.

Klein, M., Coles, M., and Donchin, E. (1984). People with absolute pitch process tones without producing a P300. *Science, 223,* 1306–1308.

Kutas, M., McCarthy, G., and Donchin, E. (1977). Augmenting mental chronometry: The P300 as a measure of stimulus evaluation time. *Science, 197,* 792–795.

Ladish, C. and Polich, J. (1989). P300 and probability in children. *Journal of Experimental Child Psychology, 48,* 212–223.

Martin, L., Barajas, J., Fernandez, R., and Torres, E. (1988). Auditory event-related potentials in well-characterized groups of children. *Electroencephalography and Clinical Neurophysiology, 71,* 375–381.

McCarthy, G. and Donchin, E. (1981). A metric for thought: A comparison of P300 latency and reaction time. *Science, 211,* 77–80.

Neshige, R., Barrett, G., and Shibasaki, H. (1988). Auditory long latency event-related potential in Alzheimer's disease and multi-infarct dementia. *Journal of Neurology and Neurosurgical Psychiatry, 51,* 1120–1125.

Newton, M., Barrett, G., Callanan, M., and Towell, A. (1989). Cognitive event-related potentials in multiple sclerosis. *Brain, 112,* 1637–1660.

Niwa, S., Ohta, M., and Yamazaki, K. (1983). P300 and stimulus evaluation process in autistic subjects. *Journal of Autism and Developmental Disorders, 13,* 33–42.

Patterson, J., Michalewski, H., and Starr, A. (1988). Latency variability of the components of auditory event-related potential to infrequent stimuli in aging, Alzheimer-type dementia, and depression. *Electroencephalography and Clinical Neurophysiology, 71,* 450–460.

Paul, D.D. and Sutton, S. (1972). Evoked potential correlates of response criterion in auditory signal detection. *Science, 177,* 362–364.

Pearce, J., Crowell, D., Tokioka, A., and Pacheco, G. (1989). Childhood developmental changes in the auditory P300. *Journal of Childhood Neurology, 4,* 100–106.

Picton, T.W. and Hillyard, S.A. (1974). Human auditory evoked potentials II: Effects of attention. *Electroencephalography and Clinical Neurophysiology, 36,* 191–199.

Polich, J. (1986). Attention, probability, and task demands as determinants of P300 latency from auditory stimuli. *Electroencephalography and Clinical Neurophysiology, 63,* 251–259.

Polich, J. (1989b). Frequency, intensity, and duration as determinants of P300 from auditory stimuli. *Journal of Clinical Neurophysiology, 6,* 277–286.

Polich, J. (1989a). P300 from a passive auditory paradigm. *Electroencephalography and Clinical Neurophysiology, 74,* 312–320.

Polich, J. (1987a). Response mode and P300 from auditory stimuli. *Biological Psychology, 25,* 61–71.

Polich, J. (1987b). Task difficulty, probability, and interstimulus interval as determinants of P300 from auditory stimuli. *Electroencephalography and Clinical Neurophysiology, 68,* 311–320.

Polich, J., Ehlers, C., Otis, S., Mandell, A., and Bloom, F. (1986). P300 latency reflects the degree of cognitive decline in dementing illness. *Electroencephalography and Clinical Neurophysiology, 63,* 138–144.

Polich, J., Howard L., and Starr, A. (1985a). Stimulus frequency and masking as determinants of P300 latency in event-related potentials from auditory stimuli. *Biological Psychiatry, 21,* 309–318.

Polich, J., Howard, L., and Starr, A. (1985b). Effects of age on the P300 component of the event-related potential from auditory stimuli: Peak definition, variation, and measurement. *Journal of Gerontology, 40,* 721–726.

Polich, J.M. and Starr, A. (1983). Middle-, late-, and long-latency auditory evoked potentials. In E.J. Moore (ed.), *Bases of auditory brainstem evoked responses.* New York: Grune & Stratton, Inc.

Pratap-Chand, R., Sinniah, M., and Salem, F. (1988). Cognitive evoked potential (P300): A metric for cerebral concussion. *Acta Neurological Scandinavica, 78,* 185–189.

Pritchard, W.S. (1981). Psychophysiology of P300. *Psychological Bulletin, 89,* 506–540.

Ritter, W., Simson, R., Vaughan, Jr., H.G., and Friedman, D. (1979). A brain event related to the making of a sensory discrimination. *Science, 203,* 1358–1361.

Rodin, E., Khabbazeh, Z., Twitty, G., and Schmaltz, S. (1989). The cognitive evoked potential in epilepsy patients. *Clinical Electroencephalography, 20,* 176–182.

Roth, W.T., Ford, J.M., and Kopell, B.S. (1978). Long-latency evoked potential and reaction time. *Psychophysiology, 15,* 17–23.

Ruchkin, D.S. and Sutton, S. (1978a). Latency characteristics and trial-by-trial variations of emitted cerebral potentials. In J.E. Desmedt, *Cognitive components in cerebral event-related potentials and selective attention.* Basel, Switzerland: Karger.

Ruchkin, D.S. and Sutton, S. (1978b). Emitted P300 potentials and temporal uncertainty. *Electroencephalography and Clinical Neurophysiology, 45,* 268–277.

Ruchkin, D.S., Sutton, S., Kietzman, M.L., and Silver, K. (1980). Slow wave and P300 in signal detection. *Electroencephalography and Clinical Neurophysiology, 50,* 35–47.

Ruchkin, D.S., Sutton, S., and Tueting, P. (1975). Emitted and evoked P300 potentials and variation in stimulus probability. *Psychophysiology, 12,* 591–595.

Sara, G., Kraiuhin, C., Gordon, E., Landau, P., James, L.,

Howson, A., and Meares, R. (1988). The P300 event related potential component in the diagnosis of dementia. *Australian and New Zealand Journal of Medicine, 18*, 657–660.

Selinger, M., Prescott, T., Shucard, D. (1989). Auditory event-related potential probes and behavioral measures of aphasia. *Brain and Language, 36*, 377–390.

Slaets, J. and Fortgens, C. (1984). On the value of P300 event-related potentials in the differential diagnosis of dementia. *British Journal of Psychiatry, 145*, 652–656.

Snyder, E., Hillyard, S.A., and Galambos, R. (1980). Similarities and differences among the P3 waves to detected signals in three modalities. *Psychophysiology, 17*, 112–122.

Squires, K.C. and Hecox, K.E. (1983). Electrophysiological evaluation of higher level auditory processing. *Seminars in Hearing, 4*, 415–433.

Squires, K., Petuchkowski, S., Wickens, C., and Donchin, E. (1977). The effects of stimulus sequence on event-related potentials: A comparison of visual and auditory sequences. *Perception and Psychophysics, 22*, 31–40.

Squires, K.C., Squires, N. K., and Hillyard, S.A. (1975). Decision-related cortical potentials during an auditory signal detection task with cued observation intervals. *Journal of Experimental Psychology: Human Perception and Performance, 1*, 268–279.

Squires, K.C., Wickens, C., Squires, N., and Donchin, E. (1976). The effects of stimulus sequence on the waveform of the cortical event-related potential. *Science, 153*, 1142–1145.

Squires, N.K., Duncan-Johnson, C.C., Squires, K.C., and Donchin, E. (1977). Cross-modal sequential effects on the P300 component of the event-related potential. *Psychophysiology, 14*, 96.

Squires, N.K., Squires, K.C., and Hillyard, S.A. (1975). Two varieties of long-latency positive waves evoked by unpredictable auditory stimuli in man. *Electroencephalography and Clinical Neurophysiology, 38*, 387–401.

Sutton, S. (1979). P300—Thirteen years later. In H. Begleiter (ed.), *Evoked brain potentials and behavior*. New York: Plenum Press.

Wood, C. and Wolpaw, J. (1982). Scalp distribution of human auditory evoked potentials II. Evidence for overlapping sources and involvement of auditory cortex. *Electroencephalography and Clinical Neurophysiology, 54*, 25–38.

Woods, D., Hillyard, S., Courchesne, E., and Galambos, R. (1980). Electrophysiological signs of split-second decision-making. *Science, 207*, 655–657.

CHAPTER 10

THE EFFECTS OF PERIPHERAL HEARING LOSS ON THE AUDITORY BRAINSTEM RESPONSE

CYNTHIA G. FOWLER
JOHN D. DURRANT

Peripheral hearing loss can have a significant effect on the auditory brainstem response (ABR) because the morphology and latencies of the component waves of the ABR are dependent on the effective spectrum of the eliciting stimuli. The effective spectrum is determined by the interaction of the characteristics of the stimuli, the transducer, and the auditory system. Stimulus parameters, such as waveform and overall intensity, determine the spectrum of the electrical signal driving the earphone or other transducer. The frequency response of the transducer further shapes the spectrum of the stimulus before it reaches the auditory system.

The effective spectrum of the stimulus is finally determined by the mechanisms of the auditory periphery involved in the coupling of sound energy to the hair cells. The effective spectrum, therefore, is influenced by the transfer characteristics of the ear canal, the middle ear (Durrant, 1983), and the inner ear. The effects in the inner ear include the cochlear mechanics, micromechanics of the organ of Corti, and hair cell transduction process(es) that lead to activation of the first order neurons of the acoustic nerve. Peripheral auditory pathology may involve any of these mechanisms/systems and, thereby, may alter the effective spectrum of the stimulus, leading to significant and variable effects on the components of the ABR. The resultant ABR depends on the interaction of the degree, configuration, and type of the hearing loss and the input spectrum of the stimulus. These effects can have a significant impact on the diagnostic outcome of the ABR (ASHA, 1988).

The primary focus of this chapter is the use of the ABR for otoneurologic diagnosis. For diagnostic applications, the effects of conductive and cochlear pathology must be recognized because conductive pathology can overlie cochlear or retrocochlear pathology in any given case (e.g., the dizzy patient, the patient with multiple sclerosis, or the comatose individual). Similarly, cochlear pathology may overlie retrocochlear pathology (e.g., presbycusis and an acoustic neuroma). The effects of different types of hearing loss on the ABR, therefore, must be known to distinguish conductive, cochlear, and retrocochlear cases; this is especially true in the absence of clear identification of wave I (Chisin, Gafni, and Sohmer, 1983).

CONDUCTIVE PATHOLOGY

A conductive pathology primarily attenuates the sound reaching the cochlea, producing significant latency shifts and waveform changes in the ABR that are consistent with the effects of decreasing stimulus intensity level in normal subjects (e.g., Chisin, Gapany-Gapanavicius,

Portions of this manuscript were funded by the Medical Research Service of the Veterans Health Services and Research Administration (CGF) and the Ben Franklin Partnership of the Commonwealth of Pennsylvania (JDD). We would like to extend our appreciation to Charlene Mikami, M.A.. for contributions to this chapter.

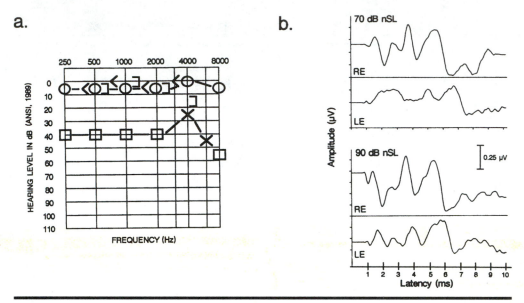

FIGURE 10.1.   Audiogram (a) and auditory brainstem responses (b) obtained in a 22-year-old female with surgically confirmed glomus tumor, presenting preoperatively with a significant conductive hearing loss in the left (involved) ear.

Gafni, and Sohmer, 1983). An example of the waveform differences between normal hearing and conductive pathology is given in Figure 10.1, in which the left ear ABR shows the prolonged latencies and reduced amplitudes of all the waves, consistent with a stimulus that is effectively 30 dB less intense at the cochlea than in the normal right ear. As the conductive component increases, the waves prior to wave V become less well defined and may be absent. Consequently, the I–V interpeak interval may not be determined for cases in which a conductive component exists, unless efforts are made to enhance wave I via high-level stimulation (as illustrated by Figure 10.1), extratympanic recording, or bone conduction stimulation. The interpeak interval decreases slightly with decreasing stimulus intensity level (Stockard, Stockard, Westmoreland, and Corfits, 1979; Durrant, 1986), suggesting the need to allow for the level effect.

The effect of different degrees of conductive hearing loss on the latencies of wave V of the ABR is shown in Figure 10.2. The lowest line in the figure shows an example of the normal wave V latencies for

click levels from 10 to 80 dB nSL[1] (normalized sensation level from a group of normal hearing subjects). A family of latency-intensity level (L-I) functions was constructed by shifting the normal L-I function along the intensity level axis in 20 dB steps. These functions represent the progressive parallel latency shift of the normal function that occurs as the degree of the conductive hearing loss increases. The L-I function in a conductive case, therefore, is expected to parallel the normal function, but be displaced by the degree of the hearing loss (Fria, 1980). For relatively large losses, the L-I functions have the illusion of becoming steeper and converging toward the normal L-I function, reminiscent of those functions observed in cases of sensory loss (see below). The validity of the concept of a parallel latency shift in conductive pathology is supported by

[1]Sensation Level (SL) is defined as "the pressure level of the sound in decibels above its threshold of audibility for the individual subject or for a specified group of subjects" (Sonn, 1969, p. 45). The prefix "n" is included to clarify that a group of normal-hearing subjects is used as the referent.

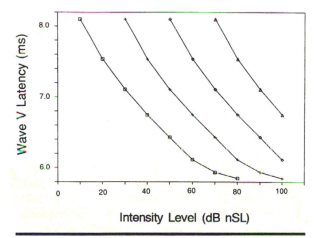

FIGURE 10.2. Hypothetical latency-intensity level functions for click-elicited wave V in conductive hearing losses of 0 (the normative function), 20, 40, and 60 dB, respectively.

various studies (e.g., Borg, Lofqvist, and Rosen, 1981; Chisin, Gapany-Gapanavicius, Gafni, and Sohmer, 1983; Fria and Sabo, 1980; McGee and Clemis, 1982; van der Drift, van Anten, and Brocaar, 1989; Yamada et al., 1975).

The classification of the type of hearing loss as conductive by using the L-I shift data has produced mixed results. Only 55% correct identification of pure conductives was realized with the ABR by van der Drift et al. (1989). Still, there was 94% correct indentification of a conductive component when cochlear and mixed cases were combined, and there were relatively low percentages of misclassifications of "normal" and "cochlear" cases as conductive (2 and 20%, respectively). The difficulty in distinguishing conductive and cochlear pathology arises from the parallel latency shift introduced by some types of cochlear hearing loss, as discussed later.

The L-I shift data have also been used to estimate behavioral threshold in cases of conductive hearing loss. Both the click-evoked ABR threshold and the magnitude of the shift of the L-I function correlate highly with the average pure tone threshold from 2000–4000 Hz. The regression analysis for the behavioral and ABR thresholds yields a linear regression

whose slope is essentially unity with standard errors of less than 10 dB (van der Drift et al., 1989).

In flat conductive losses, significant changes in the ABR waveform beyond level-dependent effects are not expected. Whereas this premise is difficult to test directly, indirect support is provided by Borg and Lofqvist (1982b). They demonstrated that the absolute differences in wave V latencies elicited by condensation and rarefaction clicks were similar in cases of conductive hearing loss and normal hearing.

The effect of the configuration of the conductive hearing loss also must be taken into account. Gorga, Reiland, and Beauchaine (1985) reported ABR findings in a case of high-frequency sloping conductive hearing loss. The L-I function in this case for the involved ear was steeply sloping (unlike the functions in Figure 10.2), much as in the case of a sensory impairment. As discussed below, these results reflect the differing contribution of apical versus basalward regions of the organ of Corti according to the sensitivity of low- and high-frequency hearing, respectively. Again, independent of etiology, the recorded waveform depends not only on the effective stimulus level but also on the effective stimulus spectrum, as determined by the degree and configuration of the hearing loss.

The evaluation of the ABR is more straightforward if conductive lesions are identified or resolved before the ABR data are collected. Otoscopic examination can identify excessive cerumen or foreign objects in the ear canal, potential ear canal collapse, and possible middle ear pathology. Thus, preliminary otoscopic examination, immittance testing, and air and bone conduction thresholds are highly recommended to reduce the amount of guesswork involved in the interpretation of the ABR (ASHA, 1988). Additionally, slippage of the earphones during the testing can produce a variable test-related conductive impairment that can be remedied if it is recognized (Noffsinger and Fowler, 1982).

BONE CONDUCTION STIMULI

Another approach to the identification of conductive pathology is similar to the approach used in conventional audiometry; that is, the comparison is made between air conduction thresholds and bone conduction thresholds obtained with standard bone conduction vibrators (see Schwartz, Larson, and DeChicchis, 1985). The latency of the bone conduction ABR has been reported to be later than the latency of the air conduction ABR at equal intensity levels (Weber, 1983). The latency differences have been partially attributed to the apparent differences in the response characteristics of the transducers (Mauldin and Jerger, 1979), suggesting significant differences in the effective spectra of bone conduction versus air conduction clicks. Recent information, however, suggests that the bone vibrator is not the low pass transducer it appears to be based upon the output measured in force on an artificial mastoid. The effective output (i.e., sensation level) actually increases with frequency (Dirks and Kamm, 1975; Gorga and Thornton, 1989). Durrant, Nozza, Hyre, and Sabo (1989), therefore, using equal sensation levels, were able to obtain comparable click-evoked ABRs using the Radioear B71 bone vibrator with mastoid placement and the Telephonics TDH-39 earphone in normal-hearing subjects up to 65 dB SL, namely the saturation limits of the bone vibrator. Thus, despite the clear perceptual differences in the air and bone conduction clicks, resulting from acousticomechanical differences between the two tranducers and coupling to the ear, the spectra reaching the cochlea are more alike than different when the stimuli are matched for sensation levels.

The limits of bone conduction testing, therefore, may be no more problematic in ABR than in conventional audiometry. The inherent problems with bone conduction testing include sensitivity to vibrator placement, individual subject differences in air and bone conduction thresholds, and the tendency for the bone vibrator to ring more than the earphone. An additional technical problem is that the bone vibrator generates more electrical artifact than the earphone because the bone vibrator requires a much higher driving voltage for the same sensation level as compared to the earphone. Further difficulties may occur with forehead placement of the bone vibrator. The intensity level is reduced approximately 10 dB in forehead placement as compared to mastoid placement (Studebaker, 1967), and there may be an additional propagation-like delay as the stimulus travels through the skull (Boezeman, Kapteyn, Visser, and Snel, 1983; Durrant et al., 1989).

Despite the limitations, the direct measurement of bone conduction thresholds may be the only option for obtaining ABR information in certain cases, such as congenital atresia, and may serve as a useful adjunct to air-conduction ABR testing in cases of suspected conductive hearing losses. Bone conduction testing has also proven valuable in newborn screening programs (Hooks and Weber, 1984). Monitoring head trauma and other intensive care patients who may have middle ear involvement, is another possible application.

An alternative to the direct measurement of bone conduction thresholds is an indirect measurement using a modification of the Sensorineural Acuity Level (SAL) procedure. In the SAL measurement, the behavioral air conduction threshold is measured in quiet and in the presence of bone-conducted noise. The amount of noise heard causes an increase in the masked threshold as compared to the threshold in quiet; the amount of threshold shift, then, provides an estimation of the amount of the conductive component (Jerger and Tillman, 1960). The ABR version of this test has been described by Hicks (1980) and Webb and Greenberg (1983). The wave V threshold for clicks or tone pips replaces the behavioral response, and there is a prescribed protocol for manipulating the masking noise. Suffice it to say, the results of this test appear to be equivalent to the results of testing bone conduction thresholds directly in mild to moderate hearing losses. The derived bone conduction thresholds were within 10 dB of the behavioral thresholds in 74% of the cases overall, although prediction was poorest in cases of mixed hearing loss (Webb and Greenberg, 1983). The major limitations of the modified SAL method are the substantial amount of time involved and the inherent difficulties in obtaining thresholds with ABR.

COCHLEAR HEARING LOSS

The most common diagnostic application of the ABR is the evaluation of patients with unilateral or asymmetrical sensory hearing loss. In these cases, differences in latencies of wave V between ears may exceed normal limits, and the dilemma is whether the prolongation is due to a cochlear or retrocochlear pathology. Knowledge of the configuration and degree of the hearing loss, thus, is very important in the interpretation of the ABR. Although there are various formulas suggested in the literature for compensating for the latency delay from a given hearing loss, no one predictive approach has worked well enough to gain universal acceptance. The best approach is to evaluate the ABRs with an understanding of the types of changes a cochlear hearing loss can impose and to make every effort to identify wave I.

The most common stimulus used for neurodiagnostic purposes is the unfiltered click. The rise time of a click is sufficiently rapid to synchronize the discharges of a large population of neurons, and thus, to yield a large, well-formed ABR with all its component waves. The relatively long stimulus rise times required for frequency specific stimuli reduce the synchrony of firings in the neural contributions to the waveforms. Whereas the resulting waveform degradation may not be significant in the normal hearing subject, the effects may be more deleterious in the hearing impaired subject, because the presence of a hearing loss compromises identification of the waveforms. Any further degradation of the ABR by the stimulus, then, is to be avoided. The presence of all the waves (or at least I, III, and V) is desired for the most definitive interpretation of the ABR. The absolute latencies of waves (wave V in particular) contribute significantly to the interpretation of the ABR, but the I–V interval may be the single most important measure.

Although a click theoretically has energy at all frequencies, the spectrum reaching the basilar membrane is shaped by the transducer and the filter characteristics of the external and middle ears (Durrant, 1983). A TDH-49 earphone, for example, has a resonance peak at about 4000–6000 Hz (2000–4000 Hz for the TDH-39). This resonance peak and the superior synchronization of traveling wave motion in the base of the cochlea lead to ABR latencies that are biased by the status of high frequency neurons. Further, the traveling wave passes over the base first and its velocity is highest in the base, thus yielding shorter latencies for the high frequencies than for the low frequencies. Because clinic norms are generally based on the responses from normal hearing subjects, the norms reflect the latencies from cochlear/neural units responding near 4000 Hz for moderately intense stimuli (Don and Eggermont, 1979).

The presence of the high frequency emphasis of the click-evoked ABR does not preclude the presence of low frequency activity; the low frequency activity is simply not reflected in the click response due to phase cancellation of the output of neurons arising in the more apical regions (Kiang, 1975). With the use of more frequency-specific stimuli (e.g., filtered clicks or tone bursts), selective masking of the response, or other conditions (e.g., pathology) that eliminate the basalward contribution, more apical contributions will emerge with concomitant changes in wave morphology and increased latency. Thus, the morphology of the ABR elicited from high frequency neural units includes waves I–V for derived frequency bands down to approximately 2000 Hz (Don and Eggermont, 1979). Below 2000 Hz, waves I, II, and IV are significantly reduced in amplitude or are absent. The latencies of the waves are progressively lengthened as the frequency decreases.

Sharply sloping, severe, high-frequency losses cause the ABR to resemble the ABR from a lower frequency stimulus in normals. The waves prior to wave V may be reduced in amplitude or lost, and the component waves may have prolonged latencies (Bauch and Olsen, 1988; Coats and Martin, 1977; Gorga et al., 1985; Møller and Blegvad, 1976; Jerger and Mauldin, 1978). The prolonged latencies result from both the added time for the traveling wave to reach healthy regions of the cochlea and the effective reduction in stimulus intensity because the most effective stimulating frequencies are removed from the stimulus spectrum. The elimination of fibers from the basal end of the cochlea, which respond with the shortest latencies, results in an eighth nerve action potential generated more apically, and therefore, later than normal (Aran, Darrouzet, and Erre, 1975; Elberling and Salomon, 1976). The L-I function shifts to the right, as a result, and the prolonged latencies are simply transmitted up the brainstem pathways, reflected as a delay in the latency of wave V. These effects are shown in Figure 10.3, in which the severe-to-profound high-frequency hearing loss caused the prolongation of all the component waves. At 80 dB nSL, wave I occurs at 2.57 ms, III at 4.65 ms, and V at 6.57 ms, all of which are approximately 0.5 ms beyond the normal limits. The I–V

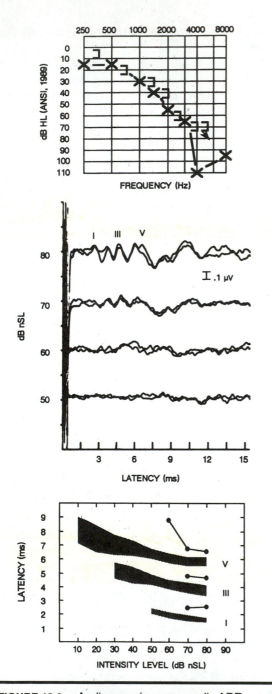

FIGURE 10.3. Audiogram (upper panel), ABR waveforms (middle panel), and latencies of waves I, III, and V (lower panel) plotted against the norms for a subject with a severe-to-profound, high-frequency, sensory hearing loss.

interwave latency, however, remains within normal limits at 4.00 ms.

Despite the fact that a cochlear hearing loss does not prolong the I–V latency difference, the loss may not produce an equal effect on all the component waves of the ABR. Specifically, the I–V latency difference may be shortened relative to normal (Coats and Martin, 1977; Elberling and Parbo, 1987; Keith and Greville, 1987) because the frequencies within the stimulus that are effective for eliciting the response are shifted downward. The I–V interval is correspondingly shortened, as the I–V interval for lower frequency tone pips is shorter than for higher frequency tone pips (Fowler and Noffsinger, 1983). Additionally, in a cochlear hearing loss, the I–III latency may be prolonged (with concomitant shortening of the III–V interval), without prolonging the I–V latency (Fowler and Noffsinger, 1983). In a patient with a unilateral cochlear hearing loss, therefore, the ABR may display a shorter I–V latency for the suspect ear than in the normal ear. If the interpretation of the ABR is done without the benefit of an audiogram, the wrong ear may be labeled abnormal based on the I–V interval.

If the hearing loss is flat or only mildly sloping and mild to moderate in severity, then the effect of the hearing loss on the ABR for high level stimuli is substantially reduced. The latencies are essentially equivalent to those collected at the same intensity level in normal hearing subjects (Selters and Brackmann, 1977), as long as the stimuli are approximately 20 dB above the threshold at 4000 Hz. For high level stimuli, the L-I functions for these subjects are consistent with those of normal hearing subjects. The divergence of the function for cochlear-impaired subjects from the function for normals occurs with slightly prolonged latencies only within about 20 dB of threshold. The amplitude of the waves may be slightly smaller than in normal hearing subjects, presumably because of the loss of some neural contributions. An example of the L-I function for a patient with a moderate, essentially flat hearing loss is given in Figure 10.4. At 80 dB nSL, wave I occurs at 1.78 ms, III at 4.12 ms, and V at 5.91 ms, all of which are within normal limits. The I–V interwave latency difference is 4.15 ms, and is also within normal limits. Wave V is beyond the normal limits only at 60 dB nSL, which is the threshold response.

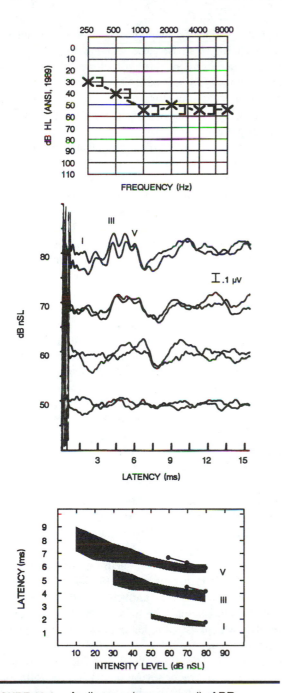

FIGURE 10.4. Audiogram (upper panel), ABR waveforms (middle panel), and latencies of waves I, III, and V (lower panel) plotted against the norms for a subject with an essentially flat, moderate, sensory hearing loss.

Hearing losses confined to the low frequencies have no appreciable effect on click-evoked ABR latencies. If the hearing in the high frequencies is normal or near normal, then the high-frequency bias of the ABR hides the presence of a low-frequency loss. The waveform and amplitude- and latency-intensity level functions are within normal limits. The L–I function for a patient with a mild, low frequency, sensory hearing loss is given in Figure 10.5. At 80 dB nSL, wave I occurs at 1.61 ms, III at 3.77 ms, and V at 5.63 ms, yielding a I–V interwave latency difference of 4.02 ms. All of these values are within the normal limits down to threshold.

The data presented in Figure 10.6 summarize the overall effects expected from the presence of cochlear hearing loss (Durrant, Dickter, and Ronis, 1982). Groups were constituted with six or more subjects with comparable types and degrees of unilateral peripheral impairment, wherein responses had been tested at common levels for both ears. Members of each group thus served as their own controls. The ABRs from these subjects were averaged to form grand mean responses for each ear and point-wise standard errors were calculated to form ±1 standard error traces, thus defining "bands" of high probability for the occurrence of each point of the ABR. The results for subjects with mild high-frequency losses, given moderately high levels of stimulation, reveal no significant abnormalities in the ABR waveform or interaural latency differences. For severe high-frequency sensory losses, however, differences are evident even when the stimulus was 10 dB higher (not shown) in the pathologic ear, requiring some correction factor in the interpretation. As lower frequencies also become involved, abnormalities become progressively more striking (Bauch and Olsen, 1988) and substantial waveform/latency abnormalities and interaural differences may be unavoidable. Borg and Lofqvist (1982a) presented a group of audiograms demonstrating the audiometric limits beyond which the ABR could not be elicited with click stimuli.

Lastly, predominantly low-frequency losses do not significantly alter the ABR waveform or cause interaural latency differences. In the low-frequency group shown in Figure 10.6, however, differences were seen in the standard error traces due to the inclusion of data from one subject. This subject had substantially larger responses

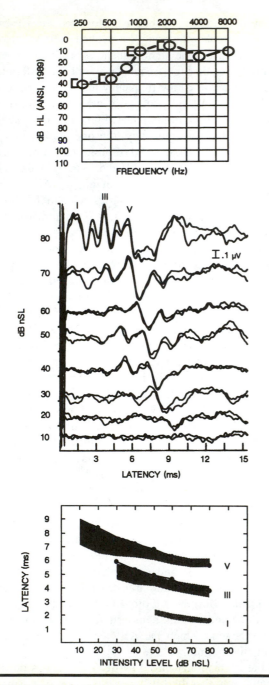

FIGURE 10.5. Audiogram (upper panel), ABR waveforms (middle panel), and latencies of waves I, III, and V (lower panel) plotted against the norms for a subject with a mild, low-frequency, sensory hearing loss.

with stimulation of the involved ear than with stimulation of the normal ear. Because imaging studies failed to demonstrate retrocochlear pathology, elimination of these data was not justified. Nevertheless, this subject's data did not significantly affect the central tendencies of the pathological vs. control ear data, again suggesting no significant differences.

Of all the recording parameters that affect the ABR (see Chapter 6), only stimulus phase produces effects in hearing-impaired subjects that cannot be predicted on the basis of the responses from normal-hearing subjects. Although stimulus polarity is a nonpathologic variable, the effect of stimulus polarity on the ABR of cochlear-impaired subjects may be variable and/or exaggerated. The effect of phase on the responses of normal-hearing subjects has been debated in the literature, with some studies reporting earlier responses to rarefaction than to condensation phases of the stimulus (Ornitz and Walter, 1975; Stockard et al., 1979) and shorter latencies to condensation phases in other studies (Coutin, Balmaseda, and Miranda, 1987), or no differences for the two phases (Rosenhamer, Lindström, and Lundborg, 1978; Tietze and Pantev, 1986). The different findings result from the use of predominately normal hearing subjects whose ABRs are dominated by high frequency fiber responses. The phase effects are low frequency phenomena (Fowler and Swanson, 1985) that are not clearly evident in the normal raw ABR.

The latency differences due to stimulus phase are pronounced in subjects with high frequency hearing losses (Borg and Loqvist, 1982b; Coats and Martin, 1977; Stockard et al., 1979) because of the downward shift in frequency dominance when the high frequencies are removed by the hearing loss. Borg and Lofqvist (1981) suggested that the latency difference between responses to rarefaction and condensation stimuli could be used to indicate the high-frequency cutoff in steeply sloping hearing losses; the inverse of the time difference between wave V peaks to rarefaction and condensation clicks was highly correlated with the cutoff frequency (at 50 dB HL). A follow-up study confirmed that the absolute value of the wave V latency difference for rarefaction and condensation stimuli increased as the cutoff frequency for the hearing loss decreased, although the exact cutoff could not be identified. The inability to identify an exact cutoff

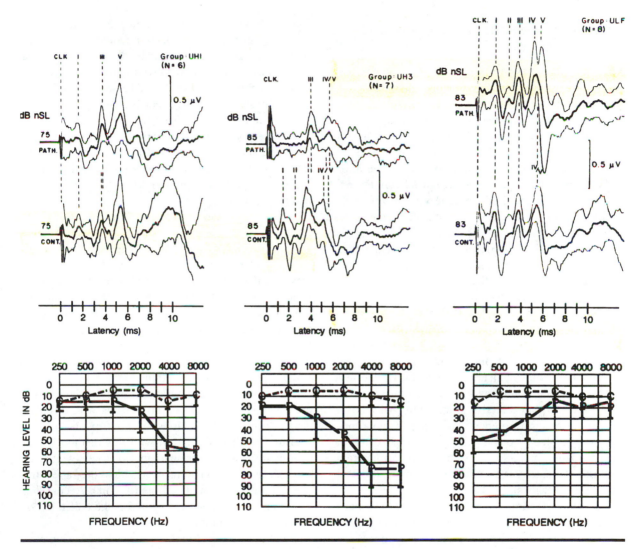

FIGURE 10.6.   Composite auditory brainstem responses (upper panels, thick trace) and mean audiograms (lower panels) of subjects with unilateral sensorineural hearing losses whose ABRs were averaged to form the composites. The thin traces above and below each composite (i.e., mean of the individual subjects' averages) represent the ±1 standard error. (Note: Although the point-wise standard deviation actually was calculated, each subject's data are means; this, by definition, is a measure of standard.) Shown are the data from groups characterized by relatively mild (UH1), more severe high-frequency (UH3), and mild low-frequency (ULF) losses. P or path.—pathologic ear; C or cont.—control (normal) ear.

may be partially due to the unknown status of the neurons bordering the damaged region of the cochlea. The absolute difference between the condensation and rarefaction latencies was used because only 19 of the 29 subjects exhibited a shorter latency for rarefaction than for condensation stimuli (Borg and Lofqvist, 1982b). The reason for the lack of consistency in which stimulus phase produced the shorter latency is not evident.

ACCOUNTING FOR COCHLEAR-IMPOSED LATENCY DELAYS

Several methods have been proposed to account for the latency delay introduced by cochlear hearing losses when attempting to screen for retrocochlear lesions. These methods unfortunately have not reached universal acceptance because of their poor predictive ability for an individual subject/patient. Interactive or overriding effects occur with the severity and configuration of the hearing loss, age, gender, and head size. For example, the dominant effect on wave V latency for mild to moderate losses is age, whereas the dominant effect for severe to profound losses is the degree of the loss (Hyde, 1985). Even when all of these effects are taken into account, they explain less than one-third of the variability in the prediction of ABR latencies (Mitchell, Phillips, and Trune, 1989).

Identification of wave I, and thus the I–V interval, may help determine the amount of wave V delay that can be accounted for by peripheral causes. The difficulty of this method of interpretation is the frequent loss of wave I with cochlear pathology due to an effective low-frequency emphasis in the stimulus spectrum and/or reduction in effective stimulus intensity level. Alternative methods to elicit wave I may be appropriate, such as electrocochleography or an ear canal or extratympanic membrane electrode in conjunction with the standard vertex placement (Durrant, 1986; Ferraro and Ferguson, 1989).

Various corrections for wave V latency have been suggested to account for the degree of peripheral loss. One method is to subtract a predicted delay in wave V latency of 0.1 ms for each 10 dB increase in hearing loss above 50 dB at 4000 Hz; an interaural wave V latency difference that exceeds 0.2 ms is then considered abnormal (Selters and Brackmann, 1977). A second method of correction is an initial subtraction of the average conductive component at 1000, 2000, and 4000 Hz (if any), and a subtraction of 0.1 ms for each 5 dB increase in hearing loss above 55 dB at 4000 Hz; an interaural wave V latency difference exceeding 0.3 ms is considered abnormal (Hyde and Blair, 1981). These correction factors may be representative of a group of subjects, but variability for individual subjects is too great to warrant extensive reliance on this method. Further, these correction factors were derived on patients with auditory thresholds of ≤75 dB HL at 2000 and 4000 Hz, and with stimuli of 83–85 dB nSL. In reality, many patients referred for an ABR will have worse thresholds and these correction factors will not apply. The use of stimuli up to 100 dB nSL may increase the pool of testable patients. Extreme caution, however, should be exercised in the use of stimulus levels >100 dB nSL as the peak equivalent SPL of the stimulus is >130 dB (e.g., see data of Stapells, Picton, and Smith, 1982).

The configuration of the hearing loss can have a greater effect on the latency of the ABR than the degree of the loss, although the two are not independent measures (Jerger and Mauldin, 1978). A contour index was calculated from the dB difference in thresholds from 1000 to 4000 Hz; the steeper the contour, the greater the delay in wave V, but no audiometric contour could explain a latency of >7.0 ms (for stimuli up to 90 dB nSL). These data suggest the need for further audiological or medical work-up on patients whose wave V latencies exceed 7.0 ms.

As an alternative to predicting latency delays, reference data can be collected on persons with different degrees and configurations of confirmed cochlear hearing loss. The limitation with this method is that hearing losses do not group themselves neatly into categories, and duration of the hearing loss may affect the condition of the stimulated neural units. Accounting for gender and age as well would make collection of reference data prohibitive.

Finally, tone pip stimuli or ipsilateral masking may be of benefit diagnostically (Eggermont and Don, 1980; Fowler and Noffsinger, 1983; Kileny, Schlagheck, and Spak, 1986). Masking can exclude the frequency region in a normal ear that is eliminated by cochlear pathology in a pathological ear, such that theoretically similar areas of the cochlea contribute to the ABR in both ears. Tone pips can target similar, relatively normal cochlear bands in normal and pathological ears in an attempt to produce comparable responses. In both cases, the goal is to equalize the cochlear component in normal and pathological ears in order to attribute any latency delay to neural pathology. These methods, however, are limited by the persistent basalward dominance of the response (Fowler and Leonards, 1985) even when a restricted band of frequencies is stimulated. Also cochlear/neural units may be damaged sufficiently to disrupt the ABR but not sufficiently to be evident in the behavioral threshold to pure tones. In order to use tone pips effectively for diagnostic purposes, more work is needed to show the practical use of tone burst stimuli restricted to normal hearing areas. Further information on the use of frequency specific stimuli is given in the next chapter.

THRESHOLD DERIVATION—CONSIDERATIONS

Although the primary emphasis of this chapter has been on the neuro-diagnostic applications of the ABR in cases of peripheral hearing loss, several comments are warranted regarding threshold considerations. As discussed earlier, unfiltered click stimuli reflect a high frequency bias in the ABR and consequently are of limited benefit in deriving audiometric information. For conductive hearing losses, click-evoked responses correlate best with the average pure tone thresholds from 2000–4000 Hz (van der Drift et al., 1989).

Similarly, the click-evoked response in sensory hearing losses reflects the high frequency bias, agreeing with the average of the frequencies between 2000 and 4000 Hz (Bauch and Olsen, 1988) or 1000, 2000, and 4000 Hz (Jerger and Mauldin, 1978). An example of a threshold estimation in three subjects with cochlear hearing losses is given in Figures 10.3, 10.4, and 10.5. In Figure 10.3, the ABR threshold for the patient with a severe-to-profound high-frequency hearing loss is 60 dB nSL, which agrees with the threshold from 2000–3000 Hz. The better thresholds from 250–1500 Hz and the worse thresholds from 4000–8000 Hz are not identified with the click stimuli. In Figure 10.4, the ABR threshold for the patient with the moderate flat hearing loss is also 60 dB nSL, which agrees with the thresholds from 1000–8000 Hz. Because all the thresholds are relatively similar, the click provided a good estimate of the auditory thresholds for this subject. In Figure 10.5, the ABR threshold for the subject with a mild low-frequency hearing loss is 20 dB nSL, which agrees with the averaged thresholds from 1000–4000

Hz. In this case, the low-frequency hearing loss was not identified through the use of click stimuli.

The range of accuracy of ABR estimates of behavioral threshold can be quite large. The ABR threshold estimates for a group of 275 ears produced a standard deviation of 15 dB, yielding a range of 60 dB for 95% accuracy of threshold prediction for a given subject (Jerger and Mauldin, 1978). Jerger and Mauldin suggested a formula of the ABR threshold multiplied by 0.6 to predict the average threshold of 1000, 2000, 4000 Hz. The prediction of the average behavioral threshold using ABR with click stimuli did not vary with the contour of the audiogram, which is fortunate given the unavailability of that information for most of the patients for whom the ABR threshold technique is necessary.

The behavioral threshold of normal-hearing subjects is dependent on a number of factors related to temporal integration. The behavioral threshold improves with increasing click rate and the number of clicks presented (Yost and Klein, 1979). The behavioral threshold also varies as a function of the duration of the stimulus used, such that the threshold improves by 8–10 dB for each decade increase in stimulus duration under 200 ms. The slope of the threshold power integration function for subjects with conductive hearing losses is the same as for normals, whereas the slope for cochlear-impaired subjects is generally less than for normals. Although this relation was the basis for development of the behavioral brief tone audiometry test, it is too variable to be significant diagnostically in distinguishing normal or conductive pathology from cochlear or retrocochlear pathology (Olsen and Carhart, 1966; Olsen, Rose, and Noffsinger, 1974).

In normal-hearing subjects, ABR thresholds are higher than behavioral thresholds, at least partially because of the influence of temporal integration and the difference between typical audiometric tones and testing procedures and ABR threshold estimation procedures. The ABR, as an onset response, does not yield lower thresholds with increased stimulus duration, whereas the audiometric threshold takes advantage of temporal integration in yielding lower thresholds than would have been measured if the short ABR stimuli had been used. In subjects with cochlear pathology, the reduced slope of the behavioral integration function may decrease the gap between the threshold of the ABR and the behavioral threshold (Gorga, Beauchaine, Reiland, Worthington and Javel, 1984). Unfortunately, a constant value cannot be subtracted from the ABR threshold in the prediction of the behavioral threshold because the brief tone effect is different for each patient.

SUMMARY AND CONCLUSIONS

This chapter has focused on the effects of peripheral hearing loss on the diagnostic interpretation of the ABR. All activity that reaches the level of wave V generation has been modified by the filtering of the stimulus through the transducer and the auditory system, including normal and pathologic conditions of the external, middle, and inner ears. The diagnostic interpretation of the ABR, therefore, is an educated guess based on knowledge of the interactive effects of hearing loss and stimulus characteristics plus the information that can be derived from the ABR, including absolute and relative latencies and the L-I function. Interpretive errors can arise because different auditory disorders do not produce necessarily unique effects on the ABR, and because disorders do not occur in isolation.

The methods proposed in the literature for predicting ABR latency delays caused by peripheral hearing losses must be used cautiously with an understanding of the underlying conditions that result in the latency prolongations. Every effort should be made to elicit wave I because the I–V interval is modified less by peripheral hearing losses than the absolute latencies are. Alternative stimuli, including tone pips and ipsilateral masking, may be used. Bone conduction stimulation may be appropriate in some cases. Formulas predicting the amount of delay for a given hearing loss may provide guidelines whereby the ABRs of individual patients may be judged. Reference data may be collected from subjects with different types, configurations, and degrees of hearing loss. Notwithstanding these approaches, future research must delineate accurate methods to separate the effects of conductive, cochlear, and neural pathology. Until then, the best ABR strategy is to choose the stimuli and form the diagnostic impression based on a thorough knowledge of the stimulus and the audiologic information.

REFERENCES

Aran, J. M., Darrouzet, J., and Erre, J. P. (1975). Observation of click-evoked compound VIII nerve responses before, during, and over seven months after kanamycin treatment in the guinea pig. *Acta Otolaryngologica, 79*, 24–32.

ASHA Audiologic Evaluation Working Group on Auditory Evoked Potential Measurements (1988). *The Short Latency Auditory Evoked Potentials.* Rockville, MD: American Speech-Language-Hearing Association.

Bauch, C. D. and Olsen, W. O. (1988). Auditory brainstem responses as a function of average hearing sensitivity for 2000–4000 Hz. *Audiology, 27*, 156–163.

Boezeman, E. H. J. F., Kapteyn, T. S., Visser, S. L., and Snel, A. M. (1983). Comparison of the latencies between bone and air conduction in the auditory brain stem evoked potential. *Electroencephalography and Clinical Neurophysiology, 56*, 244–247.

Borg, E. and Lofqvist, L. (1982a). A lower limit for auditory brainstem response (ABR). *Scandinavian Audiology, 11*, 277–278.

Borg, E. and Lofqvist, L. (1982b). Auditory brainstem response (ABR) to rarefaction and condensation clicks in normal and abnormal ears. *Scandinavian Audiology, 11*, 227–235.

Borg, E. and Lofqvist, L. (1981). Auditory brainstem response (ABR) to rarefaction and condensation clicks in normal hearing and steep high-frequency hearing loss. *Scandinavian Audiology, 13*, 99–101.

Borg, E., Lofqvist, L., and Rosen, S. (1981). Brainstem response (ABR) in conductive hearing loss. *Scandinavian Audiology, 13*, 95–97.

Chisin, R., Gafni, M., and Sohmer, H. (1983). Patterns of auditory nerve and brainstem-evoked responses (ABR) in different types of peripheral hearing loss. *Archives of Otorhinolaryngology, 237*, 165–173.

Chisin, R., Gapany-Gapanavicius, B., Gafni, M., and Sohmer, H. (1983). Auditory nerve and brainstem-evoked responses before and after middle ear corrective surgery. *Archives of Otorhinolaryngology, 238*, 27–31.

Coats, A. C. and Martin, J. L. (1977). Human auditory nerve action potentials and brain stem evoked responses: Effects of audiogram shape and lesion location. *Archives of Otolaryngology, 103,* 605–622.

Coutin, P., Balmaseda, A., and Miranda, J. (1987). Further differences between brain-stem auditory potentials evoked by rarefaction and condensation clicks as revealed by vector analysis. *Electroencephalography and Clinical Neurophysiology, 66,* 420–426.

Dirks, D. D. and Kamm, C. (1975). Bone-vibrator measurements: Physical characteristics and behavioral thresholds. *Journal of Speech and Hearing Research, 18,* 242–260.

Don, M. and Eggermont, J. J. (1979). Reconstruction of the audiogram using brain-stem responses and high pass noise masking. *Annals of Otology, Rhinology, and Laryngology, Supplement 578,* 1–20.

Durrant, J. D. (1986). Combined ECochG-ABR versus conventional ABR recordings. *Seminars in Hearing (Electrocochleography), 7,* 289–305.

Durrant, J. D. (1983). Fundamentals of sound generation. In E. J. Moore (ed.), *Bases of auditory brainstem evoked responses,* pp. 15–49. New York: Grune & Stratton.

Durrant, J. D., Dickter, A. E., and Ronis, M. L. (1982). *Composite brain stem evoked potentials in cases of unilateral hearing loss.* Midwinter Meeting of the Association for Research in Otolaryngology. St. Petersburg Beach, Florida (January, 1982).

Durrant, J. D., Nozza, R. J., Hyre, R. J., and Sabo, D. L. (1989). Masking level difference at relatively high masker levels: Preliminary report. *Audiology, 28,* 221–229.

Eggermont, J. J. and Don, M. (1980). Analysis of the click-evoked brainstem potentials in humans using high-pass noise masking. II. Effects of click intensity. *Journal of the Acoustical Society of America, 68,* 1671–1675.

Elberling, C. and Parbo, J. (1987). Reference data for ABRs in retrocochlear diagnosis. *Scandinavian Audiology, 16,* 49–55.

Elberling, C. and Salomon, G. (1976). Action potentials from pathological ears compared to potentials generated by a computer model. In R. J. Ruben, C. Elberling, and G. Salomon (eds.), *Electrocochleography,* pp. 439–456. Baltimore, MD: University Park Press.

Ferraro, J. A. and Ferguson, R. (1989). Tympanic ECochG and conventional ABR: A combined approach for the identification of Wave I and the I–V interwave interval. *Ear and Hearing, 10,* 161–196.

Fowler, C. G. and Leonards, J. S. (1985). Frequency dependence of the binaural interaction component of the auditory brainstem response. *Audiology, 24,* 420–429.

Fowler, C. G. and Noffsinger, D. (1983). The effects of stimulus repetition rate and frequency on the auditory brainstem

response in normal, cochlear-impaired, and VIII nerve/brainstem-impaired subjects. *Journal of Speech and Hearing Research, 26,* 560–567.

Fowler, C. G. and Swanson, M. R. (1985). *Correlate of the masking level difference in the ABR.* American Speech-Language-Hearing Association Convention, Washington, D. C. (November, 1985).

Fria, T. J. (1980). The auditory brain stem response: Background and clinical applications. *Monographs in Contemporary Audiology, 2,* 1–44.

Fria, T. J. and Sabo, D. L. (1980). Auditory brainstem responses in children with otitis media with effusion. *Annals of Otology, Rhinology, and Laryngology, Supplement 68,* 190–195.

Gorga, M. P., Beauchaine, K. A., Reiland, J. K., Worthington, D. W., and Javel, E. (1984). The effects of stimulus duration on ABR and behavioral thresholds. *Journal of the Acoustical Society of America, 76,* 616–619.

Gorga, M. P., Reiland, J. K., and Beauchaine, K. A. (1985). Auditory brainstem responses in a case of high-frequency conductive hearing loss. *Journal of Speech and Hearing Disorders, 50,* 346–350.

Gorga, M. P. and Thornton, A. R. (1989). The choice of stimuli for ABR measurements. *Ear and Hearing, 10,* 217–230.

Hicks, G. E. (1980). Auditory brainstem response. Sensory assessment by bone conduction masking. *Archives of Otolaryngology, 106,* 392–395.

Hooks, R. G., and Weber, B. A. (1984). Auditory brain stem responses of premature infants to bone-conducted stimiuli: A feasibility study. *Ear and Hearing, 5,* 42–46.

Hyde, M. L. (1985). The effect of cochlear lesions on the ABR. In J. T. Jacobson (ed.), *The auditory brainstem response,* pp. 133–146. San Diego, CA: College Hill Press.

Hyde, M. L. and Blair, R. L. (1981). The auditory brainstem response in neuro-otology: Perspectives and problems. *Journal of Otolaryngology, 10,* 117–125.

Jerger, J. and Mauldin, L. (1978). Prediction of sensorineural hearing level from the brain stem evoked response. *Archives of Otolaryngology, 104,* 456–461.

Jerger, J. and Tillman, T. (1960). A new method for the clinical determination of sensorineural acuity level (SAL). *Archives of Otolaryngology, 71,* 948–955.

Keith, W. J. and Greville, K. A. (1987). Effects of audiometric configuration on the auditory brain stem response. *Ear and Hearing, 8,* 49–55.

Kiang, N. Y.-S. (1975). Stimulus representation in the discharge patterns of auditory neurons. In D. B. Tower (ed.), *The nervous system,* vol. 3, pp. 81–96. New York: Raven Press.

Kileny, P., Schlagheck, G., and Spak, C. (1986). *Site of lesion ABR testing with tonal stimuli.* American Speech-Language-Hearing Association Convention, Detroit (November, 1986).

Mauldin, L. and Jerger, J. (1979). Auditory brain stem evoked responses to bone-conducted signals. *Archives of Otolaryngology, 105,* 656–661.

McGee, T. J. and Clemis, J. D. (1982). Effects of conductive hearing loss on auditory brainstem response. *Annals of Otology, Rhinology, and Laryngology, 9,* 304–309.

Mitchell, C., Phillips, D. S., and Trune, D. R. (1989). Variables affecting the auditory brainstem response: Audiogram, age, gender and head size. *Hearing Research, 40,* 75–85.

Møller, K. and Blegvad, B. (1976). Brain stem responses in patients with sensorineural hearing loss. *Scandinavian Audiology, 5,*115–127.

Noffsinger, D. and Fowler, C. G. (1982). Brain stem auditory evoked potentials. Applications in clinical audiology. *Bulletin of the Los Angeles Neurological Societies, 47,* 43–54.

Olsen, W. O. and Carhart, R. (1966). Integration of acoustic power at threshold by normal hearers. *Journal of the Acoustical Society of America, 40,* 591–599.

Olsen, W. O., Rose, D. E., and Noffsinger, D. (1974). Brief-tone audiometry with normal, cochlear, and eighth nerve tumor patients. *Archives of Otolaryngology, 99,* 185–189.

Ornitz, E. M. and Walter, D. O. (1975). The effect of sound pressure waveform on human brain stem auditory evoked responses. *Brain Research, 92,* 490–498.

Rosenhamer, H. J., Lindström, B., and Lundborg, T. (1978). On the use of click-evoked electric brain stem responses in audiological diagnosis. I. The variability of the normal response. *Scandinavian Audiology, 7,* 193–205.

Schwartz, D. M., Larson, V. D., and DeChicchis, A. R. (1985). Spectral characteristics of air and bone conduc-

tion transducers used to record the auditory brain stem response. *Ear and Hearing, 6,* 274–277.

Selters, W. A. and Brackmann, D. E. (1977). Acoustic tumor detection with brain stem electric response audiometry. *Archives of Otolaryngology, 103,* 181–187.

Sonn, M. (1969). *Psychoacoustical Terminology.* Portsmouth, RI: Raytheon Company.

Stapells, D. R., Picton, T. W., and Smith, A. D. (1982). Normal hearing thresholds for clicks. *Journal of the Acoustical Society of America, 72,* 74–79.

Stockard, J. E., Stockard, J. J., Westmoreland, B. F., and Corfits, J. L. (1979). Brainstem auditory-evoked responses: Normal variation as a function of stimulus and subject characteristics. *Archives of Neurology, 36,* 823–831.

Studebaker, G. A. (1967). The standardization of bone-conduction thresholds. *Laryngoscope, 77,* 823–835.

Tietze, G. and Pantev, Ch. (1986). Comparison between auditory brain stem responses evoked by rarefaction and condensation step functions and clicks. *Audiology, 25,* 44–53.

van der Drift, J. F., van Anten, G. A., and Brocaar, M. P. (1989). Brainstem electric response audiometry: Estimation of the amount of conductive hearing loss with and without use of the response threshold. *Audiology, 28,* 181–193.

Webb, K. C. and Greenberg, H. J. (1983). Bone-conduction masking for threshold assessment in auditory brain stem response testing. *Ear and Hearing, 4,* 261–266.

Weber, B. A. (1983). Masking and bone conduction testing in brainstem response audiometry. *Seminars in Hearing, 4,* 343–352.

Yamada, T., Yagi, T., and Yamane, H., et al. (1975). Clinical evaluation of the auditory evoked brainstem response. *Auris, Nasus, Larynx, 2,* 97–105.

Yost, W. A. and Klein, A. J. (1979). Thresholds of filtered transients. *Audiology, 18,* 17–23.

CHAPTER 11

ELECTROPHYSIOLOGIC MEASURES OF FREQUENCY-SPECIFIC AUDITORY FUNCTION

DAVID R. STAPELLS
TERENCE W. PICTON
ANDRÉE DURIEUX-SMITH

The *frequency specificity* of an audiometric measurement indicates how independent a measure at one frequency is of the measures at other frequencies. The term is usually applied to the evaluation of auditory thresholds. When frequency specificity is poor, the threshold at one frequency may be inaccurate because of responses mediated at other frequencies. A related concept is that of *frequency selectivity*, which represents the ability of the auditory system to resolve the different frequencies present in a complex sound. In general, the more frequency-selective a system, the more frequency-specific its response to a stimulus of a particular frequency. This chapter discusses some aspects of frequency specificity and selectivity in auditory evoked potentials and describes techniques which can provide useful information about a patient's hearing. In particular, we will try to convince you that the long search for a reliable evoked potential correlate of the behavioral audiogram has been more successful than is commonly believed.

BASIC PRINCIPLES

Acoustics of Brief Stimuli

Brief auditory stimuli are quite different from the long-lasting pure tones used in conventional audiometry.

Clicks produced by passing a brief square wave through an earphone have a broad frequency spectrum with a null value at the frequency equal to the reciprocal of the square-wave duration (Pfeiffer, 1974). The flatness and the upper frequency cutoff of the spectrum are determined by the transfer function of the earphone. A 100 μs square wave transduced by a TDH-49 earphone results in an acoustic wave containing equal energy from around 100 Hz to just below 8000 Hz, above which there is rapid attenuation to the predicted null at 10000 Hz (Stapells, Picton, and Smith, 1982). Brief tones have a concentration of energy at the nominal frequency of the tone and sidebands of energy at higher and lower frequencies (Burkard, 1984; Gorga and Thornton, 1989; Laukli, 1983). The spread of energy to frequencies other than the nominal frequency of the tone is termed "spectral splatter" (Durrant, 1983). Increasing the rise time of the tone decreases this splatter. Several approaches to a reasonable compromise between the brief duration of the tone and its frequency specificity are available (Davis, Hirsh, Popelka, and Formby, 1984; Gabor, 1947; Gorga and Thornton, 1989; Harris, 1978; Nuttall, 1981), but none can completely prevent spectral splatter. Because both clicks and brief tones contain energy over a range of frequencies, responses to these stimuli may be evoked by any of the frequencies present

This research was supported by the Medical Research Council of Canada, the Natural Sciences and Engineering Research Council of Canada, the Ontario Deafness Research Foundation, the U.S.P.H.S. National Institutes of Health—National Institute for Deafness and Other Communicative Disorders, and the Deafness Research Foundation. Several colleagues helped in these studies, including Marilyn Perez-Abalo, Daniel Read, Christopher G. Edwards, Linda M. Moran, Sandra C. Champagne, and Kathy Down.

in their spectrum. Although in a normal subject responses to a near-threshold brief tone will be evoked by the tone's nominal frequency, this may not always be the case in a hearing-impaired patient.

Frequency Analysis in the Cochlea

The frequency content of an auditory stimulus is analyzed in the cochlea by several mechanisms. The traveling wave results in a place coding for frequency on the basilar membrane (BM) (Békésy, 1960). The higher frequencies in the sound will vibrate only the basal regions of the BM; the lower frequencies will vibrate all the regions of the BM but mostly the apical regions. There are three important corollaries to this analysis: First, the traveling wave has a finite velocity that decreases as it moves along the BM. The wave takes approximately 5 ms to travel from the base to the apex of the human cochlea. Responses to low-frequency sounds are initiated later than those to high-frequency sounds. Second, the traveling wave is asymmetrical. High frequencies activate only the high-frequency region of the BM but low frequencies activate both basal and apical regions. Thus the traveling wave acts as a sequential low-pass filter. Third, because of the decreasing velocity of the traveling wave, the extent of BM specifically activated by a particular frequency increases as the wave moves from base to apex. The mapping of frequency to distance along the BM is approximately logarithmic.

In addition to the BM traveling wave, there may exist a "second filter" that makes the normal neuronal response more specific to one "characteristic frequency" (CF) than would be expected from initial evaluation of the mechanics of the traveling wave. This sharpening of tuning may derive from some complex interaction between the BM and the hair cells (Allen, 1988). The frequency threshold or tuning curve (FTC) of an VIIIth nerve fiber shows a low-intensity tip with a broad high-intensity region. In cochlear pathology this tip is reduced. The thresholds for activating nerve fibers are elevated, but once reached, the activation is similar to when the tips were present. However, there is a loss of frequency selectivity with similar thresholds for stimuli over a range of frequencies. As well, masking noise may

not result in as great threshold shifts as seen in normal listeners (Gorga and Worthington, 1983).

The phase locking of neuronal discharges to the periodicity of an auditory stimulus is an additional means for providing frequency information. The auditory brainstem responses (ABR) have not been extensively evaluated in the context of this type of frequency analysis. The *frequency following potential* (Huis in't Veld, Osterhammel, and Terkildsen, 1977; Moushegian, Rupert, and Stillman, 1978) may reflect the locking of brainstem neurons to low-frequency stimuli. However, since it is only evoked by low-frequency stimuli with intensities greater than 40 dB above threshold, it is not very helpful in evaluating frequency-specific thresholds and will not be further discussed.

Masking

Masking has been used in several evoked potential techniques for obtaining frequency-specific thresholds. It is therefore important to review briefly some of the present concepts of masking. The "line-busy" hypothesis proposes that the response of neurons to the masking stimulus makes them unable to respond further when the masked stimulus is presented. This theory can explain most masking phenomena, particularly the effects of adaptation to an ongoing masking stimulus (Smith, 1979). There remain, however, some phenomena that are difficult to explain in this way and require the further postulation of "suppression" (Delgutte, 1990; Geisler and Sinex, 1980; Pickles, 1982). Suppression occurs when a stimulus decreases the sensitivity of an auditory unit to another stimulus without itself activating the unit. Suppression may be similar to the processes mediating "two-tone inhibition" (Sachs and Kiang, 1968). Most studies of the mechanisms of masking have been performed in normal cochleas. Exactly how masking is changed in pathological cochleas is not well known, and it is possible that pathology may invalidate some of the assumptions underlying the use of masking to increase frequency specificity (Gorga and Worthington, 1983). A final aspect of masking that should be considered is the "spread of masking". Because of the asymmetry of the traveling wave, low-frequency stimuli are able to mask higher frequency stimuli but not vice versa (Egan and Hake, 1950). Suppression mechanisms appear to be largely responsible for this upward spread of simultaneous masking (Delgutte, 1990).

BRAINSTEM RESPONSES TO CLICKS

The most common stimulus in ABR measurement is a broadband click. While few frequency-specific auditory threshold data can be gained from the responses to clicks alone, such information is available if the clicks are presented with various masking stimuli. This section initially discusses responses to nonmasked clicks, and then the use of high-pass noise, pure-tone, and notched noise maskers.

Nonmasked Clicks

Although the ABR to broadband clicks cannot provide accurate information about hearing threshold levels at different frequencies, it nevertheless provides useful audiometric information. The threshold for the click-evoked potential can give a rough idea of the overall threshold for hearing, while the latency-intensity function for wave V can provide some insight into the etiology of a hearing loss.

Several reports have indicated that the click-ABR threshold correlates best with hearing threshold at 2000–4000 Hz (Coats and Martin, 1977; Drift, Brocaar, and Zanten, 1987; Jerger and Mauldin, 11978; Yamada, Kodera, and Yagi, 1979; Yamada, Yagi, Yamane, and Suzuki, 1975). Figure 11.1 shows click-ABR threshold results compared to the average of 2000 and 4000 Hz pure-tone behavioral thresholds obtained for 161 ears of 82 cochlear-impaired patients. An EEG filter bandpass of 30–3000 Hz and a 15 ms sweep were employed. These results demonstrate that any particular click-ABR threshold may represent a wide range (20–80 dB) of pure-tone thresholds. The less-than-unity slope of the regression line (0.55 dB increase in click-ABR threshold per 1 dB increase in the pure-tone average) indicates that greater losses in the 2000–4000 Hz region are not matched by equally large click-ABR elevations (Kileny and Magathan, 1987). This is probably due to signifi-

cant contributions from more-sensitive lower frequency (500–1000 Hz) regions.

The click-ABR wave V latency-intensity function provides some information concerning the nature of the hearing loss. Specifically, functions with latencies which are within normal limits at higher stimulus intensities but prolonged at lower intensities are most often associated with cochlear losses. Conductive impairments usually result in a shift of the entire function to the right to an extent equivalent to the conductive

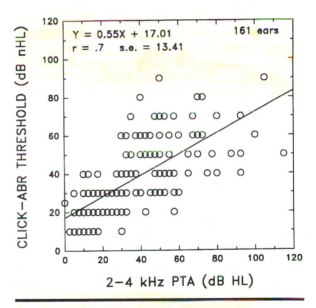

FIGURE 11.1.   Threshold estimation using the ABR to nonmasked clicks. Shown are the click-ABR thresholds versus the pure-tone average (PTA) of the 2000 and 4000 Hz behavioral thresholds, obtained from 161 ears of 82 cochlear-impaired adults. Patients with conductive impairments and patients with retrocochlear involvement were excluded. Brainstem responses were recorded using a 30–3000 Hz EEG bandpass, a 15 ms analysis time, and two or more replications of 2000 trials each. Clicks were presented at 61/s. Depending upon the click-ABR threshold, corresponding PTAs show a wide (20–80 dB) range. The 0.55 slope of the linear regression (solid line) indicates that click-ABR threshold does not grow as fast as does the 2000 to 4000 Hz PTA.

impairment, although similar patterns are also produced by steep high-frequency cochlear losses as well as retrocochlear dysfunction (Stapells, Picton, Pérez-Abalo, Read, and Smith, 1985). Importantly, click-ABRs provide an evaluation of the VIIIth nerve and brainstem auditory pathways.

There are several disadvantages to limiting the evaluation to nonmasked clicks. Normal thresholds and latency-intensity functions for click-evoked ABRs can be recorded from ears having significant losses between 500 and 6000 Hz (Picton, Ouellette, Hamel, and Smith, 1979; Stapells, 1989; Yamada et al., 1979). Furthermore, the residual low-frequency sensitivity in a patient with a severe high-frequency loss cannot be adequately assessed with these responses. Finally, the click-evoked ABR cannot provide the information about hearing at different frequencies that is necessary for the proper fitting of hearing aids. High-pass noise and notched noise have therefore been used to improve the frequency specificity of the click-evoked brainstem potential.

Derived Responses Obtained Using Clicks in High-Pass Noise

High-pass noise was initially introduced in 1962 by Teas, Eldridge, and Davis. The traveling wave in the cochlea and the response pattern of single auditory nerve fibers show a very steep high-frequency edge. Noise in the high-frequency regions can therefore mask the responses of high-frequency fibers without affecting fibers with lower characteristic frequencies. With low-pass masking, on the other hand, there is a spread of masking into the higher frequencies.

The ABR remains relatively unchanged in the presence of masking noise that has been high-pass filtered as low as 4000 Hz. Lowering the cutoff frequency further causes the earlier waves I to IV to disappear, leaving only wave V clearly recognizable (Don and Eggermont, 1978; Thümmler, Tietze, and Matkei, 1981) (Figure 11.2). The latency of wave V increases as the response is limited to more and more apical regions of the BM by decreasing the cutoff frequency of the high-pass noise. Nevertheless, high-pass noise cutoffs as low as 500 Hz still result in a clear wave V with

a latency about 4 ms later than the latency in the unmasked response (Don and Eggermont, 1978; Picton, Stapells, and Campbell, 1981; Thümmler et al., 1981).

Subtraction of the response in high-pass noise at one cutoff frequency from the response at a higher cutoff frequency leaves a "derived response" to the frequencies between the two cutoff settings. This process is illustrated in Figure 11.2. Derived responses representing a full intensity series for each audiometric frequency are obtained using high-pass noise masking cutoffs from 4000 to 500 Hz (Figure 11.3). This technique was first applied to human electrocochleography by Elberling (1974) and has subsequently been used to analyze the human ABR (Burkard and Hecox, 1983; Don and Eggermont, 1978; Don, Eggermont, and Brackman, 1979; Eggermont and Don, 1980, 1982; Kramer, 1992; Kramer and Teas, 1982; Nousak and Stapells, 1992; Parker and Thornton, 1978a, b, c; Picton et al., 1981) The basic assumption of this technique is that the response evoked through the region of the cochlea that has lower frequencies than the cutoff of the high-pass noise is unaffected by the masking noise. Although there is little spread of masking from high- to low-frequency regions in the cochlea related to the traveling wave, there are definite interactions both in the cochlea and the brainstem between sounds of different frequencies. Nevertheless, the derived responses obtained using this technique have definite frequency specificity as demonstrated by masking within the frequency band of the derived response (Parker and Thornton, 1978b), by evaluating patients with hearing losses at specific frequencies (Don et al., 1979), and by cochlear nerve single fiber recordings in cats (Evans and Elberling, 1982).

As the center frequency of the narrow-band derived response decreases, there are changes in the latency and morphology of the response. Wave V latency increases by approximately 4 ms as the center frequency decreases from 4000 to 500 Hz (Figures 11.2, 11.3 and 11.4). The higher frequency (2000 and 4000 Hz) waveforms show small early responses (waves I and III) at high intensities, but below 2000 Hz the waveforms show only a broad wave V component. At 70 dB nHL, the derived responses from the 2000 and 4000 Hz re-

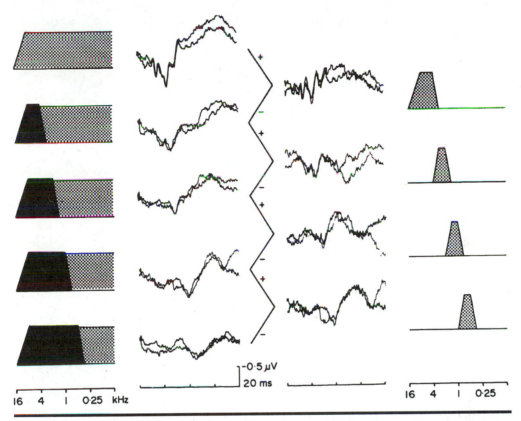

FIGURE 11.2. Derived brainstem responses obtained using high-pass masking. On the left of the figure are shown the brainstem responses to 70 dB nHL clicks presented at a rate of 39/s either alone or in the presence of high-pass masking with the cutoff settings at 4000, 2000, 1000, and 500 Hz. Each tracing represents the average of 2000 responses recorded from the vertex to mastoid. In this figure, and all subsequent figures, waveforms are plotted with negativity at the vertex being represented by an upward deflection. The diagrams to the left of the tracings represent the spectra of the click (dotted area) and the masking noise (black area). On the right are shown the derived responses obtained by sequential subtraction of the responses obtained using decreasing filter settings for the high-pass noise. On the far right of the figure are shown diagrammatically the narrow-band frequency areas that theoretically activate the derived responses. Note the decreased replicability of the derived responses compared to the original high-pass noise-masked waveforms.

gions of the cochlea are most similar in latency and morphology to the nonmasked response, suggesting that the basal region of the cochlea provides the greater contribution to the high-intensity nonmasked response recorded from a normal subject. The contribution of different frequency regions to the nonmasked response can be estimated from the amplitudes of the narrow-band derived responses. This analysis indicates that center frequencies from 500 to 4000 Hz contribute equally to the amplitude of wave V in response to high-intensity nonmasked clicks (Figures 11.2, 11.3, and 11.4), that is, little change in amplitude is seen as a

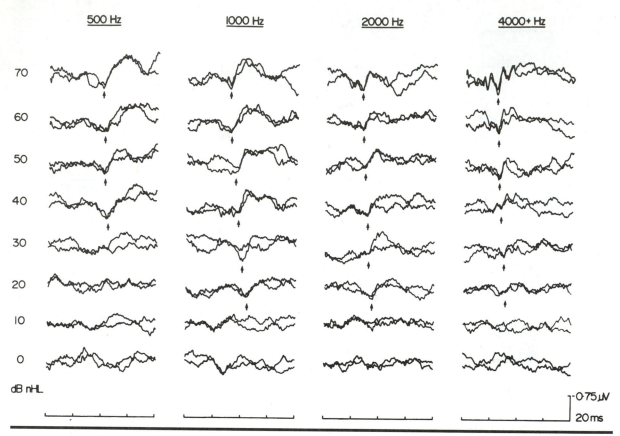

500 Hz   1000 Hz   2000 Hz   4000+ Hz

70

60

50

40

30

20

10

0

dB nHL

0·75 μV

20 ms

FIGURE 11.3.   Derived response intensity series. These derived responses were obtained from the same normal-hearing subject illustrated in the previous figure. They represent the derived responses at each of the frequency bands obtained using clicks that decreased in intensity from 70 to 0 dB nHL. There is a recognizable wave V (arrows) at 500 Hz down to 40 dB and at other frequencies down to 20 dB nHL.

function of center frequency (Don and Eggermont, 1978). The early studies of these derived brainstem responses reported that thresholds were predicted within 10–25 dB of pure-tone behavioral threshold at 1000, 2000, and 4000 Hz and within about 30 dB for 500 and 8000 Hz (Don et al., 1979; Stapells, 1984).

There are several drawbacks to the high-pass noise/ derived response technique. First, the subtraction procedure decreases the signal-to-noise ratio of the response (Figure 11.2). Since the background noise is random, its polarity is irrelevant and subtracting one noise-waveform from another is effectively the same as

adding them together. The subtraction of the background noise thus increases the root-mean-square value of the noise by the square root of 2, or 1.4. In practical terms, if one wishes to obtain derived responses that are as reliable as the waveforms one usually records without subtraction, one must average twice as many responses. Thus the time required to obtain reliable derived responses is at least twice the time required to obtain direct responses.

Second, the procedure takes time. At any intensity one must obtain one more response than the number of frequency bands that one is observing (e.g., four de-

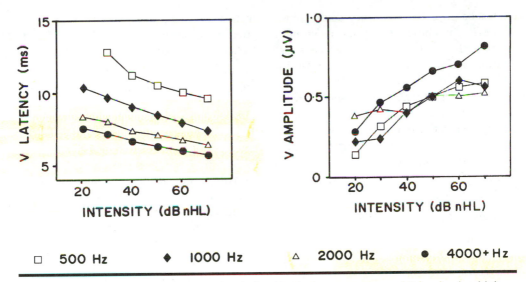

FIGURE 11.4.   Effects of intensity on the derived brainstem responses obtained using high-pass noise masking. These results represent the mean values from 10 normal subjects. The waveforms were obtained as illustrated in Figures 11.2 and 11.3. On the left are shown the average latencies of wave V in the derived response. On the right are shown the average amplitudes of wave V measured to the following negative wave.

rived responses require five separate recordings). Furthermore, if one does not have immediate computation of the derived responses, one will have to make recordings at all intensities and at all frequencies rather than those just above and below threshold at each of the frequency bands that one is examining. Thus, any technique that obtains frequency-specific responses without the need for subtraction will be more efficient than the derived-response technique.

Third, high levels of acoustic noise are required to mask the response to a click. The average intensity of white noise necessary to mask the perception of a 60 dB nHL (96 dB peak SPL) click presented at a rate of 10/s is 80 dB SPL (Stapells, 1984). Because of intersubject variability of this masking threshold, and because the threshold for masking the brainstem response may be a few dB higher than the threshold for masking the perception, we have used a noise level of 28 dB more than the nHL of the click when obtaining derived responses. These high levels of noise (118 dB SPL to mask a 90 dB click) can increase the back-

ground electrical noise in the recording: a waking subject becomes more tense when loud sounds are being presented, and a sleeping subject may wake up.

More importantly, the high levels of noise can cause temporary threshold shifts and even damage the cochlear receptors. We studied one patient with a mild/moderate low-frequency sensory hearing loss (normal at 2000 Hz and higher) who had a temporary threshold shift in the high frequencies that lasted for over a day after being exposed for approximately 5 minutes to noise levels of 118 dB SPL that were used to assess derived responses at 90 dB nHL (Stapells, 1984). We therefore recommend that white-noise intensities of greater than 108 dB SPL should not be used in patients with sensory hearing loss. This recommendation limits the intensities over which derived responses can be assessed to below 80 dB nHL.

The above disadvantages notwithstanding, the derived responses obtained using high-pass masking are probably the most frequency-specific responses available. There is no spread of energy related to the brevity of the stimulus because the frequency-determining high-pass noise is continuous during the recording. Since the steep high-frequency edge of the auditory nerve fiber response curve usually remains in pathologic cochleas, the basic technique is valid for patients with hearing loss. Due to its superior frequency specificity, the high-pass noise/derived response technique is valuable for the evaluation of the frequency specificity of responses, such as those to short-duration tones (e.g., Eggermont, 1976; Kramer, 1992; Nousak and Stapells, 1992).

Derived Responses Obtained Using Clicks and Tonal Masking

Another technique for obtaining derived responses uses tonal (or narrow-band noise) masking. The continuous pure tone would activate those neurons responding specifically to that frequency and prevent them from responding to the broadband click. Subtracting the response to the combined click and tone from the response to the click alone would yield a derived response equivalent to the tone response. Using this technique, derived responses with wave V latencies appropriate to the frequency of the tone are seen when the intensity (in SL) of the tones is 0–20 dB greater than the intensity of the click (Pantev and Pantev, 1982). When the intensity of the masking tone is increased to more than 20 dB greater than that of the click, there is evidence of spread of masking. The 500 Hz derived response has early peaks apparently related to higher frequency regions of the cochlea that are affected by the spread of masking from the 500 Hz tone into the 1000–4000 Hz frequency regions of the cochlea (Pantev and Pantev, 1982; Stapells et al., 1985). This spread of masking is not a problem when using high-pass masking derived response techniques. Both techniques involve subtraction, and therefore increase the noise levels of the recording. Masking with tones or narrow-band noise can be done at higher intensities than those possible using high-pass noise masking. However, the complexities of the spread of masking suggests that high-pass masking is at present the better approach. Tone-derived responses have been recorded using tones that are much lower in continuous intensity

than the transient stimulus that is evoking the response (Berlin and Shearer, 1981; Salt and Vora, 1990). This technique has promise but will need further validation.

Clicks in Notched Noise

Notched noise is broadband noise in which one band of frequencies has been stopped or rejected. The logic of notched noise is to restrict the responsive region of the cochlea to the frequencies within the notch. Figure 11.5 illustrates the use of notched noise with both clicks and tones. The notched noise technique has the advantage of recording frequency-specific responses directly without the need for any computation. However, it has several disadvantages. These are particularly evident when recording responses to clicks in notched noise (Laukli, 1983; Pratt, Ben-Yitzhak, and Attias, 1984; Pratt and Bleich, 1982; Thümmler and Tietze, 1984; Zanten and Brocaar, 1984).

One major problem with the technique is the spread of masking into the notch from its low-frequency edge (Figure 11.5). The spread of masking toward higher frequencies occurs with a slope that is typically somewhere between 20 and 30 dB/octave. The spread will be greater at higher intensities (Egan and Hake, 1950) and may be greater in patients with sensorineural hearing loss (Trees and Turner, 1986). Thus the actual nonmasked region within the notch will be limited by this spread of masking regardless of the actual acoustical depth of the notch.

A second problem with the clicks in the notched noise technique concerns the apparently inappropriate latencies that have been reported when notched noise is used to mask the clicks. Pratt and Bleich (1982) reported that the latency of the most prominent positive peak of the brainstem response to a click presented in notched noise did not vary with the frequency of the notch. This finding is very difficult to explain. The latency of the response should have increased as the center frequency of the notch decreased. Indeed, appropriate latency measurements have been reported in subsequent studies (Folsom and Wynne, 1986; Starr and Don, 1988; Zanten and Brocaar, 1984).

We have found results similar to those reported by Pratt and Bleich (Stapells et al., 1985). Our results in-

Clicks in Notched Noise   ## Tones in Notched Noise

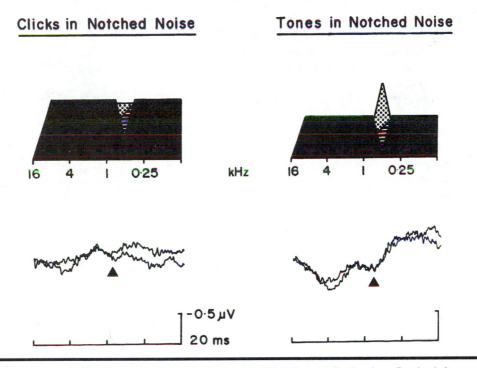

FIGURE 11.5. Auditory brainstem responses recorded using notched noise. On the left are shown the responses to clicks in notched noise and on the right the responses to brief tones in notched noise. The upper part of the figure represents diagramatically the frequency spectra of the stimuli (dotted area) and the masking noise (black area). Frequencies in these spectra are plotted from high to low frequency. This is done to make the diagrams compatible with diagrams of the traveling wave which goes from the base (high frequency) to apex (low frequency) of the cochlea. The area shaded by horizontal lines represents the spread of masking into the notch from its low frequency edge. In the lower portion of the figure are plotted the evoked potentials from a single subject to 60 dB nHL clicks on the left and 60 dB nHL 500 Hz tones (2-1-2) on the right. For both, the one-octave-wide notch was centered at 500 Hz. Each tracing represents the average of 2000 responses recorded from the vertex to mastoid. Wave V of the brainstem responses is indicated by the triangle. The response is much larger to tones than to clicks. Since the stimuli were presented at a rate of 39/s, wave V is superimposed upon a 40 Hz response that is most apparent in the tone-evoked potential, where there is a roughly sinusoidal wave with a positive peak at approximately 5 ms and a negative peak between 15 and 20 ms.

dicated that the problem lay in the intensity of the masking noise. We found that the average intensity necessary for the perceptual masking of the 60 dB nHL click was 80 dB SPL but for complete masking of the brainstem response it was 83 dB SPL. Thus, there are intensities of masking noise at which a click cannot be perceived but which can evoke a recognizable brainstem response. This indicates that there is some central masking effect that occurs in auditory centers that are beyond or parallel to those generating the brainstem response.

The complex results with clicks in notched noise can best be considered by looking at the responses obtained using levels of masking noise that were just adequate to mask the brainstem response when no notch was present (Figure 11.6, top). The middle and lower waveforms shown in Figure 11.6 illustrate the pattern of results seen in most subjects. When a 500 Hz notch was used, five out of eight subjects showed a response with two distinct positive peaks at 7.2 and 11.0 ms, two subjects showed no recognizable response at all, and one subject showed a response containing only the late positive wave at 11.3 ms. How can we explain these findings? The single subject with the single late positive wave follows what would be expected from the traveling-wave delay, the response being generated via the non-masked apical region of the cochlea. For the two subjects with no clear response, one can surmise that the spread of masking into the notch was sufficient to prevent any response from that region of the cochlea. For the other subjects, there appears to be, in addition to the response generated via the apical regions, some other response occurring at a latency equal to the wave V that was generated when a 2000 Hz notch was used—in this case all subjects showed a clear positive peak with an average latency of 7.2 ms (Figure 11.6, bottom). This earlier wave is apparently equivalent to that recorded by Pratt and Bleich who describe latencies of around 7 ms. One possible explanation for the extra early wave is that the 500 Hz notch, as well as allowing a response at the frequency region of the notch, also removed some inhibitory influence on the higher frequency regions of the cochlea. Such an influence could be explained in terms of two-tone suppression (Delgutte, 1990; Javel, McGee, Walsh, Farley, and Gorga, 1983). If this explanation is true, some part of normal masking is due to suppression mechanisms in addition to busy-line effects. This release from masking effect of the notch could be prevented by using higher levels of noise. However, at such levels one runs the risk of removing the frequency-specific response by spread of masking.

What can we then conclude about the use of clicks in notched noise as a frequency-specific stimulus? First, the noise levels must be sufficiently high to ensure appropriate masking of the electrophysiologic response when there is no notch, and to prevent any release from masking of the response to other frequencies when the notch is used. Second, when such noise levels are used,

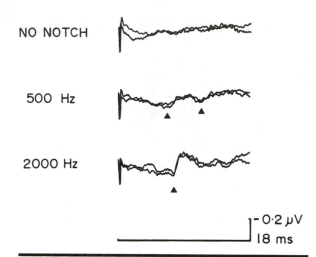

FIGURE 11.6. Brainstem responses to clicks in notched noise. These waveforms represent the responses to 60 dB nHL clicks presented at a rate of 50/s. Each tracing represents the average of 8000 trials recorded using an EEG bandpass of 25–3000 Hz. The top tracings represent the responses to the clicks in white noise at an intensity of 83 dB SPL. No clear response is recognizable. The middle tracings represents the potential evoked by the click when presented in noise containing a notch at 500 Hz that was one-octave wide and 24 dB deep. The response shows two small positive waves, one at 7.0 ms and one at 11.3 ms. The lower tracings show the response to the clicks when the noise contained a notch centered at 2000 Hz. A clear positive wave is recorded with a peak latency at 7.6 ms.

the responses may be small and difficult to recognize because of spread of masking into the notch. Third, ABR thresholds using this technique do not correlate well with pure-tone behavioral thresholds in patients with hearing loss (Pratt et al., 1984; Stapells, 1984).

A better approach to obtaining frequency-specific responses is to use tones in notched noise (Picton, Ouelette, Hamel, and Smith, 1979; Purdy, Houghton, Keith, and Greville, 1989; Stapells and Picton, 1981; Stapells, Picton, Durieux-Smith, Edwards, and Moran, 1990). The brief tone allows one to concentrate the energy of the stimulus at the frequency being examined; the notched noise prevents a response to the spread of energy away from this frequency caused by the brief duration of the tone. As well as being a direct technique for measuring frequency-specific responses, the technique of tones in notched noise does not require noise levels as high as those necessary to obtain derived responses with click stimuli.

EVOKED POTENTIALS TO TONES

The most direct approach to obtaining frequency-specific thresholds is to use frequency-specific stimuli. Many researchers have therefore recorded responses to brief tones. This section considers these responses and discusses the problem of tonal spectral splatter. Several techniques are reviewed that may provide frequency-specific thresholds.

Nonmasked Tones

There are three main responses occurring within 25 ms of a brief tone: wave V, SN10, and the 40 Hz potential. Brief high-frequency tones elicit brainstem responses which are similar to those evoked by clicks (Terkildsen, Osterhammel, and Huis in't Veld, 1973, 1975). Early researchers found that responses to low-frequency tones were difficult to identify and were probably mediated by the basal regions of the cochlea (Davis and Hirsh, 1976). Subsequent research, however, showed that the brainstem response to a low-frequency stimulus was a broad vertex-positive wave that could be recorded to within 10–20 dB of threshold provided that the high-pass filter setting of the EEG amplifier was lowered to 0.5 Hz from the usual 100–150 Hz (Suzuki, Hirai, Horiuchi, 11977; Suzuki and Horiuchi, 1979). Davis and Hirsh (1979), using a high-pass filter set at 40 Hz, found the vertex-negativity following wave V to be the most prominent component of the ABR to low-frequency tones. They called this wave the "slow negative wave at 10 ms" or SN10. Stapells and Picton (1982) investigated the effects on the brainstem response to 500 Hz tones of varying the cutoffs of the EEG high-pass filters from 10 to 100 Hz. They recorded the largest brainstem responses—a broad vertex-positive wave—using a high-pass filter setting of 10 Hz. The use of increased high-pass filter settings, particu-

larly when combined with high roll-off slopes, resulted in responses of lower amplitude and a distortion of the response so as to accentuate the vertex-negative wave (V' or SN10) following wave V. Results of this study recommended using a low (10–20 Hz) high-pass filter setting on the amplifier (Stapells and Picton, 1981). This low filter setting allows for the recording of the large slow-wave ABR component underlying and integral to the V–V' deflection. This slower ABR component appears to be more important for threshold estimation purposes than the faster (>300 Hz) components (Suzuki, Kobayashi, and Takagi, 1986; Takagi, Suzuki, and Kobayashi, 1985).

Brief tones differ from clicks in two important characteristics: rise time and frequency content. Two kinds of brief tones are commonly used in ABR measure—those with rise times comprising a constant number of cycles, and those with rise times lasting a constant time regardless of the frequency of the stimulus. Figure 11.7 demonstrates the spectral differences between these two types of tones. The advantage of the former is that the spectra of tones with different frequencies are equivalent when plotted on a logarithmic frequency axis; that is, the bandwidth of the energy in the tone, expressed in octaves, is constant across frequency. Davis and his colleagues (Davis et al., 1984) have recommended tones having rise and fall times of 2 cycles each and plateau durations of 1 cycle—the "2-1-2" tone (Figure 11.7, top). The advantage of the constant rise time tone is that once the traveling wave delays have been accounted for, the initiation of the auditory impulse occurs at an approximately equivalent time for each frequency.

The rise time of a stimulus affects both the latency and the amplitude of the brainstem response (Brinkmann and Scherg, 1979; Burkard, 1990; Folsom and Aurich, 1987; Hecox and Deegan, 1983; Hecox, Squires, and Galambos, 1976; Stapells and Picton, 1981). The longer the rise time of the stimulus, the longer the latency of wave V. Brinkmann and Scherg (1979) have introduced the concept of a "virtual trigger time", which represents the point in the rise time of a stimulus at which the majority of nerve fibers innervating the generators of the brainstem response are activated. This virtual trigger time is a function of the rise

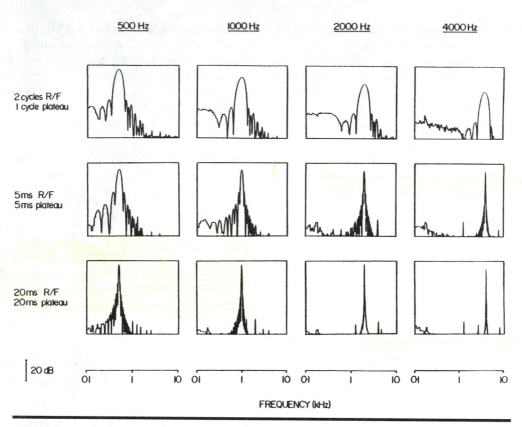

FIGURE 11.7.   Effects of rise and fall time, plateau duration, and frequency on the acoustic power spectra of tones. Spectra in the top row are for tones with constant number of cycles: 2 cycles rise (R), 1 cycle plateau, and 2 cycles fall (F). Spectra in middle and bottom rows are for stimuli with constant rise, plateau, and fall times. Bottom row tones (20-20-20 ms) are appropriate for recording the slow cortical responses and do not elicit a clear ABR. All stimuli were presented at 111 dB peak-to-peak equivalent SPL. [From Stapells, 1984.]

time, the intensity, and the frequency of the stimulus. Increasing the rise time of a tone while keeping the slope of the rise constant causes no significant alteration in the latency or amplitude of the brainstem response after a critical duration is reached (Kodera, Marsh, Suzuki, and Suzuki, 1983; Suzuki and Horiuchi, 1981). This critical duration is approximately 2 ms for 2000 Hz tones and 4 ms for 500 Hz tones. For tonal stimuli, the amplitude of brainstem responses decreases with increasing rise times, the major changes occurring when rise times exceed 5 ms (Stapells and Picton, 1981) The latency of wave V in response to a brief tone shows complex varia-

tions with the rise time, frequency, and intensity of the tone (Jacobson, 1983; Stapells and Picton, 1981). A high-intensity, low-frequency tone with a rapid rise time has extensive spectral splatter and evokes a dominant early response through the high-frequency regions of the cochlea.

A change in rise time from 2 to 5 ms causes an increase in wave V latency of approximately 0.5 ms for 4000 Hz tones but a 1.5 ms change for 500 Hz tones (Stapells and Picton, 1981). The change in latency of wave V caused by varying the rise time of a tone is composed of both a specific rise-time effect and an effect of decreasing spectral splatter with longer rise times. The latter effect is most evident for high-intensity low-frequency tones.

Changing the frequency of the tone causes very significant changes in the brainstem response. These effects can be seen in Figure 11.8, which shows the responses of one subject to tones of 500 and 2000 Hz. The peak latency of wave V is longer in response to

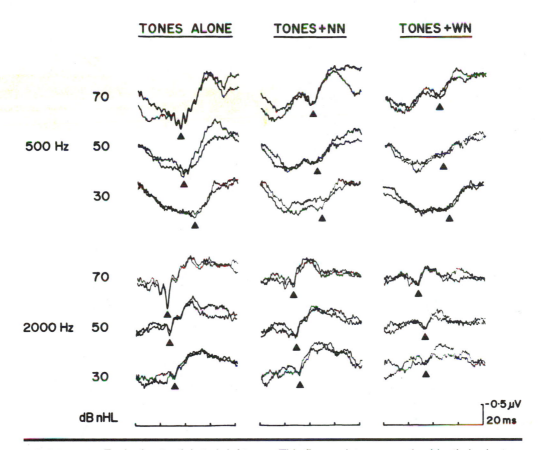

FIGURE 11.8.   Evoked potentials to brief tones. This figure plots a normal subject's brainstem responses to brief tones presented at a rate of 39/s with rise and fall times equal to two cycles of the frequency and plateau durations of one cycle. Each tracing represents the average of 2000 responses recorded from the vertex to mastoid. In the top half of the figure are the evoked potentials to 500 Hz tones and in the bottom half of the figure are the responses to 2000 Hz tones. Three conditions are given at each intensity: responses to tones presented ALONE, tones presented in notched noise (NN), and tones presented in white noise (WN). The filled triangles indicate wave V in the brainstem response. At high stimulus intensities, the masking noise decreases the amplitude of the responses at both frequencies and increases the latency of wave V to 500 Hz tones. There is little change in the latency of the response at 2000 Hz. A 40 Hz response can be seen together with wave V in the responses to 500 Hz tones. This goes from positive in the first part of the tracing to negative at the end of the tracing.

low-frequency tones than to high-frequency tones. The increased latency reflects, in part, the time taken by the traveling wave to reach the low-frequency regions of the BM near the apex of the cochlea. The magnitude of this latency difference depends upon the intensity of the tone. At 120 dB peak SPL (about 90 dB nHL) a tone of 2000 Hz evokes a wave V with a latency approximately 1 ms earlier than does a 500 Hz tone, whereas at 70 dB peak SPL the latency is about 3 ms earlier (Stapells and Picton, 1981). This relationship to intensity is most easily interpreted on the basis of the spread of energy in the tone and traveling wave. The relatively early responses to high-intensity, low-frequency tones are probably mediated by the high-frequency region of the cochlea. This spread of energy away from the nominal frequency of the tones becomes subthreshold when stimulus intensity is de-

creased and the tone then evokes a response through the region of the cochlea specific to its frequency. When the spread of energy in the tone to other regions of the cochlea is prevented by notched noise masking, the latency-intensity functions for low-frequency tones are roughly parallel to those for tones of higher frequency (Stapells, 1984; Stapells and Picton, 1981). The effects of notched noise on the latency and amplitude of the brainstem response to 1000 Hz tones are illustrated in Figure 11.9. The amplitude of the brainstem response remains relatively constant across frequencies (500–4000 Hz) provided that the recording amplifiers have a sufficiently low high-pass cutoff. Indeed, there is a tendency for the response to be larger for lower frequency stimuli, regardless of whether the rise time is specified in terms of a constant number of cycles (Coats, Martin, and Kidder, 1979; Stapells,

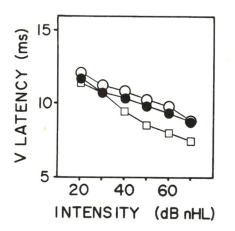
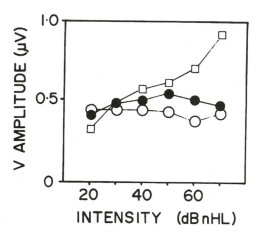

□ ALONE   ● NOTCHED NOISE   ○ WHITE NOISE

FIGURE 11.9. Brainstem responses to tones alone and in masking noise. On the left of the figure are graphed the latencies of wave V of the brainstem response to 1000 Hz tones with rise and fall times of 2 ms and plateau durations of 1 ms ("2-1-2" cycles). Tones are presented either ALONE, in NOTCHED NOISE, or in WHITE NOISE. At low intensities the latencies are similar but at high intensities the latency of the nonmasked response is shorter than the latency of the response to tones presented in masking noise. On the right of the figure are plotted the amplitudes of wave V to the following negative wave. Each of the measurements graphed represents the average of 10 normal subjects.

1984; Takagi et al., 1985) or a constant rise time (Klein, 1983a; Kodera, Yamane, Yamada, and Suzuki, 1977; Stapells and Picton, 1981; Takagi et al, 1985).

There are several means of evaluating the frequency specificity of the brainstem response to brief tones. One method is to compare nonmasked tonal responses to those obtained using notched noise. Notched noise serves to limit the responsiveness of the cochlea to regions of the BM specific to the nominal frequency of the tone (Picton et al., 1979). Notched noise significantly alters the response when tones have intensities of greater than 80 dB peak SPL (Picton et al., 1979; Stapells and Picton, 1981). At these intensities there are components in the response that are mediated through frequencies in the spectrum of the brief tone that are outside of the nominal frequency of the tone. Notched noise can also demonstrate the decreased frequency specificity of tones with short rise times (Jacobson, 1983; Stapells and Picton, 1981). Other approaches use high-pass noise to mask out the contribution of the high-frequency regions of the cochlea (Burkard and Hecox, 1983; Jacobson, 1983; Kileny, 1981; Laukli, Fjermedal, and Mair, 1988; McDonald and Shimizu, 1981). These studies demonstrate that the responses to high-intensity, low-frequency nonmasked tones are largely mediated by the basal turn of the cochlea.

Pure-tone masking has been used to assess the frequency specificity of the brainstem responses to brief tones (Folsom, 1984; Folsom and Wynne, 1987; Klein, 1983b; Klein and Mills, 1981a,b). Klein (1983b) measured the level of pure-tone masking necessary to reduce the slow wave component of the brainstem response by half. These measurements provide an inverse assessment of how much energy in the brief tone at the frequency of the masking tone is evoking the response. Klein found that frequency specificity was reasonably achieved for tones with rise and fall times of 3 ms up to intensities of 80 dB SPL, except at 250 Hz, where poor frequency specificity was seen (see Figure 11.14). Folsom (1984) measured the change in latency of wave V caused by the pure tone masking. He found that 40-dB SL filtered clicks at 1000 and 4000 Hz (three cycle rise and fall times and one cycle plateau) showed good frequency specificity, but at 60 dB SL (approximately 95

dB SPL) there was a high-frequency spread of cochlear activation. A final means of evaluating the frequency-specificity of the response to brief tones is to record these responses in patients with hearing losses that are significantly different across frequencies. There are several reports of patients whose high-frequency thresholds were significantly underestimated because responses were mediated through the spread of energy in high-frequency tones to the low-frequency regions of the cochlea where their hearing was much better (Picton, 1978; Picton et al., 1979; Purdy and Abbas, 1989; Stapells et al., 1990). Such a patient is illustrated in Figure 11.10. This difference between the ABR threshold and the threshold obtained during conventional pure-tone audiometry does not happen in patients with low-frequency hearing losses because the pure-tone audiogram in these patients may also underestimate the actual loss. As their intensity is raised, low-frequency pure tones can be heard through the basal regions of the cochlea. The steepness of a low-frequency hearing loss thus never exceeds 40 dB/octave on a pure tone audiogram (Gravendeel and Plomp, 1960; Schuknecht, 1960; Vanderbilt University Hereditary Deafness Study Group, 1968).

The frequency specificity of brief tones may be improved by employing nonlinear gating functions (Harris, 1978; Dolan and Klein, 1987; Gorga and Thornton, 1989; Nuttall, 1981). The acoustic sidelobes of "Blackman" windowed tones are approximately 20–30 dB lower compared to linear windows. In a study of gerbil VIIIth nerve action potential tuning curves, Dolan and Klein (1987) report the tuning curves for responses to linear-gated and nonlinear-gated (¼-sine) envelopes were similar and equally frequency specific, although at high probe intensities there was somewhat less frequency displacement using the nonlinear gating function. Recently, Purdy and Abbas (1989) reported no significant difference between hearing-impaired subjects' ABR thresholds for linear-windowed versus Blackman-windowed tones. Such findings may be related to the fact that the ABR reflects primarily the first 2–4 ms of a brief tone (Kodera et al., 1983; Suzuki and Horiuchi, 1981), thus the acoustic spectrum of the whole Blackman-windowed tone may not accurately

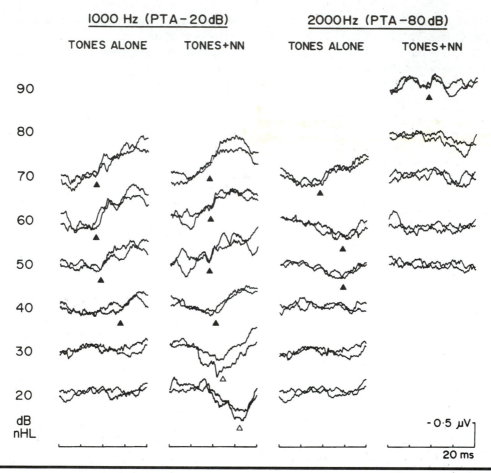

FIGURE 11.10.   Brainstem responses in a patient with a steep high-frequency hearing impairment. This patient's pure-tone audiometric thresholds (PTA) were 20 dB at 1000 Hz and 80 dB at 2000 Hz. This figure represents the brainstem responses to tones presented either ALONE or in notched noise (NN). There is little difference in the responses obtained for the 1000 Hz tones. However, the responses to 2000 Hz tones show a marked difference in threshold when the tones are presented alone or in notched noise. When the tones are presented alone responses are recognizable down to 50 dB nHL. These responses are probably mediated by the frequency spread to the 1000 Hz region of the cochlea. The nonmasked 2000 Hz response at 70 dB is very similar to the 1000 Hz (NN) response at 40 dB. Notched noise prevents this frequency spread and gives a threshold at 90 dB that is just above the threshold obtained using pure-tone audiometry. In each of the tracings recognized as a response, wave V is indicated by a filled triangle. The unusually large responses (open triangles) noted at 30 and 20 dB for the 1000 Hz tones in notched noise may represent 40 Hz potentials.

describe the "effective" spectrum. Further human ABR studies employing masking will provide further insight regarding whether the evoked potentials elicited using these nonlinear functions show better frequency specificity than linear functions.

In summary, nonmasked brief tones may not evoke frequency-specific brainstem responses. At high intensities, they may evoke responses that are mediated by regions of the cochlea that are most sensitive to frequencies other than the nominal frequency of the tone. Some of the techniques that have been used to demonstrate the lack of frequency specificity to brief tones may also be used to ensure that these responses are frequency specific. These are considered in the following sections.

Tones in Notched Noise

As we have discussed earlier, notched noise can be used to restrict the responsiveness of the cochlea to frequencies within the notch. Picton et al. (1979) recorded ABRs to tones in notched noise using rise and fall times of 1 ms and a two-octave notch width. Although the slope of the filters creating the notch was 48 dB/octave, the effective notch was reduced to about 27 dB by the spread of masking from the low-frequency edge of the notch (Figure 11.5). The advantage of using tones rather than clicks is the lower intensity of the noise necessary to mask responses outside of the notch. In this early study, SPL noise levels (before filtering) of 15 dB below the peak SPL of the tone were found to provide effective masking even in patients with steep high-frequency hearing losses. Recently, we used 2-1-2 tones and a one-octave notch and found that noise levels can be reduced a further 8 dB to 23 dB SPL below the peak SPL (20 dB below peak-to-peak equivalent SPL) of the brief tone (Stapells et al., 1990). By contrast, to mask clicks, the SPL intensity of the noise must be greater than 13 dB below the peak SPL of the click. The difference is even more striking if one considers that since the tones concentrate their energy in one frequency region, they have much lower thresholds than the broadband clicks. Normal threshold for a click is 36 dB peak SPL (Stapells, Picton, and Smith, 1982), and

for a 2-1-2 500 Hz tone is approximately 25 dB peak SPL (Davis et al., 1984; Stapells et al., 1990). Thus, for a 60 dB nHL click, masking levels of at least 83 (96-13) dB SPL are required but for a 60-dB nHL 2-1-2 500 Hz tone masking levels of 62 (85-23) dB SPL can be used (see Figure 11.5). Tones in notched noise provide a greater concentration of stimulus energy at the frequency under examination than do clicks in notched noise. This leads to a larger but not less frequency-specific response. Furthermore, because much of the frequency spread in the tone is overmasked, there is probably little effect of the suppression mechanisms that may confuse the response to clicks in notched noise.

Notched noise has different effects on the responses to tones of high and low frequencies. These are illustrated in Figures 11.8 and 11.9. Notched noise does not significantly alter the latency of wave V to tones of 2000 and 4000 Hz but it does reduce the amplitude of the response at high intensities. These effects are most easily explained by the removal of an underlying broad response to the low-frequency spread of energy in the tone. The removal of this broad component does not alter the peak latency, which is measured at the sharp deflection initiated by the well-synchronized, high-frequency region of the cochlea. However, the amplitude measured from the peak positivity to the succeeding negativity is reduced. Some degree of masking at the frequency of the notch could also contribute to the decrease in amplitude. Notched noise significantly increases the latency and decreases the amplitude of the response to high-intensity tones of 1000 and 500 Hz. This is because of the removal of the early sharp wave that is evoked by the spread of energy into the high-frequency regions of the cochlea and is superimposed upon the broad wave V evoked from the low-frequency regions. At low intensities (≤ 40–50 dB nHL), the splatter becomes subthreshold and amplitudes and latencies are similar for responses to the nonmasked tones and tones in notched noise (Stapells, 1984).

The ABR to tones in notched noise can provide an accurate assessment of the pure-tone audiogram even in patients with steep hearing losses (Munnerley, Greville, Purdy, and Keith, 1991; Picton et al., 1979; Stapells et al., 1990). In the patient presented in Figure 11.10, the 2000

Hz thresholds for the tones without masking underestimate his severe hearing loss, but tones in notched noise provide a reasonable estimate of the elevated threshold. Figure 11.11 presents ABR (tones in notched noise) versus behavioral (pure tones) threshold results for 500, 1000, 2000, and 4000 Hz, reported in our study for 20 normal-hearing and 20 hearing-impaired older children and adults (Stapells et al., 1990). On average, this technique estimated within 11.6, 6.1, 6.3, and 0.8 dB at 500, 1000, 2000, and 4000 Hz, respectively, of these individuals' pure-tone behavioral thresholds with the estimates being better in the hearing-impaired patients.

The tuning curves of auditory nerve fibers in pathologic cochleas may differ from normal by the absence of a specific tip and by a decreased fall-off of threshold toward the low frequencies. As pointed out by Gorga and Worthington (1983), this difference may interfere with the mechanisms of notched noise masking, although our experience has so far shown no evidence of this. Tones in notched noise have been used to assess hearing in infants (Alberti, Hyde, Riko, Corbin, and Abramovich, 1983; Hyde, 1985; Hyde, Matsumoto, and Alberti, 1987; Stapells, 1989; Stockard and Stockard, 1986; Stockard, Stockard, and Coen, 1983), and a recent study in our laboratory indicates the technique is at least as accurate for hearing-impaired infants as it is for adults (Stapells, Gravel, and Martin, 1993).

A simpler approach to masking the energy spread in brief tones is to use unfiltered white noise (Beattie and Boyd, 1985, Picton, Ouellette, Hamel, and Smith, 1979). White noise causes effects similar to those of notched noise, except that the amplitudes of the responses are reduced (Stapells, 1984), as illustrated in Figures 11.8 and 11.9. Although white noise has the advantage of simplicity, notched noise is more appropriate when measuring responses near threshold.

Tones in High-Pass Noise

The responses to low-frequency tones are more frequency specific when presented in high-pass masking noise. High-pass masking prevents the contribution of basal cochlear regions which could be activated either by traveling wave hydrodynamics or by the spread of energy in the spectrum of the brief tone. This approach has been used by Jacobson (1983), Kileny (1981), and Laukli (1983, 1988). Its advantage over notched noise is based on the lack of any spread of masking from high to low frequencies; therefore, very little masking occurs at the frequency of the tone. Furthermore, the overall intensity of high-pass noise is less than that of notched noise and therefore, produces less stapedius reflex effect which could result in an attenuation of hearing at low frequencies. The disadvantage of this approach is that it is inappropriate for middle- and high-frequency tones where the lack of specificity is in the opposite direction to that controlled by high-pass noise. High-frequency brief tones may evoke responses through the spread of energy into the low frequencies. This problem would be accentuated in patients with high-frequency impairments. It is possible that a compromise would be to use notched noise at the middle and high frequencies and high-pass noise for the lowest frequency to be examined (Purdy, Houghton, Keith, and Greville, 1989).

Tone-ABR from Infants

Several studies investigating the tone-ABR in infants have demonstrated that these responses are still recognizable near adult threshold levels in these patients (Alberti et al., 1983; Hyde, 1985; Hyde et al., 1987; Stapells, 1989; Suzuki, Kodera, and Yamada, 1984; Yamada, Ashikawa, Kodera, and Yamane, 1983). Tone-ABR estimates of hearing-impaired infants' audiometric thresholds appear to have the same accuracy as for adults (Hyde, 1985; Kileny and Magathan, 1987; Stapells et al., 1993; Suzuki, Kodera, and Yamada, 1984), although further data are needed. There is some question as to whether very young infants (under one month of age) show elevated ABR thresholds at 4000 Hz compared to 500 Hz (Klein, 1984), although this has not been our experience. Figure 11.12 shows the brainstem responses to 500, 2000, and 4000 Hz tones presented in notched noise recorded from a 4-month-old infant with normal middle ear function. Replicable responses are seen down to 30 dB at 500 Hz, 10 dB at 2000 Hz and 30 dB or better at 4000 Hz. As seen with click-ABRs, peak latencies are longer in young infants, and decrease with maturation. Longer analysis times, 20 to 25 ms, are therefore required to include the complete V-to-V' positive-to-negative deflection. Table 11.1 pre-

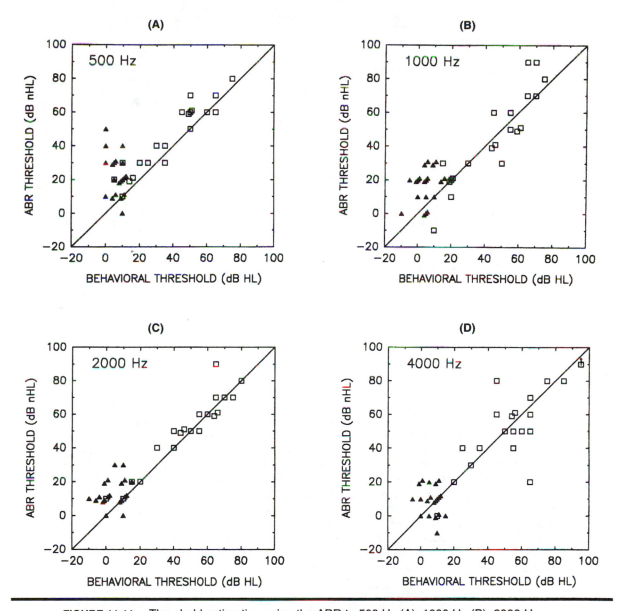

FIGURE 11.11.   Threshold estimation using the ABR to 500 Hz (A), 1000 Hz (B), 2000 Hz (C), and 4000 Hz tones (D) presented in notched noise. Shown are the ABRs to tones in notched noise threshold (dB nHL) versus pure-tone behavioral threshold (dB HL) results for 20 normal-hearing (filled triangles) and 20 hearing-impaired (open squares) older children and adults. Brief tones (2 cycles rise and fall times, 1 cycle plateau duration) were presented at 39.1/s. Noise with a one-octave wide notch centered on the tone frequency was presented 23 dB below the peak intensity of the tones. In total, 98% of the ABR thresholds are within 30 dB of the behavioral thresholds, 91% within 20 dB, and 69% within 10 dB. [Adapted from Stapells, Picton, Durieux-Smith, Edwards, and Moran, 1990.]

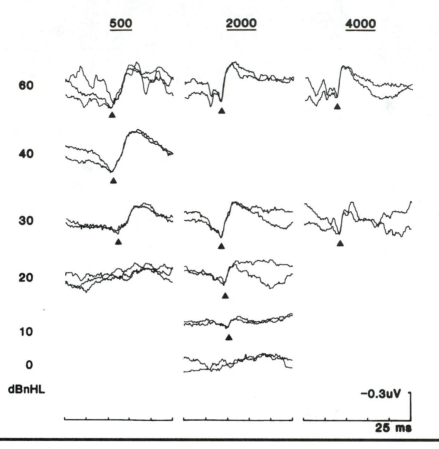

FIGURE 11.12.   Infant's ABR to tones in notched noise. Shown are a normal 4-month-old's ABRs to 500, 2000, and 4000 Hz tones presented in notched noise. The infant had normal middle-ear status on the day of test. Brief tones (2 cycles rise and fall times, 1 cycle plateau duration) were presented at 39.1/s. Noise with a one-octave wide notch centered on the tone frequency was presented 23 below the peak intensity of the tones. Each tracing represents the average of 2000 trials recorded using an EEG bandpass of 30–3000 Hz. Waveforms judged to contain a response are identified by a triangle at the location of wave V. This infant's ABR thresholds are 30 dB nHL for 500 Hz tones and 10 dB nHL for 2000 Hz tones; threshold for 4000 Hz tones was not completed but is 30 dB nHL or better.

sents tone-ABR results obtained from a group of 49 normal infants (83 ears) with normal middle ear status, tested longitudinally between ages 2 weeks and 18 months. As is clear from these results, infants' tone-evoked brainstem responses are detectable at low intensities. Our minimum response levels for screening purposes are currently 30–40 dB nHL at 500 Hz, and 30 dB nHL at 1000, 2000, and 4000 Hz (Stapells, 1989;

Stapells et al., 1993). Most normal infants show responses at even lower intensities.

ABR to Bone-Conducted Tones

The ABR can also be elicited by tonal stimuli presented through a bone oscillator, allowing for the evaluation of cochlear sensitivity when conductive impairments may

TABLE 11.1.   Detectability of normal infants' ABRs to air-conducted tones.[1]

Frequency (Hz)	Intensity dB nHL			
	40	*30*	*20*	*10*
500	98%	83%	67%	41%
	(55)	(47)	(46)	(17)
2000	100%	100%	100%	80%
	(20)	(29)	(37)	(41)
4000	100%	100%	100%	85%
	(13)	(19)	(30)	(33)

[1]Numbers in parentheses are number of ears assessed. Results from a total of 49 infants (83 ears), aged 2 weeks to 18 months. Only data from ears with normal middle ear status are included. 1000 Hz was not assessed.

be present (Stapells and Ruben, 1989). Studies of these responses in infants, currently underway in our laboratories, suggest maturational differences with bone conduction. Presented at equal intensities relative to adult behavioral threshold, 500 Hz bone-conducted tones evoke brainstem responses in infants which are shorter in latency than those of adults (Foxe and Stapells, 1993; Kramer, 1992; Nousak and Stapells, 1992; Stapells and Ruben, 1989). Further, the 500 minus 2000 Hz wave V latency difference for infants is shorter for recordings to bone-conducted versus air-conducted tones (Stapells and Ruben, 1989; Foxe and Stapells, 1993). These findings suggest either (i) poorer frequency specificity for bone-conducted versus air-conducted tones, (ii) a maturational effect on the intensity of bone-conducted tones, such that these tones are more effective in infants (particularly at 500 Hz), or (iii) a combination of both. Adults' brainstem responses to these bone-conducted tones appear to be frequency specific, at least those recorded in response to low-intensity tones (Kramer, 1992), and our results suggest the same is true in infants (Nousak and Stapells, 1992). Infant-adult ABR differences for bone-conduction stimuli may thus be related to changes in effective intensity.

Infants' responses to 500 Hz bone-conducted tones are present at lower intensities (relative to adult behavioral threshold) than are responses to 2000 Hz bone-conducted tones. In a group of 48 infants without sensorineural loss, 100 percent of the ears tested produced responses to 20 dB nHL 500 Hz bone-conducted

tones, while only 83 percent produced responses to 2000 Hz bone-conducted tones presented at this intensity (Stapells and Ruben, 1989). The 500 Hz results are different from those seen for air-conducted tones (Table 11.1), and support the suggestion that bone-conducted stimuli are more effective in infants (Foxe and Stapells, 1993).

An example of the clinical utility of brainstem response recordings to bone-conducted tones is shown in Figure 11.13, which depicts the responses to 500 Hz air and bone-conducted tones recorded from a 6-month-old infant with unilateral aural atresia. The atretic ear's responses to the air-conducted stimuli demonstrate the moderate-severe/severe threshold elevation seen with atresia; the responses to the bone-conducted tones (presented to the temporal bone on the same side as the atretic ear), however, indicate that the cochlea of his atretic ear responds to low-intensity bone-conducted stimuli. These results are consistent with the conductive impairment resulting from aural atresia.

MIDDLE LATENCY RESPONSES

Another approach to obtaining frequency-specific thresholds is to use tonal stimuli with less frequency splatter. The simplest way to decrease frequency-splatter is increase the rise time and duration of a tone. Unfortunately, the brainstem responses are evoked only by the onset of a longer tone and this procedure does not increase the specificity of the response. How-

MASKED AIR   MASKED BONE

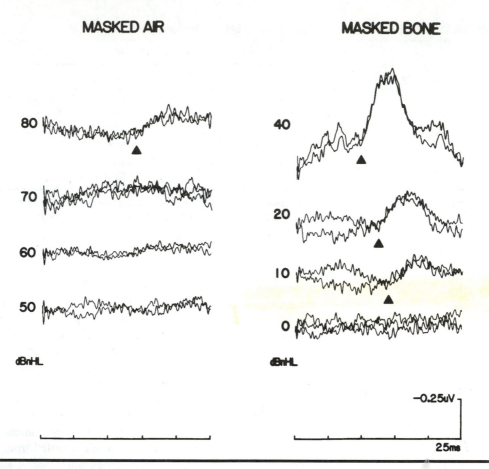

FIGURE 11.13.   Tone-evoked ABRs from a 6-month-old infant with unilateral external auditory meatal atresia. This infant's ABR to air-conducted clicks showed a threshold of 70 dB nHL for the atretic ear, 30 dB nHL or better for the normal ear. Shown are the responses to air-conducted (left) and bone-conducted (right) 500 Hz tones. The bone oscillator was placed on the infant's temporal bone just above his atretic ear. The normal ear contralateral to the atretic ear was masked using white noise (88 dB SPL) for both the air- and bone-conducted tones. Ipsilateral notched noise masking was not employed. Waveforms judged to contain a response are identified by a triangle at the location of wave V. The responses to 500 Hz air-conducted tones show a threshold of 80 dB nHL, about 50–60 dB above the normal ABR threshold to 500 Hz tones. His responses to the 500 Hz bone-conducted tones are present down to 10 dB nHL. The results are consistent with a 50–60 dB conductive impairment, with normal cochlear sensitivity at 500 Hz. [Data adapted from Stapells and Ruben, 1989.]

ever, the auditory middle latency responses (MLR) appear to integrate a significantly longer duration of the tone into the response. The transient MLRs have long been used as a means for objective audiometry (see review by Mendel, 1977). Several studies in adults have demonstrated reasonable accuracy of threshold prediction using the transient MLRs (Kavanagh, Harker, and Tyler, 1984; Kileny and Shea, 1986; Musiek and Geurkink, 1981; Palaskas, Wilson, and Dobie, 1989). Our results indicate the transient MLR is susceptible to patient electrophysiologic noise and thresholds are variable (Stapells, 1984). Furthermore, the MLR is of uncertain value for threshold estimation purposes in pediatric populations, because many studies have shown absent MLRs in normal infants up to 10 years of age (e.g., Kileny, 1983; Kraus, Reed, Smith, Stein, and Cartee, 1985; Stapells, Galambos, Costello, and Makeig, 1988).

Galambos and his colleagues (Galambos, Makeig, and Talmachoff, 1981) showed that the human MLR may be optimally recorded at stimulus rates near 40/s. At these rates, the response is a steady-state response with a waveform that is periodic at the rate of stimulation, allowing it to be accurately and efficiently analyzed using frequency-based (Fourier analysis) techniques (Picton, Vajsar, Rodriguez, and Campbell, 1987; Stapells, Linden, Suffield, Hamel, and Picton, 1984; Stapells, Makeig, and Galambos, 1987). This "40 Hz" response represents the superimposition of wave V and the middle latency responses (Galambos, Makeig, and Talmachoff, 1981; Plourde, Stapells, and Picton, 1991; Stapells et al., 1988). This steady-state MLR can provide fairly accurate auditory thresholds at different tonal frequencies (Picton, 1987; Rodriguez, Picton, Linden, Hamel, and Laframboise, 1986; Stapells et al., 1987). The 40 Hz response is particularly helpful in demonstrating thresholds for low-frequency stimuli (250–1000 Hz). It therefore nicely complements the brainstem response which is more easily recognized at the higher frequencies. Indeed, a reasonable approach is to record both the 40 Hz response and the brainstem response simultaneously by presenting stimuli at a rate of 40/s and by using a recording bandpass that allows both the brainstem and middle latency responses to be recorded.

The 40 Hz response can also be elicited by amplitude-modulated (AM) tones (Kuwada, Batra, and Maher, 1986; Picton, Skinner, Champagne, Kellett, and Maiste, 1987). An AM tone is perhaps the most frequency-specific of any rapidly repeating stimuli. This stimulus has energy only at the carrier frequency and at sidebands separated from the carrier by the frequency of the modulation.

Unfortunately, the amplitude of the 40 Hz response is decreased by sleep (Linden, Campbell, Hamel, and Picton, 1985) and this may decrease the accuracy of threshold-estimation (Picton et al., 1987). As well, the 40 Hz MLR is difficult to record in young infants (Stapells et al., 1988).

ELECTROPHYSIOLOGICAL MEASURES OF SUPRATHRESHOLD AUDITORY FUNCTION

As we have shown, techniques such as tones in notched noise or the derived responses to clicks in high-pass noise can provide an electrophysiologic estimate of the audiogram. An important question to consider is how necessary is the audiogram in the evaluation and management of patients with hearing impairment. The major use of the threshold audiogram is to infer a patient's ability to discriminate sounds at suprathreshold levels. Measures of absolute sensitivity provide only the initial evaluation of a patient's auditory capabilities (Patterson, Nimmo-Smith, Weber, and Milroy, 1982). In clinical audiology, measures of speech discrimination and other measures of suprathreshold audition evaluate a patient's impairment and the effects of amplification. In evoked potentials, it may be as important to have some direct means of assessing a patient's ability to discriminate frequencies as it is to determine at what levels he or she can detect pure tones.

Frequency Selectivity

Frequency selectivity is the ability of the auditory system to resolve the frequencies present in a complex sound. Although usually associated with frequency-specific threshold changes, changes in frequency selectivity can be seen without corresponding alterations of threshold, and vice versa (Harrison, 1988). The frequency threshold or tuning curve (FTC), obtained by recording the response to a probe stimulus of one frequency in the presence of a stimulus of another frequency, provides a direct indication of the frequency regions responding to specific stimuli, and an indirect measure of the frequency resolving capability of the system. Electrophysiologic FTCs have commonly been measured from single auditory nerve fibers as well as compound VIIIth nerve action potentials (e.g., Harrison, 1988; Mills and Schmiedt, 1983).

Human ABR frequency tuning curves have been obtained from normal adults (Folsom and Wynne, 1987; Klein, 1983b; Klein and Mills, 1981a), adults with temporary threshold shift (Klein and Mills, 1989*b*), and normal infants (Folsom and Wynne, 1987). Figure 11.14 depicts normal-hearing adults' ABR tuning curves reported for 250, 500 and 1000 Hz probe tones (Klein, 1983*b*, Figure 11.14A); for 3600 Hz probe tones (Klein and Mills, 1981*a*, Figure 11.14A); for 1000, 4000 and 8000 Hz probe tones (Folsom and Wynne, 1987, Figure 11.14B); and for 2000 Hz probe tones obtained in our laboratories (Figure 11.14C). Probes were presented at 70 dB peak-to-peak equivalent (pe) SPL (ex-

cept the 3600 Hz FTC, which was obtained for 60 dB pe SPL probes). The FTCs shown in Figure 11.14 are qualitatively similar to those obtained for VIIIth nerve fibers: FTCs for higher-frequency probes are asymmetric and sharper than those for lower-frequency probes; a steep high-frequency slope and a high-intensity low-frequency tail region are evident for higher-frequency probe FTCs. With the exception of the FTC to 250 Hz probes, the FTCs demonstrate a relatively sharp low-intensity tip region near the frequency

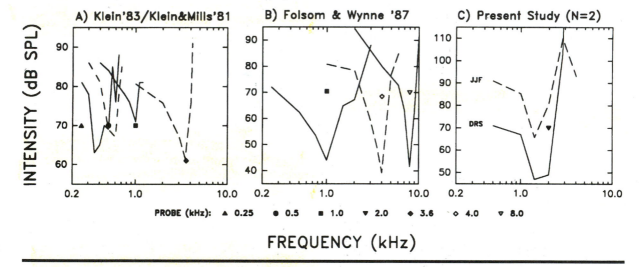

PROBE (kHz):   ▲ 0.25   ● 0.5   ■ 1.0   ▼ 2.0   ◆ 3.6   ◇ 4.0   ▽ 8.0

FIGURE 11.14. ABR Frequency Tuning Curves (FTC). Shown are ABR tuning curves reported for normal adults for 250, 500 and 1000 Hz probe tones with 3 ms rise and fall times (no plateau) (A); for 3600 Hz probe tones with a 0.75 ms rise and fall time (no plateau) (A); for 1000, 4000 and 8000 Hz probe tones with 3-cycle rise and fall times and 1-cycle plateau (B); and for 2000 Hz probe tones with 4 ms rise and fall times and a 1 ms plateau, obtained in our laboratories (C). The intensities (dB peak-to-peak equivalent SPL) and frequencies (kHz) of the probes are indicated by the symbols. Probes were presented at or close to 70 dB peak-to-peak equivalent (pe) SPL (except the 3600 Hz FTC, which was obtained for 60 dB pe SPL probes). FTC points represent the masker intensity predicted to produce a 50% decrease in the nonmasked wave V amplitude. The FTC for the 3600 Hz probe (A) was obtained by calculating the mean of 5 individuals' FTCs presented in Figure 4 of Klein and Mills (1981*a*). FTCs for higher-frequency probes are asymmetric and sharper than those for lower-frequency probes. A steep high-frequency slope and a high-intensity low-frequency tail region are evident for higher-frequency probe FTCs. With the exception of the FTC to 250 Hz probes, the FTCs demonstrate a relatively sharp low-intensity tip region near the frequency of the probe. The 250 Hz ABR FTC (A) is broad and tuned off-frequency to about 350 Hz. The large differences in absolute levels of the FTCs may be due to the use of differing stimulus envelopes, different ABR recording procedures, and/or differing response criteria. [Data adapted from Klein, 1983*b*; Klein and Mills, 1981*a*; Folsom and Wynne, 1987.]

of the probe. The 250 Hz ABR FTC is broad and tuned off-frequency to about 350 Hz (Klein, 1983*b*). The large differences in absolute levels of the FTCs obtained between these studies may be due to the use of differing stimulus envelopes, different ABR recording procedures, and/or differing response criteria. A drawback of the FTC technique is the length of time required to obtained reliable data from a single subject.

Frequency tuning curves obtained using the ABR demonstrate features of pathological auditory systems such as the loss of the low-intensity tip region, widening of the tuning curve, and displacement along the frequency axis of the tuning curve relative to probe frequency ("detuning"). Using the ABR FTC technique, Folsom and Wynne (1987) have demonstrated degraded ABR tuning curves for higher frequency probes in infants compared to adults, suggesting these young subjects have poorer frequency resolving capabilities for higher frequencies.

Frequency Discrimination

The brain's response to shifts in the frequency of a tone may possibly provide some insight into its ability to discriminate between different frequencies or to perceive frequency changes. Several different responses have been recorded. Eggermont (1976) reported an electrocochleographic response to the change in the frequency of a tone, and Arlinger and Jerlvall (1981) described an early brainstem response. Several studies have considered the slow cortical (N1-P2) responses to frequency changes (e.g., Arlinger, Jerlvall, Ahren, and Holmgren, 1976; Clynes, 1969).

Recently we have recorded a steady-state middle latency response to the sinusoidal modulation of the frequency of a tone (Picton, Dauman, and Aran, 1987; Picton, Skinner, Champagne, Kellett, and Maiste, 1987). Figure 11.15 illustrates this response. The frequency of a 1000 Hz tone was modulated between 950 and 1050 Hz (10%) at a rate of 39.1 Hz. The response to this modulation was recorded between vertex and mastoid using a sweep duration of 128 ms. The tracings in the top left of the figure show a reliable though somewhat noisy sinusoidal response to the modulation.

The steady state responses can be evaluated at the exact frequency of the stimulation through Fourier

analysis, which gives the amplitude and phase of the response at that particular frequency (Regan, 1982). This is far more efficient than averaging since it considers the response independently of "noise" at other frequencies. The results of Fourier analysis can be plotted on polar coordinates as shown in the middle column of the figure. In the figure, the ellipse represents the confidence limits for the mean response (Picton, Vajsar, Rodriguez, and Campbell, 1987). The probability that the true mean exists outside of the ellipse is 0.05.

The response can be recorded at levels close to the psychoacoustic threshold for detecting the frequency modulation. In the right column of the figure are shown the responses (evaluated using Fourier analysis) obtained as the depth of modulation is decreased to near-threshold levels. In this particular subject the response accurately predicts the threshold for detecting the modulation. In a group of 8 subjects the EP threshold was on average 3% higher than the psychoacoustic threshold.

This response is not yet ready for clinical use. The effects of age and state of arousal need to be assessed. Nevertheless, it or some similar response may provide a means to assess the suprathreshold discrimination of sounds in patients with normal and abnormal hearing, with and without amplification. This objective assessment of suprathreshold hearing may become more important than an accurate evaluation of threshold.

CONCLUSIONS

This final section considers the experiments on frequency specificity with reference to the introductory principles of the chapter. The masking procedures used with brief stimuli are related to frequency analysis in the cochlea by the concept of place specificity. Some recommendations are proposed on the basis of recording efficiency—a parameter that derives from the principles of averaging. Finally, some comments are made about these recommendations in the context of clinical audiometry.

Frequency and Place

The frequency specificity of the EP is intimately related to the place specificity in the cochlea where the response is initiated (Starr and Don, 1988). Frequency

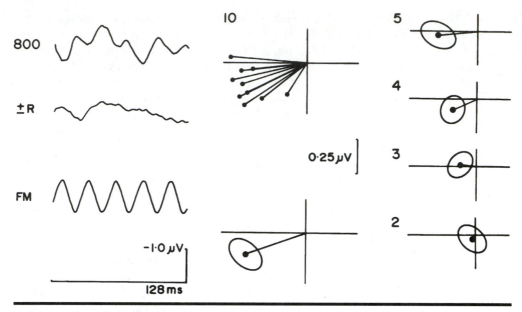

FIGURE 11.15. Evoked potentials to frequency modulation. The left column of this figure shows the potentials evoked by a continuous tone the frequency of which was modulated at a rate of 39.1 Hz. The responses were recorded between the vertex and right mastoid using an EEG bandpass of 5–100 Hz. The upper tracing represents the average of 800 responses. The middle tracing represents the (±) reference. The lower tracing represents the frequency modulation of the tone from 950 Hz to 1050 Hz. This amount of modulation is considered to be 10%. In the middle column are shown the responses measured using Fourier analysis. The upper plot shows the vectors for 10 measurements obtained during the recording of the average waveform shown in the left column. The amplitude of the response equals the length of the vector from the origin and the phase of the response equals the angle made by the vector with the horizontal axis. The phase delay of the signal relative to the frequency modulation signal is plotted rather than the phase at the onset of the recording. The lower plot shows the ellipse that represents the 95% confidence limits for the mean vector. The probability that the mean of the measurements occurs outside of this ellipse is 0.05. In the right column of the figure are shown the results of Fourier analysis when the frequency modulation was 5, 4, 3 and 2%. At 5, 4 and 3% the response is significantly different from zero (i.e., the ellipse does not contain the origin). At 2% the response is not significantly different from zero. This subject's psychoacoustic threshold for detecting the frequency modulation was 3%.

specificity and place specificity can, however, lead to quite different results. The pure-tone audiograms of patients without any functioning cells beyond the first turn of the cochlea do not show an absence of hearing but only a mild to moderate hearing loss in the low frequencies. The traveling wave allows the low frequencies to be received by regions of the cochlea nor-mally specialized for high-frequency hearing. Evoked potential techniques that obtain their frequency specificity by masking are in fact place specific. In these particular patients, place-specific measurements show a severe hearing loss at low frequencies that is not present in the pure-tone audiogram. In trying to prevent the spread of energy in the spectrum of the click or brief tone from evoking a response, the masking has also removed the spread of energy in the traveling wave which allows low-frequency sounds (without any spectral splatter) to be received by high-frequency regions in the cochlea. Responses obtained using brief tones without masking do not have this problem. They will give quite similar results to the pure-tone audiogram provided that the spread of energy in the brief tone is less than the spread of activation that results from the traveling wave. The main difficulty with this approach is that there is a spread of energy in the tones from high to low frequencies as well as from low to high. High-frequency thresholds on the pure-tone audiogram may therefore be significantly underestimated when the high-frequency hearing loss has a steepness of greater than the approximately 30 dB/octave spread of energy in a brief tone. It is interesting to note that the spread of energy in brief tones is within the recommended standards for clinical audiometers that was set on the basis of the traveling wave effects (ANSI, 1973). Clinical audiometers, however, far exceed these standards and allow us to detect very steep high-frequency hearing losses. The information available through place-specific threshold techniques is much more helpful than that available through frequency-specific techniques. The pure-tone audiogram can be reasonably accurately derived from the place-specific thresholds, but not vice versa.

Recommendations

When considering the best approach to obtaining frequency-specific thresholds by means of auditory EPs, one must assess the frequency specificity and recording efficiency of the response, as well as the reliability of the response in the patient group to be evaluated. The middle latency and slow cortical responses are not currently reliable for threshold estimation purposes in infants and children, thus the auditory brainstem responses are the measure of choice. Efficiency reflects how quickly a reasonable signal-to-noise ratio can be obtained so that a response (or its absence) may be recognized. Efficiency is increased by increasing the size of the response and by decreasing the amplitude of the background noise (Picton,

Linden, Hamel, and Maru, 1983). Although the technique of measuring derived brainstem responses with high-pass noise is probably the most frequency-specific of the procedures that we have reviewed, its efficiency is low because of the increased electrical noise in the recording caused by the subtractions. Furthermore, the technique is limited at high intensities by the high levels of acoustic noise required.

Our recommendation, therefore, is to record the ABR to brief tones in notched noise (see Stapells, 1989 for protocols). A brief tone (either linear 2-1-2 cycles or nonlinear windows), a noise level 20 dB SPL below the peak-to-peak equivalent SPL of the tone, and a notch with a width of one octave and a depth of at least 20 dB is preferable. Since the efficiency of the measure is improved by recording responses of larger amplitude, notched noise rather than white noise is recommended. Furthermore, it is best to present the stimuli at a rate of about 40/s. At this rate wave V and the 40 Hz response are superimposed and the overall response is larger. The bandpass of the amplifier should therefore be approximately 20–2000 Hz to allow both wave V and the 40 Hz components to be recorded. Finally, we recommend that the click-evoked ABR be recorded, at least to high-intensity clicks, as well as evaluating frequency-specific thresholds. The click responses provide necessary information about the integrity of the VIIIth nerve and brainstem auditory pathways; their threshold provide a general idea of auditory sensitivity.

Some Final Thoughts

It is presently possible to measure frequency-specific thresholds in patients by means of the ABR. Certain caveats should be recognized. First, although it is reasonably objective, the technique is unlikely to attain the accuracy to which we are accustomed when behaviorally testing older patients. One should expect in most patients to have a range of accuracy of –10 to +20 dB with regard to the pure-tone audiogram. Second, patients with brainstem disorders may not have measurable responses even though they still have sufficient auditory function to mediate hearing. If there is suspicion of a discrepancy between ABR thresholds and auditory behavior, one should consider the use of electrocochleography to assess cochlear function. The recording of oto-acoustic emissions would provide a further evaluation of cochlear function (Kemp, Ryan, and Bray, 1990; Lonsbury-Martin, and Martin, 1990). Third, the presence of ABRs does not necessarily indicate normal perception. The auditory system may be able to generate brainstem EPs but not the more complex patterns that allow the full perception of speech and

music. In audiology, the pure-tone audiogram is helpful in the initial evaluation of the patient, but speech tests and other tests of suprathreshold audition are necessary when evaluating impairment or therapeutic improvement. Having found the audiogram, EP researchers should now consider objective electrophysiologic tests of such suprathreshold features as frequency resolution, loudness, and speech discrimination.

REFERENCES

Alberti, P.W., Hyde, M.L., Riko, K., Corbin, H., and Abramovich, S. (1983). An evaluation of BERA for hearing screening in high-risk neonates. *Laryngoscope, 93*, 1115–1121.

Allen, J.B. (1988). Cochlear signal processing. In A.F. Jahn and J. Santos-Sacchi (eds.), *Physiology of the ear*, pp. 243–270. New York: Raven Press.

American National Standards Institute (1973). Specifications for audiometers. ANSI S3.6-1969 (R1973), 1–22.

Arlinger, S. and Jerlvall, L. (1981). Early auditory electric responses to fast amplitude and frequency tone glides. *Electroencephalography and Clinical Neurophysiology, 51*, 624–631.

Arlinger, S.D., Jerlvall, L.B., Ahren, T., and Holmgren, E.C. (1976). Slow evoked cortical responses to linear frequency ramps of a continuous pure tone. *Acta Physiologica Scandinavia, 98*, 412–424.

Beattie, R.C. and Boyd, R.L. (1985). Early/middle evoked potentials to tone bursts in quiet, white noise and notched noise. *Audiology, 24*, 406–419.

Békésy, G. von (1960). *Experiments in hearing*. New York: McGraw-Hill.

Berlin, C.I. and Shearer, P.D. (1981). Electrophysiological simulation of tinnitus. In D. Evered and G. Lawrenson (eds.), *Tinnitus*. Ciba Foundation Symposium 85. London: Pitman Books.

Brinkmann, R.D. and Scherg, M. (1979). Human auditory on- and off-potentials of the brainstem. *Scandinavian Audiology, 8*, 27–32.

Burkard, R. (1984). Sound pressure level measurement and spectral analysis of brief acoustic transients. *Electroencephalography and Clinical Neurophysiology, 57*, 83–91.

Burkard, R. (1990). The effects of noiseburst risetime and level on the gerbil BAER. *Proceedings of the 13th Midwinter Research Meeting of the Association for Research in Otolaryngology*. St. Petersburg Beach, FL, pp. 155–156.

Burkard, R. and Hecox, K. (1983). The effect of broadband noise on the human brainstem auditory evoked response. II. Frequency specificity. *Journal of the Acoustical Society of America, 74*, 1214–1223.

Clynes, M. (1969). Dynamics of vertex evoked potentials: The R-M brain function. In E. Donchin and D.B. Lindsley (eds.), *Averaged Evoked Potentials*, pp. 363–374. Washington, DC: NASA SP-191.

Coats, A.C. and Martin, J.L. (1977). Human auditory nerve action potentials and brain stem evoked responses. *Archives of Otolaryngology, 103*, 605–622.

Coats, A.C., Martin, J.L., and Kidder, H.R. (1979). Normal short-latency electrophysiological filtered click responses from vertex and external auditory meatus. *Journal of the Acoustical Society of America, 65*, 747–758.

Davis, H. and Hirsh, S.K. (1976). The audiometric utility of the brain stem response to low-frequency sounds. *Audiology, 15*, 181–195.

Davis, H. and Hirsh, S.K. (1979). A slow brain stem response for low frequency audiometry. *Audiology, 18*, 445–461.

Davis, H., Hirsh, S.K., Popelka, G.R., and Formby, C. (1984). Frequency selectivity and thresholds of brief stimuli suitable for electric response audiometry. *Audiology, 23*, 59–74.

Delgutte, B. (1990). Physiological mechanisms of psychophysical masking: Observations from auditory-nerve fibers. *The Journal of the Acoustical Society of America, 87*, 791–809.

Dolan, T. and Klein, A. (1987). Effect of signal temporal shaping on the frequency specificity of the action potential in gerbils. *Audiology, 26*, 20–30.

Don, M. and Eggermont, J.J. (1978). Analysis of the click-evoked brainstem potentials in man using high-pass noise masking. *Journal of the Acoustical Society of America, 63*, 1084–1092.

Don, M., Eggermont, J.J., and Brackmann, D.E. (1979). Reconstruction of the audiogram using brainstem responses and high-pass noise masking. *Annals of Otology, Rhinology and Laryngology, Supplement, 57*, 1–20.

Drift, J.F.C. van der, Brocaar, M.P., and Zanten, G.A. van (1987). The relation between the pure-tone audiogram and the click auditory brainstem response threshold in cochlear hearing loss. *Audiology, 26*, 1–10.

Durrant, J.D. (1983). Fundamentals of sound generation. In E.J. Moore (ed.), *Bases of auditory brain-stem evoked responses*. New York: Grune & Stratton.

Egan, J.P. and Hake, H.W. (1950). On the masking pattern of a simple auditory stimulus. *Journal of the Acoustical Society of America, 22*, 622–630.

Eggermont, J.J. (1976). Electrocochleography. In W.D. Keidel and W.D. Neff (eds.), *Handbook of sensory physiology, Vol. V, Part 3*, pp. 625–705. Berlin: Springer.

Eggermont, J.J. and Don, M. (1980). Analysis of the click-evoked brainstem potentials in humans using high-pass noise masking. II. Effects of click intensity. *Journal of the Acoustical Society of America, 68*, 1671–1675.

Eggermont, J.J. and Don, M. (1982). Analysis of the click-evoked brainstem auditory electric potentials using high-pass noise masking and its clinical application. *Annals of the New York Academy of Sciences, 388*, 471–486.

Eggermont, J.J. and Odenthal, D.W. (1974). Frequency selective masking in electrocochleography. *Revue de Laryngologie, 95 (7–8)*, 489–496.

Elberling, C. (1974). Action potentials along the cochlear partition recorded from the ear canal in man. *Scandinavian Audiology, 3*, 13–19.

Elberling, C. (1976). Simulation of cochlear action potentials recorded from the ear canal in man. In R.J. Ruben, C. Elberling, and G. Salomon (eds.), *Electrocochleography*. Baltimore, MD: University Park Press.

Evans, E.F. and Elberling, C. (1982). Location-specific components of the gross cochlear nerve action potential. An assessment of the validity of the high-pass masking technique by cochlear nerve fiber recording in the cat. *Audiology, 21*, 204–227.

Folsom, R.C. (1984). Frequency specificity of human auditory brainstem responses as revealed by pure-tone masking profiles. *Journal of the Acoustical Society of America, 75*, 929–924.

Folsom, R.C. and Aurich, C.D. (1987). Auditory brainstem responses from human adults and infants: Influences of stimulus onset. *Audiology, 26*, 117–122.

Folsom, R.C. and Wynne, M.K. (1986). Auditory brain stem responses from human adults and infants: Restriction of frequency contribution by notched-noise masking. *Journal of the Acoustical Society of America, 80*, 1057–1064.

Folsom, R.C. and Wynne, M.K. (1987). Auditory brain stem responses from human adults and infants: Wave V tuning curves. *Journal of the Acoustical Society of America, 81*, 412–417.

Foxe, J.J. and Stapells, D.R. (1993). Normal infant and adult auditory brainstem responses to bone-conducted tones. *Audiology, 32*, 95–109.

Gabor, D. (1947). Acoustical quanta and the theory of hearing. *Nature (London), 159*, 591–595.

Galambos, R. and Hecox, K.E. (1978). Clinical applications of the auditory brain stem response. *Otolaryngologic Clinics of North America, 11*, 709–722.

Galambos, R., Makeig, S., and Talmachoff, P.J. (1981). A 40 Hz auditory potential recorded from the human scalp. *Proceedings of the National Academy of Sciences (U.S.A), 78*, 2643–2647.

Geisler, C.D. and Sinex, D.G. (1980). Responses of primary auditory fibers to combined noise and tonal stimuli. *Hearing Research, 3*, 317–334.

Gorga, M.P. and Thornton, A.R. (1989). The choice of stimuli for ABR measurements. *Ear and Hearing, 10*, 217–230.

Gorga, M.P. and Worthington, D.W. (1983). Some issues relevant to the measurement of frequency-specific auditory brainstem responses. *Seminars in Hearing, 4*, 353–362.

Gravendeel, D.W. and Plomp, R. (1960). Perceptive bass deafness. *Acta Otolaryngologica, 51*, 548–560.

Harris, F.J. (1978). On the use of windows for harmonic analysis with the discrete Fourier transform. *Proceedings of the Institute of Electrical and Electronic Engineers, 66*, 51–83.

Harrison, R.V. (1988). *The biology of hearing and deafness*. Springfield, IL: Charles C. Thomas.

Hecox, K. and Deegan, D. (1983). Rise-fall time effects on the brainstem auditory evoked response: Mechanisms. *Journal of the Acoustical Society of America, 73*, 2109–2116.

Hecox, K.E., Squires, N.K., and Galambos, R. (1976). Brainstem auditory evoked responses in man. I. Effect of stimulus rise-fall time and duration. *Journal of the Acoustical Society of America, 60*, 1187–1192.

Huis in't Veld, F., Osterhammel, P., and Terkildsen, K. (1977). The frequency selectivity of the 500 Hz frequency following response. *Scandinavian Audiology, 6*, 35–42.

Hyde, M.L. (1985). Frequency-specific BERA in infants. *Journal of Otolaryngology Suppl., 14*, 19–27.

Hyde, M.L., Matsumoto, N., and Alberti, P.W. (1987). The normative basis for click and frequency-specific BERA in high-risk infants. *Acta Otolaryngologica (Stockholm), 103*, 602–611.

Jacobson, J.T. (1983). Effects of rise time and noise masking on tone pip auditory brainstem responses. *Seminars in Hearing, 4*, 363–372.

Javel, E. (1981). Suppression of auditory nerve responses. I: Temporal analysis, intensity effects, and suppression contours. *Journal of the Acoustical Society of America, 69*, 1735–1745.

Javel, E., McGee, J., Walsh, E.J., Farley, G.R., and Gorga, M.P. (1983). Suppression of auditory nerve responses. II: Suppression threshold and growth, iso-suppression contours. *Journal of the Acoustical Society of America, 74*, 801–813.

Jerger, J. and Mauldin, L. (1978). Prediction of sensorineural hearing level from the brain stem evoked response. *Archives of Otolaryngology, 104*, 456–461.

Kavanagh, K.T., Harker, L.A., and Tyler, R.S. (1984). Auditory brainstem and middle latency responses. II. Threshold responses to a 500 Hz tone pip. *Annals of Otology, Rhinology, and Laryngology, 93 (Supplement 108)*, 8–12.

Kemp, D.T., Ryan, S., and Bray, P. (1990). A guide to the effective use of otoacoustic emissions. *Ear and Hearing, 11*, 93–105.

Kileny, P. (1981). The frequency specificity of tone-pip evoked auditory brainstem responses. *Ear and Hearing, 2*, 270–275.

Kileny, P. (1983). Auditory evoked middle-latency responses: Current issues. *Seminars in Hearing, 4*, 403–413.

Kileny, P. and Magathan, M.G. (1987). Predictive value of ABR in infants and children with moderate to profound hearing impairment. *Ear and Hearing, 8*, 217–221.

Kileny, P. and Shea, S.L. (1986). Middle-latency and 40 Hz auditory evoked responses in normal-hearing subjects: Click and 500 Hz thresholds. *Journal of Speech and Hearing Research, 29*, 20–28.

Klein, A.J. (1983a). Properties of the brain-stem response slow-wave component. I. Latency, amplitude, and threshold sensitivity. *Archives of Otolaryngology, 109*, 6–12.

Klein, A.J. (1983b). Properties of the brain-stem response slow-wave component. II. Frequency specificity. *Archives of Otolaryngology, 109*, 74–78.

Klein, A.J. (1984). Frequency and age-dependent auditory evoked potential thresholds in infants. *Hearing Research, 16*, 291–297.

Klein, A.J. and Mills, J.H. (1981a). Physiological (waves I and V) and psychophysical tuning curves in human subjects. *Journal of the Acoustical Society of America, 69*, 760–768.

Klein, A.J. and Mills, J.H. (1981b). Physiological and psychophysical measures from human with temporary threshold shift. *Journal of the Acoustical Society of America, 70*, 1045–1053.

Kodera, K., Marsh, R.R., Suzuki, M., and Suzuki, J-I. (1983). Portions of tone pips contributing to frequency-selective auditory brain stem responses. *Audiology, 22*, 209–218.

Kodera, K., Yamane, H., Yamada, O., and Suzuki, J-I. (1977). Brain stem response audiometry at speech frequencies. *Audiology, 16*, 469–479.

Kramer, S.J. (1992). Frequency specific auditory brainstem responses to bone-conducted stimuli. *Audiology, 31*, 61–71.

Kramer, S.J. and Teas, D.C. (1982). Forward masking of auditory nerve and brainstem responses using high-pass noise maskers. *Hearing Research, 8*, 317–337.

Kraus, N., Reed, N., Smith, D.I., Stein, L., and Cartee, C. (1985). Auditory middle latency responses in children: Effects of age and diagnostic category. *Electroencephalography and Clinical Neurophysiology, 62*, 343–351.

Kuwada, S., Batra, R., and Maher, V.L. (1986) Scalp potentials of normal and hearing-impaired subjects in response to sinusoidally amplitude-modulated tones. *Hearing Research, 21*, 179–192.

Laukli, E. (1983). High-pass and notch noise masking in suprathreshold brainstem response audiometry. *Scandinavian Audiology, 12*, 109–115.

Laukli, E. (1983). Stimulus waveforms used in brainstem response audiometry. *Scandinavian Audiology, 12*, 83–89.

Laukli, E., Fjermedal, O., and Mair, I.W.S. (1988). Low-frequency auditory brainstem response threshold. *Scandinavian Audiology, 17*, 171–178.

Linden, R.D., Campbell, K.B., Hamel, G., and Picton, T.W. (1985). Human auditory steady state potentials during sleep. *Ear and Hearing, 6*, 167–174.

Lonsbury-Martin, B.L. and Martin, G.K. (1990). The clinical utility of distortion-product emissions. *Ear and Hearing, 11*, 144–154.

McDonald, J.M. and Shimizu, H. (1981). Frequency specificity of the auditory brain stem response. *American Journal of Otolaryngology, 2*, 36–42.

Mendel, M.I. (1977). Electroencephalic tests of hearing. In S.E. Gerber (ed.), *Audiometry in infancy*, pp. 151–181. New York: Grune & Stratton.

Mills, J.H. and Schmiedt, R.A. (1983). Frequency selectivity: Physiological and psychophysical tuning curves and suppression. In J.V. Tobias and E.D. Schubert (eds.), *Hearing research and theory. Volume 2*, pp. 233–336. New York: Academic Press.

Moore, E. J. (1983). Effects of stimulus parameters. In E.J.

Moore (ed.), *Bases of auditory brain-stem evoked responses*. New York: Grune & Stratton.

Moushegian, G., Rupert, A.L., and Stillman, R.D. (1978). Evaluation of frequency-following potentials in man: Masking and clinical studies. *Electroencephalography and Clinical Neurophysiology, 45,* 711–718.

Munnerley, G.M., Greville, K.A., Purdy, S.C., and Keith, W.J. (1991). Frequency-specific auditory brainstem responses; relationship to behavioural thresholds in cochlear-impaired adults. *Audiology, 30,* 25–32.

Musiek, F.E. and Geurkink, N.A. (1981). Auditory brainstem and middle latency evoked response sensitivity near threshold. *Annals of Otology, Rhinology, and Laryngology, 90,* 236–240.

Nousak, J.K. and Stapells, D.R. (1992). Frequency specificity of the ABR to bone-conducted tones in infants and adults. *Ear and Hearing, 13,* 87–95.

Nuttall, A.H. (1981). Some windows with very good sidelobe behavior. *IEEE Transactions in Acoustics, Speech, and Signal Processing, 29,* 84–91.

Palaskas, C.W., Wilson, M.J., and Dobie, R.A. (1989). Electrophysiologic assessment of low-frequency hearing: Sedation effects. *Otolaryngology—Head and Neck Surgery, 101,* 434–441.

Pantev, Ch. and Pantev, M. (1982). Derived brain stem responses by means of pure-tone masking. *Scandinavian Audiology, 11,* 15–22.

Parker, D.J. and Thornton, A.R.D. (1978*a*). Derived cochlear nerve and brainstem evoked responses of the human auditory system. *Scandinavian Audiology, 7,* 1–8.

Parker, D.J. and Thornton, A.R.D. (1978*b*). Frequency specific components of the cochlear nerve and brainstem evoked responses of the human auditory system. *Scandinavian Audiology, 7,* 53–60.

Parker, D.J. and Thornton, A.R.D. (1978*c*) The validity of the derived cochlear nerve and brainstem evoked responses of the human auditory system. *Scandinavian Audiology, 7,* 45–52.

Patterson, R.D., Nimmo-Smith, I., Weber, D.L., and Milroy, R. (1982). The deterioration of hearing with age: Frequency selectivity, the critical ratio, the audiogram, and speech threshold. *Journal of the Acoustical Society of America, 72,* 1788–1803.

Pfeiffer, R.R. (1974). Consideration of the acoustic stimulus. In W.D. Keidel and W.D. Neff (eds.), *Handbook of sensory physiology, Vol. 1: auditory system. anatomy and physiology (Ear).* New York: Springer-Verlag.

Pickles, J.O. (1982). *An introduction to the physiology of hearing.* New York: Academic Press.

Picton, T.W. (1978). The strategy of evoked potential audiometry. In S.E. Gerber and G.T. Mencher (eds.), *Early diagnosis of hearing loss,* pp. 297–307. New York: Grune & Stratton.

Picton, T.W. (1987). Human auditory steady state responses. In C. Barber and T. Blum (eds.), *Evoked potentials III,* pp. 117–124. Boston, MA: Butterworth.

Picton, T.W., Dauman, R., and Aran, J.-M. (1987). Réponses évoquées en "régime permanent" chez l'homme par la modulation sinusoidale de fréquence. *Journal of Otolaryngology, 16,* 140–145.

Picton, T.W., Linden, R.D., Hamel, G., and Maru, J.T. (1983). Aspects of averaging. *Seminars in Hearing, 4,* 327–340.

Picton, T.W., Ouellette, J., Hamel, G., and Smith, A.D. (1979). Brainstem evoked potentials to tonepips in notched noise. *Journal of Otolaryngology, 8,* 289–314.

Picton, T.W., Skinner, C.R., Champagne, S.C., Kellett, A.J.C., and Maiste, A.C. (1987). Potentials evoked by the sinusoidal modulation of the amplitude or frequency of a tone. *Journal of the Acoustical Society of America, 82,* 165–178.

Picton, T.W., Stapells, D.R., and Campbell, K.B. (1981). Auditory evoked potentials from the human cochlea and brainstem. *Journal of Otolaryngology (Supplement 9), 10,* 1–41.

Picton, T.W., Vajsar J., Rodriguez, R., and Campbell, K.B. (1987). Reliability estimates for steady state evoked potentials. *Electroencephalography and Clinical Neurophysiology, 68,* 119–131.

Picton, T.W., Woods, D.L., Baribeau-Bräun, J., and Healey, T.M.G. (1977). Evoked potential audiometry. *Journal of Otolaryngology, 6,* 90–119.

Plourde, G., Stapells, D.R., and Picton, T.W. (1991). The human auditory steady-state potentials. *Acta Otolaryngologica (Stockholm) Supplement, 491,* 153–160.

Pratt, H., Ben-Yitzhak, E., and Attias, J. (1984). Auditory brain stem potentials evoked by clicks in notch-filtered masking noise: Audiological relevance. *Audiology, 23,* 380–387.

Pratt, H. and Bleich, N. (1982). Auditory brain stem potentials evoked by clicks in notch-filtered noise. *Electroencephalography and Clinical Neurophysiology, 53,* 417–426.

Purdy, S. and Abbas, P.J. (1989). Auditory brainstem response audiometry using linearly and Blackman-gated tonebursts. *ASHA, 31,* 115–116.

Purdy, S.C., Houghton, J.M., Keith, W.J., and Greville, K.A. (1989). Frequency-specific auditory brainstem responses. Effective masking levels and relationship to behavioural thresholds in normal hearing adults. *Audiology, 28*, 82–91.

Regan, D. (1982). Comparison of transient and steady-state methods. *Annals of the New York Academy of Sciences, 388*, 45–71.

Rodriguez R., Picton, T.W., Linden D., Hamel, G., and Laframboise, G. (1986). Human auditory steady state responses: Effects of intensity and frequency. *Ear and Hearing, 7*, 300–313.

Sachs, M.B. and Kiang, N.Y.S. (1968). Two-tone inhibition in auditory nerve fibers. *Journal of the Acoustical Society of America, 43*, 1120–1128.

Salt, A.N. and Vora, A.R. (1990). Cochlear threshold assessment using tone-derived action potentials. *Audiology, 29*, 135–145.

Schuknecht, H.F. (1960). Neuroanatomical correlates of auditory sensitivity and pitch discrimination in the cat. In G.L. Rasmussen and W.E. Windle (eds.), *Neural mechanisms of the auditory and vestibular systems*. Springfield, IL: Thomas.

Smith, R.L. (1979). Adaptation, saturation, and physiological masking in single auditory-nerve fibers. *Journal of the Acoustical Society of America, 65*, 166–178.

Stapells, D.R. (1984). *Studies in evoked potential audiometry*. Doctoral dissertation, University of Ottawa, Ontario, Canada.

Stapells, D.R. (1989). Auditory brainstem response assessment of infants and children. *Seminars in Hearing, 10*, 229–251.

Stapells, D.R., Galambos, R., Costello, J.A., and Makeig, S. (1988). Inconsistency of auditory middle latency and steady-state responses in infants. *Electroencephalography and Clinical Neurophysiology, 71*, 289–295.

Stapells, D.R., Gravel, J.S., and Martin, B. (1993). ABR thresholds to tones in notched noise obtained from infants and young children with sensorineural hearing loss. *Proceedings of the 16th Midwinter Meeting of the Association for Research in Otolaryngology, 16*, 59.

Stapells, D.R., Linden, R.D., Suffield, J.B., Hamel, G., and Picton, T.W. (1984). Human auditory steady state potentials. *Ear and Hearing, 5*, 105–113.

Stapells, D.R., Makeig, S., and Galambos, R. (1987). Auditory steady-state responses: Threshold prediction using phase coherence. *Electroencephalography and Clinical Neurophysiology, 67*, 260–270.

Stapells, D.R. and Picton, T.W. (1981). Technical aspects of brainstem evoked potential audiometry using tones. *Ear and Hearing, 2*, 20–29.

Stapells, D.R., Picton, T.W., Durieux-Smith, A., Edwards,

C.G., and Moran, L.M. (1990). Thresholds for short-latency auditory evoked potentials to tones in notched noise in normal-hearing and hearing-impaired subjects. *Audiology, 29*, 262–274.

Stapells, D.R., Picton, T.W., Pérez-Abalo, M., Read, D., and Smith, A. (1985). Frequency specificity in evoked potential audiometry. In J.T. Jacobson (ed.), *The auditory brainstem response*, pp. 147–177. San Diego, CA: College-Hill Press.

Stapells, D.R., Picton, T.W., and Smith, A.D. (1982). Normal hearing thresholds for clicks. *Journal of the Acoustical Society of America, 72*, 74–79.

Stapells, D.R. and Ruben, R.J. (1989). Auditory brain stem responses to bone-conducted tones in infants. *Annals of Otology, Rhinology and Laryngology, 98*, 941–949.

Starr, A. and Don, M. (1988). Brain potentials evoked by acoustic stimuli. In T.W. Picton (ed.), *Human event-related potentials. EEG Handbook (revised series, volume 3)*, pp. 97–157. Amsterdam: Elsevier.

Stockard, J.E. and Stockard, J.J. (1986). Clinical applications of brainstem auditory evoked potentials in infants. In R.Q. Cracco and I. Bodis-Wollner (eds.), *Evoked potentials*, pp. 455–462. New York: Alan R. Liss.

Stockard, J.E., Stockard, J.J., and Coen, R.W. (1983). Auditory brain stem response variability in infants. *Ear and Hearing, 4*, 11–23.

Suzuki, J-I., Kodera, K., and Yamada, O. (1984). Brainstem response audiometry in newborns and hearing-impaired infants. In A. Starr, C. Rosenberg, M. Don, and H. Davis (eds.), *Sensory evoked potentials. 1. An international conference on standards for auditory brainstem response (ABR) testing*, pp. 85–93. Milan, Italy: CRS Amplifon.

Suzuki, T., Hirai, Y., and Horiuchi, K. (1977). Auditory brainstem responses to pure tone stimuli. *Scandinavian Audiology, 6*, 51–56.

Suzuki, T. and Horiuchi, K. (1977). Effect of high-pass filter on auditory brainstem responses to tone pips. *Scandinavian Audiology, 6*, 123–126.

Suzuki, T. and Horiuchi, K. (1981). Rise time of pure-tone stimuli in brain stem response audiometry. *Audiology, 20*, 101–112.

Suzuki, T., Kobayashi, K., and Takagi, N. (1986). Effects of stimulus repetition rate on slow and fast components of auditory brain-stem responses. *Electroencephalography and Clinical Neurophysiology, 65*, 150–156.

Takagi, N., Suzuki, T., and Kobayashi, K. (1985). Effect of tone-burst frequency on fast and slow components of auditory brain-stem response. *Scandinavian Audiology, 14*, 75–79.

Teas, D.C., Eldridge, D.H., and Davis, H. (1962). Cochlear responses to acoustic transients: An interpretation of whole-nerve action potentials. *Journal of the Acoustical Society of America, 34*, 1438–1459.

Terkildsen, K., Osterhammel, P., and Huis in't Veld, F. (1973). Electrocochleography with a far field technique. *Scandinavian Audiology, 2*, 141–148.

Terkildsen, K., Osterhammel, P., and Huis in't Veld, F. (1975). Far-field electrocochleography. Frequency specificity of the response. *Scandinavian Audiology, 4*, 167–172.

Thümmler, I. and Tietze, G. (1984). Derived acoustically evoked brainstem responses by means of narrow-band and notched-noise masking in normal-hearing subjects. *Scandinavian Audiology, 13*, 129–137.

Thümmler, I., Tietze, G., and Matkei, P. (1981). Brain-stem responses when masking with wide-band and high-pass filtered noise. *Scandinavian Audiology, 10*, 255–259.

Trees, D.E. and Turner, C.W. (1986). Spread of masking in normal subjects and in subjects with high-frequency hearing loss. *Audiology, 25*, 70–83.

Vanderbilt University Hereditary Deafness Study Group. (1968). Dominantly inherited low-frequency hearing loss. *Archives of Otolaryngology, 88*, 242–250.

Yamada, O., Ashikawa, H., Kodera, K., and Yamane, H. (1983). Frequency-selective auditory brain-stem response in newborns and infants. *Archives of Otolaryngology, 109*, 79–82.

Yamada, O., Kodera, K., and Yagi, T. (1979). Cochlear processes affecting wave V latency of the auditory evoked brain stem response. *Scandinavian Audiology, 8*, 67–70.

Yamada, O., Yagi, T., Yamane, H., and Suzuki, J.-I. (1975). Clinical evaluation of the auditory evoked brain stem response. *Auris-Nasus-Larynx, 2*, 97–105.

Zanten, G.A. van and Brocaar, M.P. (1984). Frequency specific auditory brainstem responses to clicks masked by notch noise. *Audiology, 23*, 253–264.

PART THREE

PEDIATRIC ASSESSMENT

CHAPTER 12

NEURODEVELOPMENT AND AUDITORY FUNCTION IN PRETERM INFANTS

ALAN SALAMY
JOS EGGERMONT
LYNNETTE ELDREDGE

INTRODUCTION

Study of the preterm infant offers an intriguing opportunity to observe, although indirectly, ongoing maturational processes in the central nervous system. Perhaps at no other time in the course of development do changes occur so rapidly that primitive behaviors can be tied to physioanatomic transformations. Complicating our understanding of such events, however, is a considerable array of medical conditions imposed by premature birth. Differential rates of development across the various yet interdependent subsystems (cardiac, respiratory, immune, motor, etc.) pose certain problems when prematurely expelled from the womb which may threaten the very survival of the neonate. Often compounded by numerous external factors, including disease as well as the necessary interventions themselves, determining the impact on one or any combination of outcome measures presents a most challenging task.

The aim of this chapter is to review briefly some key aspects of neurogenesis in order to increase awareness of phenomena actively taking place in the perinatal period and manifest in the adaptations and organization of the preterm infant. Keeping these maturational changes in mind, an attempt is made to integrate this knowledge with information of the evolving auditory system and hearing function. In this capacity, evoked potentials (EPs) serve as the interface between brain and sensory experience. Despite the proliferation of sophisticated neuroimaging techniques (e.g., computed tomography, magnetic resonance imaging, etc.) during the last decade, the electroencephalogram and associated EPs still provide an inexpensive, noninvasive means of appraising the functional integrity of the brain in the newborn and young infant. The resolution of EPs remains orders of magnitude greater then other dynamic methods of brain assessment, such as positron emission tomography and single photon emission tomography. That is to say, neurophysiologic events occurring in milliseconds can be examined in contrast to many seconds required by other biochemical procedures. Moreover, this can be accomplished without exposing the infant to various intensities of radiation. This very favorable quality permits the frequent and repeated use of EP recordings in patient populations and is well suited for longitudinal research often required for accurate evaluation of the preterm and "high risk" infant.

NEUROBIOLOGY OF CNS DEVELOPMENT

A rudimentary nervous system is apparent early in human embryogenesis. Neurulation, the process whereby the nervous system is formed, is evident by the third week of gestation. Cell proliferation proceeds at a phenomenal rate averaging up to 250,000 new neurons per minute until an asymptote is reached during the second trimester. Mitosis for nerve cells rapidly declines thereafter. At birth virtually all the neurons of the mature central nervous system (CNS) are present and the brain approximates 25 percent (350 grams) of the adult volume. Growth and development of the neuropil and supportive infrastructure, particularly in the neocortex, however, extends well into postnatal life with most of the mass added by the fourth year (Kostovic and Rakic, 1980; Cowan, 1979; Blinkoff and Glazer, 1968).

By the onset of the second month post-conception, neuronal migration from periventricular proliferate zones is well underway. The destination of these cells ultimately gives rise to the various divisions of the CNS (Nowakowski and Rakic, 1981). Active movement of cells into the brainstem is complete by the second month of gestation, whereas migration into the cerebral cortex and other structures continues for several months after birth in the term infant (Chi, Dooling, and Gilles, 1977; Friede, 1975; Sarnat, 1984). The final location of nerve cells determines the type and extent of connections that will eventually be achieved. Specialization and diversification of neural function is also established at the target sites. This sequence of events adheres to a strict timetable largely governed by gestational age. Intrinsic (faulty genetic coding) or extrinsic (environmental toxins, fetal infection, etc.) disruption of this pattern has been linked to malformations of the cerebral cortex. Learning and behavioral disorders, including dyslexia and schizophrenia as well as craniofacial anomalies, seizures, mental retardation, hydrocephalus and ethanol exposure, have also been associated with disturbances in cell position (concentrations of heterotopic neurons) (Koveman and Scheibel, 1983; Galaburda, Sherman, and Geshwind, 1983).

Once in the appropriate place, the nerve cell begins the intricate process of differentiation. Axonal outgrowth commences almost immediately. Following some delay, dendrites project from the opposite pole of the neuron branching from terminal segments (Nowakowski, 1987; Berry, 1974). The appearance of dendritic spines and the formation of synaptic contacts takes place relatively late in gestation. The perinatal period from the 28th week extending into infancy and early childhood exhibits intense synaptogenesis and elaboration of pre- and post-synaptic circuits (Jacobson, 1978; Purves and Lichtman, 1985). The number of synapses constantly changes throughout the life span. Figure 12.1 illustrates the course of synaptogenesis in the human visual cortex. Following an abrupt increase during the third trimester, there is a plateau from birth to two months of age when a sharp

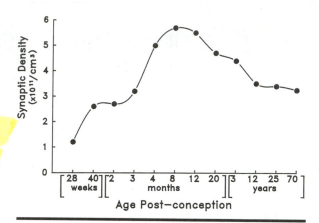

Synaptic Elaboration

FIGURE 12.1.   Changes in synaptic density across the life span in the human visual cortex, typical of other regions of the nervous system (curved spline interlopation). Adapted from P.R. Huttenlocher, C. deCourten, L.J. Garey, and H. Van der Loos, *Neuroscience Letters, 33,* 247–252, 1982.

ascent peaking between eight and eleven months is observed gradually waning into senescence. The complexity of dendritic networks parallels synaptic expansion in early postnatal life as shown in Figure 12.2.

The temporal succession for the emergence and ontogeny of specific cell types (pyramidal, basket, stellate, other interneurons), their neuronal processes, and the interrelationships among the various elements, is rigidly predetermined for each CNS structure. In the fetal human cortex, for example, axodendritic synapses evince by the onset of the second trimester, progress from superficial to deep layers and are typically excitatory in nature. Axosomatic synapses as well as axodendritic spine synapses occur primarily during the third trimester and early postnatal period and are generally inhibitory (Jacobson, 1978; Purves and Lichtman, 1985; Purpura, 1975). Deviations in the number, distribution, or geometry of dendritic spines, ultimately representing synaptic contacts, or local atrophy of the axonal plexus has been observed in developmental disorders such as Down's Syndrome and mental retardation of unknown etiology (Purpura, 1971).

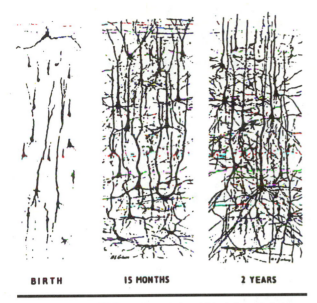

BIRTH   **15 MONTHS**   **2 YEARS**

FIGURE 12.2. Elaboration of dendritic feltwork from birth to two years postnatal age in the human cerebral cortex. From J. Dobbing, In D.F. Roberts and A.M. Thompson, *The biology of human fetal growth, Vol XV, 145*, 1976.

It must be kept in mind that different aspects of neurogenesis take place somewhat independently, yet simultaneously and interactively. The nervous system is constantly undergoing reorganization. Degenerative and regressive events involving cell death, retraction of axonal processes and elimination of synapses occur concurrently throughout development (Berry, 1974). Myelination also respects a definite chronological order. Starting early in the second trimester, after cell multiplication and migration have ended, the deposition of a lipid-protein material, arranged in concentric layers around nerve axons, persists well into adulthood (Purpura, 1975; Yakovlev and Lecours, 1967; Longworthy, 1933). Myelination essentially abides by an ontogenetic and phylogenetic succession according to the origin and type of neuron. Figure 12.3 depicts the timetable for myelination of selected nervous structures. The onset and termination of myelination in the auditory pathway including the acoustic nerve, trapezoid body, lateral lemniscus and brachium of the infe-

rior colliculi is most active between 22–24 weeks gestation (Yakovlev and Lecours, 1967). The roots of the eighth nerve, both divisions, are among the earliest of the sensory tracts to show myelin lamellae ordinarily completing their cycle by the end of the fifth fetal month. The cortical auditory system, however, does not conclude its cycle until beyond the first year postpartum. Using birthweight as the criterion for prematurity, Rourke and Riggs (1969) found the secondary acoustic pathway to be poorly sheathed in infants below 1500 grams.

Unlike the auditory system, the visual pathway from the retina to the calcarine fissure myelinates very rapidly in a relatively short spurt soon after birth. The corpus callosum, on the other hand, does not even commence ensheathment until about the fourth month, while the intracortical neuropil of the frontal, parietal, and temporal association areas of the forebrain do not become fully myelinated until the third or forth decade of adult life. The course of myelination for the various fibers correlates well with the functional capacity of each structure or region in the overall organization of the brain and neurobehavioral development.

Damage to the nerve cell perikaryon produces a characteristic degradation in myelin composition. Diverse insults such as anoxia, toxins, narcotics, nutritional deficiencies, or ionizing radiation can also induce demyelination. Conductile failure or diminished propagation velocity interferes with polysynaptic transmission precluding repetitive firing (synaptic block). Myelin loss may therefore result in severe neurologic symptoms as seen in a variety of degenerative diseases (e.g., multiple sclerosis, leukodystrophies, etc.) (Reinis and Goldman, 1980).

BIOELECTRIC BRAIN DEVELOPMENT

Although a primary physiologic province of myelin is to accelerate neural conduction, impulse traffic nevertheless takes place in pre- and unmyelinated fibers. Indeed, the development of electrical potential and excitability of nerve cell membranes precedes synaptic formation and axonal transmission. Brain electrical activity has been recorded *in utero* by the third fetal month. Intermittent but spontaneous subcortical

REGIONAL MYELINATION
FOR SELECTED CNS STRUCTURES

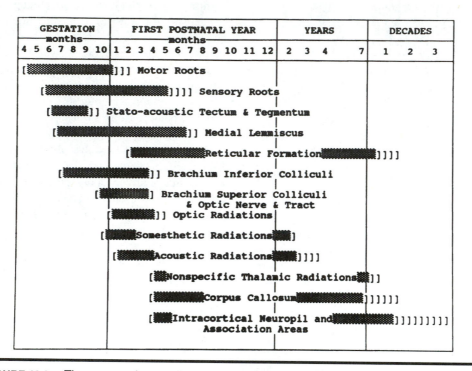

FIGURE 12.3. The progressive myelination of selected central nervous system structures in man as based on the intensity of staining. Horizontal bar (shaded) indicates onset and course of myelination and vertical brackets indicate the age range to maturity. Adapted from P.I. Yakovlev and A-R. Lecours, In A. Minkowski (ed.), *Regional development of the brain in early life*, 1967. Oxford: Blackwell Scientific Publications, Ltd.

rhythms were detected as early as the seventeenth day of gestation in the human embryo (Williams, Karacan, and Hursch, 1974).

Of course, interneuronal communication cannot occur prior to the biosynthesis of neurotransmitter substances. Over 26 "neurohumors", mostly composed of amino acids, have been identified as neurotransmitters in the CNS and many others are thought to participate in the transfer of impulses between neurons. Yet, in man, little is known about the creation of these substrates during maturation. In the rat, norepinephrine, dopamine, and serotonin are present before or soon after the genesis of the neurons for which they will serve as chemical

mediators, e.g., the locus coeruleus and raphaé nuclei. Later developing cell populations such as the nucleus of the lateral lemniscus, the dorsal cochlea nuclei, and Golgi type II neurons do not exhibit evidence of enkephalin and γ-aminobutyric acid respectively for several days after the cessation of cell proliferation (Lauder and Krebs, 1968). Interruption in the production of transmitters has been implicated in pathologic conditions resulting from asphyxia. Psychotrophic drugs (methylamphetamine, chlorpromazine), opiates (methadone), and stress during critical periods in development have been tied to regional changes (increases, decreases) in serotonin, diminished synaptosomal uptake of monoamines, and altered catecholamine synthesis in laboratory animals (Lauder and Krebs, 1968). Behavioral and teratologic consequences may readily be inferred from modifications in neurotransmitters.

Since neurologic maturation appears to proceed at about the same pace whether in an intrauterine or extrauterine environment (some exceptions noted), changes in the electroencephalogram (EEG) are commonly accepted as representing the cumulative effects of brain development. The premature infant may therefore serve as a convenient model of CNS electrogenesis. The scalp-recorded EEG largely reflects post-synaptic potentials generated along the vertically oriented apical dendrites of neocortical pyramidal neurons. As such, the sequential modification of electrical patterns is thought to mirror the establishment of new synapses and intracortical circuits (Dreyfus-Brisac, 1979; Parmelee, Wenner, Akiyama, and Flescher, 1967; Parmelee and Stern, 1972; Ellingson, 1964).

Prior to 26 weeks, conceptional age, the EEG is described as a single undifferentiated pattern characterized by polymorphic irregular activity. After 28 weeks, some periodicity and sleep organization can be discerned. From 29–31 weeks, bursts of theta predominate the EEG wave-train. In this phase, rapid eye movement (REM) sleep becomes firmly established. Between 32–36 weeks, distinct sleep stages are still often difficult to distinguish but discontinuous slow waves in the absence of REMs gradually increase. Periods of relative silence with clusters of slow waves define the "tracé" alternant. This is the prevailing pattern in the full term neonate at birth and portends the onset of quiet or nonREM sleep (NREM). The ability to sustain NREM indicates the emergence of inhibitory function attributable to cortical influences on brainstem control centers. Indirectly, this intimates the activation of axosomatic and spine synapses. Above 36 weeks three unequivocal EEG patterns associated with unique states of consciousness, active sleep (REM), quiet sleep (NREM), and waking, can easily be identified. The relative proportions of each state change with advancing age. Other noteworthy developmental transitions include the disappearance of the tracé alternant between 40–44 weeks, well-defined central sleep spindles are observed by six weeks, a precursor to the onset of occipital alpha (3–4 Hz) is seen by three

months of age and initiation of the sleep cycle by NREM for the first time (Williams et al., 1974; Parmelee, Stern, and Harris, 1972; Dehkharghani, 1984; Berg and Berg, 1979). Despite wide individual variations in the timing and waveform morphology of the developing EEG, marked deviations from these milestones have profound implications for normal CNS processing and the biochemical valence in the brain (Adrien, 1976; Jouvet, 1967). The sleep-waking cycle constitutes the principal behavioral repertoire of the newborn, which rarely goes undisturbed in infants receiving intensive care. Continuous exposure to light, auditory stimulation, and multiple caretaking procedures are unavoidable in the nursery setting (Hack, 1983). Abnormalities in the EEG (e.g., seizures, asymmetries, maturational lag) are important indices of neurologic dysfunction and state organization in early life (Parmelee and Stern, 1972; Berg and Berg, 1979).

SENSORY EVOKED POTENTIALS

While the tonic potential flux of the ongoing EEG may reflect both global and focal brain development or pathology, it provides little information regarding specific sensory processes. Although Hans Berger in 1929 was credited with being the first to identify and categorize certain spontaneous cerebral potentials (e.g., alpha, theta, delta, beta, etc.), historically, reports of "feeble electrical currents" emanating from the brain had actually been published by Richard Caton as early as 1875. According to the description of Caton's data, he was, in fact, monitoring sensory evoked potentials. Evoked potentials (EPs), evoked responses, or event-related potentials, terms often used interchangeably, are distinguishable from the more or less random oscillations detected by Berger and his contemporaries in that they are temporally related to the onset of a given stimulus. An EP may therefore be regarded as that observable change in electrical potential in any region of the central nervous system following sudden peripheral or central stimulation (Chang, 1959). Peripheral stimulation usually means an external pulse delivered to a sensory end organ, such as a click or brief tone, a flash of light or current applied transcutaneously to a large nerve. Central stimulation refers to direct electrical or chemical activation of spinal or brain tissue. The correlation between a given sensory signal and the ensuing electrical response of the brain was firmly established in the mid and late 1930's (Adrian, 1936; Davis, Davis, Loomis, Harvey, and Hobart, 1939). Today these potential fluctuations can be recorded either intra- or extracellulary from single neurons or small groups of cells, from nuclei and nerve tracts deep in the brain, epicortically and, of course, from the surface of the scalp. As such the EP technique has greatly assisted the neurophysiologist in tracing sensory impulses through specific afferent systems to their destinations in the cortex. Even transcranial EPs picked up through the intact skull show a topological distribution in accordance with the sensory pathways being activated (Gastaut, Regis, Lyagoubi, Mano, and Simon, 1968). However, because the sensory EP as recorded from the scalp is relatively small (<1–15 µV) with respect to the background EEG, which may range from 20–200 µV, the accurate mapping of the minute current fields set up by deliberate stimulation of a sensory transducer had to await the development of special purpose computers, or "averagers". With these devices, repetitive samples of EEG are automatically summated. Electrical activity unrelated to the onset of a stimulus tends to cancel with successive samples while the response initiated by the stimulus, the EP, reinforces itself. In this way the signal-to-noise ratio can be sufficiently resolved to permit quantification of the EP. With the aid of advanced computers, EP methodology has emerged from its beginnings as a means of assessing sensory transmission to a potent investigative technique for the understanding of brain function, integrity and maturation.

The average EP presents itself as a complex series of polarity reversals which may endure for over 500 milliseconds (ms). Each deflection varies somewhat depending on the modality activated and on the locus from which it was recorded. Although there is some specificity of response following somatosensory, visual, or auditory stimulation, a certain degree of similarity across modalities is also apparent. Each segment of the EP waveform may contain one or more physiologically related or independent components of varying amplitude and duration. Over the years numerous classification systems have been advanced to describe

the various undulations of the EP (Williams, Morlock, Morlock, and Tobin, 1964; Ciganek, 1961; Allison, 1962). These schemes usually involve dividing the wavefront into predefined segments and labeling the individual peaks/waves according to latency and/or polarity (e.g., N1, negativity at 100 ms, P3 or P300, positivity at 300 ms, etc.). The acoustic EP is typically partitioned into early (1–10 ms), middle (10–50 ms) and late (50–500 ms), components. Each subdivision represents the passage of impulses (volume conducted and propagated) from the cochlea and eighth nerve through brainstem and diencephalic structures to their cortical terminals (see Figure 12.4). The different components not only reflect excitation at discrete stations along the auditory pathway but mediate distinct psychophysiological operations as well. In this regard, the EP has been further segregated according to its pre-

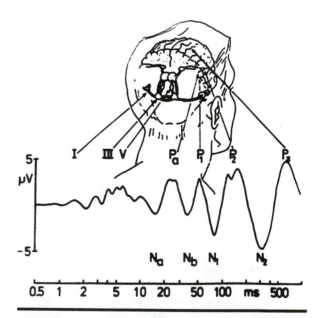

FIGURE 12.4. Auditory evoked potentials including the ABR (waves I, III, V) occurring in the first 10 ms, the middle latency components (Na, Pa, Nb), from 15–50 ms, and the slow vertex potentials (P1-P3) from 60–500 mec., displayed in a logarithmically compressed fashion. The putative generator source for the positive waves is indicated above.

sumed functional significance (Rockstroh, Elbert, Birbaumer, and Lutzenberger, 1982). Table 12.1 differentiates the exogenous components, those controlled by external events, from the endogenous components, those regulated by internal aspects of brain activity. Note that roughly the first 60 ms largely reflect input from the thalamic radiations and carry sensory-specific information. These components are generally more localized over primary receiving areas. Because the auditory cortex (tucked under Heschl's gyrus) is relatively inaccessible to surface electrodes, the EP shows a more prominent central and frontal rather then temporal distribution (Goff, Allison, and Vaughn, 1978). The longer latency components, on the other hand, are more diffusely represented over the entire scalp and are thought to originate from nonspecific reticular and thalamic afferents ultimately reaching all parts of the cerebral mantle. These components are considered to be polysensory in that they can be elicited by stimulation in any modality. Some of the later occurring waves (>200 ms) are thought to convey perceptual, cognitive or motor information arising from intracortical origin.

Although the precise source of the individual waves

as well as the interrelationships among them has yet to be worked out, there is little doubt as to the contribution of the ascending relay nuclei from the first central synapse, olivary complex, nuclei of the lateral lemniscus, inferior colliculi, medial geniculate bodies, and sensory receiving cortex to the elaboration of the early and middle auditory components [see Chapter 2 for greater detail]. In contrast, identification of the probable generators of the later components has been much more elusive (Goff et al., 1978; Picton, Hillyard, Krausz, and Galambos, 1974). In general, the longer the latency, the greater the likelihood of interaction with distant structures involving short and long association bundles, projection fibers, and commissural tracts.

Several studies of preterm infants describe a long-latency surface negative wave as the most salient feature of evoked activity seen at or before 25 weeks post-conception (Ellingson, 1970, Ohlrich and Barnet, 1972; Barnet, Ohlrich, Weiss, and Shanks, 1975; Weitzman and Graziani, 1968; Hrbek, Karlberg, and Olsson, 1973). While the underlying morphophysiological mechanisms remain speculative, this pattern is consistent with a model whereby presynaptic

TABLE 12.1.   Classification of evoked potentials.

Exogenous	Endogenous
Short Latency, <60–100* ms	Long Latency, >60–100* ms to several seconds
Modality specific with respect to scalp distribution	Modality nonspecific, diffuse scalp distribution
Represent activity in classical sensory pathways	Represent nonspecific sensory pathways
Response parameters depend upon physical properties of the stimulus, e.g., intensity/duration	Independent of physical stimuli, may be evoked by low level or absent stimuli
Relatively independent of psycho-physiological state	Highly influenced by subject state, psychological set, etc.
Good intersubject reliability	Very idiosyncratic
Reflect integrity and organization of sensory receptors, pathways and brain structures involved	Associated with perceptual, cognitive or motor processes

*Somewhat modality dependent

excitatory drive produces dendritic depolarization of the large pyramidal cells of the neocortex (Creutzfeldt, Watanabe, and Lux, 1966). With advancing age, the EP waveform is rapidly transformed into multiple biphasic components in keeping with the emergence of dendritic and somatic excitatory/inhibitory connections. Prior to 30 weeks post-conception, the ultrastructure of the apical (excitatory) dendrites is undergoing continuous augmentation and is developmentally more advanced than its basilar (inhibitory) dendritic counterpart. The apical shafts, however, are still devoid of spines. As these neuronal elements expand the EP becomes correspondingly complex (Purpura, 1975; Robinowicz, 1964). Because the late components are easily influenced by a wide range of organismic and extrinsic variables, clinical utility regarding the integrity and development of the auditory system in the neonate and young infant has focused on the early components.

MATURATION OF THE ABR AND THE ONSET OF AUDITORY FUNCTION

Initially described over two decades ago as a series of minute, positive deflections or "far-field potentials" occurring within 8 ms of an abrupt acoustic stimulus, these submicrovolt signals comprise the early components of the acoustic EP which now define the auditory brainstem response or ABR (Jewett, 1969; Jewett and Williston, 1971). While the gross anatomical structures responsible for the generation of the ABR are fairly well understood, the molecular substrate and complex interactions that produce the successive waves remain obscure. There is little question, however, that the first six waves represent, to some extent, the compound action potential along the proximal and distal segments of the eighth nerve (waves I and II), and the sequential and concurrent activation of the cochlear nuclei, superior olives, nuclei of the lateral lemniscus, and the inferior colliculi. The later waves, III–VI, originating from multiple brainstem generators, involve fast and slow conducting fibers of varying diameter (Møller and Janetta, 1981; Hashimoto, Ishiyama, and Yoshimoto, 1981).

Thus the ABR can provide a wealth of information concerning the functional capacity and development of the caudal auditory pathway. The ABR is currently accepted as the method of choice for assessing cochlear sensitivity in the neonate, young infant and otherwise "hard to test" populations.

Over the years, maturational trends for the various parameters of the ABR have been amply documented in the literature (Hecox and Galambos, 1974; Salamy and McKean, 1976; Starr, Amlie, Martin, and Sanders, 1977). Much emphasis has been placed on response latency and interwave intervals because of their dependency on age and stimulus intensity and their high within and between subject reliability. Typically the latency of wave I is taken as an index of peripheral conduction and the wave V–I interwave interval as an estimate of central (brainstem) conduction time. Figure 12.5 illustrates the changes in ABR morphology including the decrease in peak latency as a function of age from 32 weeks to 3 years post-conception. The most striking effects are seen prior to term age. Not only shifts in latency but improved separation and definition of the individual waves, increments in component magnitude, and overall response stability are readily observed. Figure 12.6 depicts these rapid transformations between 31 and 37 weeks in a single preterm infant. Maturation of axonal elements, principally myelogenesis and fiber diameter enlargement, are commonly offered to explain the age-related latency decrements. As alluded to earlier, myelination of the subcortical auditory pathway is relatively advanced by the 25th gestational week. Alteration of this process through experimental manipulation in laboratory animals or certain disease states in humans is known to prolong latencies and interwave differences. Amochaev, Johnson, Salamy, and Shah, (1979), showed that reduction of myelin density through trietheline-induced intoxication in the rat led to a significant slowing of all ABR components. Further, the "quaking" mouse, an autosomal recessive neurologic mutant characterized by a specific disturbance in myelin metabolism, exhibits vastly delayed ABRs (Shah and Salamy, 1980). Figure 12.7 illustrates this latency lag in a quaking mouse relative to a normal litter-mate control. Comparisons between the concentration of cerebroside, which is exclusively a myelin lipid, in the inferior colliculi and the V–II latency difference in the rat reveals a negative,

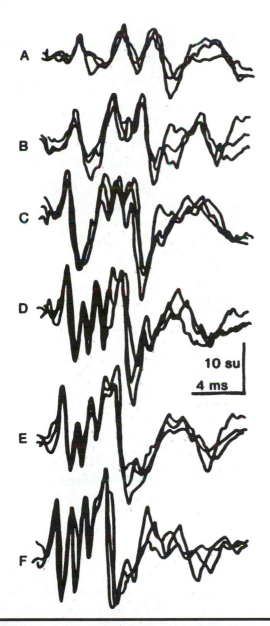

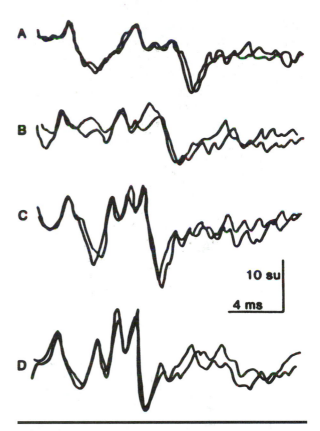

FIGURE 12.6. Longitudinal changes in the ABR for a single preterm infant at 31 (A), 33 (B), 35 (C) and 37 (D) weeks postconception. From A. Salamy, Maturation of the auditory brainstem response from birth through childhood. *Journal of Clinical Neurophysiology, 1, 3*, 1984.

FIGURE 12.5. Maturational changes in the ABR as a function of post-conceptional age. 32 weeks (A), 35 weeks (B), 40 weeks (C), 3 months (D), 1 year (E) and 3 years (F). Each trace represents the averaged response from a different individual in each age group. From A. Salamy, Maturation of the auditory brainstem response from birth through childhood. *Journal of Clinical Neurophysiology, 1, 3*, 1984.

curvilinear relationship with age from 15–50 days as shown in Figure 12.8 (Shah, Bhargava, Johnson, and McKean, 1978). In man, demyelination due to multiple sclerosis is known to adversely affect all ABR latencies and interwave intervals (Robinson and Rudge, 1977; Stockard and Rossiter, 1977; Starr and Achor, 1975).

While the implication of normal myelogenesis in latency reduction is clear, the contribution of other maturational processes active during this time must also be considered. Recall that auditory function begins well before birth in humans. Fetuses of 25–29 weeks show eye blink reflexes to acoustic stimuli de-

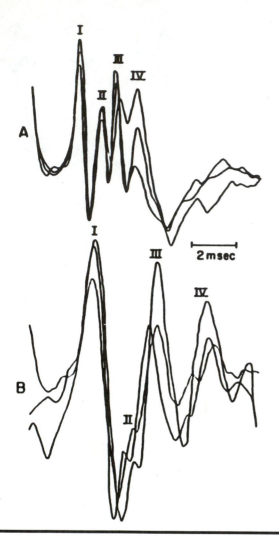

FIGURE 12.7.   Prolonged ABR latencies and interwave intervals in a "quaking" mouse (B) relative to a normal littermate control (A). Reprinted from *Neuroscience, 3*, S.N. Shah, V. Bhargava, and C.W. McKean, Maturational changes in early auditory evoked potentials and myelination of the inferior colliculus in rats, pp. 561–563, Copyright 1978, with kind permission from Pergamon Press Ltd, Headlington Hill Hall, Oxford OX3 0BW, UK.

livered to the abdominal wall of the mother (Birnholz and Benacerraf, 1983). Modification of fetal heart rate to auditory signals starts in the 20th week of gestation becoming more reliable by the 24th week (Bench and

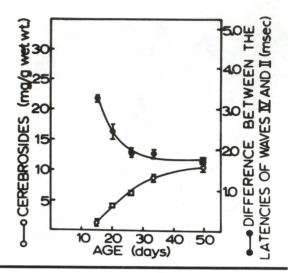

FIGURE 12.8.   Inverse relationship between the concentration of cerebroside (open circles) in the inferior colliculi of the rat and II–IV interwave interval of the ABR (closed circles) over a 50 day period. Reprinted from *Neuroscience, 5*, S.N. Shah and A. Salamy, Auditory evoked farfield potentials in myelin-deficient mutant quaking mice, pp. 2321–2323, Copyright 1980, with kind permission from Pergamon Press Ltd, Headlington Hill Hall, Oxford OX3 0BW, UK.

Metz, 1974). These findings are consistent with the appearance of the ABR and the N1-P2 slow vertex potential in premature infants around 25 weeks (Weitzman and Graziani, 1968; Starr et al., 1977). At this time the cochlea has attained its final size. Before becoming operational, however, differentiation of the hair cells, which begins in the first half of the basal turn, initially progressing toward the base and reaching the apex about two weeks later, must be complete. The inner hair cells and most of their afferent synaptic connections with the auditory nerve take on an adult-like appearance prior to that of cochlear function. The outer hair cells and efferent synapses descending from the brainstem do not become evident until after cochlea activation (Lavinge-Rebillard and Pujol, 1988). Walsh and McGee (1986) maintain that the number of lamina surrounding auditory nerve fibers in the kitten require six months to reach maturity. They found that the decrease in wave I latency and changes in myelination followed independent timetables and concluded that the latter was inconsequential in the development of EP's in the auditory nerve. According to Eggermont (1988), if one postulates an exponential increase in fiber length, presumably correct for the early stages of myelination, a hyperbolic decrease in latency would be expected during this phase. Alternately, a linear escalation in fiber diameter will result in a logarithmic increase in conduction velocity. Thus latency would be inversely proportional to the logarithm of the diameter. In either case, latency change is more in line with the decrement actually observed for wave I.

Eggermont has formulated a simple model of EP development based on the following assumptions:

1. Latency changes for the various components of the EP reflect maturation of structures preceding, that is, inferior to, the putative generator site, for example, wave V is contingent upon cochlear, auditory nerve, and lower brainstem development, etc.

2. Myelination, synaptic density, and synaptic efficacy (available transmitter at pre- and post-synaptic terminals and synchronicity of quanta release) accounts for most of the maturational effects in the auditory system as measured by EPs.

3. Each process results in an exponential decline in component latencies but with a different time course or rate of development.

4. Many maturational events proceed in parallel.

5. The resulting changes in EP latency can be described as a sum of gradually decaying exponentials.

By plotting latency values as deviations from adult norms with respect to conceptional age, Eggermont was able to demonstrate the utility of this approach. In Figure 12.9, data for wave I, wave V, and the I–V interval as compiled from the literature are treated in this way. Since an exponential function becomes a straight line on semi-log coordinates, the deviation from the adult latency is displayed on logarithmic axes. As can be seen in Figure 12.9A, the regression line intersects with the age axis at about 60 weeks. In practical terms, this indicates that the latency difference between infants and adults vanishes for wave I around 45–50 weeks post-conception. The slope of the regression line reflects the rate of maturation or the time constant, in this case about 6 weeks, for this process. A regression line based

on the sum of two or more exponential functions, however, is curvilinear as revealed for wave V and the I–V interval (Figures 12.9B, 12.9C) also ploted in a semi-log fashion. Time constants of 5 and 74 weeks for wave V and 3.3 and 60 weeks for the I–V interval are observed. Note that a third exponential function with still a longer time constant is required for a more complete description of the data above 200 weeks post-conception. Eggermont (1985, 1986, 1988, 1989) has established these to be on the order of 3 years and 3–5 years respectively for wave V and the I–V interval.

Latency decrements in the I–V interval are thought to reflect maturation of brainstem structures free of peripheral influences which would affect waves I and V in a comparable manner. While the rate of maturation for the slower process is identical to that of wave V, the residual fast process has a time constant somewhat shorter than that of wave I. This intimates that the I–V delay may encompass some aspect of cochlea evolution or a fast and slow component of brainstem development.

Thus, interpolation of the maturational period from birth to adulthood with exponential functions reveals time constants of about 6 weeks for the cochlea as expressed in wave I latency, 5 weeks and 1–1.5 years for wave V and the I–V interval reflecting brainstem and perhaps some cochlea maturation (Eggermont, 1988; Eggermont and Salamy, 1988a). Preterm infants show slightly slower growth curves for waves V and I but not for the V–I latency difference, most likely resulting from temporary latency increments produced by middle ear effusions.

Curve fitting procedures have also been applied to the middle latency auditory response and the slow vertex potential. Figure 12.10A depicts the time constants for the P2 (55 weeks) and N2 (44 weeks) cortical components plotted with the I–V interval. The rate of change for these measures roughly approximates that of the ABR (Eggermont, 1988). In contrast, the Na and Pa components of the middle latency response have considerably shorter time constants (8 and 29 weeks respectively), which may be an artifact of the truncated age range of available data but does not obscure sharp maturational differences between the two waves (Eggermont, 1989). From our knowledge of the morphological changes that accompany maturation, it may be concluded that the observed exponentials represent

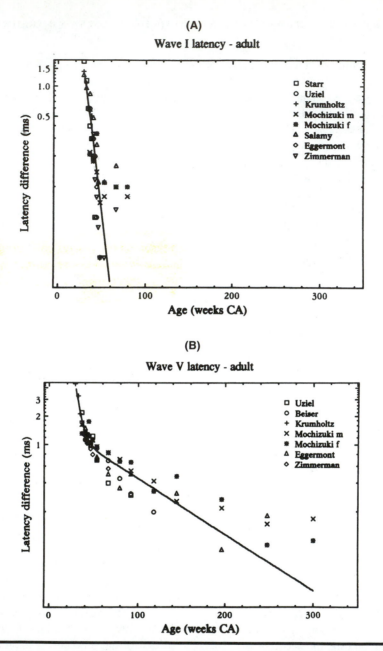

(A)

Wave I latency - adult

(B)

Wave V latency - adult

FIGURE 12.9. Time-constants for maturation of wave I (A), wave V (B), and the I–V interval (C) of the ABR. Exponentials based on differences from adult values as a function of conceptional age plotted on a semi-log scale. Data are mean values derived from various publications indicated by the first author, male (m) and female (f) subjects after Mochizuki. Eggermont data from Eggermont and Salamy (1988*b*). The exponential regression line is drawn in: y=163 exp (−0.16x), time constant 6,22 weeks for wave I (A). For wave V and the I–V interval the data do not fall along a straight line and necessitate two or more exponential functions: y=1468 exp (−0.210x)+1.72 exp (−0.013x), time constants respectively 4.76 and 74.1 weeks for wave V (B), and Y=16705 exp (−0.303x)+1.89 exp (−0.017x), time constants 3.3 and 59.5 weeks for the I–V interval (C).

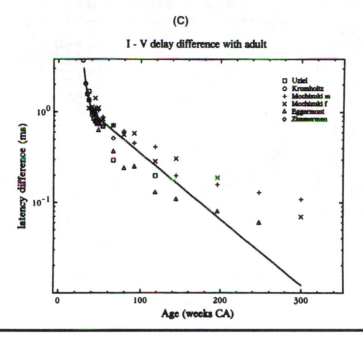

FIGURE 12.9. Continued

two underlying developmental processes: myelination and enhanced synaptic density/efficacy, or any combination thereof characterized by the short and long time constants. This theorem succinctly describes all maturational aspects of the auditory EP from the cochlea to the cerebral cortex (Eggermont, 1988; Eggermont and Salamy, 1988b).

Rate of change alone, however, provides only a partial explanation. The age at which adult latencies are achieved is also an important consideration. This information can be ascertained from the intercept with the time axis of the respective exponential functions at a prespecified value of the latency difference (e.g., 1%). Table 12.2 provides a brief chronology of morphological, physiological, and behavioral events associated with the development of hearing in humans. Note that the point of maturity tends to increase for more central generators.

MEDICAL COMPLICATIONS AND THE ABR

There is little doubt that the ABR provides valuable information regarding hearing loss and aids in the diagnosis of punctate as well as generalized neurologic

lesions in neonates and infants. However, its relationship to more systemic disorders, particularly those common to premature birth, remains uncertain. While some investigators have found ABR abnormalities associated with specific disease states such as asphyxia, hyperbilirubinemia, acidosis and hypoxia, intracranial hemorrhage, apnea, etc., others have not (Perlman, Feinmesser, Shomer, Tamari, Wax, and Pevsner, 1983; Lenhardt, McAstor, and Bryant, 1984; Barden and Peltzman, 1980; Kileny, Connelly, and Robertson, 1980; Goldstein, Krumholtz, Felix, Shannon, and Carr, 1977; Despland and Galambos, 1980; Marshall, Reichart, Kerley, and Davis, 1980; Henderson-Smart, Pettigrew, and Cambell, 1983). In these studies the exact source of the ABR deviations could not always be determined in that such clinical conditions rarely occur in isolation and concurrent medical events were not controlled. Attempts to examine combinations of risk factors has also produced ambiguous results. Cox, Hack, and Metz (1981) found "low risk" and unselected premature infants to be equivalent in terms of the ABR. We (Salamy, Mendelson, Tooley, and Chaplin, 1980a,b), observed striking differences between healthy

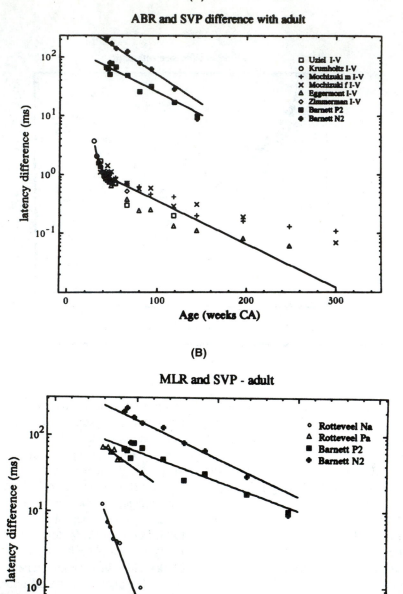

(A)

ABR and SVP difference with adult

- □ Uziel I-V
- ○ Krumholtz I-V
- + Mochizuki m I-V
- × Mochizuki f I-V
- △ Eggermont I-V
- ◇ Zimmerman I-V
- ■ Barnett P2
- ✦ Barnett N2

(B)

MLR and SVP - adult

- ○ Rotteveel Na
- △ Rotteveel Pa
- ■ Barnett P2
- ✦ Barnett N2

FIGURE 12.10. Time-constants for maturation of the I–V interval and the slow vertex potential as described above (A). Similar comparisons for the middle latency and cortical potentials (B). Note that the Na and Pa waves mature at a different rate then the SVP, which is comparable to the Pa component. The regression lines are: y=499 exp (–0.023x) for N2; y=149.5 exp (–0.018x) for P2; y=197 exp (–0.035x) for Pa and y=477 exp (–0.128x) for Na.

TABLE 12.2.   Chronology for auditory development.

3 MONTHS	First afferent nerve endings to inner and outer hair cells can be seen. No sign of myelination.
4 MONTHS	Inner hair cells are fully developed.
5 MONTHS	Outer hair cells developed in basal and middle turn, efferents contact base of outer hair cells at 14 weeks. Myelination of most nerve fibers has begun. Modification of fetal heart rate by external auditory stimuli is possible.
6 MONTHS	The cochlea attains its final size but maturation is not yet complete at 22 weeks as myelination of spiral lamina fibers and efferent outer hair cell synapses are incomplete. The cochlear microphonic and summating potential appear. Auditory brainstem responses can be recorded. Slow vertex potentials evince.
7 MONTHS	The fetus makes movements in reaction to sound. All fetuses show eye blink reflexes. The cochlea is functionally mature.
8 MONTHS	The cochlea is complete and adult like.
9 MONTHS	The cochlear microphonic and summating potential are mature. The middle ear becomes functionally mature.
1 MONTH after birth	The auditory nerve response reaches maturity.
5 YEARS	The auditory brainstem response essentially matches the adult.
10–14 YEARS	The middle latency response and slow vertex potential mature.
15–20 YEARS	The P-300 component is mature.

and "high risk" infants on a number parameters of the ABR which persisted for some time after discharge from the hospital. Our study sample included very low birthweight (<1500g) infants who suffered multiple insults. While it may be taken as axiomatic that preterm birth compounded by perinatal complications resulting in protracted illness may adversely affect the CNS and subsequent outcome including the ABR and hearing capacity, prediction of developmental risk is not quite so simple. Over the years three fundamental approaches have been utilized toward this end:

1. The search for a "preeminent" factor such as birthweight, Apgar score, gestational age, or a single medical occurrence, for instance, anoxia, respiratory distress, etc., in hopes of arriving at a clear-cut relationship with some outcome variable (Drillen, 1961; Lubchenco, Delivoria-Papadopouls, and Searls, 1972; Broman, 1979).

2. General inventories and physical measures, specific behaviors, including habituation, sensory, perceptual processes, etc., or IQ type tests (Lewis, 1976; Field and Sostek, 1983; Lipsitt and Field, 1982; Hunt, 1976).

3. Compilation of long lists of perinatal, intrapartum, and postnatal events thought to be implicated in developmental disorders (Prechtl, 1986; Wigglesworth, 1968; Nesbitt and Aubry, 1969). At present, it must be concluded that prediction, by any means, is weak and unreliable at best (Hunt, 1986; McCall, Hogarty, and Hurlburt, 1972).

A principal tenant of infant assessment is that the appropriate response to various stimuli or test items depends upon the level of maturity of the CNS. In the case of high risk infants, this may be extended to include an intact nervous system as well. Of course the integrity of the CNS can only be inferred from performance measures or diagnostic designations. While the

EEG and cortical EP yield a more direct estimate of CNS function, they are easily modulated by a host of psychophysiological variables, including state of consciousness, and may therefore be difficult to interpret in infant populations. Since the ABR is resistant to such influences, it can furnish a special measure of neurophysiological maturation in early life.

The belief that medical complications in infancy can bias eventual outcome, nevertheless, continues to attract interest, particularly in view of the presumed lingering consequences of neonatal intensive care. Thus more recent inquiries into the causes of poor outcome have sought to discern from among survivors of the tertiary care nursery those infants at risk for aberrant development (Hobel, Hyvarinen, Okada, and Oh, 1973; Littman, 1979; Littman and Parmelee, 1978; Sigman and Parmelee, 1979). Although relatively small but significant correlations are often reported, the amount of variance explained is usually minimal. In these attempts to relate outcome to obstetrical or neonatal events, risk histories are simply tabulated. The number of abnormal or less then optimal responses are then tallied with the idea that sheer plurality is indicative of subsequent handicaps. Typically, all medical conditions are either equally weighted or assigned arbitrary values based upon assumed risk. Our approach to improving prediction was to develop a classification system contingent upon the cumulative effects of medical complications sustained in early life. Our goal was to formulate a comprehensive scale representing a wellness-illness continuum which would enable us to characterize a given individual with respect to his/her NEONATAL STATUS by a single objectively derived score.

NEONATAL STATUS AND LONG TERM OUTCOME

Preterm birth per se does not appear to alter the rate of CNS development. Organ systems yet too immature to function properly, however, are often seriously affected, which in turn may impact on neural integrity. To determine the contribution of medical involvement and maturation effectively, as well as meaningfully appraise the influence of risk factors, all must be taken into account. Existing multi-factor scoring systems tacitly presuppose an additive model as the risk index. These procedures do not actually consider the degree or duration of illness but merely enumerate the incidence of clinical maladies. As such they fail to manage numerous inexorably interrelated events adequately. In order to classify infants with respect to perinatal medical complications, several indicies reflective of the extent of treatment and life support requirements in early life were utilized (Salamy, Davis, Eldredge, Wakeley, and Tooley, 1988). These included the number of days spent under intensive care, total number of X-rays during hospitalization, days of assisted ventilation (mechanical ventilation or continuous positive airway pressure), number of samples taken for blood gas analysis, number of days on antibiotics, and the number of units of blood used for transfusions. Table 12.3 summarizes these variables which represent length of care and medical procedures and are, themselves, highly correlated. Principal components analysis was therefore employed to reduce the redundancy or dimensionality associated with neonatal intensive care and very low birthweight. With this technique, the original set of variables is transformed into new, uncorrelated (orthorgnal) variables referred to as "principal components". Each component represents a combination of the original variables arranged in descending order according to the percentage of variance explained. Thus the first few components to be extracted are the most informative. In our study, a single component that accounted for over 80% of the variance was retained. This hypothetical factor concisely summarized the original set of variables and was entitled neonatal status (NS). Component scores (calculated as a sum of the product of the subject's original measurements and the component loadings converted to standard scores) were generated for NS and assigned to each of 250 very low birthweight infants requiring intensive care in the nursery. Most subjects were enrolled in the Pediatric Follow-up Clinic at the University of California, San Francisco. In this program very low birthweight infants routinely receive a complete medical, physical, and psychometric examination at six-month intervals throughout the first two years of life and annually thereafter. This includes a standard neurologic exam in which the severity of motor distur-

TABLE 12.3. Neonatal status originable variables.

1. Days in intensive care
2. Number of X-rays
3. Days of assisted ventilation
4. Number of blood gases taken
5. Days on antibiotics
6. Number of blood units transfused

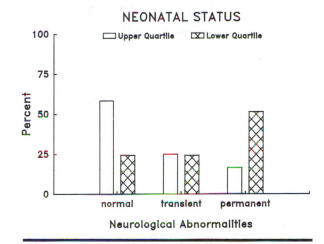

FIGURE 12.11. Frequency of transient and persistent neurological abnormalities in upper or first "Neonatal Status" (NS) quartile (open box) and lower or fourth quartile (crosshatched box). From A. Salamy, S. Davis, L. Eldredge, A. Wakeley and W.H. Tooley, *Early Human Development, 17*, 233–243, 1988.

bances are graded as follows: transient abnormalities of the first year only; mild, persistent disorders of tone or reflexes beyond the first year; moderate impairment of function but ambulatory, and severe dysfunction (non-ambulatory). Standardized tests of cognitive ability are also regularly administered including the Bayley Mental Development Index at 3,9,15 and 21 months corrected age, and the Stanford-Binet Intelligence Scale at 33 and 45 months (2.75 and 3.75 years respectively). All subjects ranged from 24–34 weeks gestation (mean=28, SD=2.11) and had birth weights from 520–1500 grams (mean=1036, SD=226).

By virtue of the individual NS scores, subjects could be characterized in terms of their neonatal course. That is to say, very low birthweight infants relatively free of disease could be assessed against those who experienced complications, graded by severity, in early life. The study population was then divided into NS quartiles for the purpose of making comparisons across the dependent measures by age. In this way a truly high risk subgroup of infants from the ranks of intensive care survivors was identified. In short, those subjects falling into the lower 25% of the NS distribution could be distinguished from all others in several respects. They sustained significantly more neurologic anomalies persisting beyond the first year (Chi square=18.39, p<0.005). Figure 12.11 contrasts the incidence of transient and permanent neurologic abnormalities between the upper (first) and lower (fourth) NS quartiles. There were essentially no statistical differences between the upper three quartiles. The likelihood of suffering neurologic sequelae was substantially increased (Contingency coefficient=0.44, Chi square=31.73, p<0.001) for infants who sustained intracranial hemorrhage (ICH) which occurred with

greater frequency in the lower quartile group (Chi square=36.07, p<0.001). The percentages of subjects in the upper and lower quartiles with ICH (collapsed over grade) are given in Figure 12.12. It should be noted that even in the absence of ICH, enduring neurologic problems were still significantly related to NS (Contingency coefficient=0.34, Chi square=7.64, p<0.05).

Comparisons (ANOVA) across NS groups on intellectual performance also disclosed that only subjects falling into the lowest quartile deviated from all others (p<0.001) at all age levels. Figure 12.13 shows the striking interquartile (upper/lower) differences throughout infancy and early childhood. An average 12 point differential separated these subjects from 3 months to 3.75 years despite the elimination of all those with major neurologic and/or sensory deficits which could limit performance on accepted measures (Bayley, Stanford-Binet) of mental function. The steady decline in efficiency observed from 3 to 21 months, more pronounced for the lower quartile, may reflect greater cognitive demand placed on our very low birthweight sample with increasing age and is consistent with the findings of others

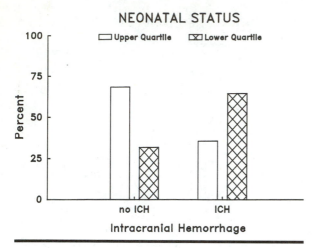

FIGURE 12.12.   Incidence of intracranial hemorrhage (ICH) in upper (open box) and lower crosshatched box) NS quartiles. From A. Salamy, S. Davis, L. Eldredge, A. Wakeley, and W.H. Tooley, *Early Human Development, 17*, 233–243, 1988.

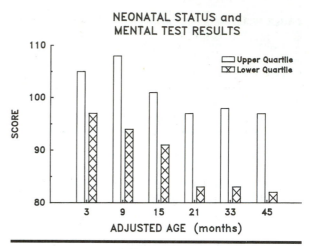

FIGURE 12.13.   Mental test results for the upper (open box) and lower (crosshatched box) NS quartiles by age. Bayley, Mental Development Index, 3–21 months; Stanford-Binet, 33–45 months.

(Hunt, 1981). Demographic variables including gestational age, Apgar scores, gender, and parental education did not contribute to any of the interquartile differences, although birthweight did maintain a low order but significant correlation with mental ability from 15 months to 3.75 years. These data indicate that medical complications incurred in the nursery may impact on long term cognitive development. Current estimates suggest that as much as 35–40% of infants with birthweights below 1500 grams exhibit learning and language disabilities of sufficient magnitude to preclude normal school progress (Hunt, 1986; Fitzhardinge, 1980). While not quite at the point of predicting individual outcome, our measure of NS effectively identified a genuinely high risk subgroup from among the ever-growing ranks of intensive care survivors.

NEONATAL STATUS, THE ABR, AND HEARING LOSS

Severe hearing loss is estimated to occur in approximately 0.01 percent of the births in the United States (Schein and Delk, 1974; Bergstrom, Hemenway, and

Downs, 1971; Simmons, 1980). In contrast, the prevalence of auditory impairment among recipients of neonatal intensive care may range from 1–28% depending on the subpopulation examined (Bergman, Hirsch, Fria, Shapiro, Holtzman, and Painter, 1985; Dura, Suter, Bessard, and Gutberlet, 1986; Sanders, Durieux-Smith, Hyde, Jacobson, Kileny, and Murnave, 1985; Abramovich, Gregory, Slemick, and Stewart, 1979; Nield, Schrier, Ramos, Platzker, and Warburton, 1986). Mild to moderate deficits are even more commonplace but difficult to document. Although numerous "risk factors" have been identified over the years, currently there is little agreement as to the best predictors (Abramovich et al., 1979; Galambos and Despland, 1980; Slack, Wright, Michaels, and Forhlich, 1986; Halpern, Hosford-Dunn, and Malachowiki, 1978). Moreover, the source of the deficit remains unknown in a large proportion (35%) of these infants (Bergman et al., 1985; Stennert, Schulte, Volrath, Brunner, and Frauenrath, 1978; Feinmesser, Lilly, and Levi, 1986). Recent studies show that traditional diagnostic criteria may be unreliable and attempt to pinpoint etiological events ineffective in infants suffering multiple, concurrent insults (Dura et al., 1986; Nield et al., 1986; Galambos, Hicks, and Wilson, 1984). There is, however, a growing recognition that infants presenting with a combination of medical complications face a much greater likelihood of sustaining auditory damage (Sanders et al., 1985; Halpern et al., 1987; Feinmesser et al., 1986). Thus, the general medical condition of the infant in the early postnatal period appears to serve as a reasonable gauge of vulnerability to hearing loss (Bergman et al., 1985; Dura et al., 1986; Sanders et al., 1985; Halpern et al., 1987). Determining the effects of any one incident from among many highly correlated conditions is simply not feasible. By classifying infants according to NS we sought to clarify the relationship between clinical

involvement and hearing loss among intensive care survivors (Salamy, Eldredge, and Tooley, 1989).

Hearing assessment consisted of screening cochlear sensitivity with the ABR in the nursery, once the infant attained a stable condition, and again at 3–6 months, 9–15 months, and 2–4 years adjusted age. Brief clicks (100 µsec) delivered monaurally at intensities of 30 to 70 dB nHL were used as the auditory stimulus. At follow-up infants and children in natural sleep also received these stimulus levels. Subjects who remained awake were presented with 70 dB clicks and if possible 40 dB clicks as well. The latency of waves I, V and the interwave difference served as the dependent measures. Behavioral (HEAR-Kit, BAM World Markets,

TABLE 12.4. Comparisons between subjects with and without sensory hearing loss in the lowest NS quartile.

| | Subjects | | | |
| | With shl | Without shl | | |
Variable	mean ± SD	mean ± SD	F ratio	P<
Gestational age (wk)	28.6 ± 2.4	26.5 ± 1.5	15.23	.0003
Birthweight	1146 ± 256	895 ± 209	12.29	.0009
Bilirubin (mg/kg)	9.90 ± 4.29	7.57 ± 1.78	7.93	.007
Creatinine (mg/dl)	1.66 ± 36	1.90 ± 73	1.11	ns
Gentamicin (total)	43.25 ± 36.3	53.23 ± 39.9	0.61	ns
Gentamicin (peak)	7.64 ± 3.54	7.19 ± 2.33	0.22	ns
Gentamicin (trough)	3.15 ± 78	2.65 ± 1.61	2.49	ns
Neonatal Status	5.00 ± 3.13	2.54 ± 1.61	14.10	.0004
Furosemide (total)	139.1 ± 130	41.5 ± 76	11.00	.001
Furosemide (days)	52.5 ± 43	19.0 ± 23	12.74	.0008
Furosemide with aminoglycosides	12.3 ± 11	4.5 ± 5.6	11.26	.0001
Vancomycin (total)	64.4 ± 125	78.9 ± 161	0.09	ns
Aminoglycosides (days)	24.3 ± 14	20.6 ± 10	0.89	ns
Apgar score (5 min)	6.25 ± 2.5	4.86 ± 2.03	4.00	.05
Boold pH (<7.2)	46.75 ± 41.7	16.7 ± 14.4	9.37	.004
Po$_2$ <50 mm Hg	133.7 ± 108	58.67 ± 50	6.39	.01

Denver CO) and otologic examinations were also performed at most follow-up visits. At three years, or sooner if a hearing loss was suspected, pure-tone audiometry (250–8000 Hz) was administered and speech detection thresholds were determined. Tympanometry was also carried out at this time.

Of the 224 infants from our high risk follow-up program participating in this phase of the research, 12, or 5%, incurred major sensory hearing loss (shl). The distribution of shl revealed that all 12 subjects fell in the lowest NS quartile (Chi square=38.03, p<0.0001, contingency coefficient=0.38) constituting 21.4% of this group. Analyses of specific risk factors implicated in auditory pathology was accomplished by comparing (ANOVAs) those subjects with and without shl exclusively in the lowest NS quartile. These results are summarized in Table 12.4. Contrary to popular belief, subjects with shl were larger, had longer gestations, and higher 5-minute Apgar scores. As expected, they received greater amounts of furosemide for longer durations with extended periods of simultaneous aminoglycoside or vancomycin administration. These medications are known to possess ototoxic properties and could have contributed to the hearing loss. Furthermore, the interaction of these drugs is thought to potentate such effects. Gentamicin, vancomycin, or tobramycin alone did not distinguish the groups nor did the highest creatinine level. The frequency of pH measurements <7.2, Po_2 values <50 mm Hg, and highest bilirubin level were statistically greater for infants with shl. The average bilirubin level, however, was distorted by a single outlier with severe liver damage. No group differences were evident when this subject was removed. Perfusion of the cochlea with blood low in pH (<7.25) and hypoxemia early in life have been shown to be important precursors to hearing loss (Neild et al., 1986; Galambos and Despland, 1980). Contrary to the view that cochlear hemorrhage secondary to ICH represents a prime cause of shl (Slack et al., 1986), there was no difference in the distribution of bleeds between those with and without shl (40% per group), although 56% of the infants with grade 3 or 4 ICH did fall in the lowest NS quartile. Chronic lung disease was the only medical condition common to all the hearing-impaired subjects. The severity of this illness, however, was essen-

tially uniform over those with and without shl in the lower quartile. Subjects in this NS quartile also consistently had later ABR latencies in the nursery (wave I, F=5.51, p<0.001, and wave V, F=9.01, p<0.0001) but not for the I–V interval. Subsequent analyses across the age span studied disclosed that only wave I latency continued to differentiate the NS groups (Figure 12.14). This finding indicates delayed conduction through the peripheral auditory apparatus, intimating a reduction in the effective stimulus reaching the cochlea or possibly sensorineural loss >40 dB in the 4–8 kHz range. These subjects also had a higher incidence of ABR abnormalities at follow-up. Cross tabulations with otoscopic examinations or tympanometry and behav-

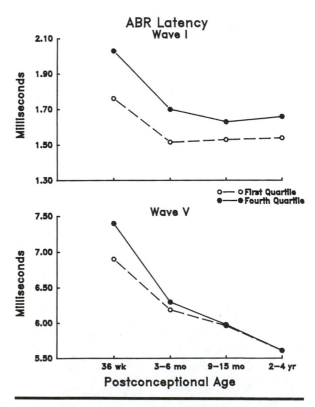

FIGURE 12.14.   Wave I and wave V latency for the upper (first) and lower (fourth) NS quartile by age. From A. Salamy, L. Eldredge, and W.H. Tooley, *Journal of Pediatrics, 14*, 849, 1989.

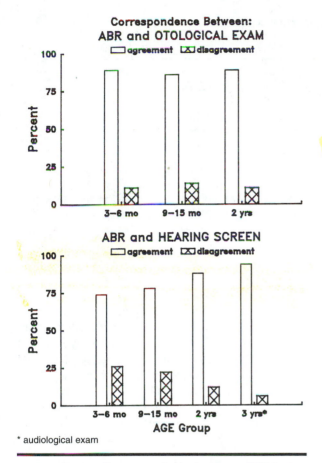

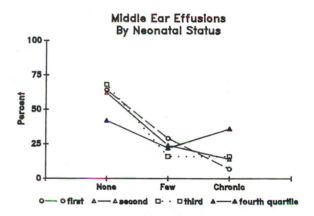

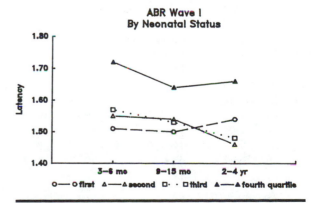

FIGURE 12.15.   Correspondence between ABR test and otologic exam results (upper graph) and ABR and hearing screening results (lower graph).

bitual middle ear effusions as well as the percentage of elevated thresholds (Table 12.5). Thus a prolonged wave I latency is likely to be associated with conductive hearing loss attributable to middle ear pathology.

These results demonstrate that protracted neonatal illness and its management, independent of specific diagnostic categories, are instrumental in promoting sensory and conductive hearing loss in very low birthweight infants. By placing subjects on a wellness-illness continuum, NS was successful in identifying a subgroup of infants at the greatest risk for hearing loss. Since auditory deficits developed after discharge from the hospital in 50% of the subjects with shl, it is im-

FIGURE 12.16.   Percentage of middle ear effusions by NS quartile (upper graph) and wave I latency by NS quartile (lower graph) over age.

ioral hearing screening results obtained at the same clinic visit showed good agreement with the ABR results (all subjects with shl were excluded from these trend analyses). Figure 12.15 portrays this correspondence by age group. For this purpose the ABR was dichotomized as normal or abnormal based on threshold if multiple intensity data were available, or the latency of wave I at 70 dB if not. A late response was defined by a wave I delay >95th percentile of age-matched control subjects with normal values at 40 dB. Figure 12.16 shows infants in the forth NS quartile to be disproportionately represented in terms of the incidence of ha-

TABLE 12.5.   Percent ABR threshold (nHL) by neonatal status quartile.

Quartile	30 dB	40 dB	50 dB	70 dB	80 dB
First	79.41	17.65	2.94	0.00	0.00
Second	58.14	32.56	6.98	2.33	0.00
Third	64.00	20.00	6.00	6.00	4.00
Fourth	43.86	14.04	3.51	29.82	8.77

Chi-square (12 df)=41.96, p<0.0001

perative that evaluation strategies continue throughout the first few years of life.

SUMMARY

Maturation of the CNS proceeds according to a rigidly predetermined timetable. Specific elements of neurogenesis follow a precise and unique course but in an integrative fashion. Certain neurobiologic changes occurring in the third trimester of human gestation are manifest, to some degree, in the behavior and organization of the preterm infant. The electroencephalogram and allied EPs recorded in early life reflect physiologic aspects of brain development during this time and yield important information about sensory capacity. Measurements derived form the ABR provide functional data on cochlea sensitivity as well as the maturation and integrity of the caudal auditory brainstem pathway. However, perinatal complications, common in preterm infants, not only elevate the likelihood for hearing impairment but often confound diagnosis and obscure crisp interpretation of ABR results. By formulating a "Neonatal Status" score to account for multiple, concurrent insults, we were able to establish an individual's standing along a hypothetical wellness-illness continuum. Multivariate statistical procedures were then applied in order to describe the nature and source of hearing loss in quantitative terms. In this way, identification of those preterm infants at the greatest risk for auditory deficits was facilitated.

REFERENCES

Abramovich, S. J., Gregory, S., Slemick, M., and Stewart, A. (1979). Hearing loss in very low birthweight infants treated with neonatal intensive care. *Archives of Diseases of Children, 54,* 421–426.

Adrian, E. D. (1936). The spread of activity in the cerebral cortex. *Journal of Physiology, 88,* 127–161.

Adrien, J. (1976). Lesion of the anterior rephe nuclei in the newborn kitten and the effects of sleep. *Brain Research, 103,* 579–583.

Allison, T. (1962). Recovery functions of somatosensory evoked responses in man. *Electroencephalography and Clinical Neurophysiology, 14,* 331–343.

Amochaev, A., Johnson, R. C., Salamy, A., and Shah, S. N. (1979). Brainstem auditory evoked potentials and myelin changes in triethylin-induced edema in young adult rats. *Experimental Neurology, 66,* 629–635.

Barden, T. S. and Peltzman, P. (1980). Newborn brainstem auditory evoked responses and perinatal clinical events. *American Journal of Obstetrics and Gynecology, 136,* 912–919.

Barnet, A. B., Ohlrich, E. S., Weiss, I. P., and Shanks, B. (1975). Auditory evoked potentials during sleep in normal children from ten days to three years of age. *Electroencephalography and Clinical Neurophysiology, 39,* 29–41.

Bench, R. J. and Metz, D. L. (1974). On the measurement of fetal auditory responses. In R. J. Bench et al. (eds.), *Sound reception in mammals,* pp. 11–22. New York: Academic Press.

Berg, K. W. and Berg, K. M. (1979). Psychophysiological development in infancy: State, sensory function and attention. In J. D. Osofsky (ed.), *The handbook of infant development,* pp. 283–343. New York: John Wiley & Sons, Inc.

Berger, H. (1929). Uber das elektrekephalogram des menschen. *Archives of Psychiatry Nervenkr, 87,* 527–570.

Bergman, M., Himmerlfarb, M.Z., Gold, M.Z., and Shannon, E. (1985). Maturation of the auditory brainstem potentials in neonates and infants. *International Journal of Pediatric Otorhinolaryngology, 9*, 69–78.

Bergstrom, L. B., Hemenway, W. G., and Downs, M. P. (1971). A high risk registry to find congenital deafness. *Otolaryngology Clinics of North America, 4*, 369–399.

Berry, M. (1974) Development of the cerebral neocortex of the rat. In G. Gottlieb (ed.), *Aspects of neurogenesis*, Vol. 2, pp. 7–67. New York: Academic Press.

Birnholz, J. C. and Benacerraf, B. R. (1983). The development of human fetal hearing. *Science, 222*, 516–518.

Blinkov, S. M. and Glazer, I. I. (1968). *The human brain in figures and tables: A quantitive handbook*. New York: Plenum Press.

Broman, S. H. (1979). Perinatal anoxia and cognitive development in early childbirth. In T. M. Field, A. M. Sostek, S. Goldberg, and H H. Sherman (eds.), *Infants born at risk, behavior and development*, pp. 29–52. New York: S. P. Medical & Scientific Books.

Caton R. (1875). The electric currents of the brain. *British Medical Journal, 2*, 278.

Chang, H. T. (1959). The evoked potentials. In J. Field, H W. Magoun, and V. F. Hall (eds.), *Handbook of physiology, neurophysiology*, Vol. 1, pp. 299–313. American Physiological Society.

Chi, J. G., Dooling, E. C., and Gilles, F. H. (1977). Gyral development of the human brain. *Annals of Neurology, 1*, 86–93.

Ciganek, L. (1961). The EEG response (evoked potential) to light stimulus in man. *Electroencephalography and Clinical Neurophysiology, 13*, 165–172.

Cowan, M. W. (1979). The development of the brain. *Scientific American, 241*, 112–133.

Cox, L. C., Hack, M., and Metz, D. A. (1981). Brainstem evoked response audiometry in the premature infant population. *International Journal of Pediatric Otorhinolaryngology, 3*, 213–224.

Creutzfeldt, O. D., Watanabe, S., and Lux, H.D. (1966). Relations between EEG phenomena and potentials of single cortical cells. I. Evoked responses after thalamic and epicortical stimulation. *Electrocephalography and Clinical Neurophysiology, 20*, 1–18.

Davis, H., Davis, A.A., Loomis, A. L., Harvey, E. N., and Hobart, G. (1939). Electrical reactions of the brain to auditory stimulation during sleep. *Journal of Neurophysiology, 2*, 500–514.

Dehkharghani, F. (1984). Application of electroencephalography and evoked potential studies in the neonatal period. In H.B. Sarnat (ed.), *Topics in neonatal neurology*, pp. 257–288. New York: Grune & Stratton, Inc.

Despland, P. A. and Galambos, R. (1980). The auditory brainstem response (ABR) is a useful diagnostic tool in the intensive care nursery. *Pediatric Research, 14*, 154–158.

Dreyfus-Brisac, C. (1979). Ontogenesis of brain bioelectrical activity and sleep organization in neonates and infants. In F. Falkner and J. M. Tanner (eds.), *Human growth, vol. 3, neurobiology and nutrition*, pp. 157–182. New York: Plenum Press.

Drillen, C. M. (1961). Longitudinal study of the growth and development of prematurely and maturely born children. Part VIII: Mental developmental at 2–5 years. *Archives of Diseases of Children, 36*, 233–240.

Duara, S., Suter, C. M., Bessard, K. K., and Gutberlet, R. L. (1986). Neonatal screening with auditory brainstem responses: Results of follow-up audiometry and risk factor evaluation. *Journal of Pediatrics, 108*, 276–281.

Eggermont, J.J. (1985). Physiology of the developing auditory system. In S.E. Trehub and B. Schneider (eds.), *Auditory development in infancy*, pp. 21–45. New York: Plenum Press.

Eggermont, J.J. (1986). Evoked potentials as indicators of the maturation of the auditory system. In V. Gallai (ed.), *Maturation of the CNS and evoked potentials*, pp. 177–182. Amsterdam: Elsevier Science Publishers.

Eggermont, J. J. (1988). On the rate of maturation of sensory evoked potentials. *Electroencephalography and Clinical Neurophysiology, 70*, 293–305.

Eggermont, J. J. (1989). The onset and development of auditory function: Contributions of evoked potential studies. *Journal of Speech and Language Pathology and Audiology, 13*, 5–27.

Eggermont, J. J. and Salamy, A. (1988a). Maturational time course for the ABR in preterm and full term infants. *Hearing Research, 33*, 35–48.

Eggermont, J. J. and Salamy, A. (1988b). Development of ABR parameters in a preterm and a term born population. *Ear and Hearing, 5*, 283–289.

Ellingson, R. (1964). Studies of the electrical activity of the developing human brain. *Progress in Brain Research, 9*, 26–53.

Ellingson, R. J. (1970). Variability of visual evoked responses in the human newborn. *Electroencephalography and Clinical Neurophysiology, 291*, 10–19.

Feinmesser, M., Lilly, T., and Levi, H. (1986). Etiology of childhood deafness with reference to the group of unknown causes. *Audiology, 25*, 65–69.

Field, T. M. and Sostek, A. V. (eds.) (1983). *Infants born at risk*. New York: Grune & Stratton.

Fitzhardinge, P. (1980). Current outcomes: ICU populations. In A. W. Brown and J. J. Volpe (eds.), *Neonatal neurologi-*

cal assessment and outcome, pp. 1–7. Columbus, OH: 77th Ross Laboratories Conference on Pediatric Research.

Friede, D. L. (1975). *Developmental neuropathology*, New York: Springer-Verlag.

Galaburda, A. M., Sherman, G. F., and Geschwind, N. (1983). Developmental dyslexia: Third consecutive case with cortical anomalies. *Society of Neuroscience Abstracts, 9*, 940.

Galambos, R. and Despland, P-A. (1980). The auditory brainstem response (ABR) evaluates risk factors for hearing loss in the newborn. *Pediatric Research, 14*, 159–163.

Galambos, R., Hicks, G. E., and Wilson, M. J. (1984). The auditory brainstem response reliably predicts hearing loss in graduates of a tertiary intensive care nursery. *Ear and Hearing, 5*, 254–260.

Gastaut, H., Regis, H., Lyagoubi, S., Mano, T., and Simon, L. (1968). Comparison of potentials recorded from the occipital, temporal and central regions of the human scalp, evoked by visual, auditory and somatosensory stimuli. *Electroencephalography and Clinical Neurophysiology, Supplement 26*, 19–28.

Goff, W. R., Allison, T., and Vaughan Jr., H. G. (1978). The functional neuroanatomy of event-related potentials. In E. Callaway, P. Tueting, and S. H. Koslow (eds.), *Event-related brain potentials in man*, pp. 1–92. New York: Academic Press.

Goldstein, P. J., Krumholtz, A., Felix, D. R., Shannon, D., and Carr, R. F. (1977). Brainstem evoked responses in neonates. *American Journal of Obstetrics and Gynecology, 135*, 622–629.

Hack, M. (1983). The sensorimotor development of the preterm infant. In A. A. Fanaroff and R. J. Martin (eds.), *Neonatal-perinatal medicine, diseases of the fetus and infant*, pp. 328–346. St. Louis, MO: The C. V. Measly Co.

Hashimoto, I., Ishiyama, Y., Yoshimoto, T., and Nemoto, S. (1981). Brainstem auditory evoked potentials recorded directly from human brain-stem and thalamus. *Brain, 104*, 841–859.

Hecox, K. and Galambos, R. (1974). Brain stem auditory evoked responses in infants and adults. *Archives of Otolaryngology, 99*, 30–33.

Henderson-Smart, D. J., Pettigrew, A. G., and Cambell, D. S. (1983). Clinical apnea and brainstem neural function in preterm infants. *New England Journal of Medicine, 308*, 353–357.

Hobel, C. J., Hyvarinen, M. A., Okada, D. M., and Oh, W. (1973). Prenatal and intrapartum high-risk screening. *American Journal of Obstetrics and Gynecology, 177*, 1–9.

Halpern, J., Hosford-Dunn, H., and Malachowski, N. (1987). Four factors that accurately predict hearing loss in high risk neonates. *Ear and Hearing, 8*, 21–25.

Hrbek, A., Karlberg, P., and Olsson, T. (1973). Development of visual and somato-sensory evoked responses in preterm newborn infants. *Electroencephalography and Clinical Neurophysiology, 34*, 225–232.

Hunt, J. V. (1976). Environmental risks in fetal and neonatal life as biological determinants of infant intelligence. In M. Lewis (ed.), *Origins of intelligence*, pp. 223–258. New York: Plenum Press.

Hunt, J. V. (1986). Developmental risk in infants. In *Advances in Special Education*, Volume 5, pp. 25–59. New York: Jai Press.

Hunt, J. V. (1981). Predicting intellectual disorders in children for preterm infants with birthweights below 1501 grams. In S. L. Friedman and M. Sigman (eds.), *Preterm birth and psychological development*, pp. 329–351. New York: Academic Press.

Jacobson, M. (1978). *Developmental neurobiology*. New York: Plenum Press.

Jewett, D. L. (1969). Averaged volume-conducted potentials to auditory stimuli in the cat. *Physiologist, 12*, 262.

Jewett, D. L. and Williston, J. S. (1971). Auditory-evoked far fields averaged from the scalp of humans. *Brain, 94*, 681–696.

Jouvet, M. (1967). Neurophysiology of the states of sleep. In G.C. Quarton, T. Melnechuk, and F.O. Schmitt (eds.), *The neurosciences, A study program*, pp. 529–544. New York: Rockefeller University Press.

Kileny, P., Connelly, C., and Robertson, C. (1980). Auditory brainstem response in perinatal asphyxia. *International Journal of Pediatric Otorhinolaryngology, 2*, 147–159.

Kostovic, I. and Rakic, P. (1980). Cytology and time of origin of interstitial neurons in the white matter of infant and adult human and monkey telencephalon. *Journal of Neurocytology, 9*, 219–242.

Koveman, J. A. and Scheibel, A. B. (1983). A neuroanatomical correlate of schizophernia. *Society of Neuroscience Abstracts, 9*, 850.

Krumholz, A., Felix, J.K., Goldstein, P.B., and McKenzie, E. (1985). Maturation of the brain-stem auditory evoked potential in premature infants. *Electroencephalography and Clinical Neurophysiology, 62*, 124–134.

Lauder, J. M. and Krebs, H. (1968). Do neurotransmitters, neurohumors and hormones specify critical periods? *Developmental Neuropsychobiology*, pp. 119–174. New York: Academic Press.

Lavigne-Rebillard, M. and Pujal, R. (1988). Hair cell intervention in the fetal human cochlea. *Acta Otolaryngologica, 105*, 398–402.

Lenhardt, M. L., McArtor, R., and Bryant, B. (1984). Effect of neonatal hyperbilirubinemia on the brainstem electric response. *Journal of Pediatrics, 104*, 281–284.

Lewis, M. (1976). The origins of intelligence. *Infancy and early childhood.* New York: Plenum Press.

Lipsitt, L. P. and Field, T. M. (1982). *Infant behavior and development: Perinatal risk and newborn behavior.* New York: Albex Corp.

Littman, B. (1979). The relationship of medical events to infant development. In. T. M. Field, A. M. Sostek, S. Goldberg, and H. H. Sherman (eds.), *Infants born at risk, behavior and development*, pp. 29–52. New York: Scientific Books.

Littman, B. and Parmelee, A. H. (1978). Medical correlates of infant development. *Pediatrics, 61*, 470–474.

Longworthy, O. R. (1933). Development of behavior patterns and myelinization of the nervous system in human fetus and infant. *Contributions to Embryology, Carnegie Institute, 24*, 1–58.

Lubchenco, L., Delivoria-Papadopouls, M., and Searls, D. (1972). Longterm follow-up studies of prematurely born infants. II: Influence of birthweight and gestational age on sequelae. *Journal of Pediatrics, 80*, 509–512.

Marshall, R. E., Reichart, J. J., Kerley, S. M., and Davis, H. (1980). Auditory function in newborn intensive care unit patients revealed by auditory brainstem potentials. *Journal of Pediatrics, 96*, 731–735.

McCall, R.B., Hogarty, P. S., and Hurlburt, N. (1972). Transitions in infant sensorimotor development on the prediction of childhood I.Q. *American Psychologist, 27*, 728–748.

Mochizuki, Y., Go, T., Ohkubo, H., and Motomura, T. (1983). Development of human brain stem auditory evoked responses and gender differences from infants to young adults. *Progress in Neurobiology, 20*, 273–285.

Møller, A. R. and Jannetta, P. J. (1981). Compound action potentials recorded intracranially from the auditory nerve in man. *Experimental Neurology, 74*, 862–874.

Nesbitt, R. E. L. and Aubry, R. H. (1969). High-risk obstetrics. II. Value of semiobjective grading system identifying the vulnerable group. *American Journal of Obstetrics and Gynecology, 103*, 972–985.

Nield, T. A., Schrier, S., Ramos, A. D., Platzker, A. C. G., and Warburton, D. (1986). Unexpected hearing loss in high-risk infants. *Pediatrics, 78*, 417–422.

Nowakowski, R. S. (1987) Basic concepts of CNS development. *Child Development, 58*, 568–595.

Nowakowski, R. S. and Rakic, P. (1981). The site of origin and route and rate of migration of neurons to the hippocampal region of the rhesus monkey. *Journal of Comparative Neurology, 196*, 129–154.

Ohlrich, E. S., and Barnet, A. B. (1972). Auditory evoked responses during the first year of life. *Electroencephalography and Clinical Neurophysiology, 32*, 161–169.

Parmelee, A.H. and Stern, E. (1972). Development of states in infants. In C. D. Clemente, D. P. Purpura, and F. E. Mayer (eds.), *Sleep and the maturing nervous system*, pp. 199–228. New York: Academic Press Inc.

Parmelee, A. H., Stern, E., and Harris, M. A. (1972). Maturation of respiration in prematures and young infants. *Neuropadiatrie, 3*, 294–304.

Parmelee, A. H. Jr., Wenner, W.H., Akiyama, Y., and Flescher, J. (1967). Electroencepholography and brain maturation. In A. Minkowski (ed.), *Symposium on regional development of the brain in early life*, pp. 459–480. Philadelphia, PA: F. A. Davis.

Perlman, M., Fainmesser, P., Sohmer, H., Tamari, H., Wax, Y., and Pevsmer, B. (1983). Auditory nerve-brainstem evoked responses in hyperbilirubinemic neonates. *Pediatrics, 72*, 658–664.

Picton, T. W., Hillyard, S. A., Krausz, H. I., and Galambos, R. (1974). Human auditory evoked potentials. I: Evaluation of Components. *Electroencephalography and Clinical Neurophysiology, 36*, 179–190.

Prechtl, H. V. (1968). Neurological sequelae of prenatal and perinatal complications. *British Medical Journal, 4*, 763–767.

Purpura, D. P. (1975). Normal and aberrant neuronal development in the cerebral cortex of human fetus and young infants. In N.A. Buchwald and A.B. Brazier (eds.). *Brain mechanisms in mental retardation*, pp. 41–169. New York: Academic Press.

Purpura, D. P. (1971). Synaptogenesis in mammalian cortex, problems and perspectives. In M. B. Sterman, D. J. McGinty, and A. M. Adinoff (eds.), *Brain development and behavior*, pp. 23–42. New York: Academic Press.

Purves, D. and Lichtman, J. W. (1985). *Principles of neural development*, Sinaner Associates, Inc.

Reinis, S. and Goldman, J. M. (1980) *The development of the brain, biological, and functional perspectives.* Springfield: Charles C. Thomas.

Robinowicz, T. (1964). The cerebral cortex of the premature infant of the 8th month. *Progress in Brain Research, 4*, 39–86.

Robinson, K. and Rudge, P. (1977). Abnormalities of the auditory evoked potentials in patients with multiple sclerosis. *Brain, 100*, 19–40.

Rockstroh, B., Elbert, T., Birbaumer, N., and Lutzenberger, W. (1982). *Slow brain potentials and behavior.* Baltimore, MD: Urban & Schwarzenberg.

Rorke, L. B. and Riggs, H. (1969). *Myelination of the brain in the newborn*, pp. 1–28. Philadelphia, PA: J.B. Lippincott Co.

Rotteveel, J.J., Colon, E.J., Stegeman, D.F., and Visco, Y.M. (1987). The maturation of the central auditory conduction in preterm infants until three months post term. I. Composite group averages of brain stem (ABR) and middle latency (MLR) auditory responses. *Hearing Research, 26,* 11–20.

Salamy, A., Eldredge, L., and Tooley, W. Y. (1989). Neonatal status and hearing loss in high-risk infants. *The Journal of Pediatrics, 114,* 847–852.

Salamy, A., Davis, S., Eldredge, L., Wakeley, A., and Tooley, W. H. (1988). Neonatal status: An objective scoring method for identifying infants at risk for poor outcome. *Early Human Development, 17,* 233–243.

Salamy, A., Mendelson, T., and Tooley, W.H. (1982). Developmental profiles for the brain stem auditory evoked potential. *Early Human Development, 11,* 331–339.

Salamy, A., Mendelson, T., Tooley, W. H., and Chaplin, E. R. (1980*a*). Contrasts in brainstem function between normal and high risk infants in early postnatal life. *Early Human Development, 4,* 179–185.

Salamy, A., Mendelson, T., Tooley, W. H., and Chaplin, E. R. (1980*b*). Differential development of brainstem potentials in healthy and high risk infants. *Science, 210,* 553–555,

Salamy, A. and McKean, C. M. (1976). Postnatal development of human brainstem potentials during the first year of life. *Electroencephalography and Clinical Neurophysiology, 40,* 418–426.

Sanders, R., Durieux-Smith, A., Hyde, M., Jacobson, J., Kileny, P., and Murnave, O. (1985). Incidence of hearing loss in high risk and intensive care infants. *Journal of Otolaryngology, 14,* 28–33.

Sarnat, H. B. (1984). Anatomic and physiologic correlates of neurologic development in prematurity. In H. B. Sarnat (ed.), *Topics in neonatal neurology*, pp. 1–25. New York: Grune & Stratton Inc.

Schein, J. D. and Delk, M. T. Jr. (1974). *The Deaf Population of the United States*, pp. 3–72. Silver Springs, MD: National Association of the Deaf.

Shah, S. N. and Salamy, A. (1980). Brainstem auditory potentials in myelin deficient mice. *Neuroscience, 5,* 2321–2323.

Shah, S. N., Bhargava, V. K., Johnson, R. C., and McKean, C. M. (1978). Latency changes in brainstem auditory evoked potentials associated with impaired brain myelination. *Experimental Neurology, 58,* 111–118.

Sigman, M. and Parmelee, A. H. (1979). Longitudinal evaluation of the preterm infant. In T. M. Field, A. W. Sostek, S. Goldberg, and H. H. Sherman (eds.), *Infants born at risk, behavior and development*, pp. 193–217. New York: Scientific Books.

Simmons, F. B. (1980). Diagnosis and rehabilitation of deaf newborns: Part II. *American Speech-Language-Hearing Association, 22,* 275.

Starr, A., Amlie, R. N., Martin, W. H., and Sanders, S. (1977). Development of auditory function in newborn infants revealed by auditory brainstem potentials. *Pediatrics, 60,* 831–839.

Starr, A. and Achor, L. J. (1975). Auditory brainstem responses in neurological disease. *Archives of Neurology, 32,* 761–766.

Stennert, E., Schulte, F. J., Vollrath, M., Brunner, E., and Frauenrath, C. (1978). The etiology of neurosensory hearing deficits in preterm infants. *Archives of Otorhinolarngology, 221,* 171–182.

Stockard, J. L. and Rossiter, U. S. (1977). Clinical and pathologic correlates of brainstem auditory response abnormalities. *Neurology, 27,* 316–325.

Uziel, A., Marot, M. and Germain, M. (1980). Les potentiels évoqués du nerf auditif et du tronc cérébral chez le nouveau-né et l'enfant. *Review of Laryngology, (Bordeaux) 101,* 55–71.

Walsh, E. J. and McGee, J. (1986). The development of function in the auditory periphery. In R. A. Altshuler, D. W. Hoffman, and R. P. Bobbin (eds.), *Neurobiology of hearing: The cochlea*, pp. 247–269. New York: Raven Press.

Weitzman, E. D. and Graziani, L. J. (1968). Maturation and topography of the auditory evoked response in premature infants. *Developmental Psychobiology, 1,* 79–89.

Wigglesworth, R. (1968). "At risk" registers. *Developmental Medicine and Child Neurology, 10,* 678–680.

Williams, H. L., Morlock, H. C., Morlock, J. V., and Lubin, A. (1964). Auditory evoked responses and the EEG stages of sleep. *Annals of the New York Academy of Science, 112,* 172–181.

Williams, R., Karacon, I., and Hursch, C. (1974). *Electroencephology (EEG) of human sleep.* New York: John Wiley & Sons.

Yakovlev, P. I. and Lecours, A-R. (1967). The myelogenetic cycles of regional maturation of the brain. In A. Minkowski (ed.), *Regional development of the brain in early life*, pp. 3–64. Oxford: Blackwell Scientific Publishers Ltd.

Zimmerman, M.C., Morgan, D.E., and Dubno, J.R. (1987). Auditory brain stem evoked response characteristics in developing infants. *Annals of Otology, Rhinology, and Laryngology, 96,* 291–299.

CHAPTER 13

NEWBORN AND INFANT AUDITORY BRAINSTEM RESPONSE APPLICATIONS

JOHN T. JACOBSON
JAMES W. HALL, III

INTRODUCTION

The effective audiologic diagnosis and management of the pediatric population requires the integration of information obtained from a variety of sources. Because of the limitations associated with conventional behavioral audiometry in neonates and very young infants, there is a general consensus that the use of objective measures is prerequisite to ensure valid estimates of auditory sensitivity (Jacobson and Morehouse, 1984; Durieux-Smith and Jacobson, 1985; Durieux-Smith, Picton, Edwards, et al., 1985).

The use of auditory evoked potentials (AEPs) and in particular, the auditory brainstem response (ABR), represents an accepted clinical technique in pediatric hearing evaluation. The ease and reliability with which the ABR is measured has resulted in its rapid proliferation. As a diagnostic tool, the ABR has focused on two unique yet ancillary applications. The first involves the study of the peripheral auditory mechanism, including the middle ear system, the cochlea, and its related pathology. The ability to identify, quantify, and accurately characterize auditory deficits in patients who are difficult to test continues to represent a major application of the ABR. Because this technique can be used to determine the magnitude and type of hearing defect, it is especially suitable for infants with unsuspected or unconfirmed hearing loss who are unable to respond appropriately to behavioral stimuli. Clinical comparisons between electrophysiologic and behavioral test thresholds in older infants and children have resulted in threshold levels within 10 dB HL (Sasama, 1990).

Additionally, the ABR technique is suitable for infant hearing screening and has been recommended as the test of choice by the Joint Committee on Infant Hearing (1991). Thus, congenitally deaf newborns or those infants identified with lesser degrees of hearing impairment by ABR can benefit from early auditory intervention, habilitative management, and longitudinal, objective monitoring.

The second primary ABR application embraces the area of neurodiagnostics and the ability to monitor the functional integrity of the central auditory pathway objectively. Currently, the ABR is the most accurate electrophysiologic measure for the identification of posterior fossa lesions and provides a powerful technique during the surgical management of brainstem lesions. Fortunately, these applications are rare in children. Further, the ABR has also been used successfully in a variety of other neurotologic abnormalities in the operating arena and the intensive care unit. Finally, common disorders observed in infants in which ABR has been used with supplementary diagnostic support include hypoxic ischemic encephalopathy, respiratory distress, closed head injuries, intraventricular hemorrhage and neurodegenerative diseases. Thus, ABR has a permanent role in the areas of neonatology and pediatric otology.

Although ABR has become the objective test of choice for pediatric auditory assessment, the absence of acceptable clinical standards remains a major limitation, particularly in the preterm and high risk infant (Cox, Hack, and Metz, 1981, 1982, 1984; Salamy, 1984; Murray, Javel, and Watson, 1985; Lary, Briassoilis, deVries, et al., 1985; Fawer, Dubowitz, Levene, et al., 1983; Cox, 1985). Before test results can be considered valid and interpreted with clinical confidence, a normative data base must be established as a benchmark from which all other responses are compared. In any diagnostic technique such as the ABR, technical and procedural variables must be sufficiently limited or controlled before normative data can be universally applied. Unfortunately, the task is frequently difficult given the variables that may act either independently or synergistically during pediatric ABR assessment. In this chapter we describe those technical and subject related variables that affect ABR application in the pediatric patient.

A caveat is appropriate at this juncture. ABR test results should not be considered in isolation; nor is the technique intended to usurp a thorough history, physical examination, and other supplementary laboratory tests. Rather, the results of this technique should be considered in concordance with other auditory, neurotologic, and imaging evidence. The multi-site neural generators of this subcortical event and ABR insensitivity to pathology that does not impinge upon the brainstem auditory pathway are major limitations that must be integrated into the final diagnostic analysis.

MEASUREMENT AND ANALYSIS

ABR measurement is not restricted to ideal environments. As a result, testing is often conducted in settings that are hostile to electrophysiologic evaluations. For example, testing newborns in the neonatal intensive care unit (NICU) can involve excessive noise, competing electrical monitoring equipment and infant developmental status, as well as medical and nursing interruption. Despite the best of intentions and quality control, there will always be some ABR records that are compromised by electrical and myogenic artifact. To date, no universal guidelines exist that are applicable in every testing situation. However, there are several procedural modifications and manipulations that can be incorporated into routine protocol that will assist in the clarification and interpretation of complex ABR traces.

Because a wide variety of pathologic and stimulus-recording factors directly affect ABR interpretation, a thorough understanding of normative response variability is required. In the estimation of normal auditory sensitivity and confirmation of neurotologic integrity, analysis of the ABR involves three response properties. They include the measurement of absolute and relative wave peak latency, and to a lesser degree, amplitude, and morphology of the wave peak component.

Response Characteristics

Morphology. Unlike the five to seven wave peaks that are characteristic of an adult recording, only three prominent wave components are typically discernable in the term newborn (Despland and Galambos, 1980; Jacobson, Morehouse, and Johnson, 1982; Jacobson, Seitz, Mencher, et al., 1981; Salamy and McKean, 1976; Starr, Amlie, Martin, et al., 1977). Figure 13.1 illustrates the ABR differences for a normal hearing newborn and that of an adult. Even the most cursory comparison illustrates the distinctive morphologic differences between the two. The emergence of the ABR is commonly reported between the 26th and 30th week of the gestational period, but only at high click intensity presentation levels (Galambos and Hecox, 1978; Starr et al., 1977; Stockard, Stockard, and Coen, 1983; Stockard and Westmoreland, 1981). Between three and four months of age, wave II is readily identifiable and waves IV and V begin to show signs of progressive peak separation (Hecox and Jacobson, 1984). By the end of the first year of life, the morphology of the infant response approximates that of the adult.

The morphology of an ABR is subject to changes due to maturation, pathology, and stimulus and recording variables (Jacobson et al., 1982; Rowe, 1978; Stockard, Stockard, Westmoreland, et al., 1979). As a result, ABR waveform components are not precise indicators of auditory pathology. However, certain characteristics such as the presence or absence of wave peaks provide gross indications of auditory pathology. For example, the presence of only waves I and II in a technically correct ABR measurement suggests marked dysfunction in the pontine region of the brainstem.

Latency. The ABR wave peak components are most often described in terms of their latency characteristics.

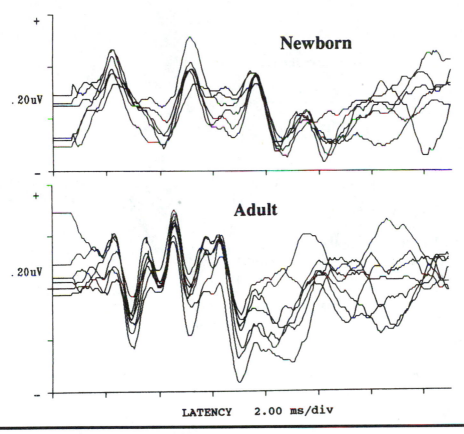

FIGURE 13.1.   A series of 6 auditory brainstem response (ABR) waveforms, each obtained from the same ear of a newborn (6-week-old term male—top) and that of an adult (bottom). Positivity is upward in this and all subsequent figures. Each trace represents the sum of 2000 click stimuli at 60 dB nHL.

Absolute wave latency is the duration in milliseconds (ms) between signal presentation and the measured peak. The relative period between two waves is most commonly called the interwave interval (IWI) or the interpeak latency (IPL). Absolute and relative ABR latencies typically calculated from a newborn are displayed in Figure 13.2A.

Latency of the ABR is affected by a number of variables, most notably, development of the auditory system and stimulus intensity. The absolute latencies of all waves increase with decreasing stimulus intensity. In a healthy term infant, waves I and V latencies are about 2.0 and 7.0 ms respectively, for a 60 dB nHL click stimulus. These latency values are extremely variable and change as a function of maturation until about 18 to 24 months of age. In general, latencies reduce with increasing age although the rate of decrease is dependent on both the specific wave (e.g., peripheral or central site of generation) and physiologic condition (e.g., synaptic efficiency, myelination, dipole orientation). Generally, the more rostral the wave generator site, the longer the developmental time course (Hecox and Burkard, 1982). That is, wave I latency reaches adult levels earlier than more centrally generated wave peak components (waves III, IV, and V). A detailed description of the effects of age on latency follows in

(A)

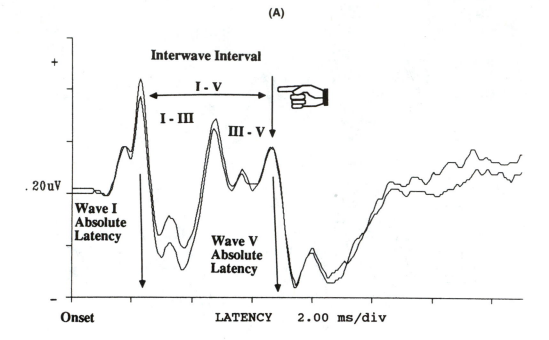

(B)

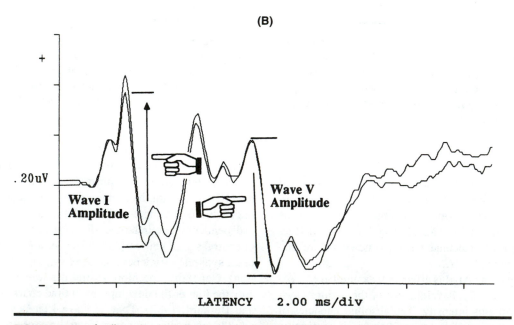

FIGURE 13.2. Auditory brainstem response (ABR) waveforms obtained from a three-year-old male. Each trace represents the sum of 2000 click stimuli at 85 dB nHL. (A) latency measurement criteria; (B) amplitude measurement criteria.

this chapter, as well in Chapter 12, Salamy et al., *Neurodevelopment and Auditory Function in Preterm Infants.*

In comparison, relative latency offers insight into functional integrity of the auditory brainstem pathways. The advantage of IWIs is that they are less variable and more sensitive than absolute peak latency to CNS pathologies (Eggermont and Salamy, 1988). Both conductive and sensory hearing loss will generally prolong the absolute latency of all wave peak components. In contrast, lesions of the acoustic nerve and brainstem pathway tend to prolong wave peaks generated beyond wave I (at the distal segment of the acoustic nerve). Therefore, increases in interwave latency values (i.e., I–III, III–V, I–V) tend to distinguish between peripheral and central abnormalities. Although greater variability in ABR measures have been reported for younger rather than older infants (Morgan, Zimmerman, and Dubno, 1987), a high correlation between ears is found in all age groups (Salamy, 1984; Gorga, Reiland, Beauchaine, et al., 1987). Finally, Cone-Wesson, Kurtzberg, and Vaughan (1987) reported that about 15% of high risk infants present with prolonged interwave intervals on evaluation. Infants with this manifestation include those suffering from post-infectious and post-anoxic encephalopathy, myelinopathy, and other neurologic insult (Hecox and Cone, 1981; Kileny, Connely, and Robertson, 1980).

Amplitude. Response amplitude is usually described in microvolts (μV) and is a vertical measure from either the voltage baseline having a zero reference to the wave peak or more commonly, as the difference between the peak of a wave and its following trough (Figure 13.2B). Amplitude will tend to decrease as stimulus intensity decreases, although the degree of wave peak amplitude reduction varies (Durieux-Smith et al., 1985; Hecox and Galambos, 1974; Picton, Stapells, and Campbell, 1981). At or near term, the newborn wave V amplitude approximates the wave I amplitude (Jacobson et al., 1982; Salamy, McKean, and Buda, 1975; Starr et al., 1977; Stockard, Stockard, and Sharbrough, 1978). Decreases in wave amplitude are usually consistent with hearing loss or neurotologic disease. In extreme cases of neurodegenerative disorders or severe-to-profound hearing loss, wave peaks may be unmeasurable. A typical amplitude recording from a newborn using a 70 dB nHL click stimulus at a rate of 10/sec is about 0.35 and 0.40 μV for waves I and V, respectively (Durieux-Smith et al., 1985).

Although amplitude measures have been used as a supplementary response parameter in ABR analysis, they have not gained clinical acceptance due to their inherent variability. As an alternative, Starr and Achor (1975) were first to suggest the use of the amplitude ratio as a clinical alternative to absolute amplitude measures. The wave V/I amplitude ratio is most often used clinically because waves I and V are prominent at an early age, are easily identifiable and represent two distinct anatomical generator sources; that is, peripheral versus central. The ratio compares activity in the auditory nerve and more rostral regions of the brainstem (Hecox and Burkard, 1982). The amplitude ratio is affected by stimulus intensity, presentation rate, electrode type, scalp location and age (Pratt and Sohmer, 1976; Cone, Hecox, and Finitzo-Hieber, 1977; Hecox and Cone, 1981; Salamy, McKean, Petett, et al., 1978). For example, as age increases, the amplitude ratio increases until about the first year of life when it reaches adult value (Salamy, Mendelson, and Tooley, 1982). In an early study, Salamy, Fenn, and Bronshvag (1979) contended that the amplitude ratio was capable of distinguishing high-risk infants from healthy infants especially at about 1 year of age. However, Eggermont and Salamy (1988) found large standard deviations in their earlier data and conceded that the use of V/I ratio as a parameter to differentiate term from preterm infants was no longer applicable. Variations in response amplitude have been attributed to a number of biologic factors including dipole wave orientation, volume conduction, impedance properties, and neural synchrony (Hecox and Burkard, 1982).

While the adult V/I amplitude ratio often exceeds 2.0 (Stockard et al., 1978), the newborn amplitude ratio is about 1.0 (Hecox, Cone, and Blaw, 1981; Jacobson et al., 1982). Amplitude ratios less than 0.5 have been identified in a group of infants diagnosed with severe perinatal asphyxia (Hecox and Cone, 1981).

Response Analysis. Two general analysis strategies are employed in newborn hearing screening with ABR.

With the first strategy, a *pass* outcome is defined by the presence of a reliable response (presence of repeatable wave components), and a *fail* outcome as no response, at predetermined intensity levels (e.g., 35 dB nHL). Traditionally, this appears to be a common analysis approach (e.g., Duara, Suter, Bessard, et al., 1986; Durieux-Smith and Jacobson, 1985; Galambos, Hicks, and Wilson, 1982; Marshall, Reicher, Kerley, et al., 1980; Swigonski, Shallop, Bull, et al., 1987; Dennis, Sheldon, Toubas, et al., 1984; Cox et al., 1982). As illustrated by infant A in the top two traces in Figure 13.3, the major clinical advantage and appeal of the presence vs. absence analysis approach is its simplicity. Relatively little expertise in waveform analysis is required and normative data are not necessary. Some investigators further simplify the newborn ABR screening measurement and analysis approach by determining response presence or absence for only one ear (e.g., Duara et al., 1986; Galambos et al., 1982; Swigonski et al., 1987; Weber, 1983). With this approach, the ear that is tested is deter-

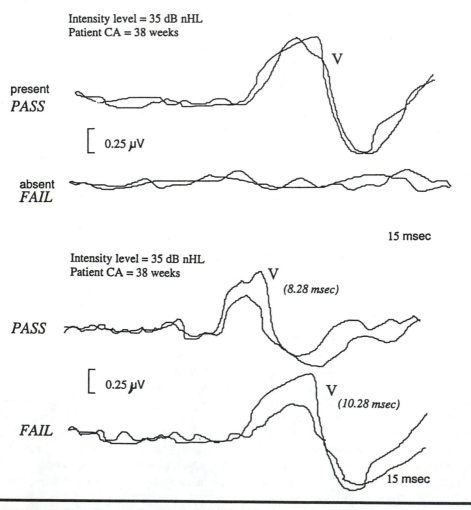

FIGURE 13.3. Two common approaches for analysis of auditory brainstem response (ABR) waveforms in newborn hearing screening.

mined by convenience (the exposed ear). See Chapter 15, Weber and Jacobson, *Newborn Hearing Screening,* for further explanation.

The strategy of stimulating only one ear and defining outcome on the basis of the presence or absence of a response presents two distinct limitations for newborn hearing screening. First, one-half of all infants with unilateral hearing loss may not be detected when just one ear is tested. There is now ample evidence that unilateral hearing loss, especially for the right ear, may lead to academic and communicative problems (Bess, 1985). Second, the simple presence of a response, without regard to wave V latency, does not rule out the possibility of high frequency sensory or mild conductive hearing loss. Comparison of ABR latency-intensity functions and audiometric configurations in adults with sensory hearing loss confirms the disadvantage of the wave V presence vs. absence strategy (Hall, 1992; Yamada, Kodera, and Yagi, 1979). That is, patients with high frequency sensory deficits may have a reliable wave V at screening intensity levels. A wave V peak will typically be present, although abnormally delayed in latency, at screening intensity levels when hearing sensitivity for lower frequency regions (1000 Hz or below) is reasonably normal. The ABR wave V latency-intensity function for such patients will tend to slope upward markedly at lower intensity levels as the response becomes dependent on more apical regions of the cochlea.

A more precise ABR analysis approach in newborn hearing screening is to first verify that a reliable response is present at the screening stimulus intensity level, and then to compare wave V latency with age-matched normative data (Figure 13.3). This approach requires more skill in response interpretation, mainly the ability to identify wave V, and access to appropriate normative data. Moreover, the measurement parameters used in the ABR screening protocol should be consistent with those used in collection of the normative data. Consistency is probably most important for earphone type, stimulus intensity, stimulus rate, and high pass filter setting parameters. Clearly, accurate calculation of the infant's age (conceptional or gestational) is also essential for proper analysis of wave V latency. Assuming these precautions have been taken,

most investigators consider an ABR wave V abnormal if latency exceeds a specific statistical criterion above the age-matched normal mean value, such as +2.5 standard deviations or the 95% confidence limit. This process is illustrated in the lower two records of Figure 13.3. Relevant data are shown for two infants, including age, the stimulus intensity level, and ABR wave V latency. In comparing wave V latency for each of these infants' age appropriate normative data, it is apparent that infant B would pass the hearing screening and infant C would fail.

ABR ACQUISITION

Generally, changes in ABR latency, amplitude ratios, and waveform morphology are directly affected by subject characteristics (i.e., physical status) and stimulus and recording parameters used in testing. Accurate clinical decisions must be based on a knowledge and understanding of normal response variability.

The establishment of norms for neonates and infants introduces special problems since prematurity and physical status may synergistically affect test outcome. The results of a physically compromised infant has been shown to affect test measurement (Cox et al., 1981, 1984; Salamy et al., 1980; Cox, 1985; Eggermont and Salamy, 1988). For example, Eggermont and Salamy (1988) reported that differences in mean absolute latency values in preterm infants (N=178) were significantly longer than for full-term infants (N=465) up to 2 years of age; however, relative latencies and amplitude ratios were not dissimilar between their experimental groups. Similar absolute and relative wave latency findings were reported by Lauffer and Wenzel (1989) and Samani, Peschiulli, Pastorini, et al., (1990) who also observed greater latency variability in preterm newborns. Further, because mild hearing loss is difficult to detect and may be prevalent in this population, auditory status is another influencing factor that must be taken into consideration.

The following comments describing normative aspects of pediatric ABR assessment are limited to the use of auditory click stimuli. Unfiltered clicks are most often used in auditory and neurologic ABR recordings. Stimuli are produced by driving a transducer (headphone) with a rectangular voltage pulse and duration of about 100 microseconds (μs). Due to the rapid onset of a click, it is an optimal stimulus for eliciting neural synchronization but lacks frequency specificity. Tone bursts (see Chapter 3, Hyde, *Signal Processing and Analysis*) offer a more concentrated energy-density spectrum that allows better audiometric estimations; however, because tone bursts have longer rise/fall times than clicks, they reduce synchronous neural discharge activity. Thus, a compromise must be struck based on the specific needs of the diagnostic evaluation. Generally, clicks are used in neurotologic assessment and in the estimation of high frequency hearing sensitivity. Although other click-generated techniques (e.g., "derived" responses, notched noise, and other masking paradigms) have been employed, short duration tone bursts are most often used to estimate frequency sensitivity from the apical regions of the basilar membrane. As indicated elsewhere in this book (see Hyde, Chapter 8, *The Slow Vertex Potential*), other AEPs, chiefly the late or slow vertex response may offer more frequency specificity in determining audiometric configuration, although they too have age specific limitations.

Subject Variables

Age. Although changes in the ABR have been reported in older adults (Hyde, 1985; Jerger and Hall, 1980; Kjaer, 1980) the effects of age is the primary subject variable in infants. Latency differences are so pronounced that establishing age-specific normative data is recommended on a weekly basis during the preterm period, biweekly between term and about three months, and monthly thereafter until 18 to 24 months of age.

The effects of maturational change on infant ABR measures are well documented (Adelman, Levi, Linder, et al., 1990; Lauffer and Wenzel, 1989; Eggermont and Salamy, 1988; Gorga et al., 1987; Gorga, Kaminski, Beauchaine, et al., 1989; Hecox, 1975; Morgan et al., 1987; Zimmerman, Morgan, and Dubno, 1987; Schulman-Galambos and Galambos, 1975, 1979; Schwartz, Pratt, and Schwartz, 1989; Starr et al., 1977; Fria and Doyle, 1984; Rotteveel, Colon,

Notermans, et al., 1986; Despland, 1985; Jacobson et al., 1982; Cevette, 1984). As summarized in Figure 13.4, response latency decreases with age whereas wave amplitude increases, particularly those waves generated from more rostral neural generator sites. The ABR has been identified in premature infants as early as the 26th gestational week at high stimulus intensities (Starr and Acher, 1977), although typically, the response may only consist of a wave I peak component. Galambos and associates (1984) observed the presence of replicable ABR traces in one or both ears in 83 percent of a group of premature newborns tested at 30 weeks gestational age (GA). This percentage increased proportionally and by term (40th wk GA), 91 percent of all infants tested produced ABRs at 30 dB nHL. The remaining 9 percent failure rate was attributed to either transient or permanent hearing loss or neurologic sequelae.

The recognition that the various wave peaks are differentially affected by maturation has led to the establishment of age-specific norms for the newborn and infant population. Wave V latency decreases nonlinearly from term ultimately reaching adults equivalency between 12 and 24 months (Gorga et al., 1989; Hecox and Galambos, 1974; Salamy et al., 1979; Salamy and McKean, 1976; Zimmerman et al., 1987). Despite conflicting reports (Folsom and Wynne, 1987), wave I latency approximates adult value by the third month of age although the specific time course varies among studies (Jacobson et al., 1982; Kaga and Tanaka, 1980; Salamy and McKean, 1976; Schwartz et al., 1989; Zimmerman et al., 1987; Gorga et al., 1989). For example, Schwartz et al. (1989) found, in a group of 20 preterm infants aged 35 to 38 weeks PCA, no significant difference in wave I latency compared to adult values. They support the concept of peripheral auditory maturity and central auditory immaturity as reflected by latency prolongation of waves III and V relative to the adult response.

In a comprehensive study of age-related ABR measures, Gorga and colleagues (1987) investigated 585 stable infants with normal hearing who ranged from 33 to 44 post-conceptional age (PCA) in weeks. ABR data were divided into six two-week age groups. Generally, these authors found orderly decreases in latency with increasing age. The latency of waves I and V and the

AUDITORY BRAINSTEM RESPONSE

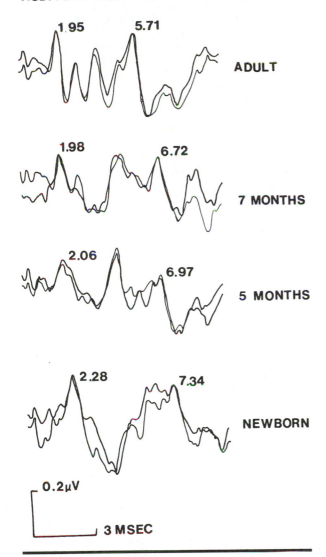

FIGURE 13.4. Auditory brainstem response (ABR) traces representing the maturation of the auditory system. Note the latency shifts and emerging of wave components with increasing age.

84 percent of 585 babies had ABR 30 dB nHL thresholds in both ears. Normative data reported by Gorga and colleagues for absolute latency I and V and interwave intervals (i.e., I–III, III–V, I–V) as a function of age are shown in Tables 13.1, 13.2 and 13.3 respectively.

Gorga et al. (1989) reported nonsignificant wave I latency changes in 535 children ranging from 3 months to 3 years of age suggesting early maturation of the response. However, consistent with previous data, they observed a systematic decrease in mean wave V latency during the first 24 month period. They reported mean wave V latencies that were about 0.6 ms shorter for the 33 to 36 month group (5.63 ms at 80 dB nHL) compared to the 3 to 6 month group (6.25 ms). Also, similar differences were observed when the 3 to 6 month group was compared to term infants (6.81 ms). For the I–V latency, a similar latency relationship existed. A mean difference of about 0.5 ms was observed between the three age groups (term: 5.09 ms; 3–6 months: 4.65 ms; 33–36 month: 4.12 ms). These differential effects on latency have been attributed to a number of variables including improvements in peripheral status (Durieux-Smith et al., 1985; Goldstein, Krumholz, Felix, et al., 1979; Salamy et al., 1978) and central status, specifically, myelination, and synaptic

TABLE 13.1. Normative Data: Means and standard deviations of wave I latency as a function of age (33 to 44 wks conceptional age) at 80 dB nHL.

Age Group (Weeks)	M (ms)	SD
33–34	1.779	0.304
35–36	1.781	0.261
37–38	1.741	0.208
39–40	1.718	0.234
41–42	1.691	0.192
43–44	1.652	0.150

From Gorga et al. (1987). ABRs from graduates of an intensive care nursery: Normal patterns of response. *Journal of Speech and Hearing Research, 30,* 311–318. Reprinted with the permission of the American Speech-Language-Hearing Association.

interwave intervals all produced systematic statistically significant decreases. Additionally, they reported that 89 percent of their sample (1,249 ears) demonstrated ABR thresholds of at least 30 dB nHL and that

TABLE 13.2. Normative Data: Means and standard deviations of wave V latency as a function of age (33 to 44 wks conceptional age) and intensity.

Level (dB nHL)	Age Group (Weeks)	M (ms)	SD
20	33–34	9.718	0.562
	35–36	9.609	0.666
	37–38	9.565	0.744
	39–40	9.355	0.567
	41–42	9.310	0.541
	43–44	9.156	0.528
40	33–34	8.479	0.493
	35–36	8.418	0.536
	37–38	8.290	0.510
	39–40	8.110	0.489
	41–42	8.075	0.350
	43–44	7.944	0.507
60	33–34	7.615	0.411
	35–36	7.576	0.429
	37–38	7.450	0.438
	39–40	7.300	0.396
	41–42	7.197	0.294
	43–44	7.082	0.327
80	33–34	7.054	0.394
	35–36	7.019	0.375
	37–38	6.939	0.419
	39–40	6.816	0.381
	41–42	6.687	0.294
	43–44	6.532	0.317

From Gorga et al. (1987). ABRs from graduates of an intensive care nursery: Normal patterns of response. *Journal of Speech and Hearing Research, 30,* 311–318. Reprinted with the permission of the American Speech-Language-Hearing Association.

TABLE 13.3. Normative Data: Means and standard deviations of interwave interval latencies as a function of age (33 to 44 wks conceptional age) at 80 dB nHL.

Interpeak Interval	Age Group (Weeks)	M (ms)	SD
I–III	33–34	2.863	0.283
	35–36	2.848	0.269
	37–38	2.803	0.307
	39–40	2.704	0.266
	41–42	2.744	0.220
	43–44	2.650	0.255
III–IV	33–34	2.411	0.259
	35–36	2.390	0.250
	37–38	2.345	0.260
	39–40	2.379	0.246
	41–42	2.242	0.207
	43–44	2.210	0.212
I–V	33–34	5.274	0.356
	35–36	5.240	0.357
	37–38	5.171	0.401
	39–40	5.090	0.359
	41–42	4.996	0.296
	43–44	4.882	0.310

From Gorga et al. (1987). ABRs from graduates of an intensive care nursery: Normal patterns of response. *Journal of Speech and Hearing Research, 30,* 311–318. Reprinted with the permission of the American Speech-Language-Hearing Association.

efficiency (Eggermont, 1985; Goldstein et al., 1979; Hecox and Burkhard, 1982; Jacobson, 1985; Morgan et al., 1987; Salamy et al., 1978). Tables 13.4, 13.5, and 13.6 display the absolute latencies of waves I and V and relative latencies (i.e., I–III, III–V, I–V) as a function of age.

Studies by Fria and Doyle (1984) and Eggermont (1983) indicate two exponential wave latency maturational curves exhibiting independent slope functions.

The first segmental curve component represents a steep latency function completed by the 50th week PCA. A slower, moderate curve slope follows the initial function ending about the second year of life. All prominent wave peaks show similar rapid maturation with the more rostral responses (waves III and V) characterized by the additional second curve slope. Fria and Doyle calculated wave slope ratios as a function of age. They found that all ratios were independent of age during the first stage suggesting that both peripheral and central changes contribute to latency maturation. However, Eggermont and Salamy (1988) and Gorga et al. (1989) refuted the two exponential model description of wave V latency in full term infants. Eggermont and Salamy (1988) studied 465 full-term and 178

TABLE 13.4. Normative Data: Means and standard deviations of wave I latency as a function of age (3 to 36 months) at 80 dB nHL.

Age Group (Months)	M (ms)	SD
3–6	1.594	0.171
6–9	1.592	0.161
9–12*	1.592	0.177
12–15	1.593	0.169
15–18	1.578	0.145
18–21	1.551	0.116
21–24	1.572	0.169
24–27	1.532	0.139
27–30	1.588	0.194
30–33	1.588	0.157
33–36	1.557	0.152

From Gorga et al. (1989). ABRs from children three months to three years of age: Normal patterns of response II. *Journal of Speech and Hearing Research, 32*, 281–288. Reprinted with the permission of the American Speech-Language-Hearing Association.

*Kolmogorov-Smirnov D-statistic significant at the 0.05 level.

TABLE 13.5. Normative Data: Means and standard deviations of wave V latency as a function of age (3 to 36 months) and intensity.

Level (dNHI_N)	Age Group (Months)	M (ms)	SD
20	3–6	8.717	0.526
	6–9	8.591	0.612
	9–12	8.310	0.537
	12–15	8.280	0.601
	15–18	8.329	0.609
	18–21	8.219	0.624
	21–24	8.052	0.582
	24–27	8.301	0.457
	27–30	7.981	0.417
	30–33	8.115	0.528
	33–36	8.103	0.684
40	3–6	7.426	0.358
	6–9	7.276	0.375
	9–12	7.009	0.366
	12–15	6.999	0.454
	15–18	6.949	0.381
	18–21	6.949	0.356
	21–24	6.794	0.334
	24–27	6.888	0.291
	27–30	6.753	0.333
	30–33	6.789	0.323
	33–36	6.815	0.378
60	3–6	6.734	0.331
	6–9	6.563	0.286
	9–12	6.310	0.290
	12–15	6.295	0.333
	15–18	6.242	0.245
	18–21	6.190	0.180
	21–24	6.138	0.287
	24–27	6.088	0.224
	27–30	6.082	0.283
	30–33	6.073	0.310
	33–36	6.062	0.307
80	3–6	6.253	0.321
	6–9	6.101	0.265
	9–12	5.899	0.268
	12–15	5.913	0.273
	15–18	5.845	0.267
	18–21	5.736	0.194
	21–24	5.712	0.262
	24–27	5.711	0.187
	27–30	5.602	0.223
	30–33	5.675	0.267
	33–36	5.678	0.273

From Gorga et al. (1989). ABRs from children three months to three years of age: Normal patterns of response II. *Journal of Speech and Hearing Research, 32*, 281–288. Reprinted with the permission of the American Speech-Language-Hearing Association.

preterm infants, and found no difference in brainstem maturation as reported by the I–V latency between infant groups but did find differences in absolute latencies. They attributed these differences to possible mild conductive hearing loss and damage to the cochlea due to the administration of ototoxic medications in the preterm population.

Because of these measurable differences in the rate of wave maturation, IWIs also show age dependencies with the greatest changes occurring between 30 weeks GA and term (Despland and Galambos, 1980; Fawer and Dubowitz, 1982; Salamy et al., 1975; Stockard and Westmoreland, 1981). Figure 13.5 demonstrates the effects of age on the ABR interwave intervals. At term, wave I–V latency is about 5.0 ms (Gorga et al., 1987; 1989; Jacobson et al., 1982). The IWI will continue to decrease systematically until wave V reaches adult value. Gorga et al. (1989) reported a 0.5 ms decrease in IWI latency from term to 3 to 6 months of age and a further reduction of about 0.5 ms from 6 months to adult value. Thus, the effects of age on latency dictate specific norms for reliable clinical assessment.

TABLE 13.6. Normative Data: Means and standard deviations of interwave interval latencies as a function of age (3 to 36 months) and intensity.

Interpeak Latency Difference	Age Group (Months)	M (ms)	SD
I–III	3–6	2.523	0.215
	6–9	2.416	0.225
	9–12	2.313	0.235
	12–15	2.313	0.149
	15–18	2.258	0.157
	18–21	2.259	0.238
	21–24	2.168	0.206
	24–27	2.278	0.172
	27–30	2.099	0.137
	30–33	2.210	0.157
	33–36	2.171	0.197
III–V	3–6	2.128	0.215
	6–9	2.082	0.215
	9–12	1.992	0.199
	12–15	2.006	0.219
	15–18	1.999	0.163
	18–21	1.992	0.189
	21–24	1.959	0.195
	24–27	1.912	0.182
	27–30	1.915	0.155
	30–33	1.904	0.180
	33–36	1.937	0.174
I–V	3–6	4.653	0.287
	6–9	4.502	0.270
	9–12	4.306	0.285
	12–15	4.320	0.240
	15–18	4.252	0.224
	18–21	4.182	0.227
	21–24	4.140	0.248
	24–27	4.197	0.171
	27–30	4.015	0.215
	30–33	4.117	0.226
	33–36	4.121	0.251

From Gorga et al. (1989). ABRs from children three months to three years of age: Normal patterns of response II. *Journal of Speech and Hearing Research, 32*, 281–288. Reprinted with the permission of the American Speech-Language-Hearing Association.

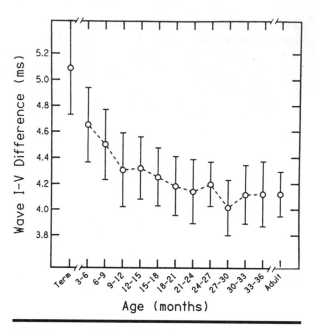

FIGURE 13.5. Auditory brainstem response (ABR) means and standard deviations for the I–V interwave interval (IWI) values plotted as a function of age at 80 dB nHL.

From Gorga et al. (1989). ABRs from children three months to three years of age: Normal patterns of response II. *Journal of Speech and Hearing Research, 32*, 281–288. Reprinted with the permission of the American Speech-Language-Hearing Association.

Healthy and premature high risk infants differ significantly, adding to the complexity of normative data collection (Salamy et al., 1980). For example, in premature infants, the rate of latency reduction for wave V is about 0.2 to 0.3 ms/wk as GA increases from 30 to 40 weeks and about 0.1 to 0.2 ms/wk for wave I (Despland and Galambos, 1980; Fawer and Dubowitz, 1982; Hecox and Burkard, 1982). To avoid maturational effects that may further complicate newborn assessment, it is recommended that ABR testing should be deferred until the infant is medically stable, off ototoxic medications, breathing unassisted and can be tested in an open crib. For an indepth review of the auditory maturational effect on the ABR, see Chapter 12, Salamy et al., *Neurodevelopment and Auditory Function in Preterm Infants.*

Gender. In the newborn, gender is not a significant factor in ABR response measures (Mochizuki, Go, Ohkubo, et al., 1982). Stockard et al. (1979) tested 77 normal term babies and found no statistical gender differences in IWIs. These findings were confirmed by Jacobson et al. (1982) who reported ABR results for 124 newborns between term and two months of age. They found no significant latency changes attributable to gender and suggested that for this age category, response measurement could be merged for clinical assessment without statistical variance. Other clinical support comes from a larger study by Durieux-Smith and colleagues (1985) who tested 434 newborns ranging in age from 32 to 56 weeks GA and found no difference in ABR latency or amplitude between gender. Conflicting data have been reported (Sanders, Duncan, and McCullough, 1979; Cox et al., 1981; Pauwels, Vogeleer, Clement, et al., 1982), although differences in peripheral hearing and neurologic status, transducers, and correct GA estimates may contribute to these apparent gender differences.

Temperature. The effects of decreasing body temperature will tend to prolong absolute and relative latency and decrease response amplitude. Typically, temperature is not a concern for most practical applications of newborn and infant ABR. However, for the premature infant where hypothermia may be encountered, core temperature must be closely monitored. Stockard et al. (1978) reported that a reduction in mean esophageal temperature less than 35°C produced IWI prolongation and associated amplitude decreases. These findings have been confirmed by others (Hall, Bull, and Cronau, 1988; Marshall and Donchin, 1981; Picton et al., 1981) and are similar to those demonstrated in the rat (Schorn, Lennon, and Bickford, 1977). Therefore, a knowledge of core body temperature is recommended when testing newborns and infants who may be monitored during surgery, on life support systems, or are generally physically compromised (e.g., shock).

Hearing Status. A prime clinical feature in pediatric ABR analysis is the identification of wave I. Because of its stability under most diverse conditions, this component latency serves as a benchmark of peripheral integrity. The absolute latency values of waves I and V provide information about the functional status (i.e., hearing sensitivity, auditory pathology) of the auditory pathway. The relationship between electrophysiologic and behavioral threshold has been established. Lary et al. (1985) and van Zanten, Brocaar, Fetter, et al. (1988) have shown that mildly elevated ABR click threshold levels decrease with increasing PCA in infants born prematurely. Galambos et al. (1982) reported that ABR click thresholds reach maturity by the first year of life, whereas Kaga and Tanaka (1980) found threshold differences in children up to 3 years of age.

The relationship between ABR and perceptual hearing threshold was examined by Sasama (1990) in a total of 115 infants and children ranging in age from less than 6 month to 3.5 years. All infants were suspected to have hearing impairment. A total of 103 were confirmed as hearing-impaired. Sasama observed an 86 percent agreement between ABR and behavioral thresholds in the hearing-impaired group whereas normal hearing children showed threshold distribution patterns that corresponded to that of normal hearing adults.

In a comprehensive comparison of click ABR and audiometric measures, Hyde, Riko, and Malizia (1990) examined the results of 1,367 ears in 713 children at risk for hearing loss. ABR measurement was conducted when infants ranged between 3 to 12 months whereas behavioral pure tone follow-up audiometry was conducted at 3 to 8 years of age. The authors reported excellent ABR accuracy for detecting average sensory hearing loss at 2000 and 4000 Hz in excess of 30 dB.

Middle Ear Pathology. The exact incidence of middle ear pathology in neonates is not known, but effusion and other forms of pathology are not uncommon in the intensive and special care nursery population. Depending on criteria and population studied, reported rates of middle ear abnormalities have ranged from 10 to over 30 percent (Balkany, Berman, Simmons, et al., 1978). Predisposing factors include sepsis, prolonged supine position, mechanical ventilation, reduction in swallowing activity and the normal anatomic features of neonates that influence eustachian tube function. Transient or permanent middle ear abnormalities are often cited as a factor of hearing screening outcome (Hall, Kripal, and Hepp, 1988; Hall, 1992; Stein, Ozdamar, Kraus, et al., 1983) and probably do contribute in some degree to the differences in failure rate among studies. Unrecognized middle ear pathology that resolves spontaneously between the time of newborn hearing screening in the hospital and the first follow-up audiologic assessment, for example at 3 to 6 months, contributes to over-referrals or *false-positive* ABR screening outcomes; that is, initial screening failures in infants without permanent hearing impairment.

One of the more recognized 1990 Joint Committee (Joint Committee, l991) risk criteria is the presence of head and neck, particularly external ear, deformities. An infant with congenital aural atresia, for example, is readily identified as at risk for auditory impairment because the deformity is quite obvious. These infants are likely to have serious, perhaps maximum (60 to 65 dB), conductive hearing impairments that remain permanent without surgical treatment. Fortunately, there are established clinical protocols for otologic, radiologic, and audiologic evaluation and management of congenital aural atresia (Hall et al., 1986; Jahrsdoerfer and Hall, 1986; Hall and Ghorayeb, 1991). With surgery (external and middle ear reconstruction), near normal hearing sensitivity can usually be restored.

More problematic, in terms of identification and management, are infants with normal-appearing external ears, yet middle ear pathology. Should an effort be made to identify these infants and, if so, how? The answer depends entirely on the philosophy and overall objectives of the hearing screening program. A screening program that is designed to identify only those infants with sensory, presumably permanent, hearing impairment would rely on a test protocol that passes infants with mild conductive hearing loss. The rationale underlying this approach is that minimal conductive hearing loss will not significantly influence speech-language development. On the other hand, when the objective of a screening program is to detect any hearing impairment, without regard to possible long-term effects on communication, the protocol should be sufficiently sensitive to identify mild persistent and even progressive conductive hearing losses.

If a newborn hearing screening protocol calls for ABR recording at 35 dB nHL and a rather simple analysis strategy, wherein response presence is considered a *pass* and response absence is considered a *fail,* then it is likely that some infants with middle ear pathology will *pass* the screening and remain undetected. Clearly, a relatively high proportion of infants with mild conductive hearing impairment will *pass* the screening, whereas none with moderate-to-severe conductive hearing impairment will *pass* with this response analysis approach. Two other common screening protocols, however, are likely to identify virtually all infants with middle ear pathology that results in conductive hearing impairment. The first of these, described previously in this chapter (*Response Analysis*), relies on analysis of ABR wave V latency in determining whether the screening outcome is a *pass* or a *fail.* The dominant effect of conductive hearing impairment on ABR is to delay absolute latency values (Figure 13.6). Essentially, the effective intensity level of the stimulus (the intensity actually reaching the cochlea) is reduced by the degree of the conductive component, at least in the 1000 to 4000 Hz region. As an example, with even a very mild conductive loss of 20 dB the intensity of the click stimulus activating the cochlea is only 15 dB (35 dB stimulus minus 20 dB attenuation induced by the conductive loss). Naturally, latency of ABR wave V for the 15 dB effective stimulus level will be markedly prolonged in comparison to a 35 dB intensity level in an ear without conductive loss.

The second screening approach that will usually detect even mild conductive hearing impairment utilizes a high-intensity click stimulus (e.g., 75 dB nHL), as well as a low level (e.g., 35 dB nHL) stimulus level. At the higher level, there will be for most infants a clear wave I in the ABR waveform. By comparing wave I latency with normative data, conductive hearing impairments will in most cases be readily detected (Fria, 1985; Fria and Sabo, 1980; van der Drift, Brocaar, and van Zanten, 1988). Management of infants with ABR evidence of conductive hearing impairment can vary. Some clinicians might favor medical consultation and perhaps management before

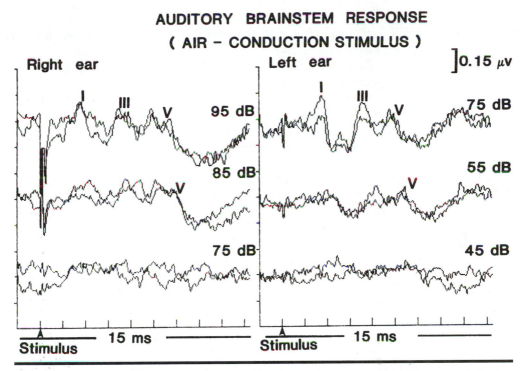

FIGURE 13.6.   Auditory brainstem response (ABR) waveforms recorded with air conduction stimulation from a two month old infant with congenital aural atresia on the right and a normal appearing external ear on the left. With right ear stimulation at 95 dB nHL, latency values for wave V (7.50 ms) and wave I (2.76 ms) were markedly delayed, consistent with severe conductive hearing impairment. Left ear stimulation also produced delayed absolute ABR wave latencies suggesting the presence of a conductive component.

hospital discharge. Others might defer this action until the conductive hearing impairment is confirmed by a comprehensive follow-up assessment consisting of ABR latency intensity functions, bone conduction ABR recordings, tympanometry, and perhaps, behavioral audiometry. With any newborn hearing screening program, it is important to rule out potentially treatable middle ear pathology before initiating amplification and other forms of audiologic management.

Activity Level.   A critical assessment for the accurate evaluation of the newborn is the activity level at the time of testing. Clinical experience has shown that significantly different outcomes can be predicted from the same newborn when asleep or quietly resting versus in

an active state (Jacobson and Spahr, 1990). Although sleep has little effect on the ABR in adults (Amadeo and Shagass, 1973; Sohmer, Gafni, and Chisin, 1978), the level of consciousness likely increases the false-positive rate observed in the newborn. Artifacts introduced into the record due to movement may contaminate and even obscure the morphology of the wave configuration, making proper wave peak identification challenging (Weber, 1983).

In an attempt to determine the influence of movement artifact on the newborn ABR, McCall and Ferraro (1991) reported the results of 52 stable neonates at risk for hearing loss. McCall and Ferraro divided neonates into three activity levels and found significantly different pass-fail findings. Using a 30 dB click intensity, they reported failure rates of 37 and 10 percent for the active versus asleep groups, respectively. They recommend that test failure under active conditions should be repeated under quiet conditions to eliminate the question of movement artifact. Figure 13.7 shows a series of ABR traces recorded from a seven-month-old infant tested in natural sleep. Using sleep as the acceptable criterion, these *textbook* waves are readily obtainable and their reproducibility should be the goal of every clinician.

The alternative to testing during natural sleep is the use of sedation. Although sedation definitely has a place in ABR testing, we do not advocate the use of sedation in the neonate or the very young infant population. Since the physical health of most high risk neonates is compromised, the use of sedation may be medically contraindicated. Further, the administration of sedation must occur under medical supervision, and at a minimum, oxygen monitoring is required. Obviously, this is not always possible outside a medical setting. Thus, we recommend for infants less than seven

months of age that a simple series of steps be used whenever testing. They include sleep deprivation, testing to coincide with feeding and testing in a quiet, darkened environment. It is best to contact the parent/caregiver and provide both written and verbal instructions immediately prior to testing to insure the importance of a cooperative infant. However, even in the best of circumstances, infants do not always cooperate. When all "tricks" have failed, we encourage rescheduling of the infant rather than providing potentially misleading and spurious test results.

STIMULUS VARIABLES

Intensity. Any change in stimulus intensity will directly affect response latency and amplitude. Generally, as intensity is increased, wave component latency decreases whereas amplitude increases. Figure 13.8 illustrates typical changes in latency and amplitude as intensity is attenuated. The wave V latency shifts with intensity at a rate of about 0.035 ms/dB (Jacobson et

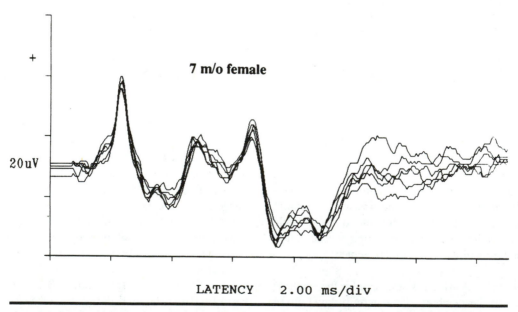

FIGURE 13.7. A series of auditory brainstem response (ABR) traces obtained from a seven-month-old infant tested in natural sleep. Each trace represents the sum of 2000 click stimuli at 85 dB nHL.

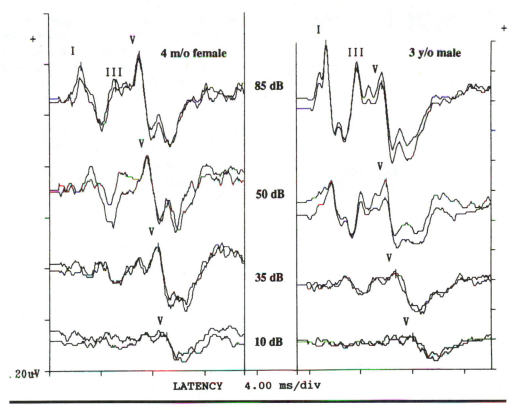

FIGURE 13.8.   The effects of intensity on the auditory brainstem response (ABR) obtained from a four-month-old infant (left) and a three-year-old child (right). Latency increases and amplitude decreases systematically as a function of decreasing intensity. Wave morphology also changes dramatically with decreased intensity.

al., 1982; Hecox and Galambos, 1974; Schulman-Galambos and Galambos, 1975). In a healthy term infant, wave V latency is observed at about 6.8 to 7.0 ms for a 60 dB nHL click stimulus.

The rate of wave I latency change with intensity has been more controversial. Stockard et al. (1979) imply two *transitional zones* for infant wave I measurement. Between 70 and 60 dB and 40 to 30 dB nHL, the magnitude of wave I latency shift is greater than that of wave V. Due to this differential effect between peripheral and central transmission, they reported a reduction in IWI as intensity is decreased. In contrast, other investigators (Jacobson et al., 1982; Salamy, 1984) reported similar latency shifts for waves I and V

resulting in a constant IWI as a function of intensity. The differences reported in IWI latency may be explained by the measurement of wave I. At higher intensities, wave I will often exhibit a bifid peak separation differing by as much as 0.4 ms (Jacobson et al., 1981). If peak selection is not consistent at varying intensity levels, calculation of the IWI may remain problematic.

As shown in Figure 13.9, the slope of wave V latency has been used as a clinical tool to evaluate the degree and pathology of the hearing loss (Hecox, 1975; Picton and Smith, 1978). This latency-intensity (L-I) function is described in terms of latency change per dB attenuation and measured in μs. In term infants, the L-I function is approximately 40 μs/dB (Galambos and

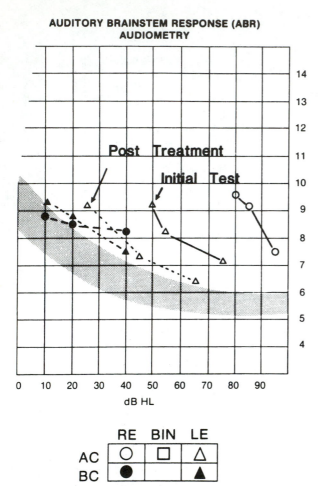

AUDITORY BRAINSTEM RESPONSE (ABR) AUDIOMETRY

Post Treatment

Initial Test

0   10   20   30   40   50   60   70   80   90

dB HL

	RE	BIN	LE
AC	○	□	△
BC	●		▲

FIGURE 13.9. Auditory brainstem response (ABR) latency-intensity (L-I) functions for a two-month infant with congenital aural atresia on the right and a normal appearing external ear on the left. Waveforms for this patient were shown in Figure 13.6. Note the shift in the (L-I) function for both ears, greater on the right ear. This pattern is consistent with middle ear pathology and conductive hearing impairment. The presence of conductive hearing impairment is confirmed by the normal (L-I) functions for bone conduction stimulation.

Hecox, 1978; Hecox, 1975). Slope configuration greater than 60 μs/dB has been associated with predominantly high frequency sensory hearing loss (Hecox and Jacobson, 1984).

Rate.   A change in the stimulus repetition rate will affect the latency, amplitude, and morphology of individual wave components. For infants, an increase in rate will shift wave latency while reducing amplitude (Salamy et al., 1978; Stockard et al., 1979; Zimmerman et al., 1987). Despland and Galambos (1980) have reported that infants as young as 32 weeks GA will respond to click stimuli at rates as high as 80/sec.

The effects of rate are displayed in Figure 13.10. An infant of less than eight months would be expected to produce a wave V shift of about 0.8 to 1.0 ms for a 70/sec rate shift whereas wave I will increase by 0.4 ms (Picton et al., 1981). Durieux-Smith and associates (1985) observed latency shifts of 1.3 ms between 11 and 61/sec for 30 week GA premature newborns and shifts of 0.6 ms for a group of 4 month old infants generating a mean slope of 38 μsec/wk. Zimmerman et al. (1987) studied 22 full-term normal newborns with GA of 39, 40, and 41 weeks for the first 6 months of life. These authors used three rates of click stimuli (11, 33, and 66/sec) to monitor ABR latency. They showed statistically significant increases in latency for wave I and wave V latency differences on the same order as reported by Picton et al. As a consequence, increasing repetition rate will result in an increase in the IWI latency and it is likely that the differences will be more pronounced for premature infants (Picton et al., 1981; Zimmerman et al., 1987).

Wave amplitude is also affected by changes in repetition rate. Wave V shows the least change, maintaining approximately 85% of its original amplitude at rates up to 80/sec (Picton, Taylor, Durieux-Smith, et al., 1986). In comparison, wave I amplitude is dramatically diminished by rate increase (Durieux-Smith et al., 1985). This difference in wave amplitude reduction results in an increase V/I amplitude ratio. To date, studies of increased rate in newborns have not produced any indications of habituation (Salamy and McKean, 1976), fatigue (Schulman-Galambos and Galambos, 1975), or refractoriness (Salamy, 1984). See Chapter 12, Salamy et al., *Neurodevelopment and Auditory Function in Preterm Infants* for developmental patterns associated with various effects on wave amplitude.

Clinically, rate plays an important role in the assessment of the pediatric population. As rate increases, the

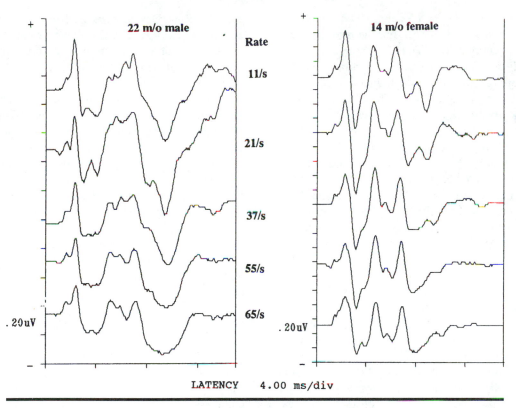

FIGURE 13.10. Auditory brainstem response (ABR) rate study. Traces were obtained from a 22-month-old infant (left) and a 14-month-old infant (right) at 11, 21, 37, 55, and 65/sec. Note the overall latency shift for all wave peak components as rate increases.

required time to record an equivalent number of averaged traces is reduced. Time is obviously a critical factor in the evaluation of an unsedated or uncooperative infant. For example, at a rate of 10/sec, it requires approximately 13 minutes to average 2000 responses for two ears, replicating trials. However, at 37/sec, a common rate for newborn screening or threshold measures, about four minutes is necessary to perform the same task. Rates of 20 to 40/sec have been reported most efficient for wave I and V identification (Picton, Liden, Hasmel, et al., 1983).

Polarity. During response averaging, stimuli may be presented with either constant initial polarity (i.e., condensation or rarefaction) or alternating polarity. In the absence of clinical standards and problems observed in earphone polarity from various manufacturers (Cann and Knott, 1979), it is advantageous to determine the acoustic profile of the stimulus at the tympanic membrane rather than the electrical drive to the transducer. Initial positive pressure or inward movement of the eardrum is caused by condensation stimulus polarity. A rarefaction stimulus will initially move the eardrum outward by a negative pressure. Only the corresponding basilar membrane movement associated with rarefaction polarity is reported to excite primary auditory neurons (Kiang, Watanabe, and Thomas, 1965). See Chapter 4, Gorga et al., *Stimulus Calibration in AEP Measurements,* for a descriptive method of polarity measurement.

There is general agreement concerning the effects of stimulus polarity on wave morphology in neonates

(Chiappa, Gladstone, and Young, 1979; Picton et al., 1981; Stockard et al., 1979). For the most part, when using conventional (e.g., TDH-39) earphones, alternating polarity tends to reduce electric artifact that affects wave I measurement, although almost exclusively at high intensity stimulus levels. There is less consensus about polarity influence on wave latency. The more rostral the generation of the wave component, the less sensitive the effects of stimulus polarity (Ornitz, Mo, Olson, et al., 1980; Terkildsen and Osterhammel, 1981). For example, in adults with normal hearing, wave I usually produces earlier latencies to rarefaction stimuli (Coats and Martin, 1977; Stockard et al., 1978, 1979) whereas wave V latency response differences are negligible. With a stable wave V latency, extended IWI's have been reported in newborns to rarefaction click stimuli (Stockard et al., 1979).

Recently, these polarity assumptions have been challenged. Schwartz et al. (1989) in a group of 20 preterm infants demonstrated that condensation clicks resulted in reduced ABR amplitudes when compared to rarefaction stimuli among infants. They also reported that polarity (i.e., condensation versus rarefaction) had no significant effect on response latency for either waves I, III, or V. Based on their findings, a cautious approach toward polarity selection is mandated. Logically, the need for independent norms for different click stimulus polarity should be based on clinic experience and specific diagnostic needs.

Transducers.   Until recently, conventional audiometric earphones were used routinely in AEP measurement. For neonates and infants, testing was usually accomplished by removing the earphone cushion and either supporting the TDH-39/49 within the crib or bassinet (e.g., folded blanket or hand-held). This technique introduces a number of problems including potential ear canal collapse, unpredictable oscillations in the frequency spectrum (low-frequency leakage), intensity variation of the click signal and no effective ambient noise attenuation. These variables lead to both measurement and interpretation errors and likely contribute to a high false-positive rate in newborn hearing screening studies (Gorga, Reiland, and Beauchaine, 1988; Hall et al., 1988; Horton, Rubin, Reiland, et al., 1985; Jacobson et al., 1990; Ruth, Dey-Sigman, and Mills, 1985; Schwartz et al., 1989). Gorga et al. (1988) have estimated that as many as half of all newborn hearing screening failures may be attributed to ear canal collapse secondary to conventional earphone placement.

To compensate for these technical problems, insert earphones (tube phones) have been used successfully in the neonate population. With the commercial introduction of the Etymotic insert foam plugs and other methods of insert probe tip modification, the problem of ear canal collapse appears alleviated (Killion, 1984). Previous findings in adults have shown that when the duration of signal transmission due to tube length is compensated, an insert and a circumaural earphone produced similar ABR latency measures (Beauchaine, Kaminshi, and Gorga, 1987). Due to differences in transducers, it is essential to establish new normative data when insertion transducers are employed. Clinical experience (Jacobson and Jacobson, 1987) in newborns and infants has shown that a simple correction factor does not always compensate for latency differences as similarly demonstrated in adults. Increases in sound pressure levels obtained in smaller canal enclosures likely increase SPL resulting in shortened latency expectations.

Bone Vibrators.   We recommend bone conduction stimulation during follow-up ABR evaluation of auditory sensitivity (not for routine screening) when air-conduction stimulation produces a response consistent with conductive hearing impairment, (i.e., delayed absolute latencies). Although adequate bone conduction stimulation can be presented anywhere on the head, the two most common vibrator placements are the mastoid bone and the frontal bone (forehead). Frontal placement produces more reliable threshold results but mastoid placement is traditionally used, probably because it permits a higher effective intensity level to reach the cochlea.

There are several commercially available bone conduction vibrators, including the Radioear models B-70A, B-71 and B-72. Among these, the B-72 produces significantly greater acoustic radiation than the B-71. Recent clinical reports have also described the Pracitronic model KH 70, a German bone vibrator with a relatively smoother and wider frequency response (Dolan and Morris, 1990; Frank and Crandell, 1986). Numerous authors note that bone vibrator output declines in the high-frequency region which is important for click stimulation (Yang, Rupert, and Moushegian, 1987; Yang, Stuart, Stenstrom, et al., 1991; Weber, 1983; Mauldin and Jerger, 1979; Schwartz and Berry, 1985). Output levels from three commercially available bone vibrators were compared with those of two air conduction earphones (TDH-49 and a hearing aid transducer plus insert plug) by Schwartz, Larson, and De Chiccicca (1985). The air conduction transducers produced a relatively flat frequency response, whereas each of the bone conduction vibrators had energy predominantly in the 2000 Hz region, with maximum output not exceeding 35 dB HL. Of the three bone vibrators, the B-70 permitted greater output. The preceding information on bone vibrators may not accurately reflect their potential for ABR measurement (Gorga and Thornton, 1989). The reduction of bone vibrator output for higher frequencies, when expressed in units of force, may not necessarily correspond to reduced effective intensity level in this audiometric region. That is, effective output of the bone vibrator is actually greater in the higher frequency region.

Other problems shared by bone vibrators are excessive distortion and inter-subject variability. The distortion, which is more pronounced with higher frequencies, reduces or may even eliminate frequency specific ABR stimulation (Harder, Arlinger, and Kylen, 1983). The static force of bone vibrator placement is another often overlooked factor in the effectiveness of bone conduction stimulation. Variability in bone vibrator force is due to inconsistencies in placement site, the pressure with which the vibrator is held to the skull, and skull impedance (Arlinger and Kylen, 1977). In a recent study, Stuart, Yang, and Stenstrom (1990) demonstrated that changes in bone vibrator placement within the temporal bone region of newborn infants produced significantly different effects on ABR wave V latency. In comparison to air-conduction stimulation, the bone-conduction stimulation mode results in a decrease in effective intensity of approximately 40 to 45 dB. That is, if a bone vibrator is plugged into the earphone stimulus jack of an evoked response system, the actual

output even at a maximum attenuator dial or instrument intensity reading of 95 dB may be only 55 dB nHL or less.

There is convincing evidence that bone conduction ABR is a clinically feasible technique in infants (Hall, 1992; Hooks and Weber, 1984; Stapells and Ruben, 1989; Stuart et al., 1990; Yang et al., 1987; Yang et al., 1991). Contrary to expectations for adult subjects, latencies for ABR waves I, III and V are shorter in infants' bone-conduction than air-conduction stimuli (Yang et al., 1987). A possible explanation for this finding relates to the pattern of cochlear development in the newborn. In the immature cochlea, responsiveness to low frequency stimuli develops initially in the basal regions, the location for high frequency responsiveness in the adult cochlea (Rubel and Ryals, 1983).

Cornacchia, Martini, and Morra (1983) studied bone conduction ABR in infants (16 to 20 months), and young adults. Alternating clicks were presented to the forehead via bone-conduction with a Radioear B-70A vibrator. As expected, ABR latencies in general were greater for adults than infants. Interestingly, the study showed the convergence of wave V latency values for adults versus children with decreasing intensity of the air-conduction, but not bone-conduction stimuli. That is, bone-conduction latency-intensity functions were parallel for adults and infants. However, for air-conduction stimuli, there was an adult versus infant wave V latency difference of 0.58 ms at high-intensity levels, but a difference of only 0.08 msec at 20 dB nHL. In contrast, however, Gorga et al. (1989) found parallel wave V latency-intensity functions for adults (N=20) versus infants (N=1,120) over the range from 20 to 80 dB HL.

There is clinical evidence that bone conduction ABR assessment can be useful in circumventing the masking dilemma associated with behavioral pure tone hearing assessment (Hall, Brown, Tompkins, and Gray, 1986; Hall, 1992; Jahrsdoerfer, Yeakley, Hall, et al., 1986; Jahrsdoerfer and Hall, 1986; Scherg, 1980; Tompkins, Hall, Jacobson, et al., 1991). The main premise underlying this clinical application is that a wave I component observed from an electrode located on or near the ear ipsilateral to the stimulus confirms contribution of the stimulated ear to the response, whether or not masking is presented to the non-test ear. Analysis of the waveform simultaneously recorded with an electrode on the ear contralateral to the stimulus is also helpful. If in the contralateral waveform there is no peak corresponding to the ipsilateral wave I (in the same latency region), one has further assurance that the presumed ipsilateral component is indeed wave I (Figure 13.11).

In summary, bone-conduction stimulation in clinical ABR measurement is underutilized, particularly in

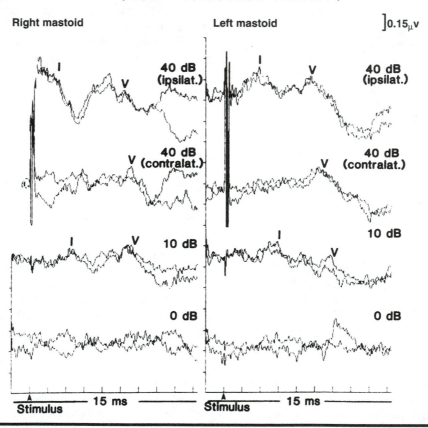

AUDITORY BRAINSTEM RESPONSE
(BONE – CONDUCTION STIMULUS)

FIGURE 13.11. Auditory brainstem response (ABR) waveforms recorded with bone conduction stimulation from a two-month-old infant with congenital aural atresia on the right and a normal-appearing external ear on the left. Air conduction ABR waveforms for this patient were shown in Figure 13.6 and the patient's ABR L-I functions were shown in Figure 13.8. With right and left ear stimulation at 95 dB nHL, there was a clear and reliable wave I component with an ipsilateral inverting electrode, whereas no wave I component with an simultaneous contralateral inverting electrode recording. This is evidence that the bone-conduction waveforms are due to stimulation of the test ear, rather than crossover to the nontest ear, even though masking was not used in the nontest ear.

infants and children. There are probably a variety of reasons for this trend. The first is the limitation in maximum effective intensity level (about 50 to 55 dB nHL) for bone-conduction stimulation. Second, problems encountered in recording a clear bone-conduction ABR in adult subjects may have led to the assumption that bone-conduction ABRs are not clinically feasible or useful for assessing sensory hearing sensitivity in infants and young children. In fact, in normal-hearing infants and young children who tend to have better than average sensory hearing sensitivity in the 1000 to 4000 Hz region compared to adults, the dynamic intensity range for bone-conduction ABR stimuli may be substantially larger. Further, a distinct wave I component can often be consistently recorded with a bone-conducted stimulus in these younger subjects.

Another possible limitation has to do with the electromagnetic energy radiating from bone vibrators and the resultant stimulus artifact in ABR recordings. This is intensified when the mastoid is used for bone vibrator placement and as a site for the inverting electrode in combination with a single polarity (i.e., rarefaction or condensation) versus alternating polarity click stimulus. Two simple technical modifications can minimize these problems. Stimulus artifact can be reduced by use of earlobe or ear canal electrodes and an alternating polarity click (Hall, 1992).

Finally, the masking dilemma and the need for contralateral masking is cited in discussions of problems associated with bone conduction ABR measurement (Weber, 1983). The head offers little or no attenuation (10 dB or less) for bone-conduction stimulation, at least in adult subjects. As a result, stimuli presented via bone conduction to one mastoid may equally activate each cochlea. Some authors (see Chapter 15, Weber and Jacobson, *Newborn Hearing Screening*) have stated rather categorically that the nontest ear must be routinely masked in ABR assessment by air conduction or bone conduction, in order to rule out a contribution to the response from unintended stimulation of the better hearing, nontest ear. However, the presence of a clear wave I component within the normal latency region from the electrode array ipsilateral to the stimulus, or a wave V of normal latency is strong evidence that the ABR is not due to stimulation of the nontest ear. Thus,

the likelihood of obtaining ear specific bone conduction ABR data is enhanced in infants and may contribute importantly to audiologic and medical management.

Recording Variables

Filters. The recording of ABR activity is affected by both physiologic and electrodynamic events. One major stumbling block in most electrophysiologic recordings is that subcortical synchronized neural discharge patterns are several magnitudes smaller than random EEG, thus obscuring the activity of interest. In order to compensate for this voltage mismatch, bandpass filtering has been introduced as one method of improving the signal-to-noise ratio during routine measurement. The degree of improvement is dependent on the spectra of the signal and the noise component (Hyde, 1985). During adult ABR neurodiagnostic evaluation using click stimuli, band-pass settings of 100 to 1500 or 3000 Hz are usually adequate for definitive results. However, high-pass filter settings of 20 to 30 Hz are required for audiologic applications of low-frequency, low-intensity stimuli (Stapells and Picton, 1981; Suzuki, Harai, and Horiuchi, 1977; Suzuki, Sakabe, and Miyashita, 1982). Although a narrowing of band-pass filter settings (e.g., high-pass filter cutoff >150 Hz) may be used in cases of severe myogenic artifact and electrical interference, there is a concomitant distortion of ABR latency and amplitude (Campbell and Leandri, 1984; Laukli and Mair, 1981) and a major reduction of the wave V spectral energy content (Kavanagh, Domico, Franks, et al., 1988; Kevanishvili and Aphonchenko, 1979). Using suggested reduced high-pass cutoff filter settings, wave V amplitude may increase by as much as 20%.

Compared to the adult ABR, the spectral content of an infant ABR response, particularly at high intensities, has greater low-frequency energy (Rubel, 1985). Therefore it is common practice to extend the high-pass filter setting downward from 100 to 20 or 30 Hz during infant recording to enhance wave V amplitude (Hall et al., 1985; Hyde, 1985; Kavanagh et al., 1988). On the average, click ABR thresholds for normal infants can improve by 3 dB using a 30 Hz filter setting (Stapells, 1990).

Scalp distribution. Differential pre-amplifiers are most commonly used in ABR measurement as a method of improving the signal-to-noise ratio. A differential recording requires input at a minimum of three electrodes, the *non-inverting,* the *inverting,* and the *common.* Since ABR activity is generated at subcortical levels, volume conducted and monitored at the scalp as far-field potentials, the frequently used terms *active* and *reference* are not applicable in this context and are discouraged. See Chapter 1, Jacobson, *Prelude to Auditory Evoked Potentials,* and Chapter 2, Møller, *Neural Generators of Auditory Evoked Potentials,* for an overview of volume conduction in electrophysiologic monitoring.

It is reasonable to assume that correct electrode placement would maximize the largest amplitude and most reliable ABR peak measurement. With newborns and infants, a single channel recording using a *vertical* electrode montage is most common, although 2-channel recordings have also been advocated (Schwartz and Schwartz, 1991). The wave V response is characteristically recorded between the vertex (Cz) or forehead (Fz) and either the mastoid or earlobe ipsilateral to the stimuli, although a noncephalic site may produce greater amplitude wave V recordings. Wave I in contrast is most robust when measured in a horizontal (i.e., earlobe to earlobe) configuration (Terkildsen and Osterhammel, 1981). Hecox and Burkard (1982) have shown that a horizontal montage will produce a larger wave V amplitude 40 percent more often than a vertical montage for infants less than eight months old, whereas wave I amplitude is larger in 70 percent of the cases. Multi-channel evoked potential systems allow greater flexibility with regard to electrode placement and recording sites and under certain circumstances, provide additional information not demonstrated using conventional single channel recordings.

Test Environment. The location for ABR recording is predicated on the rationale for testing (screening, threshold assessment, or neurotologic evaluation), infant status and the facility. Most often, the ideal site (an electrically shielded audiologic test suite) is not feasible since practical considerations usually dictate less than optimum settings. For example, high-risk infants on life support systems cannot be transferred out of special care facilities, thus requiring the testing of neonates to be accomplished in hostile environments. Ambient noise levels are typically in excess of 60 dBA and may be higher when infants are confined to isolettes (Bess, Peek, and Chapman, 1979; Jacobson and Mencher, 1981; Mjoen, Langlset, Tangsrud, et al., 1982; Mitchell, 1984). When using intensity levels less than ambient noise level, latency prolongations, and thresholds elevations should be anticipated (Richmond, Konkle, and Potsic, 1986).

Another primary environmental concern is electrical interference frequently found in NICU facilities caused by line noise (60 Hz) and other electric monitoring devices. Typically, high-risk infants are in isolettes with respiratory monitors and cardiac catheters. Temperature is controlled with either lights or warming blankets. All electrical devices are potential hazards for electrophysiologic assessment. If testing is critical and cannot be postponed until the infant can be moved to a more favorable setting, recommendations include technical alterations (e.g., insert earphones) to minimize the effects of noise and the use of an isolation transformer to compensate for electrical interference. Under such conditions, a cautious approach to interpretation is recommended.

Analysis Window. The recording of ABR activity in normal adults is usually limited to the first 10 ms poststimulus onset. However, there are several intervening factors that must be taken into account when threshold sensitivity is required. For example, the use of low-frequency tone bursts which excite apical regions of the cochlea tend to produce wave V response latency in excess of 10 ms (see Chapter 11, Stapells et al., *Electrophysiologic Measures of Frequency-Specific Auditory Function*). Auditory pathology, especially conductive hearing loss which prolongs absolute wave peak latencies, may obscure peak detection since measurable wave components can exceed the 10 ms analysis window. Additionally, when premature infants are tested prior to full-term adjusted age, incomplete maturation of the auditory system will introduce significantly delayed peak latency responses (see Chapter 12, Salamy et al., *Neurodevelopment and Auditory Function in Preterm Infants.*

The consensus of the clinical community recommends the use of 15 or 20 ms analysis latency epochs for routine newborn and infant application (Hall and Tucker, 1988; Jacobson et al., 1982; Ruth et al., 1985). Schwartz and Schwartz (1991) have recommended this latency expansion because: 1) the interval beyond 10 ms represents a means of estimating background noise levels, and 2) there is a greater likelihood of observing waves III and V to low intensity stimulus levels with the extended window.

Contralateral Recording.   As stated earlier, conventional infant ABR recording minimally requires the use of three electrodes. The most commonly used electrode placement for infants is a vertical montage with recording electrodes attached between either the vertex or forehead and the earlobe or mastoid of the stimulated ear. In the newborn and infant, this montage typically allows the on-line collection of three primary wave peaks; however, on occasion, ipsilateral recordings may be obscured and peak identification limited. Under these conditions, the use of simultaneous contralateral recordings have been recommended. Figure 13.12 illustrates the differences demonstrated in ipsilateral versus contralateral recordings from an infant ABR trace. As correctly pointed out by Stapells and Mosseri (1991) the terms *ipsilateral* and *contralateral* do not refer to the generators of the response but rather the site of the inverting electrode to the stimulated ear.

The maturation of the contralateral response does not follow the same time course as that of the ipsilateral recording (Edwards, Durieux-Smith, and Picton, 1985; Hatanaka, Shuto, Tosuhara, and Kobayashi, 1988; Salamy, Eldredge, and Wakeley, 1985; Hatanaka, Yasuhara, Hori, and Kobayashi; 1990). Typically, as age increases, contralateral wave recordings decrease in latency, and although amplitudes increase with age, responses are of such small magnitude they are more difficult to identify than their ipsilateral counterparts. Recently, Stapells and Mosseri (1991) recorded ipsilateral and contralateral responses from 37 infants aged 2 weeks to 20 months. Although contralateral response measures were consistent with previous reports, these investigators felt that due to smaller amplitudes, contralateral recordings were limited in their contribution to threshold measures, particularly prior to 9 months of age. Contralateral response measures were encouraged,

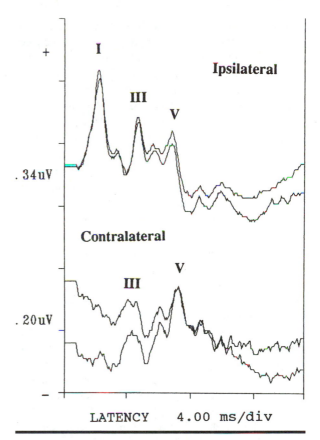

FIGURE 13.12.   Ipsilateral versus contralateral auditory brainstem response (ABR) recordings. Traces were obtained from a seven-month-old infant. Each trace represents the sum of 2000 click stimuli at 85 dB nHL. Note the absence of wave I on the contralateral recorded side.

however, when wave V peak latency was ambiguous. Stapells and Mosseri concluded that the observed differences of the ipsilateral and contralateral responses were likely due to dipole orientation of similar generators.

Electrode Types.   There are several different types of EEG electrodes used in infant evoked potential recording. Among the many varieties, a simple method of classification is either disposable or nondisposable. Within each category, several types exist and each are useful depending on subject status, recording conditions and evoked potential of interest. The nondisposable type usually consists of either a cup, flat disk, or needle electrode. Common to the cup (usually having a hole in the center for injection of conductive cream) or disk is an outer diameter of 4 to 10 mm that is attached to the scalp. These reusable electrodes are connected by an insulated lead wire to a connector plug. A useful modification of the cup is the *clip* electrode. Either one or two cup electrodes are connected in a fashion similar to a clothes pin and *clipped* on the earlobe. Depending on hospital policy, needle electrodes, which by their nature are invasive, are either immediately disposed of after use or gas sterilized and used repeatedly. In infant auditory monitoring, needle electrodes are least used and generally restricted for special applications (e.g., intraoperative or intensive care unit monitoring, or with burn victims). It is important to remember that needle electrodes always carry the added risk of infection. The proper handling and discarding (follow hospital policy) of such materials cannot be stressed sufficiently. In contrast, disposable electrodes may be metal, cloth, or plastic. They usually contain a self-adhesive surface and may contain a conductive gel. Cloth or plastic electrodes are usually attached to an insulated lead wire via an alligator clip. See Chapter 3, Hyde, *Signal Processing and Analysis,* for a detailed account of recording electrode properties.

There are as many ways of attaching electrodes to the scalp as there are clinicians. Every clinician seems to have his/her own special electrode cream/paste/gel, tape, and direction to place the electrodes. However, most important in any evoked potential recording is skin preparation prior to electrode placement. Most common is the use of a *prep* to remove dry superficial skin layers and/or any other oils or materials that would interfere in the impedance-conduction process. Once the prep is completed, we generally adhere to manufacturer's recommendation when applying conductive paste/creams. *Read the label!* Some conductive materials are not designed for infants.

Early in our experience, collodion was commonly used as an adhesive for cup or disk electrodes. However, because of the potential problems associated with its use (e.g., skin irritation, possible explosive hazard in confined areas when heated) most clinicians have switched to surgical tape or conductive *paste* as an alternative means of connection. With surgical tape, electrodes can be placed virtually anywhere on the scalp or skin and removed without discomfort. Certain pastes also act as a self-adhesive and once applied, electrodes are simply pushed into the paste for temporary bonding. One limitation of paste is that it tends to dry out over time, ultimately increasing contact impedance. In contrast, creams or gels present an adhesive problem for surgical tape because they remain moist.

SUMMARY

This chapter has provided an overview of normative ABR data and clinical insight based on the personal experience of the two authors. Obviously, individual experiences are influenced by a number of factors and what has worked for us may not be applicable for every reader. Information contained within this chapter should be looked on as clinical guidelines, not *gospel.* Nothing substitutes for "hands-on" experience.

REFERENCES

Adelman, C., Levi, H., Linder, N., and Sohmer, H. (1990). Neonatal auditory brain-stem response threshold and latency: 1 hour to 5 months. *Electroencephalography and Clinical Neurophysiology, 77,* 77–80.

Amadeo, M. and Shagass, C. (1973). Brief latency click-evoked potentials during waking and sleep in man. *Psychophysiology, 10,* 244–250.

Arlinger, S.D. and Kylen, P. (1977). Bone-conducted stimulation in electrocochleography. *Acta Otolaryngologica (Stockholm), 84,* 377–384.

Balkany, T.J., Berman, S.A., Simmons, M.A., and Jakef, B.W. (1978). Middle ear effusions in neonates. *Laryngoscope, 88,* 398–405.

Beauchaine, K.A., Kaminski, J.R., and Gorga, M.P. (1987). Comparison of Beyer DT48 and Etymotic insert earphones: Auditory brain stem response measurements. *Ear and Hearing, 8,* 292–297.

Bess, F.H. (1985). The minimally hearing-impaired child. *Ear and Hearing, 7,* 3–54.

Bess, F.H., Peek, B.F., and Chapman, J.J. (1979). Further observations on noise levels in infant incubators. *Pediatrics, 63,* 100–106.

Campbell and Leandri (1984). The effects of high pass filters on computer-reconstructed evoked potentials. *Electroencephalography and Clinical Neurophysiology, 34*, 125–133.

Cann, J. and Knott J. (1979). Polarity of acoustic click stimuli for eliciting brainstem auditory evoked responses: A proposed standard. *American Journal of EEG Technology, 19*, 125–132.

Cevette, M.J. (1984). Auditory brainstem response testing in the intensive care unit. *Seminars in Hearing, 5*, 57–69.

Chiappa, K.N., Gladstone, K.J., and Young, R.R. (1979). Brainstem auditory evoked responses: Studies of waveform variations in 50 normal human subjects. *Archives of Neurology, 36*, 81–87.

Coats, A.C. and Martin, J.L. (1977). Human auditory nerve action potentials and brainstem evoked responses. *Archives of Otolaryngology, 103*, 605–622.

Cone, B., Hecox, K., and Finitzo-Hieber T. (1977). The brainstem auditory evoked response in neonates: A narrative study. *Transcript of the American Academy of Ophthalmologists and Otolaryngologists, 84*, 188.

Cone-Wesson, B., Kurtzberg, D., and Vaughan, H.G. (1987). Electrophysiologic assessment of auditory pathways in high risk infants. *International Journal of Pediatric Otorhinolaryngology, 14*, 203–214,

Cornacchia, L., Martini, A., and Morra, B. (1983). Air and bone conduction brain stem responses in adults and infants. *Audiology, 22*, 430–437.

Cox, L.C. (1985). Infant assessment: Developmental and age-related considerations. J.T. Jacobson (ed.), *The auditory brainstem response*, pp. 297–316. San Diego, CA: College-Hill Press.

Cox, L.C., Hack, M., and Metz, D.A. (1984). Auditory brainstem response abnormalities in the very low birthweight infant: Incidence and risk factors. *Ear and Hearing, 5*, 47–51.

Cox, L.C., Hack, M., and Metz, D.A. (1981). Brainstem-evoked response audiometry: Normative data from the preterm infant. *Audiology, 20*, 53–64.

Cox, L.C., Hack, M., and Metz, D.A. (1982). Longitudinal ABR in the NICU infant. *International Journal of Pediatric Otorhinolaryngology, 4*, 225–231.

Dennis, J.M., Sheldon, R., Toubas, P., and McCaffee, M. (1984). Identification of hearing loss in the neonatal intensive care unit population. *American Journal of Otology, 5*, 210–205.

Despland, P. and Galambos, R. (1980). The auditory brainstem response (ABR) is a useful diagnostic tool in the intensive care nursery. *Pediatric Research, 14*, 154–158.

Despland, P. (1985). Maturational changes in the auditory system as reflected in human brainstem evoked responses. *Developmental Neurosciences, 7*, 73–80.

Dolan, T.G. and Morris, S.G. (1990). Administering audiometric speech tests via bone conduction: A comparison of transducers. *Ear and Hearing, 11*, 446–449.

Duara, S., Suter, C.M., Bessard, K.D., and Gutberlet, R.L. (1986). Neonatal screening with auditory brainstem response in the neonatal intensive care unit. *Journal of Pediatrics, 108*, 276–281.

Durieux-Smith, A. and Jacobson, J. (1985). Comparison of auditory brainstem response and behavioral screening in neonates. *Journal of Otolaryngology, 14 (Suppl. 14)*, 47–53.

Durieux-Smith, A., Picton, T., Edwards, C., Goodman, J.T., and MacMurray, B. (1985). The Crib-o-gram in the NICU: An evaluation based on brain stem electric response audiometry. *Ear and Hearing, 6*, 20–24.

Edwards, C.G., Durieux-Smith, A., and Picton, T.W. (1985). Neonatal auditory brain stem responses from ipsilateral and contralateral recording montages. *Ear and Hearing, 6*, 175–178.

Eggermont, J.J. (1983). Physiology of the developing auditory system. In S. Trehub and B. Schneider (eds.), *Auditory development in infancy*. New York: Plenum Press.

Eggermont, J.J. (1985). Evoked potentials as indicators of auditory maturation. *Acta Otolaryngologica (Suppl), 421*, 41–47.

Eggermont, J.J. and Salamy, A. (1988). Development of ABR parameters in a preterm and a term born population. *Ear and Hearing, 9*, 283–289.

Fawer, C.L. and Dubowitz, L.M.S. (1982). Auditory brainstem responses in neurologically normal preterm and fullterm newborn infants. *Neuropediatrics, 13*, 200–206.

Fawer, S.F., Dubowitz, N.D., Levene, and Dubowitz, V. (1983). Auditory brainstem responses in neurologically abnormal infants. *Neuropediatrics, 14*, 88–92.

Folsom, R.C. and Wynne, M.K. (1987). Auditory brainstem response from human adults and infants: Wave V tuning curves. *Journal of the Acoustical Society of America, 81*, 412–417.

Frank, T. and Crandell, C.C. (1986). Acoustic radiation produced by B-71, B-72, and KH 70 bone vibrators. *Ear and Hearing, 7*, 344–347.

Fria, T.J. (1985). Identification of congenital hearing loss with the auditory brainstem response. In Jacobson, J.T. (ed.), *The auditory brainstem response*, pp. 317–336. San Diego, CA: College-Hill Press.

Fria, T.J. and Doyle, W.J. (1984). Maturation of the auditory brainstem response (ABR): Additional perspectives. *Ear and Hearing, 5*, 361–365.

Fria, T.J. and Sabo, D.L. (1980). Auditory brainstem responses in children with otitis media with effusion. *Annals of Otology, Rhinology, and Laryngology, 89,* 200–206.

Galambos, R. and Hecox, K. (1978). Clinical applications of the auditory brainstem response. *Otolaryngological Clinics of North America, 11,* 709–722.

Galambos, R., Hicks, G., and Wilson, M.J. (1982). Hearing loss in graduates of tertiary care nursery. *Ear and Hearing, 3,* 87–90.

Galambos, R., Hicks, G.E. and Wilson, M.J. (1984). The auditory brainstem response reliably predicts hearing loss in graduates of a tertiary intensive care nursery. *Ear and Hearing, 5,* 254–260.

Goldstein, P.J., Krumholz, A., Felix, J.K., Shannon, D., and Carr, R.F. (1979). Brainstem evoked responses in neonates. *American Journal of Obstetrics and Gynecology, 135,* 622–631.

Gorga, M.P. and Thornton, A.R. (1989). The choice of stimuli for ABR measurements. *Ear and Hearing, 10,* 217–230.

Gorga, M.P., Kaminski, J.F., and Beauchaine, K.A. (1987). Auditory brainstem responses to high-frequency tone bursts in normal-hearing subjects. *Ear and Hearing, 98,* 222–226.

Gorga, M.P., Kaminski, J.R., Beauchaine, K.A., and Jesteadt, W. (1988). Auditory brainstem responses to tone bursts in normally hearing subjects. *Journal of Speech and Hearing Research, 31,* 87–97.

Gorga, M.P., Kaminski, J.R., Beauchaine, K.L., Jesteadt, W., and Neely, S.T. (1989). Auditory brainstem responses from children three months to three years of age: Normal patterns of response. II. *Journal of Speech and Hearing Research, 32,* 281–288.

Gorga, M.P., Reiland, J.K., and Beauchaine, K.A. (1988). Auditory brainstem responses from graduates of an intensive care nursery using an insert earphone. *Ear and Hearing, 9,* 144–147.

Gorga, M.P., Reiland, J.K., Beauchaine, K.A., Worthington, D.W., and Jesteadt, W. (1987). Auditory brainstem responses from graduates of an intensive care nursery: Normal patterns of response. *Journal of Speech and Hearing Research, 30,* 311–318.

Hall, J.W. (1992). *Handbook of auditory evoked responses.* Needham, MA: Allyn and Bacon.

Hall, J.W. and Ghorayeb, B.Y. (1991). Diagnosis of middle ear pathology and evaluation of conductive hearing loss. In J.T. Jacobson and J.L. Northern (eds.), *Diagnostic audiology.* Austin, TX: Pro-ed.

Hall, J.W. and Tucker, D.A. (1988). The auditory brainstem response in acute brain injury. In J.H. Owen and C.

Donohoe (eds.), *Atlas of auditory evoked responses.* Orlando, FL: Grune & Stratton.

Hall, J.W., Brown, D.P., and Mackey-Hargadine, J. (1985). Pediatric applications of serial auditory brainstem and middle latency measurements. *International Journal of Pediatric Otorhinolaryngology, 9,* 201–218.

Hall, J.W., Bull, J., and Cronau, L. (1988). The effect of hypo- versus hyperthermia on auditory brainstem response: Two case reports. *Ear and Hearing, 9,* 137–143.

Hall, J.W., Kripal, J.P., and Hepp, T. (1988). Newborn hearing screening with auditory brainstem response: Measurement problems and solutions. *Seminars in Hearing, 9,* 15–32.

Hall, J.W., Winkler, J.B., Herndon, W., and Gray, L.B. (1986). Auditory brainstem responses in young burn wound patients treated with ototoxic drugs. *International Journal of Pediatric Otorhinolaryngology, 12,* 187–203.

Harder, H., Arlinger, S., and Kylen, P. (1983). Electrocochleography with bone-conducted stimulation: A comparative study of different methods of stimulation. *Acta Otolaryngologica (Stockholm) 95,* 35–45.

Hatanaka, T., Shuto, H., Yasuhara, A., and Kobayashi, Y. (1988). Ipsilateral and contralateral recordings of auditory brainstem responses to monaural stimulation. *Pediatric Neurology, 4,* 354–357.

Hatanaka, T., Yasuhara, A., Hori, A., and Kobayashi, Y. (1990). Auditory brain stem response in newborn infants—masking effect on ipsi- and contralateral recording. *Ear and Hearing, 3,* 233–236.

Hecox, K. (1975). Electrophysiological correlates of human auditory development. In Cohen, L.B., and Salaptex P., *Infant perception: From sensation to cognition* (Vol. III). New York: Academic Press.

Hecox, K. and Burkhard, R. (1982). Developmental dependencies of the human brainstem auditory evoked response. *Annals of the New York Academy of Science, 388,* 538–556.

Hecox, K. and Cone, B.K. (1981). Prognostic importance of brainstem auditory evoked responses after asphyxia. *Neurology, 31,* 1429–1439.

Hecox, K. and Galambos, R. (1974). Brainstem auditory evoked response in human infants and adults. *Archives of Otolaryngology, 99,* 30–33.

Hecox, K. and Jacobson, J. (1984). Auditory evoked potential. In Northern J., *Hearing disorders.* Boston, MA: Little, Brown and Company.

Hecox, K., Cone, B., and Blaw, M.E., (1981). Brainstem auditory evoked response in the diagnosis of pediatric neurologic diseases. *Neurology, 31,* 832–840.

Hooks, R.G. and Weber, B.A. (1984). Auditory brain stem responses of premature infants to bone-conducted stimuli: A feasibility study. *Ear and Hearing, 5*, 42–46.

Horton, M.B., Rubin, A.M., Reiland, J.K., and Gorga, M.P. (1985). Education ICN graduates III. *Assessment of middle-ear function.* Presented at the national convention of the American Speech-Language-Hearing Association, Washington, D.C.

Hyde, M.L. (1985). Frequency-specific BERA in infants. *Journal of Otolaryngology (Toronto Suppl), 14*, 19–27.

Hyde, M.L., Riko, K., and Malizia, K. (1990). Audiometric accuracy of the click ABR in infants at risk for hearing loss. *Journal of the Academy of Audiology, 1*, 59–74.

Jacobson, J. and Mencher, G. (1981). Intensive care nursery noise and its influence on newborn hearing screening. *International Journal of Pediatric Otorhinolaryngology, 3*, 45–54.

Jacobson, J. and Jacobson, C. (1987). Principles of decision analysis in high risk infants. *Seminars in Hearing, 8*, 133–141. New York: Thieme-Stratten, Inc.

Jacobson, J.T. (ed.). (1985). *The auditory brainstem response.* San Diego, CA: College-Hill Press.

Jacobson, J.T. and Morehouse, C. (1984). A comparison of auditory brainstem response and behavioral screening in high risk and normal newborn infants. *Ear and Hearing, 5*, 247–253.

Jacobson, J.T., Jacobson, G., and Spahr, R.C. (1990). Automated and conventional ABR screening techniques in high-risk infants. *Journal of the American Academy of Audiology, 1*, 187–195.

Jacobson, J.T., Morehouse, C.R., and Johnson, M.J. (1982). Strategies for infant auditory brainstem response assessment. *Ear and Hearing, 3*, 263–270.

Jacobson, J.T., Seitz, M.R., Mencher, G.T., and Parrott, V. (1981). Auditory brainstem response: A contribution to infant assessment and management. In Mencher, G., and Gerber, S., *Early Management of Hearing Loss.* New York: Grune & Stratton.

Jahrsdoerfer, R.A. and Hall, J.W. III (1986). Congenital malformation of the ear. *American Journal of Otology, 7*, 267–269.

Jahrsdoerfer, R.A., Yeakley, J.W., Hall, J.W., Robbin, K.T., and Gray, L. C. (1985). High resolution CT scanning and ABR in congenital aural atresia—patient selection and surgical correlation. *Otolaryngology—Head and Neck Surgery, 93*, 292–298.

Jerger, J. and Hall, J.W. III. (1980). Effects of age and sex on auditory brainstem response (ABR). *Archives of Otolaryngology, 106*, 387–391.

Joint Committee on Infant Hearing, (1991). *Audiology Today, 3*, 14–17.

Joint Committee on Infant Hearing, Position Statement. (1982). *Pediatrics, 70*, 496–497.

Kaga, K. and Tanaka, Y. (1980). Auditory brainstem response and behavioral audiometry. *Archives of Otolaryngology, 106*, 564–566.

Kavanagh, K.T., Domico, W.D., Franks, R., and Han, J.C. (1988). Digital filtering and spectral analysis of the low intensity ABR. *Ear and Hearing, 9*, 43–47.

Kevanishivili, Z. and Aphonchenko, V. (1979). Frequency composition of brainstem audiometry evoked potentials. *Scandinavian Audiology, 8*, 51–55.

Kiang, N., Watanabe, T., and Thomas, E. (1965). Discharge patterns of single fibers in the cat's auditory nerve. *Research Monographs* (35). Cambridge, MA: MIT Press

Kileny, P.R., Connely, C., and Robertson, C. (1980). Auditory brainstem responses in perinatal asphyxia. *International Journal of Pediatric Otorhinolaryngology, 2*, 147–159.

Killion, M. (1984). New insert earphones for audiometry. *Hearing Instruments, 35*, 28–29.

Kjaer, M. (1980). Recognizability of brain stem auditory evoked potential components. *Acta Neurologica Scandinavia, 60*, 20–33.

Lary, S., Briassoulis, G., de Vries, L., Dubowitz, L.M.S., and Dubowitz, V. (1985). Hearing threshold in preterm and term infants by auditory brainstem response. *Journal of Pediatrics, 107*, 593–599.

Lauffer, H. and Wenzel, D. (1989). Brainstem acoustic evoked responses: Maturational aspects from cochlea to midbrain. *Neuropediatrics, 21*, 59–61.

Laukli, E. and Mair, I.W.S. (1981). Early auditory-evoked responses: Filter effects. *Audiology, 20*, 300–312.

Marshall, N.K. and Donchin, E. (1981). Circadian variations in the latency of brainstem responses and its relation to body temperature. *Science, 212*, 356–358.

Marshall, R.E., Reichert, T.J., Kerley, S.M., and Davis, H. (1980). Auditory function in newborn intensive care unit patients revealed by auditory brainstem potentials. *Journal of Pediatrics, 96*, 731–735.

Mauldin, L. and Jerger, J. (1979). Auditory brainstem evoked responses to bone-conducted signals. *Archives of Otolaryngology, 105*, 656–661.

McCall, S. and Ferraro, J.A. (1991). Pediatric ABR screening: Pass-fail rates in awake versus asleep neonates. *Journal of the American Academy of Audiology, 2*, 18–23.

Mitchell, S.A. (1984). Noise pollution in the neonatal intensive care nursery. *Seminars in Hearing, 5*, 17–24.

Mjoen, S., Langlset, A., Tangsrud, E., and Sundby, A. (1982). Auditory brainstem responses (ABR) in pre-term infants. *Acta Paediatrica Scandinavia, 71*, 711–715.

Mochizuki, Y., Go, T., Ohkubo, H., and Motomura, T. (1982). Development of human brainstem auditory evoked-potentials and gender differences from infants to young adults. *Progressive Neurobiology, 20*, 273–285.

Morgan, D.E., Zimmerman, M.C., and Dubno, J.R. (1987). Auditory brainstem evoked response characteristics in the full-term newborn infant. *Annals of Otolaryngology, Rhinology, and Laryngology, 96*, 142–151.

Murray, A.D., Javel, E., and Watson, C.S. (1985). Prognostic validity of auditory brainstem evoked response screening in newborn infants. *American Journal of Otolaryngology, 6*, 120–131.

Northern, J. (ed.) (1987). Hearing in infants. *Seminars in Hearing, 8*, 133–141. New York: Thieme-Stratten, Inc.

Ornitz, E., Mo, A., Olson, S., and Waller, L. (1980). Influence of click sound pressure direction on brainstem responses in children. *Audiology, 19*, 245–254.

Pauwels, H.P., Vogeleer, M., Clement, P.A.R., Rousseeuw, P.J., and Kaufman L. (1982). Brainstem electric response audiometry in newborns. *International Journal of Pediatric Otorhinolaryngology, 4*, 317–323.

Picton, T.W. and Smith, A.D. (1978). The practice of evoked potential audiometry. *Otolaryngology Clinics of North America, 11*, 263–282.

Picton, T.W., Linden, R.D., Hasmel, G., and Muru, J.T. (1983). Aspects of averaging. *Seminars in Hearing, 4*, 327–340.

Picton, T.W., Stapells, D.R., and Campbell, K.B. (1981). Auditory evoked potentials from the human cochlea and brainstem. *Journal of Otolaryngology, 10 (Suppl. 9)*, 1–41.

Picton, T.W., Taylor, M.J., Durieux-Smith, A., and Edwards, C.G. (1986). Brainstem auditory evoked potentials in pediatrics. In Aminoff, M.J. (ed.), *Electrodiagnosis in clinical neurology*. New York: Churchill Livingstone.

Pratt, H. and Sohmer H. (1976). Intensity and rate functions of cochlear and brainstem evoked responses to click stimuli in man. *Archives of Otorhinolaryngology, 212*, 85–93.

Richmond, K.H., Konkle, D.F., and Potsic, W.P. (1986). ABR screening of high-risk infants: Effects of ambient noise in the neonatal nursery. *Otolaryngology—Head and Neck Surgery, 94*, 552–557.

Rotteveel, J.J., Colon, E.J., Notermans, S.L.H., Stoelinga, G.B.A., Visco, Y., and de Graaf, R. (1986). The central auditory conduction at term date and three months after birth: II. Auditory brainstem response. *Scandinavian Audiology, 15*, 11–19.

Rowe, M.J. (1978). Normal variability of the brainstem auditory evoked response in young and old adult subjects. *Electroencephalography and Clinical Neurophysiology, 44*, 459–470.

Rubel, E.W. (1985). Strategies and problems for future studies of auditory development. *Acta Otolaryngologica (Supp), 421*, 114–128.

Rubel, E.W. and Ryals, B.M. (1983). Development of the place principle: Acoustic trauma. *Science, 219*, 512–514.

Ruth, R.A., Dey-Sigman, S., and Mills, J.A. (1985). Neonatal ABR hearing screening. *The Hearing Journal, 38*, 39–45.

Salamy, A. (1984). Maturation of the auditory brainstem response from birth through early childhood. *Journal of Clinical Neurophysiology, 1*, 293–329.

Salamy, A., Eldredge, L., and Wakeley, A. (1985). Maturation of contralateral brain-stem responses in preterm infants. *Electroencephalography and Clinical Neurophysiology, 62*, 117–123.

Salamy, A., Fenn, C.B. and Bronshvag, M. (1979). Ontogenesis of human brainstem evoked potential amplitude. *Developmental Psychology, 12*, 519–526.

Salamy, A. and McKean, C.M. (1976). Postnatal development of the human brainstem potentials during the first year of life. *Electroencephalography and Clinical Neurophysiology, 40*, 418–426.

Salamy, A., McKean, C.M., and Buda, F.B. (1975). Maturational changes in auditory transmission as reflected in human brainstem potentials. *Brain Research, 96*, 361–366.

Salamy, A., McKean, C.M., Pettett, C., and Mendelson, T. (1978). Auditory brainstem recovery processes from birth to adulthood. *Psychophysiology, 15*, 214–220.

Salamy, A., Mendelson, T., and Tooley, W.H. (1982). Developmental profiles for the brainstem auditory evoked potential. *Early Human Development, 6*, 331–339.

Salamy, A., Mendelson, T., Tooley, W.H., and Champlin, E.R. (1980). Contrasts in brainstem function between normal and high-risk infants in early postnatal life. *Early Human Development, 4*, 179–185.

Samani, F., Peschiulli, G., Pastorini, S., and Fior, R. (1990). An evaluation of hearing maturation by means of auditory brainstem response in very low birthweight and preterm newborns. *International Journal of Pediatric Otorhinolaryngology, 19*, 121–127.

Sanders, R.A., Duncan, P.G., and McCullough, D.W. (1979). Clinical experience with brain stem audiometry performed under general anesthesia. *Journal of Otolaryngology, 8*, 24–31.

Sasama, R. (1990). Hearing threshold investigations in infants and children. *Audiology, 29,* 76–84.

Scherg, M. (1980). Cochlear and brainstem evoked potentials: Quantitative determination of hearing impairment in children. *Scandinavian Audiology (Suppl.), 11,* 135–144.

Schorn, V., Lennon, V., and Brickford, R. (1977). Temperature effects on the brainstem auditory evoked responses (BAERs) of the rat. *Proceedings of the San Diego Biomedical Symposium, 16,* 313–318.

Schulman-Galambos, C. and Galambos, R. (1975). Brainstem auditory evoked responses in premature infants. *Journal of Speech and Hearing Research, 18,* 456–465.

Schulman-Galambos, C. and Galambos, R. (1979). Brainstem response audiometry in newborn hearing screening. *Archives of Otolaryngology, 105,* 86–90.

Schwartz, D.M. and Berry, G.A. (1985). Normative aspects of the ABR. In J.T. Jacobson (ed.), *The auditory brainstem response,* pp. 65–67. San Diego, CA: College-Hill Press.

Schwartz, D.M. and Schwartz, J.A. (1991). Auditory evoked potentials in clinical pediatrics. In W.F. Rintelmann (ed.), *Hearing assessment.* Austin, TX: Pro-ed.

Schwartz, D.M., Larson, V., and DeChiccicca, A.R. (1985). Spectral characteristics of air and bone transducers used to record the auditory brainstem response. *Ear and Hearing, 6,* 274–277.

Schwartz, D.M., Pratt, R.E., and Schwartz, J.A. (1989). Auditory brain stem responses in preterm infants: Evidence of peripheral maturity. *Ear and Hearing, 10,* 14–22.

Sohmer, H., Gafni, M., and Chisin, R. (1978). Auditory nerve and brain stem responses: Comparison in awake and unconscious subjects. *Archives of Neurology, 35,* 228–230.

Stapells, D.R. (1990). Auditory brainstem response assessment of infants and children. *Seminars in Hearing, 10,* 229–250.

Stapells, D.R. and Mosseri, M. (1991). Maturation of the contralaterally recorded auditory brain stem response. *Ear and Hearing, 3,* 167–173.

Stapells, D.R. and Picton, T.W. (1981). Technical aspects of brainstem evoked potential audiometry using tones. *Ear and Hearing, 2,* 20–29.

Stapells, D.R. and Ruben, R.J. (1989). Auditory brainstem responses to bone conducted tones in infants. *Annals of Otology, Rhinology and Laryngology, 98,* 941–949.

Starr, A. and Achor, L.J. (1975). Auditory brainstem responses in neurological disease. *Archives of Neurology, 32,* 761–768.

Starr, A., Amlie, R.N., Martin, W.H., and Sanders, S. (1977).

Development of auditory brainstem potentials. *Pediatrics, 60,* 831–839.

Stein, L.K., Ozdamar, O., Kraus, N., and Paton, J. (1983). Follow-up of infants screened by auditory brainstem response in the neonatal intensive care unit. *Journal of Pediatrics, 103,* 447–453.

Stockard, J.E. and Westmoreland, B.F. (1981). Technical considerations in the recording and interpretation of the brainstem auditory evoked potential for neonatal neurologic diagnosis. *American Journal of EEG Technology, 21,* 31–54.

Stockard, J.E., Stockard, J.J., Westmoreland, B.F., and Corfits, J.L. (1979). Brainstem auditory evoked response. Normal variations as a function of stimulus and subject characteristics. *Archives of Neurology, 36,* 823–831.

Stockard, J.E., Stockard, J.J., and Coen, R.W. (1983). Auditory brainstem response variability in infants. *Ear and Hearing, 4,* 11–23.

Stockard, J.J., Stockard, J.E., and Sharbrough, F.W. (1978). Non-pathologic factor influencing brainstem auditory evoked potentials. *American Journal of EEG Technology, 18,* 177–209.

Stuart, A., Yang, E.Y., and Stenstrom, R. (1990). Effect of temporal area bone vibrator placement on auditory brainstem response in newborn infants. *Ear and Hearing, 11,* 363–369.

Suzuki, T., Harai, Y., and Horiuchi, K. (1977). Auditory brainstem responses to pure tone stimuli. *Scandinavian Audiology, 6,* 51–56.

Suzuki, T., Sakabe, N., and Miyashita, Y. (1982). Power spectral analysis of auditory brainstem responses to pure tone stimuli. *Scandinavian Audiology, 11,* 25–30.

Swigonski, N., Shallop, J., Bull, M.J., and Lemons, J.A. (1987). Hearing screening of high risk newborns, *Ear and Hearing, 8,* 26–30.

Terkildsen, K. and Osterhammel, P. (1981). The influence of reference electrode position on recordings of the auditory brainstem responses. *Ear and Hearing, 2,* 9–14.

Tompkins, S.M., Hall, J.W., Jacobson, J.T., and Jahrsdoerfer, R.A. (1991). Poster presentation at the American Academy of Audiology, Denver, CO.

van der Drift, J.F.C., Brocaar, M.P., and van Zanten, G.A. (1988). Brainstem response audiometry: I. Its use in distinguishing between conductive and cochlear hearing loss. *Audiology, 27,* 260–270.

van Zanten, G.A., Brocaar, M.P., Fetter, W.P.F., and Baerts, W. (1988). Brainstem electric response audiometry in preterm infants. *Scandinavian Audiology (Suppl.), 30,* 91–97.

Weber, B.A. (1983). Masking and bone conduction testing in

brainstem response audiometry. *Seminars in Hearing, 4*, 343–352.

Yamada, O., Kodera, K., and Yagi, T. (1979). Cochlear processes affecting wave V latency of the auditory evoked brainstem response: A study of patients with sensory hearing loss. *Scandinavian Audiology, 11*, 53–56.

Yang, E.Y., Rupert, A.L., and Moushegian, G. (1987). A developmental study of bone conduction auditory brain stem response in infants. *Ear and Hearing, 8*, 244–251.

Yang, E.Y., Stuart, A., Stenstrom, R., and Hollett, S., (1991). Effect of vibrator to head coupling force on the auditory brainstem response to bone conducted clicks in newborn infants. *Ear and Hearing, 12*, 55–60.

Zimmerman, M.C., Morgan, D.E., and Dubno, J.R. (1987). Auditory brain stem evoked response characteristics in developing infants. *Annals of Otology, Rhinology, Laryngology, 96*, 291–299.

CHAPTER 14

NEONATAL INTENSIVE CARE UNITS: THE IMPACT ON HEARING SCREENING

CYNTHIA J. LYNN
SUSAN E. DENSON

The term "neonatology" was coined by Alexander Schaffer in 1960 (Cone, 1985). Rapid changes have occurred since then, with the development of intensive care nurseries around the world to treat conditions occurring exclusively in the neonatal period, defined as the first 28 days of life.

EVOLUTION OF THE CURRENT CARE SYSTEM

When the American Pediatric Society was founded in 1888, there was little interest in the neonate (Silverman, 1990). More than 95% of all infants were delivered at home. Early deaths were viewed as an expected reproductive loss by families and doctors, while prolonging the lives of very small or malformed infants was often seen as inhumane.

In contrast, efforts to reduce neonatal mortality in France had begun in the 1870s. These efforts were motivated by economic considerations as the country needed workers and soldiers to replace the lives lost in the Franco-Prussian War. French obstetricians were the leaders in developing incubators and special care techniques for premature infants. These infants were brought to special facilities where nurses provided warmth, careful feeding, cleanliness, and efforts to minimize exertion. These nursing routines were successful in reducing neonatal mortality.

The first paper on prematurity, presented to the American Pediatric Society in 1893, described a design for a closed incubator. Doubts about efforts to keep these small babies alive were expressed, but despite disparaging attitudes, programs for the care of these infants were organized. In 1935, the American Pediatric Society began efforts to stimulate research into problems of the neonate. By the 1940s standard care included isolation, thermal stability, nutrition, and skilled nursing care (O'Donnell, 1990).

Not all advances resulted in good outcome. Routine use of oxygen was implemented in the 1940s with hopes of improving survival and reducing brain damage from hypoxia. The routine delivery of oxygen was found to diminish apneic episodes; however, this oxygen therapy was linked to devastating eye damage and blindness in 1954. This unexpected effect served as a reminder of how little was known about the neonate. As a result, research activities expanded dramatically and perinatal publications increased sharply after 1955.

Neonatal intensive care units were established in the 1950s and 1960s with the development of the intensive care concept in adult and pediatric medicine. More aggressive medical and surgical care developed in the 1960s. The limits of viability were challenged and continue to be challenged today (Ginsberg et al., 1990).

Advances in maternal care and techniques for assessing fetal health in the late 1960s and early 1970s led to joint centers for obstetric and neonatal intensive care (Figures 14.1 and 14.2). Guidelines for regional perinatal care systems were developed in 1973. These regional care systems facilitated cooperative efforts to reduce perinatal morbidity and mortality. Professional expertise, consultation, communication, and education were emphasized for the effective use of resources. The use of highly trained perinatal personnel and intensive care facilities and the assurance of cost effec-

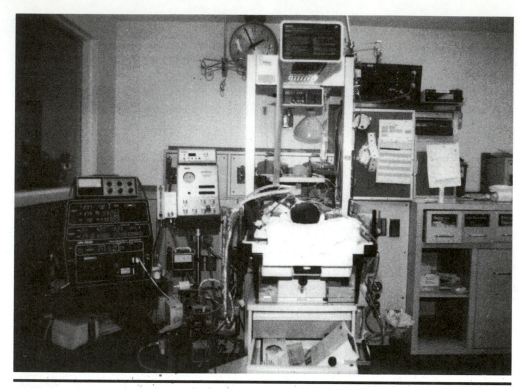

FIGURE 14.1.   A very ill newborn in the NICU on high frequency ventilation and various monitoring devices.

tiveness were proposed to insure quality care for all pregnant women and newborns (Frigoletto and Little, 1988). A summary of the historical highlights of Neonatology is presented in Table 14.1.

The availability of highly trained perinatal personnel and intensive care facilities are necessary for the most effective treatment of the small proportion of the perinatal population with the highest risks. Unfortunately, changes in the health care system are resulting in deregionalization of perinatal care, but regionalization remains the optimal approach.

NEED FOR SPECIALIZED CARE

The transition from intrauterine to extrauterine life requires many biologic and physical changes. The placenta provides many functions, including the respiratory, ex-

cretory, immunologic and nutritional functions. After delivery, the lungs must become the organ for gas exchange, the kidneys must begin to excrete wastes, the liver must neutralize and excrete toxic substances, the immune system must protect against infection, and the gastrointestinal tract must process and absorb nutrients.

Many of the problems encountered in the neonatal period are related to poor adaptation of these organ systems to extrauterine life. This poor adaptation may be a result of many factors, including complications of prematurity, intrauterine insults, congenital malformations, or an abnormal intrauterine environment. The most common diagnosis resulting in admission to a neonatal critical care unit is respiratory distress. This diagnosis occurred in 47% of the admissions to our unit in a recent year. The causes of respiratory distress include respiratory distress syndrome due to prematu-

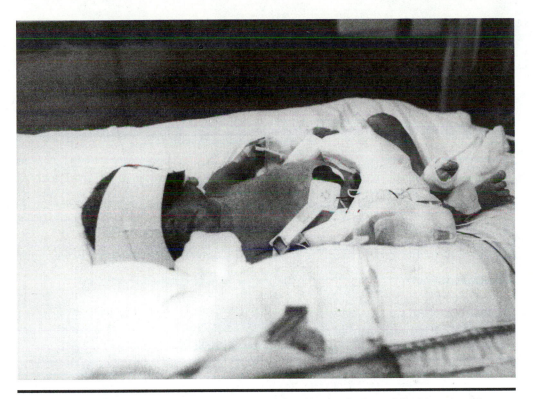

FIGURE 14.2.   A typical premature infant under phototherapy for hyperbilirubinemia with protective eye shields.

rity, meconium aspiration syndrome and persistent pulmonary hypertension usually due to intrauterine distress, diaphragmatic hernia resulting in pulmonary hypoplasia, and transient tachypnea of the newborn.

Infection, either bacterial or viral, is the diagnosis in 16% of admissions. Congenital malformations occur in 7% of admissions. The remaining 30% are admitted due to prematurity, multiple gestation, maternal substance abuse, metabolic disorders, or hematologic problems (Table 14.2).

NEONATAL MORTALITY

The neonatal mortality rate, defined as death of a newborn infant in the first 28 days, is a marker for the quality of perinatal care and has decreased as improvements have occurred in neonatal intensive care (Plesko, 1990).

Historically the mortality rate has been highest in very low birth weight infants in whom the major cause of death is pulmonary immaturity. Respiratory failure remains a significant contributor in the very premature infant (less than 700 grams), but other important causes of death include infection in 30% and congenital malformations and chromosomal abnormalities in 25%. Deaths after the neonatal period but prior to discharge from the hospital comprise 25% of all deaths in the neonatal critical care area. These deaths may be due to progressive respiratory failure or infection.

LIFELONG IMPACT OF NEONATAL PROBLEMS

Although the initial concern of families when an infant is admitted to a neonatal critical care unit is whether the infant will survive, another concern is whether there will

TABLE 14.1. History of Neonatology.

1870s	- French obstetricians developed incubators, special care techniques.
1888	- No effort was made in the United States to prolong "feeble" infants' lives.
1893	- A design for a closed incubator presented to the American Pediatric Society stirred controversy.
1935	- American Pediatric Society promoted research concerning the neonate.
1940s	- Isolation, thermal stability, nutrition, oxygen, and skilled nursing care were employed standardly.
1954	- Oxygen was linked to retinal damage and blindness.
1955	- Research activities involving neonatal issues increased.
1950–60	- Neonatal Intensive Care Units developed.
1973	- Guidelines for regional perinatal care systems developed.

TABLE 14.2. Diagnoses in the NICU.

Respiratory distress	47%
Infection	16%
Congenital malformations	7%
Prematurity, multiple births, maternal substance abuse, other	30%

TABLE 14.3. Possible Long Term Effects of Prematurity.

Increased mortality rate in first 2 years of life
Chronic lung disease
Short bowel syndrome
Failure to thrive
Neurological abnormalities
Developmental delay, mental retardation
Visual deficits, blindness, strabismus, amblyopia
Hearing deficits, deafness

be permanent sequelae (Hoffman and Bennett, 1990). Although most infants discharged from the neonatal critical care will be normal, there are certain high-risk groups that are at risk for sequelae (Mali and Tyler, 1989). Table 14.3 lists several possible consequences due to the effects of prematurity. These sequelae come in many different forms, including chronic disease, abnormalities in growth, sensorineural handicaps, and abnormal neurologic or developmental outcome (Elliman et al., 1986).

Preterm infants who survive the neonatal period have a higher mortality rate than full term infants in the first two years of life. Many of the deaths are due to chronic lung disease and infections. Failure to thrive, sudden infant death syndrome, child abuse, and inadequate maternal-infant bonding occur more frequently in these infants. Poverty-related health risks also contribute to the high mortality and morbidity of this group.

There are several chronic diseases found in this population. Bronchopulmonary dysplasia, a form of chronic lung disease, may have several manifestations. Some of these infants will be discharged from the hospital on oxygen therapy which may continue through the first year of life. Other infants with chronic lung disease will present with reactive airway disease and require extensive medical therapy (Northway et al., 1990). Some infants with necrotizing enterocolitis, an infectious complication of the gastrointestinal tract, will require major bowel resection in the neonatal period which will result in "short bowel syndrome". This leads to nutritional problems and may require long term parenteral nutrition which carries its own risks.

Physical growth of low birth weight infants may be affected by the presence of congenital anomalies, central nervous system injury, or intrauterine growth retardation. In the absence of the above problems, physical growth of most low birth weight infants (less than 2500 grams) approximates that of term infants in the second year of life. Very low birth weight infants (less than 1500 grams) may not exhibit normal growth, especially if they have chronic illness, inadequate caloric intake, or an inadequate caretaking environment.

Neurologic sequelae with motor dysfunction occur

in 9% of all low birth weight infants discharged from critical care. There are four major categories. The most common form of motor dysfunction is spastic diplegia defined as bilateral leg involvement with hypertonia and brisk reflexes. The arms are less prominently involved with poor fine motor control. Although this form of motor dysfunction initially worsens by 6–12 months, it usually resolves in early childhood. Spastic quadriparesis is a more severe form of motor dysfunction involving truncal hypotonia with spasticity of the extremities. Spastic quadriparesis progresses during late infancy and does not resolve. Hypotonia is the third type and is manifest by poor muscle tone, resulting in a delay in head control, sitting, and walking. This improves with time. The last form of motor dysfunction is spastic hemiparesis in which only one side of the body is affected. This is commonly a static lesion without progression.

Developmental delay, usually defined as a developmental quotient or IQ of less than 80, occurs in 7–10% of high-risk infants. The risk of developmental delay varies with diagnoses in the neonatal period. The groups with the highest risk include very low birth weight infants, especially those with chronic lung disease and/or post hemorrhagic hydrocephalus, infants with sepsis and meningitis, and infants with congenital malformations of the central nervous system.

Visual handicap occurs primarily in the very low birth weight infant due to the developmental status of the eye at birth. The retinal vasculature is not complete in its development until at least one month after birth at term. With increasing prematurity there is an increased amount of incompletely vascularized retina which is at risk for abnormal development. These changes become apparent at 6–8 weeks postnatal life. Retrolental fibroplasia is a condition in which the vasculature undergoes abnormal development. In the mildest forms the vasculature is abnormal and a circumferential ridge develops in the retina. In most infants these changes regress and ultimately vision will be normal. In the progressive form, abnormal vessels develop which may hemorrhage, resulting in scarring, traction on the retina, or detachment of the retina. Although blindness from this disorder is the most significant visual handicap, premature infants are also at risk for myopia, strabismus, and amblyopia.

THE NEONATAL CRITICAL CARE UNIT

Neonatal-perinatal medicine continues to change. Clinical applications of research studies have dramatically improved the outcome of ill newborns. Refinements in diagnostic and therapeutic techniques have occurred over the past decade. New developments such as surfactant therapy for respiratory distress syndrome have changed the management and outcome of preterm infants.

RESPIRATORY CARE

Many disorders may cause respiratory distress in the newborn, including respiratory distress syndrome, transient tachypnea of the newborn, meconium aspiration syndrome, and pneumonia. The treatments are similar with oxygen supplementation the initial therapy in all.

Assisted ventilation is frequently needed for infants with severe lung disease. Respiratory failure, the inability to remove carbon dioxide by respiratory efforts, is the most common reason for assisting ventilation. Hypoxemia, despite delivery of 100% oxygen, and apnea are other indications for artificial ventilation.

Respiration can be assisted by ventilation via bag and mask, endotracheal tube and bag, or endotracheal tube and a mechanical ventilator. Infants requiring ventilatory assistance must be monitored closely because of the many complications that can occur. A pneumothorax, pulmonary hemorrhage, displaced or obstructed endotracheal tube, mechanical failure of the ventilator, or disconnected tubing may result in acute deterioration.

Alternative forms of ventilation have become available recently, including high-frequency jet ventilation and high-frequency oscillator ventilation. Extracorporeal membrane oxygenation, known as ECMO, is another alternative form of support during respiratory failure. Perfusion and gas exchange are obtained by cardiopulmonary bypass through a membrane oxygenator while the infant's lungs are allowed to recover.

Respiratory distress syndrome, common in preterm infants, is characterized by inadequate lung production of surfactant. Surfactant is a surface-active phospholipid that maintains the stability of the airways. The administration of surfactant through the endotracheal tube results in improved oxygenation and ventilation

(Soll et al., 1990). The utilization of surfactant, ventilators, and alternative therapies enhances survival of acutely ill newborns with respiratory failure.

THERMAL SUPPORT

The need for temperature control for improved survival has been emphasized since the early 1900s. Infants were shown to have better survival rates in a warmer environment, probably due to decreased oxygen consumption and carbon dioxide production. Newborns gain weight more rapidly if they are kept in a warm environment, since maintaining body heat consumes calories and may limit growth.

Preterm infants are especially prone to hypothermia. They do not have a significant amount of brown fat, which is the main source of heat production in the newborn. In addition, the small preterm infant has a large surface area to volume ratio and a thin layer of subcutaneous fat, increasing heat transfer to the environment. The increased heat loss and decreased ability to produce heat result in hypothermia. In order to minimize this, infants are placed in an environment to maintain their temperature. Radiant warmers are open beds with an overhead source of heat which maintains the infant's temperature. This source is often chosen for the immediate stabilization period as it allows easy access to the infant. An incubator is an enclosed unit which can also maintain the infant's temperature. These sources of heat are utilized until an infant is large enough and stable enough to maintain his/her own temperature.

NUTRITION

The full-term healthy neonate can tolerate prolonged starvation, but the low birth weight infant has limited nutritional reserves. The malnourished preterm infant is at risk for such complications as nosocomial infections.

Parenteral nutrition is commonly used in ill newborns who cannot tolerate enteral feeding. The solutions used include glucose, amino acids, lipids, electrolytes, vitamins, and minerals. The calories delivered to the infant are limited by the glucose tolerance and the volume of fluid tolerated. Central venous catheters are commonly used to deliver higher concentrations of glucose.

When enteral feeds are begun in small infants, expressed breast milk or formula is commonly given by a nasogastric tube. Feedings are begun in small amounts and advanced slowly if tolerated by the infant.

THE SENSORY ENVIRONMENT AND PARENTAL INTERACTION

Sensory stimulation is likely to play a role in neurologic and physical maturation. Studies have revealed that fewer apneic episodes and increased weight gain result if premature infants are touched, rocked, cuddled, or talked to daily during their hospital stay. The parents are the logical choice to help provide sensory stimulation for their premature infants. Encouragement is needed since parents often do not appreciate that their premature infant can see and hear. Also parents often have a fear that they will harm or "break" the small, fragile-appearing newborn. The intensive care unit can be quite frightening to parents because of alarms, noises, lights, and activity. If the parents are taught to interact with their infants, they may take home a more responsive infant, and they may acquire a more positive view of the infant and of their parenting skills.

Very low birth weight infants frequently remain hospitalized for many months, a few will stay beyond their first birthday. The effect of prolonged infant-parent separation is unknown. Parents are encouraged to visit as frequently as possible and to participate in their infants' care, especially with feedings and baths during the infants' prolonged hospitalization. Many NICUs have formed support groups for parents of premature infants. Parents find both support and relief in talking with each other and expressing and comparing their feelings.

MONITORING AND PERIODIC ASSESSMENT

The use of monitoring in the NICU has become an essential component of medical management. Monitoring may be either continual or periodic. Some principal types of monitoring are listed in Table 14.4 and described below. For example, all newborns admitted to the NICU are continuously monitored with cardiopul-

TABLE 14.4. Monitoring in the NICU.

Cardiopulmonary monitoring

Bedside cranial ultrasound

Ophthalmologic exams

Frequent blood tests

Hearing screening

monary monitors. This detects disorders of the heart rhythm and respiratory pattern.

Apnea is the cessation of respiration for 20 seconds or less if accompanied by bradycardia, cyanosis, or pallor. Infants less than 34 weeks are at risk for apnea of prematurity. Apnea of prematurity will occur in more than 50% of infants less than 1500 grams. Apnea of prematurity may be caused by airway obstruction, a central respiratory pause, or most frequently both. Apnea usually decreases over the first month of life but can persist longer. An infant with mild apnea that is easily reversed by theophylline or mild stimulation may be sent home on an apnea monitor when otherwise ready for discharge. The parents are instructed in cardiopulmonary resuscitation and management of an apneic episode. Monitoring is discontinued when the infant has been without apnea for 1–2 months.

Premature infants are at risk for intraventricular hemorrhage (IVH) due to the fragility of brain tissue and a rich vascular supply to the germinal matrix. Particularly vulnerable is the preterm neonate of less than 35 weeks gestation; most vulnerable is the very low birth weight infant of less than 1500 grams. IVH occurs in up to 50% of preterm infants. It usually occurs in the first 2 days of life but can occur later in the first few weeks of life. IVH can be diagnosed and followed by bedside cranial ultrasonography.

Small hemorrhages do not appear to increase the risk of neurodevelopmental handicaps over similar preterm infants without hemorrhages. Larger hemorrhages may result in post-hemorrhagic hydrocephalus, which may require ventriculoperitoneal shunt placement to relieve intracranial pressure. The risk of major handicaps is increased 3–7 times, with global abnormalities in neuromotor and cognitive development.

Premature infants less than 36 weeks are at risk for retrolental fibroplasia. Routine screening of infants at risk is performed at 6 weeks of age by an ophthalmologist. Follow-up is essential. Cryotherapy is done for advancing disease in hopes of arresting the progression of severe retrolental fibroplasia.

Blood is drawn frequently and analyzed for many components, including pH, oxygen and carbon dioxide content, hematocrit, bilirubin, signs of infection, and drug concentrations. Serum medication concentrations are monitored in order to achieve concentrations high enough to be therapeutic but below the toxic range. Medications that are commonly monitored in the NICU include the aminoglycosides, vancomycin, theophylline, and digitalis. State screens are done to assess for the presence of phenylketonuria, sickle cell anemia, hypothyroidism, galactosemia, and congenital adrenal hyperplasia.

In addition to the above noted assessments, screening for hearing loss is an important aspect of Neonatal Critical Care (Nozza, 1988). The ABR should be done prior to discharge (Murray, 1988) and appropriate follow-up recommended for all who fail the initial screening (Kramer et al., 1989).

HIGH-RISK INFANT

In 1982 (American Academy of Pediatrics, 1982) and 1990 (Joint Committee on Infant Hearing, 1991), the Joint Committee on Infant Hearing identified infants at risk for having hearing impairments. Included were those infants with a family history of hearing impairment, infants with certain infections, infants with congenital anomalies, infants of low birth weight, infants with hyperbilirubinemia, infants receiving ototoxic medication, and asphyxiated infants. Infants who require mechanical ventilation for more than 10 days are also considered at high risk for hearing impairment, as are infants with a syndrome known to include sensorineural hearing loss.

RISK FACTORS FREQUENTLY ENCOUNTERED IN THE NICU

The list of risk factors for hearing impairment as defined by the American Academy of Pediatrics includes almost all infants in a neonatal intensive care unit. Therefore, most infants admitted to an intensive care nursery should have an audiologic evaluation before discharge. The following provides a summary of risk criteria established by the recent 1990 Joint Committee report.

Birth weight less than 1500 grams (~3.3lbs).

It is well-documented that premature infants have an increased incidence of hearing loss (Kenworthy et al., 1987, Sanders et al., 1985). The incidence varies from 2%–17.5%. Premature infants have multiple health problems that increase their risk for hearing impairment. These include anoxia, hyperbilirubinemia, bacterial and viral infections, hydrocephalus, and exposure to ototoxic medications. The hearing deficit in low birth weight infants is usually sensorineural and most severe in the high frequency range. In addition, as many as 20% of premature infants with birth weights less than 1500 grams will have persistent otitis media. This increases the risk for a progressive conductive hearing impairment. Progressive post-hemorrhagic hydrocephalus is not uncommon in infants of very low birth weight and is associated with multiple handicaps including hearing loss (Boynton et al., 1986).

Cranofacial anomalies including morphologic abnormalities of the pinna and ear canal, absent philtrum, low hairline, etc.

Defects of the head and neck may have accompanying hearing deficits (Coplan, 1987). Cleft lip and/or palate is one of the most common defects of the head and neck, occurring in 1 per 600 births. The incidence of recurrent otitis media in this group is between 50% and 90%. The hearing deficit occurring with cleft lip or palate is generally conductive but there are reported cases of sensorineural and mixed losses. The presence of malformed ears, low set ears, or ear tags should prompt an otologic evaluation. Any external ear anomaly may have an associated middle ear anomaly. Craniofacial skeletal disorders are frequently associated with hearing loss. Diastrophic dwarfism is associated with a congenital sensorineural hearing loss. The hearing deficit manifested in Apert's Syndrome and Fanconi's anemia is a congenital conductive hearing loss. A congenital conductive and/or sensorineural loss

may be seen in achondroplasia, Crouzon syndrome, Marfan syndrome, and Pierre Robin sequence.

Severe depression at birth, which may include infants with Apgar scores of 0–3 at five minutes or those who fail to initiate spontaneous respiration by ten minutes or those with hypotonia persisting to two hours of age.

Asphyxia is a condition usually occurring intrapartum resulting in a compromised neonate. It occurs because of a lack of oxygen delivery to the fetus resulting from impaired placental function or umbilical cord compression. The result is death if the condition is not reversed. With intervention and resuscitation, survival is possible. The insult often results in a neonate with damage to many different organ systems (Denson, 1989). The incidence of neonates suffering asphyxia at or before birth is estimated at 2–4 per 1000 full term infants (Vannucci, 1990). The incidence is increased in small preterm infants, occurring in up to 60%. Hearing impairment occurs in 4% of infants with severe perinatal asphyxia. A high-frequency sensorineural hearing loss is most common (Gerkin, 1984).

Congenital infection known or suspected to be associated with sensorineural hearing-impairment such as toxoplasmosis, syphilis, rubella, cytomegalovirus, and herpes.

Infectious diseases are responsible for approximately 25% of profound hearing losses. One-fifth of these losses are associated with congenital infections. The major infections associated with hearing loss in the newborn include rubella, cytomegalovirus, and meningitis. Other infections causing hearing loss include herpes simplex, toxoplasmosis, and syphilis.

Toxoplasmosis, rubella, cytomegalovirus, and herpes simplex present with similar clinical symptoms. A subclinical infection may also result in hearing deficits (Alpert and Plotkin, 1986). Up to 5% of all newborns are estimated to be infected with one of these agents.

A virus in the herpes family causes cytomegalovirus infection. The virus is transmitted by intimate contact within households and from blood transfusions and organ transplants. CMV can be transmitted to the fetus transplacentally or from contact with cervical secretions during labor. Asymptomatic neonatal periods occur in over 90% of infected infants. Congenital CMV may manifest as systemic illness with hepatosplenomegaly, jaundice, petechiae and thrombocytopenia, chorioretinitis, cerebral calcification, microcephaly, and intrauterine growth retardation. Central nervous system involvement may result in severe sequelae such as psychomotor retardation and deafness. Hearing loss resulting from congenital CMV occurs in 30% of symptomatic infants and 17–56% of asymptomatic infants. The hearing impairment is caused by sensorineural damage which may be unilateral or bilateral, mild or profound. A progressive hearing loss may occur secondary to ongoing active disease.

Toxoplasma gondii is an intracellular parasite of cats. Oocysts are excreted in cat feces and may be found in contaminated undercooked meat. When a pregnant woman comes in contact with the oocysts, the toxoplasma may be transmitted to the fetus transplacentally. Clinical severity varies greatly (Sever et al., 1988). Some infected infants are asymptomatic, while severely affected fetuses may die in utero or deliver prematurely. Chorioretinitis, hydrocephalus, and intracranial calcifications occur frequently. Hearing loss occurs in up to 17% of infants infected with toxoplasma. Progressive hearing loss may occur, necessitating repeated evaluation.

Rubella is caused by a pleomorphic RNA containing virus. The only natural host for rubella is the human race. The virus can be spread by oral droplets and transplacentally. Rubella should be preventable with a fully implemented immunization program. Congenital rubella may result in multiple organ involvement, intrauterine growth retardation, spontaneous abortion, or intrauterine death. Congenital heart disease and interstitial pneumonia may occur. Thrombocytopenic purpura, hepatitis, hepatomegaly, ocular manifestations including cataracts and retinitis, and bone lesions are frequently present. Central nervous system involvement may present as lethargy, irritability or seizures. Late manifestations of congenital rubella include hearing loss and mental retardation. The hearing impairment is severe to profound sensorineural and occurs in 50% of affected infants (Wild et al., 1989). The greatest loss is in the mid-frequency range.

Herpes simplex virus is a DNA-containing virus. Two strains are recognized. Type I affects skin and mucous membranes, whereas type II primarily affects the genitalia. HSV is spread by trauma and close body contact. Type II herpes simplex virus causes most neonatal infections. It is acquired by passage through an infected birth canal or by ascension of the virus after rupture of amniotic membranes. Neonatal HSV infection may present in a variety of ways, from local skin, eye, or mouth lesions to generalized disease. Disseminated disease may involve the lungs, liver, and adrenal glands, producing a sepsis-like appearance. Mortality and morbidity are high; major sequelae include seizures, mental retardation, blindness, and deafness. Neonatal HSV infection may result in sensorineural hearing impairment with similarity to CMV (Dahle and McCollister, 1988).

Syphilis is caused by a spirochete, Treponema pallidum. Transplacental transmission to the fetus is more likely during later pregnancy but infection may be acquired during the first trimester. Congenital syphilis results in intrauterine death in 25% of fetuses and postnatal death in 25% of infected newborns. Early congenital syphilis, appearing during the first two years of life, is similar to secondary syphilis in an adult. The infected infants may be asymptomatic or have hydrops, hepatosplenomegaly, anemia, thrombocytopenia, bone involvement, skin and mucous membrane lesions, and profuse nasal discharge. Late congenital syphilis appears years after birth and results from either chronic inflammation or a hypersensitivity reaction. Skeletal changes and dental abnormalities may result. Blindness can result from corneal opacification; deafness can result from eighth nerve involvement. Hearing impairment occurs in approximately 35% of children with congenital syphilis. The prognosis is poor due to neural atrophy with poor discrimination.

Bacterial meningitis.

Bacterial meningitis develops in 1 per 2500 live births. The most common etiologies are Group B beta-hemolytic streptococcus, Escherichia coli and other gram negative rods, and rarely Listeria monocytogenes. The infant may be febrile, lethargic, irritable, or jaundiced. The mortality associated with neonatal bacterial meningitis is 20–30%. One half of the survivors have permanent sequelae resulting in significant neurologic damage (Klein et al., 1986). Seizure disorders and mental retardation have been observed following bacterial meningitis. Hearing loss occurs in 2.4–29% of survivors. Hearing loss may result from spread of infection along the middle canal and cochlear aqueduct, serous or purulent labyrinthitis, or replacement of the membranous labyrinth with fibrous tissue and new bone.

Hyperbilirubinemia at a level exceeding indication for exchange transfusion.

Bilirubin is a toxic substance derived from the breakdown of red blood cells and hyperbilirubinemia is an elevated amount of bilirubin in the blood. Kernicterus is the deposition of bilirubin in brain cells, causing a yellow discoloration of the brain. Bilirubin's toxic effects include motor and sensory deficits, mental retardation, hearing deficits, and death. Bilirubin encephalopathy is the brain damage resulting from the toxicity. It is not known at what bilirubin concentration the risk of brain damage exceeds the risk of treatment. Encephalopathy is unlikely to occur in full-term neonates with hemolytic disease if the bilirubin concentration is kept below 20 mg/dl. There is little information in low birth weight or full term neonates without hemolytic disease to base guidelines for treatment of neonates with bilirubin concentrations less than 20 mg/dl (DeVries et al., 1987, Scheidt et al., 1990). Full-term infants with a bilirubin concentration of greater than 20 mg/dl should be considered at risk for hearing loss. All low birth weight infants should be considered at risk because of elevated bilirubin concentrations as well as other risk factors. The hearing damage associated with hyperbilirubinemia ranges from mild to profound and includes bilateral and unilateral sensorineural losses.

Family history of congenital or delayed onset childhood sensorineural impairment.

A family history of the presence of any form of hearing loss other than presbycusis which begins in older age is a risk factor for hearing impairment. Hereditary deafness occurs with a large number of syndromes as well as without associated anomalies. Hereditary deafness is inherited as an autosomal dominant trait in 17% of cases. The hearing loss may or may not be present at birth but may develop later as a bilateral deficit with high frequency most severely affected. About 40% of profound childhood deafness is inherited as an autosomal recessive trait. The hearing loss is present at birth and usually most severe in the high-frequency range. There is an X-linked pattern of inheritance causing hearing impairment in males only, accounting for 3% of hereditary deafness. The hearing loss develops in early infancy and is progressive.

Multi-faceted fetal alcohol syndrome (FAS) may be best characterized within this Joint Committee criteria. FAS, whose traits are becoming increasingly recognized, describes a pattern of congenital malformations seen in children of women who abuse alcohol during pregnancy. It occurs in 1–2 per 1000 births (Jones, 1986). Prenatal and postnatal growth deficiency occurs commonly in affected infants. Craniofacial, skeletal, cardiac, renal, and other anomalies may be found. Mental retardation, learning disorders, and other behavioral aberrations are associated with FAS. These patients are prone to have recurrent serious otitis media, likely secondary to eustachian tube dysfunction. Hearing impairment may be secondary to sensorineural loss or recurrent otitis media (Church and Gerkin, 1988).

THERAPEUTIC RISKS

In addition to the risk factors infants are born with, some risks are acquired. These include risks from ototoxic medications, treatment of persistent fetal circulation, and other factors.

Ototoxic medications including, but not limited to, the aminoglycosides used for more than five days (e.g., gentamicin, tobramycin, kanamycin, streptomycin), and loop diuretics used in combination with aminoglycosides.

Permanent hearing loss from ototoxic medications is observed infrequently. The cochlea, vestibular system, or neuromuscular transmission may be affected. There are at least 96 identified ototoxic agents (Catlin, 1985). Ototoxic medications commonly used in the NICU include loop diuretics and aminoglycoside antibiotics. Aminoglycosides cause ototoxic reactions in 2–25% of adults and less frequently in children. The ototoxic reaction may be permanent or reversible. Gentamicin is more toxic to the vestibular system than to the cochlea. Tobramycin appears to be slightly less ototoxic than gentamicin, but is more toxic to the cochlea than the vestibular system. Amikacin is also primarily cochleotoxic (Finitzo-Hieber et al., 1985). Ototoxicity from aminoglycosides may be enhanced by concomitant use of the loop diuretics. Furosemide alone rarely results in permanent deafness.

Prolonged mechanical ventilation for a duration equal to or greater than ten days (e.g., persistent pulmonary hypertension).

Persistent fetal circulation, or persistent pulmonary hypertension, is primarily a disease of full-term infants. It is manifested by severe hypoxemia despite aggressive ventilator management. Persistent fetal circulation is associated with a variety of diagnoses including meconium aspiration syndrome, pneumonia, sepsis, diaphragmatic hernia, and asphyxia. There is a high mortality rate despite aggressive management, including hyperventilation and the use of pulmonary vasodilators. Sensorineural hearing loss has been identified as a sequelae (Hendricks-Munoz and Waltin, 1988). The onset may be delayed and the hearing loss progressive. The number of days of respiratory therapy has been shown to be a predictor of hearing loss in premature infants (Bergman et al., 1985). Low serum sodium has also been shown to be a predictor of hearing loss (Swigonski et al., 1987). Extended stay in the hospital has been associated with hearing loss (Duara et al., 1986). Incubator noise has been suspected of threatening hearing (Bernard and Pechere, 1984). Continuous noise is more damaging than intermittent sounds, and premature infants are confined to incubators continuously for weeks or months. The noise level in the NICU may approach dangerous levels due to multiple alarms, the ventilator sounds, and the activities of skilled workers of multiple disciplines. The premature infant may be more susceptible to damaging noise exposure than the adult, especially if potentiated by ototoxic medications.

SUMMARY

Neonatology has evolved into a very specialized area with the development of neonatal intensive care units that have the capabilities of treating previously fatal diseases. This has resulted in a lower mortality rate, but with more survivors there is a higher morbidity rate. Hearing loss is a sequelae of concern to the neonatologist and parents. Recognition of those infants at risk allows screening in the newborn nursery before discharge from the hospital. Early detection of a hearing disorder is important so that intervention may be instituted, which improves the infant's potential for a good outcome.

REFERENCES

Alpert, G. and Plotkin, S.A. (1986). A practical guide to the diagnosis of congenital infections in the newborn infant. *Pediatric Clinics of North America, 33,* 465–479.

American Academy of Pediatrics, Joint Committee on Infant Hearing (1982). Position Statement 1982. *Pediatrics, 70,* 496–497.

Bergman, I., Hirsch, R.P., Fria, T.J., et al. (1985). Cause of hearing loss in the high-risk premature infant. *Journal of Pediatrics, 106,* 95–101.

Bernard, P.A. and Pechere, J.C. (1984). Does incubator noise increase risks of aminoglycoside ototoxicity? *Audiology, 23,* 309–320.

Boynton, B.R., Boynton, C.A., Merritt, T.A., et al. (1986). Ventriculoperitoneal shunts in low birth weight infants with intracranial hemorrhage: Neurodevelopmental outcome. *Neurosurgery, 18,* 141–145.

Catlin, F.I. (1985). Prevention of hearing impairment from infection and ototoxic drugs. *Archives of Otolarngology, 111,* 377–384.

Church, M.W. and Gerkin, K.P. (1988). Hearing disorders in

children with fetal alcohol syndrome: Findings from case reports. *Pediatrics, 82,* 147–154.

Cone, T.E. (1985). *History of the care and feeding of the premature infant.* Boston, MA: Little, Brown and Company.

Coplan, J. (1987). Deafness: ever heard of it? Delayed recognition of permanent hearing loss. *Pediatrics, 79,* 206–213.

Dahle, A.J. and McCollister, F.P. (1988). Audiological findings in children with neonatal herpes. *Ear and Hearing, 9,* 256–258.

De Vries, L.S., Lary, S., Whitelaw, A.G., et al. (1987). Relationship of serum bilirubin levels and hearing impairment in newborn infants. *Early Human Development, 15,* 269–277.

Denson, S.E. (1989). Fetal asphyxia: Its impact on the neonate: An approach to understanding and anticipating complications, in *Current Perinatology,* 25–37. Springer-Verlag.

Duara, S., Suter, C.M., Bessard, K.K., et al. (1986). Neonatal screening with auditory brainstem responses: Results of follow-up audiometry and risk factor evaluation. *Journal of Pediatrics, 108,* 276–281.

Elliman, A.M., Bryan, E.M., and Elliman, A.D. (1986). Low birth weight babies at 3 years of age. *Child: Care, Health and Development, 12,* 287–311.

Finitzo-Hieber, T., McCracken, G.H., and Brown, K.C. (1985). Prospective controlled evaluation of auditory function in neonates given netilmicin or amikacin. *Journal of Pediatrics, 106,* 129–136.

Frigoletto, F.D. and Little, G.A. (1988). Guidelines for perinatal care. *American Academy of Pediatrics and American College of Obstetricians and Gynecologists.*

Gerkin, K. (1984). The high risk register for deafness. *ASHA, 26,* 17–23.

Ginsberg, H.G., Goldsmith, J.P., and Stedman, C.M. (1990). Survival of a 380-g infant. *New England Journal of Medicine, 322,* 1753–1754.

Hendricks-Munoz, K.D. and Walton, J.P. (1988). Hearing loss in infants with persistent fetal circulation. *Pediatrics, 81,* 650–656.

Hoffman, E.L. and Bennett, F.C. (1990). Birth weight less than 800 grams: Changing outcomes and influences of gender and gestation number. *Pediatrics, 86,* 27–34.

Joint Commitee on Infant Hearing 1990 (1991). Position statement. *Audiology Today, 3,* 14–17.

Jones, K.L. (1986). Fetal alcohol syndrome. *Pediatrics in Review, 8,* 122–126.

Kenworthy, O.T., Bess, F.H., Stahlman, M.T., et al. (1987). Hearing, speech, and language outcome in infants with extreme immaturity. *American Journal of Otology, 8,* 419–425.

Klein, J.O., Feigin, R.D., and McCracken, G.H. (1986). Report of the task force on diagnosis and management of meningitis. *Pediatrics, 78 (Supplement),* 959–982.

Kramer, S.J., Vertes, D.R., and Condon, M. (1989). Auditory brainstem responses and clinical follow-up of high-risk infants. *Pediatrics, 83,* 385–392.

Mali, M., Tyler, P., and Brookfield, D.S. (1989). Developmental outcome of high-risk neonates in North Staffordshire. *Child: Care, Health and Development, 15,* 137–145.

Murray, A.D. (1988). Newborn auditory brainstem evoked responses (ABRs): Longitudinal correlates in the first year. *Child Development, 59,* 1542–1554.

Northway, W.H., Moss, R.B., Carlisle, K.B., et al. (1990). Late pulmonary sequelae of bronchopulmonary dysplasia. *New England Journal of Medicine, 323,* 1793–1799.

Nozza, R.J. (1988). Recent advances in audiologic assessment. *Pediatric Infectious Disease Journal, 7 (Supplement),* S169–173.

O'Donnell, J. (1990). The development of a climate for caring: A historical review of premature care in the United States from 1900 to 1979. *Neonatal Network, 8,* 7–17.

Plesko, L. (1990). Troubling trends, infant mortality in America. *Neonatal Intensive Care, Special Issue-December,* 8–18.

Sanders, R., Durieux-Smith, A., Hyde, M., et al. (1985). Incidence of hearing loss in high risk and intensive care nursery infants. *Journal of Otolaryngology, 14 (Supplement),* 28–33.

Scheidt, P.C., Bryla, D.A., Nelson, K.B., et al. (1990). Phototherapy for neonatal hyperbilirubinemia: Six-year follow-up of the National Institute of Child Health and Human Development Clinical Trial. *Pediatrics, 85,* 455–463.

Sever, J.L., Ellenberg, J.H., Ley, A.C., et al. (1988). Toxoplasmosis: Maternal and pediatric findings in 23,000 pregnancies. *Pediatrics, 82,* 181–192.

Silverman, W.A. (1990). Neonatal pediatrics at the century mark. *Pediatric Research, 27 (Supplement),* S34–37.

Soll, R.F., Hoekstra, R.E., Fangman, J.J., et al. (1990). Multicenter trial of single-dose modified bovine surfactant extract (Survanta) for prevention of respiratory distress syndrome. *Pediatrics, 85,* 1092–1102.

Swigonski, N., Shallop, J., Bull, M.J., et al. (1987). Hearing screening of high risk newborns. *Ear and Hearing, 8,* 26–29.

Vannucci, R.C. (1990). Current and potentially new management strategies for perinatal hypoxic-ischemic encephalopathy. *Pediatrics, 85,* 961–968.

Wild, N.J., Sheppard, S., Smithells, R.W., et al. (1989). Onset and severity of hearing loss due to congenital rubella infection. *Archives of Disease in Childhood, 64,* 1280–1283.

CHAPTER 15

NEWBORN HEARING SCREENING

BRUCE A. WEBER
CLAIRE JACOBSON

INTRODUCTION

Nature of the Problem

National statistics indicate that there are approximately 3.7 million live births in the United States each year (Wegman, 1987). Within this group are more than 100,000 high-risk newborns who require the special attention provided by a neonatal intensive care unit (NICU). Among these high-risk newborns are premature babies whose problems during the neonatal period include immaturity of the lungs, central nervous system, gut, liver, kidneys, and immune system (Grogaard, 1988). This group also contains full-term babies with birth asphyxia, respiratory distress, infection, jaundice, metabolic problems, and severe congenital disorders. The number of high-risk infants in the NICU who survive significant neonatal compromise continues to increase each year.

For the most part, improved survival rates can be attributed to recent advances in medical technology and related medical management. Today, survival is not uncommon for babies born less than 24 weeks gestational age and weighing less than 750 grams. The survival rate is close to 50 percent for babies weighing between 500 and 750 grams and increases to 80 percent for babies of 750–1000 gram birth weight. Ten years ago, most infants weighing less than 1000 grams did not survive more than a few days after birth (Grogaard, 1988). Accompanying this decreased rate of mortality, however, exists a proportional increase in the number of surviving infants with adverse sequelae which place them at high risk for hearing loss.

Prevalence. The prevalence of severe to profound bilateral sensory hearing loss in the general pediatric population is most often reported to range between 1:1000 (0.1%) and 1:4000 (0.025%) (Carrel, 1977; Catlin, 1978; Frasier, 1971; Jaffe, 1977). Hearing loss of lesser degree may approximate 6:1000 (0.6%) (Carrel, 1977). These figures are often based on studies which have methodological limitations (Konkle and Jacobson, 1991), so the actual numbers of hearing-impaired children may be considerably greater. The American Speech-Language-Hearing Association (ASHA) Committee on Infant Hearing (1989) recently reviewed available data and concluded that reliable information on the incidence of significant hearing impairment in infants and young children is not available at this time. Clearly, there is a pressing need for more accurate information on the prevalence of handicapping hearing loss in young infants.

Rationale for Early Identification of Hearing Loss

The development of social and cognitive learning behavior and the acquisition of acceptable levels of educational achievement are dependent on intact peripheral and central auditory mechanisms. There is evidence to suggest that developmental delays commonly occur if even only a mild hearing loss is present (Menyuk, 1977). Hearing loss suffered during the first three years of life, whether it is congenital or acquired, conductive or sensorineural, represents a significant problem for the acquisition of language skills necessary for many aspects of development (Kenworthy et al., 1987). Identification of hearing loss at a young age allows for early consideration of amplification and placement in infant/pre-school habilitation programs. Early intervention has been shown to increase the child's readiness for mainstreaming into the regular classroom at school age, and has significant financial implications because it reduces the need for specialized classes (Downs, 1986).

In response to the need for early identification of hearing loss, a number of states have created the necessary enabling legislation to permit statewide testing. Blake and Hall (1990) have provided the most recent survey of the status of statewide policies for neonatal hearing screening. According to their report, compiled in November 1988, 14 states have legislative mandates for newborn hearing screening. Twelve other states have no legislative mandate, but have addressed the issue in some way at the state level. The remaining 24 states, plus the District of Columbia, have no mandate and have indicated that the issue has not yet been addressed at the state level. Of the 14 mandated statewide programs, 10 have implemented state-run programs, 2 programs are run privately, and the remaining 2 states are in the process of developing programs. The 14 mandated states are: Arizona, California, Connecticut, Florida, Georgia, Kentucky, Maryland, Massachusetts, Mississippi, New Jersey, Ohio, Oklahoma, Rhode Island, and Virginia. In addition, the Canadian provinces of British Columbia and Nova Scotia have province-wide neonatal hearing screening programs.

Figure 15.1 geographically illustrates by category: 1) states with legislative mandates, 2) states with no legislative mandates, but with an existing screening program at the state level, and 3) states with no mandate and no statewide policy. It should be noted that the map represents only statewide programs and excludes all of the excellent screening programs throughout the country which are confined to single hospitals.

States and provinces with active regional or statewide programs vary in the type of screening which is implemented. As the Blake and Hall survey (1990) points out, two fundamental approaches to screening are most commonly used. They are: 1) screening of high-risk infants prior to discharge, and 2) use of a high-risk registry to identify infants for recommended diagnostic follow-up after discharge. For the former, testing usu-

ally includes one or a combination of auditory brainstem response (ABR), behavioral audiometry, or crib-o-gram assessment. At present, no standardized testing protocol is universally accepted. The guidelines developed by the ASHA Committee on Infant Hearing (1989) represent a significant step in this direction.

Although some strong arguments can be made in favor of postponing initial hearing screening until after the infant has been discharged from the nursery (Downs, 1982; Alberti et al., 1985; Swigonski et al., 1987), we strongly support the concept of screening in the neonatal intensive care unit (NICU) or intermediate-care unit whenever practical. In our experience, too many infants fail to return for routine outpatient follow-up testing. As a result, many high-risk babies would never receive an early hearing screening if it were conducted strictly on an outpatient basis. Hearing screening in the NICU reduces the number of infants to be followed and permits a concentrated effort toward returning these babies for follow-up testing.

It is unlikely that statewide nursery hearing screening programs will be established in every state in the near future. Therefore, some form of early identification program will need to be developed at individual hospitals. Brooks (1990) surveyed 553 hospitals which were known to have an NICU and found that 81% of the respondents reported some form of hearing screening program in operation. Though the form of screening differed markedly among hospitals, the results of the survey indicate that many hospitals have made a commitment to newborn hearing screening.

Hearing Loss Testing Act Proposed 1991

At the time of writing this chapter, James T. Walsh, Congress member, introduced bill H.R. 2089 at the 102nd Congress, 1st Session, on April 24, 1991. This bill requires hearing loss testing for all newborns in the United States. Subsequently, it was referred to the Committee on Energy and Commerce. The *Hearing Loss Testing Act* of 1991 would require all health insurance policies that provide benefits to newborns to cover screening for hearing impairment in newborns. In addition, the bill would authorize the Secretary of Health and Human Services to establish a program to

Statewide neonatal screening programs

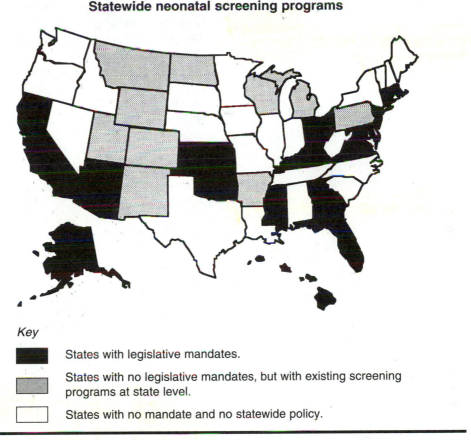

Key

States with legislative mandates.

States with no legislative mandates, but with existing screening programs at state level.

States with no mandate and no statewide policy.

FIGURE 15.1.   Map showing states with legislation for newborn hearing screening programs. (Courtesy JAAA, Vol. 1, number 2, April 1990, p. 68)

provide hearing tests to all newborns who are not covered either by Medicaid, which already covers screening for hearing loss, or by private insurance.

A 1991 cost estimate by the Congressional Budget Office (CBO) assumes that there will be 3.7 million children born in the United States in 1992 and that births will increase to 4.5 million in 1996. Based on the national survey conducted by the Agency for Health Care Policy and Research, the National Medical Expenditure Survey Estimates of the Uninsured Population in 1987, CBO assumes that 17% of those newborn children will be uninsured.

If ABR is the recommended test for hearing screening in newborns, with an average cost of $150.00 per screen, and also assuming an increase in test cost due to inflation, the CBO estimates that the program will cost the federal government approximately $90 million, increasing to $100 million by 1996.

The Purpose of Screening

Regardless of specifics of the screening procedure, the principal objective of a newborn hearing screening program is to identify hearing loss correctly in those infants who are truly hearing-impaired, while ruling out a loss in normal-hearing babies. The purpose of screening is not to specify the infant's hearing sensitivity, but rather to determine whether a hearing loss exists. Thus, the degree and nature of impairment is inconsequential in the screening process. If the result of the screening test is abnormal, additional audiological evaluation will be necessary to determine the type and degree of the impairment.

SCREENING PRINCIPLES

With the widespread adoption of newborn hearing screening across North America, there is an ever-increasing need to insure that programs carefully select test procedures that are both valid and reliable. Usually, some form of strategy is used to determine which test(s) are effective and efficient for a particular clinical situation. In order to accomplish this task, there must be a method of quantifying test performance. This process usually incorporates some aspect of clinical decision analysis which is directly concerned with the design and quantitative evaluation of testing and therapeutic strategies (Hyde, Davidson, and Alberti, 1990).

The following is a brief discussion of the principles of test selection as they apply to newborn hearing screening program. It should be noted, however, that these applications are not limited to screening programs and may be used to analyze any number of test strategies. For a more comprehensive description of the topic, the reader is referred to Fria (1985); Hyde, Davidson, and Alberti (1990); and Jacobson and Jacobson (1987).

Operating Characteristics

Because the early detection and rehabilitative management of the hearing-impaired infant is the primary goal of a newborn hearing screening program, accurate test strategies must be designed that separate hearing-impaired from normal-hearing infants. It is important to view every aspect of a newborn hearing screening program as a test which can be evaluated independently with regard to the final outcome. For example, any classification system which attempts to separate infants who are at greater risk for hearing loss is a test. If the classification system, such as the high-risk register discussed below, meets the rigors of a quantitative analysis, its use is justified in the overall testing strat-

egy. However, if the method of classification is found not to conform to some predetermined level of efficiency, it can be modified (e.g., expanded) or eliminated from the screening program. This evaluation process can be extended to every aspect of a screening program, thereby improving its overall efficiency and accountability. For purposes of discussion, the ABR will be the technique used as the screening model. Again, it must be emphasized that it is not the purpose of the ABR screening to confirm hearing loss; that is the role of the diagnostic follow-up evaluation.

Decision Matrix

Two basic questions are addressed when assessing the value of any test characteristic. They are: 1) If hearing impairment is present, what is the probability that the test outcome will be positive? 2) If hearing is normal, what is the probability that test results will be negative? The simplest model to display these characteristics is a binary 2×2 table which integrates test outcome with the presence or absence of a hearing impairment. This forms a decision matrix which is illustrated in Figure 15.2. Thus, for any screening test, there are four possible outcomes. A baby with a hearing loss can fail the test (true-positive) and a normal-hearing baby can pass the test (true-negative). Conversely, a hearing-impaired baby can pass the test (false-negative) and a normal-hearing baby can fail (false-positive). An effective screening test would produce a high true-positive rate and, conversely, a high true-negative outcome. As a result, a high percentage of hearing-impaired infants would be correctly identified and a high percentage of infants with normal hearing would pass the screen.

The probability that a hearing impaired baby will fail the test is called the test's *sensitivity*. It is determined by calculating: true-positive /(true-positive+false-negative). The probability that a normal-hearing baby will pass the screening is called the test's *specificity*. It is determined by: true-negative /(true-negative+false-positive). The ideal screening test would have perfect (100%) sensitivity and specificity, but in practice this is seldom achieved. The actual sensitivity and specificity of hearing screening can be determined by examining the relationship of the number of babies who fall in each of the four

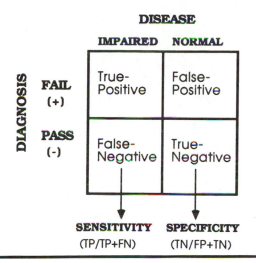

FIGURE 15.2.   Illustration of a 2 × 2 matrix commonly used to categorize test results into true-positive, true-negative, false-positive and false-negative outcomes.

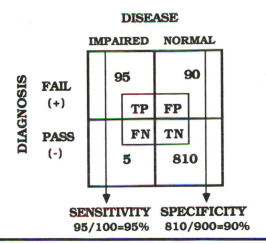

FIGURE 15.3.   Hypothetical outcome of a screening program conducted on a group of 1,000 children, illustrating test sensitivity and specificity (see text for explanation).

possible screening outcomes. Figure 15.3 gives an example of the results of ABR hearing screening on 1000 babies. In this hypothetical example, the sensitivity of the ABR screening is 95/100 or 95%, and the specificity is 810/900 or 90%. The results suggest that, in detecting a hearing impairment, ABR results were correct 95% of the time, whereas with normal hearing infants, the ABR screening was correct 97% of the time. The reciprocal characteristics for this test can also be examined. The false-negative and false-positive results, suggest that the test missed a hearing impairment 5% (5/100) of the time and normal-hearing infants failed the screening 10% (90/900) of the time.

Pass-Fail Cutoff Point

In the administration of a screening program, the audiologist has some control over the likelihood of the four different test outcomes. This, in turn, affects the sensitivity and specificity of the screening. By making the criterion for passing the screening test more stringent (e.g., requiring a detectable response at 20 dB nHL, rather than 35 dB nHL) more babies will fail the test. This more stringent criterion will increase the likelihood

that a hearing-impaired baby will fail the screening; thus, sensitivity is raised. However, this more stringent screening criterion will also increase the probability that normal-hearing babies will fail the test, so specificity is reduced. These concepts are illustrated in Figure 15.4. By altering the cutoff criterion from 35 to 50 dB nHL (less stringent), the opposite situation will occur. More hearing-impaired infants will now pass the screening, thereby decreasing the test's sensitivity. However, fewer normal-hearing infants will fail the test so specificity will be increased. It can be seen that no test can be perfectly designed. There will always remain an overlapping group that will be incorrectly identified.

A cutoff score between pass and fail is an arbitrary point which should be selected based on sound clinical evidence and a clear understanding of the screening purpose. Obviously, if identification of profound hearing impairment is the sole goal of the screening, then a high intensity (e.g., 80 dB) cutoff point is appropriate. However, if identification of milder levels of impairment are important, the cutoff point (screening intensity level) should be decreased accordingly. As mentioned above, the screening level which is finally selected will influence sensitivity and specificity.

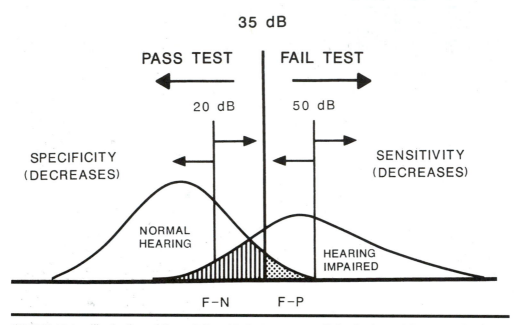

FIGURE 15.4.   Illustration of the relationship between pass/fail criteria and the concept of overlapping distribution (see text for explanation).

Test Selection

With a basic understanding of the operating characteristics of a test and its resulting interpretation, the examiner is next faced with the decision regarding which characteristic is more important: sensitivity or specificity? This is a complex issue which cannot be addressed simply. Generally, however, when it is important to confirm an acknowledged existing disease process, high test specificity is required because there is a proportionally low false-positive rate. However, if it is important to exclude a diagnostic entity, a test with high sensitivity is preferred since there will be a low false-negative rate. The latter appears to take priority in the case of newborn hearing screening. A normal-hearing child who incorrectly fails the screening will receive unnecessary follow-up testing. Though unfortunate, this is less of an error than passing a hearing-impaired infant whose loss likely will not be discovered until the age of 18–24

months (Stein, Clark, and Kraus, 1983; Stein et al., 1990).

THE HIGH-RISK REGISTER

In response to growing concern over the early identification of hearing loss, the Joint Committee on Infant Hearing (JCIH) was formed in 1969 from representatives of the Academy of Pediatrics, the Academy of Ophthalmology and Otolaryngology, and the American Speech-Language-Hearing Association. The Committee was charged with establishing recommendations for newborn hearing screening. Although the JCIH acknowledge the importance of screening, they also recognized the inherent problems associated with behavioral testing and therefore, did not support the concept of mass screening for all newborns, rather they advocated continued research in the area.

Based largely on the work of Downs and colleagues

(1964, 1969) and other longitudinal studies, in 1972 the JCIH issued a supplementary statement that endorsed the concept of a five factor high-risk register for selective testing. This statement emanated from the fact that infants who present with certain medical and genetic factors are more likely to be at risk for hearing loss. The criteria have been referred to as the ABCDs of deafness and include: A: Affected family; B: Bilirubin levels; C: Congenital rubella syndrome; D: Defects of the ears, nose, or throat; and S: Small at birth. The JCIH recommended further that infants found to be at risk should be audiologically evaluated within the first two months of life.

Subsequently, the JCIH (1982) revised the initial five factors and expanded the list to seven criteria. The two additional categories were bacterial meningitis and severe asphyxia. At the time, no single screening method was endorsed as ideal; thus, the Joint Committee suggested follow-up audiological evaluation of these infants until accurate assessments of hearing could be accomplished (JCIH, 1982)

Most recently, the JCIH (1991) issued a new position statement that has attempted to clarify and expand the current risk criteria. This statement was prompted by intensive research and new legislation (P.L. 99–457). One of the unique features of this statement is the introduction of two independent age groups: 1) *neonates* (birth–28 days), and 2) *infants* (29 days–2 years). Table 15.2 lists the risks criteria for the neonatal group including three new risk factors. Briefly they are, 1) ototoxic medications, 2) prolonged mechanical ventilation, and 3) stigmata associated with syndromes known to include sensorineural hearing loss. Table 15.2 presents the new risk criteria for the infant age group. Additional infant risk criteria which may not be present or easily identified in the neonatal period include: 1) parent/caregiver concern, 2) head trauma, 3) neurodegenerative disorders, and 4) childhood infectious disease.

The Joint Committee reports that moderate to severe sensory hearing loss can be confirmed in 2.5 to 5.0% of neonates manifesting any of the previously published risk criteria. Admittedly, not all of the new risk criteria have established performance characteristics. For example, will the introduction of new medica-

TABLE 15.1.   Risk Criteria: Neonates (birth–28 days)

The risk factors that identify those neonates who are at risk for sensorineural hearing impairment include the following:

1. Family history of congenital or delayed onset childhood sensorineural impairment.
2. Congenital infection known or suspected to be associated with sensorineural hearing impairment such as toxoplasmosis, syphilis, rubella, cytomegalovirus, and herpes.
3. Craniofacial anomalies including morphologic abnormalities of the pinna and ear canal, absent philtrum, low hairline, etc.
4. Birth weight less than 1500 grams (~3.3 lbs).
5. Hyperbilirubinanemia at a level exceeding indication for exchange transfusion.
6. Ototoxic medications including but not limited to the aminoglycosides used for more than 5 days (e.g., gentamicin, tobramycin, kanamycin, streptomycin) and loop diuretics used in combination with aminoglycosides.
7. Bacterial meningitis.
8. Severe depression at birth, which may include infants with Apgar scores of 0–3 at 5 minutes or those who fail to initiate spontaneous respiration by 10 minutes or those with hypotonia persisting to 2 hours of age.
9. Prolonged mechanical ventilation for a duration equal to or greater than 10 days (e.g., persistent pulmonary hypertension).
10. Stigmata or other findings associated with a syndrome known to include sensorineural hearing loss (e.g., Warrdenburg or Usher's Syndrome).

tions produce potential ototoxic results on newborn hearing? What deleterious auditory effects will manifest in the fetus exposed to the HIV virus? Will maternal substance abuse ultimately result in long-term auditory consequences? And most basic to the implementation of the register, will its expansion result in an increased number of infants identified with hearing loss? Although the jury remains unresolved to this point,

TABLE 15.2. Risk Criteria: Infants (29 days–2 years)

The factors that identify those infants who are at risk for sensorineural hearing impairment include the following:

1. Parent/caregiver concern regarding hearing, speech, language and/or developmental delay.
2. Bacterial meningitis.
3. Neonatal risk factors that may be associated with progressive sensorineural hearing loss (e.g., cytomegalovirus, prolonged mechanical ventilation, and inherited disorders).
4. Head trauma, especially with either longitudinal or transverse fracture of the temporal bone.
5. Stigmata or other findings associated with syndromes known to include sensorineural hearing loss (e.g., Warrdenburg or Usher's Syndrome).
6. Ototoxic medications including but not limited to the aminoglycosides used for more than 5 days (e.g., gentamicin, tobramycin, kanamycin, streptomycin) and loop diuretics used in combination with aminoglycosides.
7. Children with neurodegenerative disorders such as neurofibromatosis, myoclonic epilepsy, Werdnig-Hoffman disease, Tay-Sach's disease, infantile Gaucher's disease, Neiman-Pick disease, any metachromatic leukodystrophy, or any infantile demyelinating neuropathy.
8. Childhood infectious diseases known to be associated with sensorineural hearing loss (e.g., mumps, measles).

without longitudinal study, no clear decisions will be forthcoming. Thus, JCIH encourages further study and critical evaluation. The JCIH moreover acknowledges the continuous and compelling developments occurring in neonatal and prenatal medicine and recommends review of the risk register every three years.

The 1990 statement also addresses the question of appropriate screening protocol and follow-up. The committee recommends the use of ABR as the initial test procedure for the neonate prior to discharge from the newborn nursery but no later than 3 months of age. For the infant, screening is recommended no later than

3 months after risk factors have been identified. Neonates and infants who fail a screening should receive general medical and otologic follow-up and a comprehensive audiologic evaluation that includes the ABR, behavioral testing (>6 months) and acoustic immittance measures.

Finally, in accordance with P.L. 99–457, the Joint Committee offered early intervention guidelines for hearing-impaired infants and their families. Intervention services focus around the concept of an individualized family service plan (IFSP) and the coordination of other agencies.

PRELIMINARY CONSIDERATIONS

If a newborn hearing screening program is being contemplated, three general questions should be answered early in the planning stages: 1) How receptive is the hospital staff to the concept of hearing screening in the newborn nurseries? 2) How will hearing be measured? and 3) How will the costs involved in setting up and maintaining the desired screening program be supported? Answers to these three questions should help determine whether a screening program is feasible and, if so, what specific problem areas need to be addressed. These three topics warrant some consideration here.

Receptiveness to a Newborn Hearing Screening Program

The success of any screening program, of course, is highly dependent upon the cooperation of hospital staff and this support should not be taken for granted. The staff must be convinced of its value, so that any disruption in their already busy day is not viewed as an unwanted intrusion. It should be obvious that without the support of the physicians, nurses, and administrators, a hearing screening program has little chance of success. The importance of securing this support from the outset cannot be overstated.

How Hearing Will Be Tested

It is difficult to obtain the necessary hospital support without having a fairly specific plan for how the screening will be carried out. The nursery staff will be particularly interested in the time required to screen each baby, their required level of involvement, and the amount of disruption the screening will create in the nursery routine. Responses to these concerns will be largely determined by the type of hearing testing which will be performed. This decision will also determine staff and equipment needs. Thus, considerable attention should be given to the alternative approaches to the screening of hearing in the newborn. There are several different response measures which have been used for nursery screening, each with its own set of advantages and disadvantages. Once a decision has been made on the most appropriate measure of hearing many of the questions regarding equipment and staff needs are easier to answer. Presented below is a brief discussion of the different measures which have been used in newborn screening in the NICU.

Behavioral Observation Audiometry (BOA). In this form of hearing screening a high intensity (e.g., 90 dBA) narrow band of noise is presented by a hand-held screener positioned approximately one inch from the baby's ear. The range of acceptable responses includes cessation of activity, eye-widening, subtle changes in facial expression, crying, and gross startle responses. The determination of whether a response has occurred is highly subjective and can often be difficult for even experienced observers. There are serious concerns about the effectiveness of BOA screening. Using BOA, Plotnick and Leppler (1986) identified only two severely hearing-impaired babies among 356 newborns screened in the NICU. Assuming a very conservative 2% prevalence of a significant sensorineural hearing loss in the NICU, at least three times as many hearing-impaired babies should have been identified in the group tested. Because of the high stimulus intensity used, BOA is likely to miss a baby with a mild-moderate hearing loss. False-negative rates of 40% to 86% have been reported for BOA (Alberti et al., 1983; Durieux-Smith and Jacobson, 1985) which indicates that an unacceptably large number of babies with a significant hearing loss pass behavioral screening and are thus lost to immediate follow-up. Though BOA is no longer widely viewed as an effective screening procedure (Jacobson and Morehouse, 1984), there are still some proponents of the technique and a small hand-held

screener is currently being marketed as a convenient and inexpensive alternative to more elaborate and costly instrumentation. Because of its poor operating characteristics, BOA cannot be recommended for neonatal hearing screening.

Crib-O-Gram (COG). This hearing screening device uses sensitive motion detectors positioned under the baby's crib mattress to detect changes produced by the test stimulus. A microprocessor determines when the baby is sufficiently quiet and then presents the high-intensity stimulus (a 92 dB SPL band of noise centered at 3000 HZ). The COG apparatus records the baby's responses and indicates whether the baby has met the criteria for passing the hearing screening. Responses range from subtle changes in respiratory patterns to startle reflexes. An advantage of the COG is that it is automated, so less examiner time is required (McFarland, Simmons and Jones, 1980). However, like BOA, high stimulus intensities are needed to elicit a detectable behavioral response. As a result, the COG may miss babies with mild-moderate hearing losses. In addition, COG results are quite unreliable. Durieux-Smith et al., (1985) found that 32% of the babies tested with COG shifted from pass to fail, or vice versa, when they were retested within 48 hours. Because of these serious limitations and its poor cost effectiveness (Markowitz, 1990), there has been a significant reduction in the use of the crib-o-gram in recent years.

Acoustic Reflexes. Acoustic reflex measures, though brief and relatively simple to perform, have not received extensive consideration for use in hearing screening of newborns. This is largely because only a small percentage of babies demonstrate a detectable contralateral reflex when a conventional 220 Hz probe tone is used (Himelfarb et al., 1978). Use of ipsilateral stimulation and a 660 Hz probe tone both appear to increase the number of babies who demonstrate a response. Even so, McMillan et al. (1985) were able to elicit reflexes in only 76% of healthy full-term infants who were free of middle ear problems. The number of premature babies demonstrating an acoustic reflex would be expected to be even lower in the NICU where otitis media and neurological disorders are common. Even if an acoustic reflex can be elicited by a high intensity stimulus, its presence cannot rule out a mild or moderate hearing impairment. Because of all these problems, it seems unlikely that reflex measures will play a significant role in hearing screening in the NICU.

Auditory Brainstem Response (ABR). The Auditory Brainstem Response (ABR) or the Brainstem Auditory Evoked Response (BAER), as it is commonly referred to in pediatric and neonatology literature, was first used in the neonatal intensive care unit by Schulman-Galambos and Galambos (1975). Unlike the procedures discussed above, ABR audiometry utilizes a purely sensory response which is not directly altered by changes in the baby's arousal level. As is discussed elsewhere in this book, the ABR is highly stable, which permits detectable responses to be recorded at low stimulus intensity levels.

As a hearing screening measure, the ABR has two major limitations: 1) The raw acoustic click routinely used in neonatal screening contains frequencies predominantly in the 2000 Hz–4000 Hz range and hearing sensitivity for other frequencies is not evaluated. 2) The ABR reflects synchronous neural firing within the VIII nerve and brainstem and its presence is not evidence of a conscious response at the cortical level. In spite of these limitations, the ABR with infants has been shown to possess excellent accuracy for detecting sensorineural hearing loss in excess of 30 dB (Hyde, Riko, and Malizia, 1990).

The Middle Latency Response (MLR). The longer latency MLR is an evoked response which can be recorded with the same electrode montage as used in ABR testing. However, unlike the ABR, it is not as highly influenced by stimulus onset, so gradual onset tone bursts can be used as test stimuli. Recording MLRs to tone burst stimuli provides more frequency specific information than can be obtained with ABR testing using click stimuli. Testing of adults has shown good agreement between MLR and behavioral thresholds (Musiek et al., 1984).

Early reports which suggested that MLRs could be readily recorded from newborns (McRandle, Smith, and Goldstein, 1974) has now been widely challenged. The nervous system of the newborn does not appear to be sufficiently developed to demonstrate a clearly de-

fined MLR at the same rate of stimulation as the adult. Jerger, Oliver, and Chmiel (1988) observed that a detectable MLR was present in newborns when the rate of stimulation was 1/sec. However, its amplitude declined markedly when the rate was increased to 10/sec. Though it appears that the MLR may be elicited in newborns if very slow (1/sec) repetition rates are used, such testing is too time-consuming for clinical newborn screening.

Considering the strengths and limitations of the alternative techniques available for newborn hearing screening, ABR audiometry clearly stands as the best overall procedure presently available. Because of its current widespread use, the remainder of this chapter will assume that the ABR has been selected as the response measure for hearing screening.

Financial Support for the Program

Once a method of hearing screening has been selected, an additional major factor must be considered before steps can be taken to implement the screening program. A plan must be developed for financing the costs of the program. It is usually not difficult to get other professionals in the hospital to acknowledge the importance of early detection of hearing loss. However, few hospitals will welcome the initiation of ABR hearing screening if it is likely to create a significant financial deficit. Most audiology programs in medical settings are expected to be self-supporting, or nearly so. As a result, it is seldom possible to initiate a hearing screening program without giving careful consideration to the costs involved. Without at least a general plan for covering the costs of the program, it makes little sense to spend time dealing with the procedural aspects of ABR screening. It must be remembered that costs of the program must include such items as equipment, salaries, overhead costs, report writing, mail follow-up, and the costs of retesting babies who fail the initial screening.

The most logical source of financial support is through fees added directly to the hospital bills of the babies who are tested. However, this approach can create some problems. As a result of a nationwide prospective payment system (PPS) which was initiated in 1983, billing for services within most hospitals in the

United States has changed dramatically. Under the PPS system, prior to actual treatment, the hospital receives a set dollar amount based on the patient's admitting diagnosis. Thus, the payment to the hospital is predetermined by the patient's diagnosis related group (DRG) regardless of the actual cost of the services provide (Shakno, 1984). The system, devised originally for Medicare patients, has now been adopted by other state and federal agencies which assume responsibility for the hospital costs of many of the babies in the newborn nurseries. Commonly, over half of the babies in a nursery will be covered by one of the prospective payment systems.

The PPS approach to payment was designed to motivate hospitals to closely monitor and limit patient service. If hospital costs are kept low, the hospital will make money on a PPS patient. Conversely, if expensive services are provided during the patient's hospital stay, the hospital may well lose money because it will receive no additional compensation for these services. Not surprisingly, this approach to health care financing motivates hospitals to reduce the use of procedures which are not central to the primary health problems of the patients. This may result in pressures on the medical staff to refrain from ordering expensive elective procedures. One such procedure is ABR hearing screening.

Because of these financial constraints, it is unlikely that the entire cost of a hearing screening program can be supported through direct patient billing. Though some babies will be covered by insurance, which can be billed directly, a sizable portion of the screening costs may need to be supported from other sources. Likely alternative sources of funds are the local service clubs. Such organizations as the Sertoma Club (Weber, 1988) and the Lions Club (Ruth, Dey-Sigman, and Mills, 1985) are currently helping support newborn hearing screening programs.

When the financial aspects of a screening program have been adequately considered and a plan for funding has been worked out, the plan can be taken to the appropriate administrators for their input and approval. If there is sufficient support from the hospital administration and the medical staff, and the financial aspects of operating the program seem manageable, then some more specific procedural questions can be addressed.

SETTING UP A HEARING SCREENING PROGRAM

Initial Contacts

Once administrative support has been obtained, the initial development of a hearing screening program requires the establishment of the rationale, goals, testing methods, and follow-up criteria. Inservice meetings are useful to explain the program to administrators, medical personnel, and other support staff. Practical inservices can be conducted for staff whose daily routine is directly impacted by the screening program. The nursing staff, in particular, is key to a successful screening program. They play a critical role in selecting babies for testing and helping insure that these babies are fed and sleepy. Providing the nursing staff with information on the importance of hearing screening and early identification helps promote a supportive atmosphere.

A demonstration of the ABR testing techniques and protocols will facilitate an understanding of the new screening program. During discussions, an emphasis on program flexibility with regard to existing services and schedules will enhance program acceptance. For example, since many ABR screening programs test at cribside, it is necessary to find a quiet time in the nursery. Experience has demonstrated that evenings are the quietest and least obtrusive to perform hearing testing. An additional advantage of evening testing is that families are more often available for consultation and educational training.

The Interdisciplinary Team

A hearing screening program in the NICU will impact a number of disciplines. Whether a formalized team is created or other disciplines are involved as needed, it is important that the audiologist assumes the coordinating role because of his/her specialized training and experience in evaluating and habilitating the hearing-impaired. The audiologist should serve as the liaison and interface the program with other related services within the hospital.

There are other key individuals who are critical to the success of the screening program. Since the neonatologist has primary responsibility for the neonatal intensive care unit, it is essential that he/she is a strong proponent of the program. The neonatologist must be kept informed of the screening results and recommendations for follow-up procedures. When known, the baby's pediatrician, who will be primarily responsible for the child's health care after discharge from the hospital, should also be made aware of the screening test results and recommendations. Upon request, an otolaryngologist may perform an otologic examination of any baby who fails the hearing screening. It must be noted, however, that the roles of the otolaryngologist and the pediatrician are often not clearly defined when it comes to the medical evaluation and/or treatment of ear problems. To avoid unnecessary conflict or confusion, the audiologist coordinating the program should be aware of this "gray area" when considering a medical referral. If there is any question, it is best to consult with the physician who currently provides primary care to the infant.

The duties of the nurses in the newborn nurseries are significantly impacted by a hearing screening program. Each infant's well-being is the nurse's responsibility, and any testing interrupts the nursery routine, particularly if the testing is carried out within the nursery itself. Fortunately, nurses are usually very supportive if they are consulted before any testing, and if they understand and appreciate the importance of early detection of hearing loss. The audiologist should become familiar with the routines and schedules in the newborn nurseries and attempt to adjust hearing screening so it creates the minimum of disruption.

When a proposal for a newborn hearing screening program is presented, the hospital administrators will look closely at its cost effectiveness. If they approve the project, the administrators will assist in determining the costs, work out a billing system, approve sufficient staffing, and help secure needed space. Frequently hospital administration will expect progress reports for quality assurance and evaluation of cost-effectiveness.

Often there is a social worker or nurse clinician who is working with the baby's family. Obviously, it is essential to include him/her when conveying test results and recommendations. The social worker often serves as a coordinator for services and helps interpret test results for the family members. The social worker can also play a key role in arranging for the baby to return for outpatient visits if follow-up testing is required.

In a teaching hospital, there is a constant rotation of medical residents in the various departments. It is in the best interest of the newborn hearing screening program to provide information for the residents who relate to the newborn nurseries. This will allow them to understand the operation of the screening program better and to appreciate the need for the newborn hearing screening. This can be accomplished through the use of a protocol packet, inservices, and/or individual conversations.

Equipment

The audiologist considering the purchase of equipment for ABR hearing screening will find that there is a large selection from which to choose (Ferraro and Ruth, 1988, 1990). The wide spectrum of ABR systems range from automated screeners which deliver a simple pass/refer outcome, and thus do not require a highly trained individual to operate, to those which are highly flexible and will perform a wide range of evoked potential testing. When contemplating the purchase of ABR equipment, the audiologist should consider the following questions: 1) Is the screening program expected to provide information about a baby's neurological status as well as hearing function? 2) Who will be operating the equipment and interpreting the test results (audiologist, volunteer, auxiliary staff)? 3) How much special training will be required to operate the equipment properly? 4) Can the cost of more expensive equipment be justified considering the frequency of its use? 5) Will the equipment be used for other purposes (diagnostic and follow-up testing)? Answers to these questions should help determine if a flexible signal averager is needed or if a dedicated automated screener, to be discussed later, will suffice.

TESTING STRATEGIES

Selecting the Babies to be Screened

As mentioned at the beginning of this chapter, the Joint Committee on Newborn Hearing prepared a high-risk register containing the primary factors likely to produce a hearing loss in a newborn. This high-risk register is commonly used as the basis for selecting the babies who should receive ABR hearing screening (e.g., Ruth, Dey-Sigman and Mills, 1985; Gerkin, 1984). However, specific risk factors are often not strong indicators that a newborn may have a hearing loss. Of all the risk factors, Duara et al. (1986) found that only low birth weight, immature gestational age and extended stay in the hospital showed an independent correlation with permanent hearing loss. Halpern, Hosford-Dunn and Malachowski (1987) report that length of stay in the NICU, gestational age, craniofacial anomalies and TORCH infections predicted hearing loss with high sensitivity. Only the latter two factors are on the high-risk register. In a retrospective study, Pappas (1983) found that only 46% of children with a hearing loss would have been placed on the high-risk register.

Instead of determining if individual babies possess one or more factors on the high-risk register, an alternative approach is to focus on screening all babies who reside within the neonatal intensive care unit. Since the NICU contains very few babies who do not possess at least one factor on the high-risk register, it is recommended that all babies within the NICU be routinely screened for hearing loss. This eliminates the need to review medical records for risk factors and leaves more time for actual hearing screening.

Restricting hearing testing to the neonatal intensive care unit focuses the screening efforts on the group of babies most likely to possess a significant hearing loss. This is efficient use of limited personnel time, but it does not adequately address hearing loss which might be present in the 95% of newborns who never reside in the NICU during their hospital stay. The prevalence of a hearing loss in the full-term nursery is much lower than in the NICU (approximately 2 in a 1000 versus about 4 in a 100) (Matkin, 1984). However, the overall number of full-term nursery babies is so much larger that this group contains over half of the babies born with a handicapping sensorineural hearing loss. Thus, confining ABR hearing screening to the NICU will miss a high percentage of target babies. Clearly, every newborn hearing screening program must have a strategy for serving babies who never spend time within the NICU. This topic will be discussed later in this chapter.

Electrode Placement

The basics of ABR testing have been discussed in other chapters of this book and need not be considered in detail here. It is sufficient to say that, for ABR newborn screening, two surface recording electrodes are attached to the baby's head. The non-inverting electrode is positioned either just off the fontanel close to the top of the head (vertex) or positioned high on the forehead. The other (inverting) recording electrode is usually placed on the mastoid or earlobe ipsilateral to stimulation. An ipsilateral electrode position is important because contralateral recordings from newborns are of poor quality (Edwards, Durieux-Smith, and Picton, 1985). A third electrode (the common), which serves as the patient ground, can be positioned at most any convenient location on the baby's body. The sole of the foot, back of the hand, or opposite mastoid are common sites.

A wide variety of reusable or disposable recording electrodes are available commercially. There are also very small diameter electrodes specifically designed for use with newborns. No one electrode is the clear choice over all others. As a result, electrode selection is left to the examiner's preference based on cost and ease of use.

Even though the tenderness of the newborn's skin does not permit the use of highly abrasive electrode gels or hard scrubbing, sufficiently low electrode impedance (below 5,000–10,000 ohms) can usually be obtained without special effort. It is not unusual, however, for a baby to have high electrode impedances even after the skin has been carefully prepared. Fortunately, it is often possible to carry out ABR screening even though electrode impedances are substantially higher than desired (Eccard and Weber, 1983). There is no substitute for careful skin preparation, so testing with high electrode impedance should be a last resort which is used only when all reasonable attempts to lower the impedance have failed.

Earphone Selection

For older children and adults the TDH-39 or TDH-49 earphones with MX-41/AR cushions have been most commonly used for ABR testing. With the premature newborn, however, these two transducers are too large and heavy and may collapse the ear canal. (Hosford-Dunn et al., 1983). As an alternative, a small "walkman-type" earphone works well in newborn screening.

Though it cannot be directly coupled to an artificial ear for physical calibration, stimulus intensity levels can be based on the behavioral click thresholds of normal hearing individuals. Comparisons of ABR latencies and morphologies elicited by TDH-49 and "walkman-type" earphones (e.g., the Realistic Nova 53) have shown only minimal differences. Regardless of the earphone selected, it will be necessary to gather normative data prior to clinical testing.

A widely accepted alternative to circumaural earphones with infants is the use of insert (Etymotic ER-3A) earphones. These transducers are commercially available and have been credited with a decrease in potential ear canal collapse (Gorga, Kaminski, and Beauchaine, 1988). Jacobson, Jacobson, and Spahr (1990) have reported an improvement in the false-positive rate in newborn screening which they attribute to the use of insert earphones. As a result, they encourage the routine application of insert earphones with the newborn population.

When compared to responses elicited by conventional earphones, ABRs generated with insert earphones produce similar interwave interval latency differences and interaural symmetry (Gorga et al., 1988). The use of insert earphones, however, results in ABR absolute latency delays of 0.8–0.9 ms which relate to the length of the sound delivery tube between the transducer and the ear.

There are other factors to be considered when contemplating the use of insert earphones. If they are properly seated within the ear canal, they will attenuate ambient noise levels resulting in an improved testing condition. This is a distinct advantage when testing in the neonatal intensive care unit or other noisy environment. A further consideration is the degree of insertion into the ear canal. Because this may influence the sound pressure level of the auditory stimulus, it is recommended that each facility using insert earphones establish a consistent level of insertion and develop latency corrections for the length of the delivery tube. Finally, there is a practical advantage in using insert earphones in the NICU, or other areas where precautionary infectious measures are necessary. The use of disposable eartips eliminates any possibility of cross-contamination between infants.

Test Protocol

The stimulus parameters used for newborn ABR screening are very similar to those commonly employed in testing peripheral hearing status of older infants and children. An unfiltered click is the usual stimulus of choice because its abrupt onset makes it effective in producing a detectable response at the low screening intensity level. Clicks have their energy concentrated in the high frequencies so they provide information about peripheral hearing in the 2000 Hz to 4000 Hz range. It would certainly be desirable to obtain information about a baby's low frequency hearing as well. There are preliminary reports that frequency specific ABR information can be obtained from newborns using tone pip stimuli imbedded in band-reject noise (Hyde, 1985) or through the use of nonlinear gating functions (Kileny, 1988). However, further investigation is required to determine if the use of such stimuli significantly improves the performance of a clinical hearing screening program. That is, does the inclusion of more frequency specific stimuli result in the detection of hearing-impaired newborns who would have been missed if only clicks had been used?

In contrast with site of lesion testing, it is not critical for all component waves of the ABR to be clearly identified in newborn hearing screening. Instead, the test protocol is aimed at providing the greatest amount of information about the presence or absence of a response in the shortest possible time. As a result, stimulus rate is routinely relatively fast, between 30/sec and 40/sec, and is an odd number (e.g. 38.3/sec) to keep out of sync with the ever present 60 HZ interference and its harmonics.

If the level of contaminating interference in the nursery is so high that it obliterates any detectable response, it is permissible to reduce low pass filtering to 1500 Hz. It must be noted, however, that stimulus rate and analog filter settings both influence ABR latencies, so every screening program must establish its own latency norms for the test protocol which is selected.

The newborn infant has an immature ABR which is quite cyclic in its morphology. Any electrical interference which is not successfully filtered by the test equipment will closely approximate the newborn's 300–400 Hz cyclic ABR. Chance time-locking of this interference with the triggering of the signal averager may result in a tracing which mimics an ABR. Therefore, control (no stimulus) runs are essential in NICU screening to insure that a response to the test stimulus can be distinguished from averaged electrical background noise.

Screening Criterion

The screening criterion (the dividing line between passing and failing the test) will be dictated by the goal of the screening program. If the goal of the screening program is to detect unilateral, as well as bilateral hearing losses, it is obvious that both ears need to be tested. However, if the purpose of the screening is to rule out a bilateral hearing loss which can significantly affect speech and language development, this can be accomplished by screening only the most accessible ear. Obviously, a bilateral hearing impairment can be ruled out if a baby passes a hearing screening of a single ear. Because ABR screening is costly and time-consuming, many programs have chosen to screen a single ear. This does not imply that a unilateral hearing loss is without clinical significance. On the contrary, it is well established that a unilateral hearing loss can create cognitive and academic problems in school age children (Culbertson and Gilbert, 1986). However, it can be argued that the additional expense of testing the second ear outweighs its benefits. This argument is based on three factors: 1) A relatively small number of babies receiving ABR screening will possess a unilateral sensorineural hearing impairment. 2) If a unilateral hearing loss does exist, screening a single ear should, by chance, result in the testing of the impaired ear approximately one-half of the time. 3) If newborn hearing screening does miss a unilateral hearing loss, the resulting delay in its detection should not have a major impact on the infant's early speech and language development. If time and cost considerations are not of major importance, then both ears should be screened. However, if these practical considerations are important in maintaining the cost effectiveness of the program, screening a single ear does not appear to significantly reduce its clinical value.

A screening level of 35 dB nHL is recommended.

This level is defined as 35 dB above a previously determined behavioral click threshold for a group of normal listeners in a quiet environment. Of course, establishing the 0 dB nHL reference level in the noisy NICU would result in a grossly misleading 35 dB nHL level. In contrast to the 40 dB screening level recommended by the ASHA Committee on Infant Hearing (1989), a 35 dB screening criterion will result in a larger number of normal-hearing babies failing the screening (false positives), but this level will minimize the number of hearing-impaired babies who will pass the screening test (misses). Alberti et al. (1983) found that with a 30 dB nHL screening criterion, the failure rate three times greater than when a 40 dB level is used. Because of the importance of early detection of hearing loss, it is the authors' view that it is preferable to reduce the likelihood of missing an impaired baby at the expense of more false positive results.

Routinely, the testing conditions in the NICU are far from optimum and there are times when the recording conditions do not permit the detection of an ABR at a 35 dB nHL intensity level. The test environment is electrically and acoustically noisy. The incubators, monitors, and infusion pumps generate 60 Hz interference (along with its high-frequency harmonics) which can swamp and even mimic the small amplitude ABR. Acoustic noise in the NICU, if sufficiently high can also influence the ABR (Richmond, Konkle, and Potsic, 1986). When test conditions are particularly adverse, the absence of a response to a 35 dB stimulus would not be unexpected even from a baby with excellent hearing.

If such conditions are encountered, retesting in the NICU at a later date is indicated. Under unusual circumstances when retesting is impossible (e.g., if the baby is scheduled for immediate discharge), there is justification for using an alternative screening criterion. In such situations, one of the authors (BAW) will pass a baby if he/she demonstrates a clear response at 45 dB and the most prominent ABR component wave (routinely wave III or wave V) has a latency which falls within nursery norms for the baby's conceptual age (Weber, 1982). The rationale for this approach is that normal ABR latencies indicate that the 45 dB stimulus was sufficiently above threshold to allow the examiner to infer grossly normal peripheral hearing. It must be stressed that the presence of a detectable response at 35 dB should be the routine screening criterion and a response with normal latencies at 45 dB is accepted only when there are adverse recording conditions which cannot be corrected, and when retesting is impossible.

If response latency is used in this manner it is essential that the examiner have latency norms for different conceptual ages at 2–3 week intervals. Many sets of latency norms for premature infants have been reported in the literature. However, each testing facility should develop its own set of latency norms using its specific equipment and testing protocol.

It can be argued that if a baby fails the screening test, there is little reason to carry out testing at higher intensity levels, because the need for a retest has already been established. Nevertheless, probing for an estimate of click threshold is recommended for two reasons: 1) the baby may not return for retesting, so at the time of screening it is important to get as much information about hearing status as is reasonably possible, and 2) the baby's responsiveness at higher stimulus intensity levels provides information about the severity of the hearing loss and this information can be used to help determine how to proceed with scheduling the retesting. This topic will be discussed in some detail later in the chapter.

Use of an Automated Screener

The most common automated screener, the ALGO-1 plus, is a battery-operated microprocessor dedicated solely to newborn ABR screening (Kileny, 1988). This device uses a statistical analysis to obtain objective response detection. The screener incorporates unique design features. A disposable circumaural foam cushion with an adhesive back creates a tight seal around the infant's ear. This cushion results in an attentuation of background noise. The ALGO-1 plus has a dual artifact/rejection system which is designed to interrupt the signal averaging whenever myogenic activity or ambient noise exceed acceptable levels.

After the examiner has positioned three recording electrodes on the baby's scalp, the ALGO-1 plus is activated. It begins to automatically present click stimuli

whenever electrode impedance, ambient noise level, and movement artifacts are all within acceptable limits. The 35 dB nHL clicks are presented at a rate of 37/sec through the circumaural earphone. As the stimuli are being presented to the baby, the ALGO-1 plus is comparing the accumulated response in memory with an internal template of a neonatal ABR. When the likelihood of a response reaches a predetermined criterion level, the test stimuli automatically cease and a display panel indicates that the baby has passed the hearing screening test. If the likelihood of response (LR) is not sufficiently high at the end of 15,000 sweeps, testing is automatically halted and the display panel indicates that the baby should be referred for further testing (Kileny, 1988).

A major advantage of an automated screening device such as the ALGO-1 is that it does not require a sophisticated examiner who must be present throughout the testing. Further, an ABR screener is relatively inexpensive when compared with the cost of other ABR test units. However, a significant disadvantage of the automated screener is that its very stringent recording requirements may preclude testing in some environments. The requirements regarding acceptable electrode impedance, level of acoustic noise and muscle artifact may seldom be met in some NICU situations. The automated ABR screener is dedicated to newborn hearing screening and is not sufficiently flexible to permit other ABR applications, such as site of lesion testing. This lack of versatility may be a disadvantage for some programs.

Though an automated ABR screener has its limitations, it has been successfully integrated into different types of ABR hearing screening programs. One of the authors (CJ) uses conventional ABR test equipment in the NICU and uses the automated screener in the full-term nursery (FTN) where there is a better acoustical and electrical recording environment. Conditions are further improved by moving the baby to a quiet room adjacent to the FTN for testing.

When considering the purchase of ABR test equipment the above advantages and disadvantages of the automated screener must be weighed against those of the conventional ABR test units. Ferraro and Ruth (1988, 1990) have presented a comparison of the most common ABR test equipment.

When should ABR screening be performed?

Testing should be carried out as close to discharge or transfer as is feasible. This permits the babies to be as mature and healthy as possible at the time of test. Though babies are not discharged on a highly regular basis, it is best to set up a schedule for the ABR screening (e.g., three half days spaced out across the week). Such regular visits to the NICU minimize the chances that a baby will be discharged before testing and reduce dependence on nursery personnel for scheduling individual tests. On visits to the nursery, babies should be selected for screening based on anticipated discharge date, other procedures scheduled during the testing period, and current arousal level.

Ideally, all babies should be tested shortly after feeding when they are likely to be entering a period of quiet sleep. Most babies can be screened shortly before discharge during one of the regular visits to the nursery. However, the census in most NICUs fluctuates markedly, so to create necessary bed space, discharge plans often change with little forewarning. As a result, even with regular visits to the NICU, there must be considerable flexibility in the screening program. In the NICU, most laboratory procedures are performed during the normal work day. As discussed earlier, it is often preferable to perform hearing screening in the evening or on the weekend when the nursery is less congested.

Problems Encountered in the NICU

Just a few years ago it was possible to postpone hearing screening until the babies graduated from incubators to open basinettes. When this occurred, the babies were routinely very near full term and free from the electrical interference created by monitors and infusion pumps. The situation has changed markedly in most hospitals. A major reason for this change has been the increased concern over the financial implications of long hospital stays. As discussed earlier in the chapter, there is a strong incentive to streamline services. One way this can be accomplished is to discharge or transfer the babies as soon as possible. In the past, a baby may have been transferred from the NICU to the hospital's intermediate care nursery until he/she was ready to go home. Now a tertiary care NICU is likely to transfer the baby to an outside local newborn nursery as soon as the services of intensive care are no longer essential. As a result of this change in discharge policies, a high percentage of NICU hearing screenings must now be carried out when the baby is still very immature (34–36 weeks gestational age), in an incubator, and connected to monitors and infusion pumps. The noise levels in the incubator and the commonly high levels of accompanying electrical interference, often make it difficult to elicit a detectable ABR at the 35 dB nHL screening level (Richmond et al., 1986). Even if permission is given to temporarily turn off the incubator, the examiner must be prepared to: 1) reposition the recording electrodes to reduce impedance, 2) move the electrode cable to find a position with a minimum of interference, and 3) vary click rate to minimize the effects of cyclic interference.

TEST INTERPRETATION

It is important to remember that the presence of an ABR to a click stimulus at the screening intensity level indicates only that the baby's peripheral hearing is grossly intact for the high frequency portion of the speech range (2000 Hz–4000 Hz). Though it is reasonably safe to report that the baby has adequate peripheral hearing for speech and language development, it must be clear to all concerned that a low frequency hearing loss or central auditory problems cannot be ruled out by such ABR screening. Because the results of ABR audiometry are not directly influenced by the auditory cortex, the procedure should not be viewed as the electrophysiologic equivalent of behavioral audiometry.

Sensorineural vs Conductive Impairments

It is well documented that otitis media is more common in premature infants than in full-term infants. McLellan et al. (1962) observed pus in the middle ears of 19 of 28 (68%) infants with a birthweight between 1001 and 1500 grams. Abnormal tympanic membrane mobility is also reported to be common (22%) in premature infants (Balkany, Berman, and Simmons,

1978). Given the prevalence of middle ear problems in the NICU, it is not surprising that a high percentage of babies who fail an ABR hearing screening will do so because of the presence of a transient conductive hearing loss (Proctor and Kennedy, 1990).

It is obvious that the needs of a baby with a transient conductive hearing loss differ markedly from the needs of an infant with a permanent sensorineural impairment. To maximize the likelihood of appropriate follow-up, some effort must be made to separate the two groups of screening failures. Though tympanometry is sensitive to middle ear effusion, it is not a valid procedure with premature newborns because of their highly compliant ear canal walls, resulting in a high percentage of false negative test results (Paradise, Smith, and Bluestone, 1976). Hooks and Weber (1984), however, have demonstrated the feasibility of using bone-conducted (BC) click stimuli to record ABRs from neonates. As a result, ABRs to air-conduction and bone-conduction clicks can be compared to help differentiate transient conductive hearing impairments from permanent sensorineural hearing losses. This information is of value in determining appropriate management and follow-up. Of course, a suspected conductive impairment should be promptly brought to the attention of the appropriate physician and an attempt should be made to repeat ABR testing following treatment. If the AC and BC ABRs are in close agreement, the findings are consistent with a sensorineural hearing loss. This is viewed as a clear-cut fail of the hearing screening and no retesting need be performed prior to discharge. Because of its value in determining appropriate follow-up, it is recommended that bone-conduction ABRs be recorded from every baby who fails air-conduction screening.

When bone-conduction ABR testing is performed, the examiner must be aware that, unless masking noise is used, a normal response may be due to normal sensorineural status in the non-test ear. Without testing the other ear and/or using contralateral masking, the test results will be ambiguous. It must be further cautioned that, because of the large mass of a bone conduction oscillator, BC clicks contain more low frequency energy than AC clicks. Maximum energy is in the region of 1300 Hz, for BC clicks, compared with 2000–4000 Hz for AC clicks (Hooks and Weber, 1984;

Schwartz, Larson, and De Chicchis, 1985). As a result, it is possible for a baby with a markedly sloping high-frequency sensorineural loss to demonstrate better ABRs to the BC click; not due to a conductive hearing loss, but because of better low-frequency hearing. Such a test result would likely be mistakingly interpreted as evidence of a conductive hearing loss. The examiner must be aware of this possible explanation for better responses to BC click stimuli. Fortunately, as long as the results of BC ABR testing are used solely to provide additional information about babies who have failed the AC screening, this limitation will not result in false negative test results.

Bone conducted ABR testing has two additional practical limitations: 1) With conventional ABR test equipment, the maximum BC click output is much less than is possible for AC clicks (Schwartz et al., 1985) and 2) ABR latencies are markedly affected by the placement of the bone conduction oscillator (Yang, Rupert, and Moushegian, 1987). In spite of its limitations, ABRs to BC click stimuli have significant clinical value in a newborn hearing screening program.

Neurological Disorders

By the very nature of the newborns who require the services of the NICU, a high percentage have some form of temporary or permanent neurological dysfunction. When these disorders, such as hydrocephalus, affect the functioning of the brainstem they may alter the ABR and complicate interpretation of the test results. Thus, an abnormal or absent ABR may indicate a peripheral hearing loss or it may be the result of a neurologic dysfunction impacting the brainstem (Murray, 1988). Often these two problems cannot be separated and incorrect interpretations may result. When the examiner suspects that a neurological problem is present, e.g., when ABR component wave I is present and later waves are absent, it is appropriate to interpret the test results as they relate to a hearing impairment and also to report the nature of the observed ABR abnormality. If brainstem abnormalities have not been previously documented, further testing should be recommended to clarify the nature of the problem. This traditional view of the audiologist's role relative to neurological disorders involves being aware that they may contaminate the hearing test results, and when the ABR findings are suspicious of neurological dysfunction, reporting this suspicion so that professionals better trained in this area of diagnosis may take appropriate action.

In contrast with the traditional approach described above, it can be argued that the value of ABR screening in the NICU population goes well beyond ruling out a significant hearing impairment. Because of the expense involved it is not likely that many of the NICU babies will also receive ABR testing to evaluate brainstem status. Rather than being a potential source of contamination, some view assessing auditory brainstem status as another facet of the NICU screening program. Kileny and Robertson (1985) utilized ABR testing to screen asphyxiated newborns. They concluded that its value was twofold: it evaluated auditory sensitivity and was also sensitive to the sequelae of hypoxic encephalopathy. Hall, Kripal, and Hepp (1988) incorporate both peripheral and central components in their ABR screening program. Though such dual purpose screening clearly increases the value of the screening program, diagnosis of brainstem abnormalities in the premature infant does not fall within the expertise of most audiologists. Such an expanded role of ABR screening must not be undertaken unless the audiologist has considerable knowledge and experience in this area and has a close working arrangement with the neonatologists and pediatric neurologists.

Often the role of the audiologist in assessing nonauditory neurologic disorders is determined by whether another division within the hospital has assumed the responsibility for performing evoked potentials on neurologically impaired patients. Just as the audiologist should appropriately resist hearing testing which is not supervised by an audiologist, it is understandable why an evoked potential laboratory would oppose neurological testing by an audiologist. Even if the audiologist elects not to incorporate neurological screening with hearing testing, he/she must have a good understanding of both audiologic and neurologic determinants of response abnormalities (Hecox, 1985). Both peripheral and central factors impact the ABR and it is not possible to adequately screen for one without understanding the influences of the other.

SERVICES TO LOW-RISK NEWBORNS

The prevalence of significant hearing loss is much higher in the neonatal intensive care unit than in the full-term nursery (FTN). This can be misleading, however, because only a small percentage of newborns will ever spend time in the NICU. Stein et al. (1990) estimate that only one-third of hearing-impaired infants manifest perinatal conditions that require the specialized care of the NICU. Thus, as high as two-thirds of hearing-impaired babies may be missed if ABR hearing screening is confined to the NICU. It is clear, therefore, that every screening program should have some strategy for serving low-risk babies. Because of the expenses involved, it is not cost effective to carry out ABR screening on all newborns (Hosford-Dunn et al., 1987). Nevertheless, the focus on high-risk infants cannot result in ignoring hearing-impaired babies in the low-risk group.

Even if financial and staffing considerations restrict routine ABR hearing screening to babies in the NICU and selected babies in the FTN, there are cost-effective ways to serve the low-risk population. Increased parent awareness is an inexpensive way to increase the likelihood of detecting a hearing-impaired baby who possesses no risk factors. This can be accomplished by means of a hearing checklist card such as shown in Figure 15.5. This checklist can be included in the free packet (containing formula, diapers etc.) which the mother receives when the baby is discharged from the FTN. One side of the card explains the importance of early identification of hearing loss. The other side of the card contains developmental milestones which allow the parents to gauge whether their child is normally responsive to sound, as well as information on who to call regarding questions about the baby's hearing and how to arrange for a hearing test. Parents are urged to attach this card to the wall or refrigerator where it is regularly seen. This will serve as a frequent reminder to consider the child's responsiveness to sound.

Money to cover the cost of printing this specific hearing checklist was donated by the Friendly City Sertoma Club in Durham, NC. The club eagerly undertook this project because it permitted them to provide a significant community service for a relatively modest amount

CAN YOUR BABY HEAR?

CONGRATULATIONS ON YOUR NEW BABY! We are sure that you will receive great pride and pleasure as you watch your baby grow and mature. **The Friendly City Sertoma Club** of Durham hopes that you will use this card to track your child's development in one important area: hearing.

A large part of what your baby learns will be through hearing. Your child will learn that different sounds have different meanings and this will serve as the foundation for talking. Speech and language, however, will only occur if your baby can hear other people talk. A child with a significant hearing loss can be permanently delayed in many areas of development. Therefore, it is very important to detect a hearing loss as soon as possible to permit early treatment and training to minimize the damage it can cause.

You can help your baby by using the information on the other side of this card. Check your child's responses to sound with what is expected for a child of the same age (be sure to reduce your child's age if your baby was premature). If you find that your child falls behind what is expected call the number shown below for information on where your child's hearing can be tested. **The Friendly City Sertoma Club** wants you to know that no child is too young to have their hearing tested, so don't wait if you have concerns about hearing.

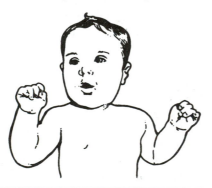

HEARING CHECKLIST

BY 3 MONTHS
Startle or cry when there are loud noises.
Show signs of waking up to loud sounds.

BY 6 MONTHS
Stop playing when there is an interesting sound.
Enjoy toys that make noise.

BY 9 MONTHS
Understand words like "NO" and "BYE BYE."
Show signs of responding to soft sounds.
Turn head to find source of interesting sounds.

BY 12 MONTHS
Try to imitate the speech sounds you make.
Can point to familiar objects when asked.

BY 15 MONTHS
Follow simple spoken instructions.
Speak simple words.

If your baby does not appear to be responding normally to sound or if you just have some questions call the staff at BEGINNINGS and they will tell you where your baby's hearing can be tested.
Call toll free: 1-800-541-HEAR
(in Durham please use 286-9797)

FIGURE 15.5. Example of a hearing checklist card, which is included in the discharge packet of all newborns who are at low risk for hearing loss. Both sides of the card are shown.

of money. The distribution of the checklist also provided the club with increased visibility in the community which is important in enhancing the success of future fundraising efforts. At the present time, the checklist is being used in the FTN at Duke University Medical Center and in six other "feeder" nurseries in the area.

FOLLOW-UP PROCEDURES

When properly administered, ABR screening can provide useful information regarding a newborn's current hearing status. It is important that a screening test be interpreted as such, and not considered to be "diagnostic" for the confirmation of permanent hearing loss. Failure of the ABR screening test does not insure that a baby has a hearing loss. It is important that the test results are interpreted clearly in the baby's medical record and appropriately conveyed to the parents. Obviously, it is inappropriate to inform parents that their child has a permanent hearing loss, based on the failure of a screening test conducted in a less-than-ideal environment.

When a baby fails the ABR screen and a hearing

loss is suspected prior to discharge, follow-up procedures should be the primary concern. An example of an appropriate follow-up system, used by one of the authors (CJ), is shown in Figure 15.6. Prior to the age of 6 months when behavioral audiometry can be incorporated into the test milieu, the infant returns for repeat ABR testing in the quiet, clinic environment. To minimize inconveniences to the family, an effort is made to schedule repeat ABR testing on the day the infant returns for other follow-up appointments, such as with the Neonatal Special Care Clinic, Eye Clinic, or Occupational/Physical Therapy. Usually, testing at an early age can be conducted in a natural sleep state, rather than requiring sedation as is necessary for an active, older

infant. Early diagnostic ABR testing is helpful in confirming functional hearing status and alleviating parental anxiety. If an infant gives normal responses on the follow-up ABR test it does not necessarily demonstrate that the NICU screening was in error. Better responses on the second test may be due to improved neurological status or the result of a resolved conductive hearing loss. If the follow-up ABR test also shows evidence of a hearing loss, a referral should be made for possible early medical intervention. Providing prompt follow-up audiologic evaluations also assists in securing needed services for amplification and training, parent education/support, and developmental follow-up programs.

If the infant passes the repeat ABR test, an appointment is scheduled to monitor auditory development in 6 months. However, if the infant fails repeat ABR testing, thresholds are established, otologic consultation is sought, and the infant is scheduled for behavioral and immittance measures at approximately 6 months corrected age. At that time, complete audiologic, rehabilitative, and otologic services are provided. The infant's physician is kept well informed of the results and recommendations. It is important that the primary care physician become involved when a hearing loss is identified. Establishing a habilitation program and securing financial assistance should be a team effort.

Though follow-up testing is a critical part of the screening process, it remains the weakest element of most programs (Jacobson, 1990). Because of the heavy dependence on parental/caregiver cooperation, loss to follow-up can be a significant problem, even when a major effort is made to maximize the return rate. Shimizu et al. (1990) went to considerable length to increase the likelihood that a baby would return for follow-up evaluation. Testing was performed free of charge, there was no fee for parking, and transportation was provided whenever needed. In addition, there were frequent phone calls and written reminders. In spite of these efforts, 26% of the babies who failed the NICU screening failed to return for their follow-up appointments. Kramer, Vertes, and Condon (1989) report a follow-up rate of only 48%. One of the greatest challenges in any newborn hearing screening program is minimizing the number of infants who fail to return for their follow-up evaluation.

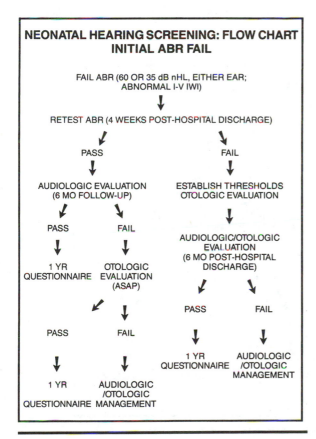

FIGURE 15.6. Illustration of a follow-up system for infants who fail the ABR screening.

Certain steps can be taken to maximize the likelihood that an infant will return for follow-up: 1) coordinating multiple appointments to occur on the same day, facilitating an easier schedule for the parents; 2) counseling the parents at the time of the original screening and sending a follow-up letter explaining the nature and importance of the testing. Parents should not be needlessly alarmed, but may be more motivated to bring the child back if they understand the implications of a possible hearing loss; 3) sending a letter to the baby's physician explaining that follow-up hearing testing has been scheduled and request that he/she stress the importance to the family of follow-up; and 4) notifying social workers and health care professionals who may be involved.

Realistically, we need to acknowledge that there will be at-risk infants who will be lost to follow-up despite our best efforts. Reasons may include a change of address making contact difficult, poor parental response, and difficulty obtaining adequate transportation. No program will be 100% successful. However, screening without follow-up is of little or no value, so every reasonable effort should be made to eliminate babies who are lost due to inadequate administration and coordination.

For the most part, follow-up services are provided only to those infants who fail initial screening. However, there is increasing evidence of delayed onset or progressive hearing loss in the high-risk newborn population (Naulty, Weiss, and Herer, 1986; Hendricks-Munoz and Walton, 1988; Allen and Schubert-Sudia, 1990). As a result, screening programs are now extending their follow-up to infants who pass initial screening. Figure 15.7 illustrates a suggested protocol for infants who

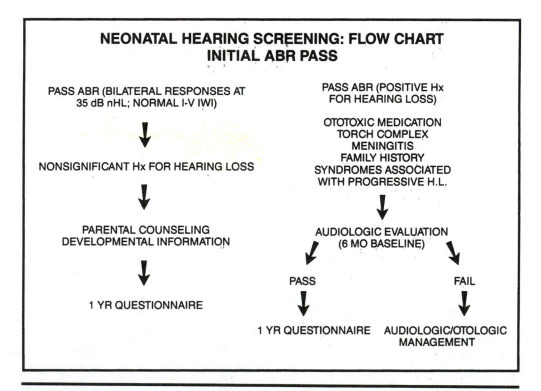

FIGURE 15.7. Illustration of a suggested protocol for infants who pass the ABR screening, yet remain at risk for hearing loss.

pass the ABR screening, yet remain at high risk for hearing loss. Decisions regarding the most appropriate form of follow-up are based on ABR screening results, the nature and degree of the babies' medical problems and family history. If a child passes the ABR screening and history is non-significant for hearing loss, routine follow-up testing is not scheduled. However, the family is sent a questionnaire inquiring about the auditory status of the child one year following discharge. If a child passes the NICU screening, but history is significant for potential delayed onset or progressive hearing loss, the child is scheduled for an ABR retest within 3 months. In addition, the infant is followed at 6-month intervals with at least behavioral audiometry and immittance measures. Either the parents/caregivers or supervising agency must assume responsibility for initiating the follow-up exam.

CONCLUSIONS AND PROJECTIONS FOR THE FUTURE

The value of hearing screening in the neonatal intensive care unit is now well established and more and more hospitals are considering initiating a program. Though an effective method of screening is now available in the auditory brainstem response, major changes are likely to occur in the years ahead. Efforts likely will be focused on improving the cost effectiveness of the screening. That is, how can the cost of identifying a hearing-impaired baby be reduced to make it financially acceptable to those hospitals which have limited resources? The automated ABR screeners are one attempt to address this problem. Another approach is to continue to look for an alternative to the time consuming, and thus costly, ABR testing procedure. Evoked oto-acoustic emissions may be such an alternative.

Evoked Oto-acoustic Emissions (EOAEs)

It has been demonstrated that acoustic responses from the cochlea can be recorded when an acoustic probe, consisting of a sound source and a miniature microphone, is sealed in the external ear canal. When a click is presented to the ear a release of acoustic energy, called evoked oto-acoustic emissions (EOAEs), can be detected from five to ten msec following stimulus onset (Kemp, 1978). Controlled studies have verified that EOAEs are not artifacts. They likely originate in the outer hair cells and can be viewed as evidence of a functioning cochlea. The response is either present or absent and, unlike the ABR, increasing the amplitude of the click stimulus does not result in a larger and more easily detectable response.

There are two strong reasons to consider EOAEs as a potential hearing screening measure for the NICU. First, responses have been detected in young infants at low intensity levels (Johnsen, Bagi, and Elberling, 1983). Bonfils, Uziel, and Pujol (1988) recorded EOAEs to a 20 dB nHL click from infants as young as two days of age. Second, EOAE screening can be completed in less time than is required for ABR testing (Stevens et al., 1990). A potential disadvantage of the technique is the requirement of a quiet test environment. In spite of this limitation, EOAEs warrant further study as a screening tool.

Recently, a study was conducted by one of the authors (CJ) to determine the feasibility of using evoked oto-acoustic emissions as a technique for early identification of hearing loss in high-risk newborns. The study compared EOAE testing with conventional ABR screening in the NICU. Using a commercially available test unit (Otodynamic LTD IL088), 225 infant ears were tested. Several practical conclusions were drawn: 1) As in ABR testing, the infant must be quiet, preferably sleeping, because myogenic artifacts contaminate the test results. 2) Successful testing requires low ambient noise levels which are seldom achieved in the NICU. This agrees with the findings of Stevens et al. (1987). 3) Using the standard probe, it is difficult to obtain and maintain a proper seal in the infants' ear canals and 4) The current EOAE equipment does not allow adequate monitoring of test conditions in a poor recording environment, such as the NICU. The results of this investigation indicate that EOAE recording techniques, though promising, have major limitations when applied to hearing screening in the NICU. Investigation into this area is in the relatively early stages, so these problems may be adequately overcome in the future. A promising new approach to oto-acoustic emissions utilizes the distortion products produced by pairs of test tones (Martin, Whitehead, and Lonsbury-Martin, 1990). By changing the frequencies of the test tones, this approach promises to provide specific information not obtainable by conventional EOAE techniques.

In the future, some form of EOAE recording may turn out to be a valuable clinical measure which will permit a quick screening of all babies at risk for hearing loss. The more time-consuming ABR testing would then be used to further evaluate those babies who do not pass the EOAE screening. At the present, however, commercially available EOAE equipment is just appearing. Clinical test protocols have not been established and normative data on infants are limited. Until the clinical value of EOAE testing in the NICU has been more fully explored, it will not seriously challenge ABR audiometry as the most attractive choice for the clinician wishing to initiate an infant hearing screening program.

REFERENCES

Alberti, P.W., Hyde, M.L., Riko, K., Corbin, H., and Abramovich, S. (1983). An evaluation of BERA for hearing screening in high-risk neonates. *Laryngoscope, 93*, 1115–1121.

Alberti, P.W., Hyde, M.L., Riko, K., Corbin, H., and Fitzhardinge, P.M. (1985). Issues in early identification of hearing loss. *Laryngoscope, 95*, 373–381.

Allen, M.C. and Schubert-Sudia, S.E. (1990). Prevention of prelingual hearing impairment. *Seminars in Hearing, 11*, 134–149.

American Speech-Language-Hearing Association Committee on Infant Hearing. (1989). Audiologic screening of newborn infants who are at risk for hearing impairment. *ASHA, 31*, 89–92.

Balkany, T., Berman, S., and Simmons, M. (1978). Middle ear effusion in neonates. *Laryngoscope, 88*, 398–405.

Blake, P.E. and Hall, J.W. (1990). The status of statewide policies for neonatal hearing screening. *Journal of the American Academy of Audiology, 1*, 67–74.

Bonfils, P., Uziel, A., and Pujol, R. (1988). Screening for auditory dysfunction in infants by evoked oto-acoustic emissions. *Archives of Otolaryngology and Head and Neck Surgery, 114*, 887–890.

Brooks, W.S. (1990). Status of nationwide neonatal hearing screening programs and procedures. Poster presentation at annual meeting of the American Academy of Audiology, New Orleans, LA.

Carrel, R.E. (1977). Epidemiology of hearing loss. In S.E. Gerber (ed.), *Audiometry in Infancy*, pp. 263–285. New York: Grune & Stratton.

Catlin, F.L. (1978). Etiology and pathology of hearing loss in children. In F.N. Martin (ed.), *Pediatric Audiology*, pp. 3–34. Englewood Cliffs, NJ: Prentice-Hall, Inc.

Culbertson, J.L. and Gilbert, L.E. (1986). Children with unilateral sensorineural hearing loss: Cognitive, academic, and social development. *Ear and Hearing, 7*, 38–42.

Downs, D.W. (1982). Auditory brainstem response testing in the intensive care unit: A cautious approach. *ASHA, 24*, 1009–1015.

Downs, M.P. (1986). The rationale for neonatal hearing screening. In E. Swigart (ed.), *Neonatal Hearing Screening*, pp. 3–20. San Diego, CA: College-Hill Press.

Downs, M.P. and Hemenway, W.G. (1969). Report on the hearing screening of 17,000 neonates. *International Audiology, 8*, 72–76.

Downs, M.P. and Sterritt, G.M. (1964). Identification audiometry for neonates: A preliminary report. *Journal of Auditory Research, 4*, 69–80.

Duara, S., Suter, C.M., Bessard, K.K., and Gutberlet, R.L. (1986). Neonatal screening with auditory brainstem responses: Results of follow-up audiometry and risk evaluation. *The Journal of Pediatrics, 108*, 276–281.

Durieux-Smith, A. and Jacobson, J.T. (1985). Comparison of auditory brainstem response and behavioral screening in neonates. *The Journal of Otolaryngology, 14*, 47–52.

Durieux-Smith, A., Picton, T., Edwards, C., Goodman, J.T., and MacMurray, B. (1985). The Crib-O-Gram in the NICU: An evaluation based on brain stem electric response audiometry. *Ear and Hearing, 6*, 20–24.

Eccard, K.D. and Weber, B.A. (1983). Influence of electrode impedance on auditory brain stem response recordings in the intensive care nursery. *Ear and Hearing, 4*, 104–105.

Edwards, C.G., Durieux-Smith, A., and Picton, T. (1985). Neonatal auditory brain stem responses from ipsilateral and contralateral recording montages. *Ear and Hearing, 6*, 175–178.

Ferraro, J.A. and Ruth, R.R. (1988). A comparison of commercial auditory evoked potential units: The economy units. *American Journal of Otology Supplement, 9*, 57–62.

Ferraro, J.A. and Ruth, R.R. (1990). A comparison of commercial auditory evoked potential units: The midpriced and luxury units. *The American Journal of Otology, 11*, 181–191.

Frasier, G.R. (1971). *The causes of profound deafness in childhood.* Baltimore, MD: The Johns-Hopkins University Press.

Fria, T.J. (1985). Identification of congenital hearing loss with the auditory brainstem response. In J.T. Jacobson (ed.), *The auditory brainstem response*, pp. 317–334. San Diego, CA: College-Hill Press.

Gerkin, K.P. (1984). The high risk register for deafness. *ASHA, 26*, 17–23.

Gorga, M.P., Kaminski, J.R., and Beauchaine, K.A. (1988). Auditory brainstem responses from graduates of an intensive care nursery using an insert earphone. *Ear and Hearing, 9*, 144–147.

Grogaard, J. (1988). High-risk neonates and long-term outcomes. In F. Bess (ed.), *Hearing impairment in children*, pp. 65–74. Parkton, MD: York Press, Inc.

Hall, J.W., Kripal, J.P., and Hepp, T. (1988). Newborn hearing screening with auditory brainstem response: Measurement problems and solutions. *Seminars in Hearing, 9*, 15–34.

Halpern, J., Hosford-Dunn, H., and Malachowski, N. (1987) Four factors that accurately predict hearing loss in "high risk" neonates. *Ear and Hearing, 8*, 21–25.

Hecox, K. (1985). Neurologic applications of the auditory brainstem response to the pediatric age group. In J.T. Jacobson (ed.), *The auditory brainstem response*, pp. 287–296. San Diego, CA: College-Hill Press.

Hendricks-Munoz, K.D. and Walton, J.P. (1988). Hearing loss in infants, with persistent fetal circulation. *Pediatrics, 81*, 650–656.

Himelfarb, M.Z., Shanon, E., Popelka, G.R., and Margolis, R.H. (1978). Acoustic reflex evaluation in neonates. In S.E. Gerber and G.T. Mencher (eds.), *Early detection of hearing loss*, pp. 109–127. New York: Grune & Stratton.

Hooks, R.G. and Weber, B.A. (1984). Auditory brain stem responses of premature infants to bone-conducted stimuli: A feasibility study. *Ear and Hearing, 5*, 42–45.

Hosford-Dunn, H., Johnson, S., Simmons, F.B., Malachowski, N., and Low, K. (1987). Infant hearing screening: Program implementation and validation. *Ear and Hearing, 8*, 12–20.

Hosford-Dunn, H., Runge, C.A., Hillel, A., and Johnson, S.J. (1983). Auditory brain stem response testing in infants with collapsed ear canals. *Ear and Hearing, 4*, 258–260.

Hyde, M.L. (1985). Frequency specific BERA in infants. *Journal of Otolaryngology, 14*, 19–27.

Hyde, M.L., Davidson, M.J., and Alberti, P. (1990). Auditory test strategy. In J. Jacobson and J. Northern (eds.), *Diagnostic Audiology*, pp. 295–322. Austin, TX: Pro-Ed.

Hyde, M.L., Riko, K., and Malizia, K. (1990). Audiometric accuracy of the click ABR in infants at risk for hearing loss. *Journal of the American Academy of Audiology, 1*, 59–66.

Jacobson, J. and Jacobson, C. (1987). Application of test performance characteristics in newborn auditory screening. *Seminars In Hearing, 8*, 133–141.

Jacobson, J.T. (1990). Issues in newborn hearing screening. *Journal of the American Academy of Audiology, 1*, 121–124.

Jacobson, J.T. and Morehouse, C.R. (1984). A comparison of auditory brain stem response and behavioral screening in high risk and normal newborn infants. *Ear and Hearing, 5*, 247–253.

Jacobson, J.T., Jacobson, C.A., and Spahr, R.C. (1990). Automated and conventional auditory brain stem screening techniques in high-risk infants. *Journal of the American Academy of Audiology, 1*, 187–195.

Jaffe, B.F. (1977). Middle ear and pinna anomalies. In B.F. Jaffe (ed.), *Hearing loss in children*, pp. 294–309. Baltimore, MD: University Park Press.

Jerger, J., Oliver, T., and Chmiel, R. (1988). Auditory middle latency response: A perspective. *Seminars in Hearing, 9*, 75–86.

Johnsen, N.J., Bagi, P., and Elberling, C. (1983). Evoked acoustic emissions from the human ear: III. Findings in Neonates. *Scandinavian Audiology, 12*, 17–24.

Joint Committee on Infant Hearing (1991). 1990 position statement. *Audiology Today, 3 (4)*, 14–9.

Joint Committee on Infant Hearing Screening Position Statement 1982. (1983). *Ear and Hearing, 4*, 3–4.

Kemp, D.T. (1978). Stimulated acoustic emissions from within the human auditory system. *Journal of the Acoustical Society of America , 64 ,*1386–1391.

Kenworthy, O.T., Bess, F.H., Stahlman, M.T., and Lindstrom, D.P. (1987) Hearing, speech, and language outcome in infants with extreme immaturity. *The American Journal of Otology, 8*, 419–425.

Kileny, P. (1988). New insights on infant ABR hearing screening. *Scandinavian Audiology , Supplement 30*, 81–88.

Kileny, P. and Robertson, C.M.T. (1985). Neurological aspects of infant hearing assessment. *The Journal of Otolaryngology, 14*, 34–39.

Konkle, D. and Jacobson, J. (1991). Detection and assessment of hearing loss in newborns, infants and young children. In W.F. Rintlemann (ed.), *Hearing assessment*, 2nd Edition, pp. 477–509. Austin, TX: Pro-Ed.

Kramer, S.J., Vertes, D.R., and Condon, M. (1989). Auditory brainstem responses and clinical follow-up of high-risk infants. *Pediatrics, 83*, 385–392.

Markowitz, R.K. (1990). Cost-effectiveness comparisons of hearing screening in the neonatal intensive care unit. *Seminars in Hearing, 11*, 161–165.

Martin, G.K., Whitehead, M.L., and Lonsbury-Martin, B.L. (1990). Potential of evoked otoacoustic emissions for infant hearing screening. *Seminars in Hearing, 11*, 186–204.

Matkin, N.D. (1984). Early recognition and referral of hearing impaired children. *Pediatrics in Review, 6*, 151–156.

McFarland, W.H., Simmons, F.B., and Jones, F.R. (1980). An automated hearing screening technique for newborns. *Journal of Speech and Hearing Disorders, 45*, 495–503.

McLellan, M.S., Strong, J.P., Johnson, O.R., and Dent, J.H. (1962). Otitis media in premature infants. *Journal of Pediatrics, 61*, 53–56.

McMillan, P., Bennett, M.J., Marchant, C.D., and Shurin, P.A. (1985). Ipsilateral and contralateral acoustic reflexes in neonates. *Ear and Hearing, 6*, 320–324.

McRandle, C.C., Smith, D.I., and Goldstein, R. (1974). Early averaged electroencephalic responses to clicks in neonates. *Annals of Otology, Rhinology, and Laryngology, 83*, 695–701.

Menyuk, P. (1977). Effects of hearing loss on language acquisition in the babbling stage. In B.F. Jaffe (ed.), *Hearing loss in children*, pp. 621–629. Baltimore, MD: University Park Press.

Murray, A.D. (1988). Newborn auditory brainstem evoked responses (ABRs): Longitudinal correlates in the first year. *Child Development, 59*, 1542–1554.

Musiek, F.E., Geurkink, N.A., Weider, D.J., and Donnelly, K. (1984). Past, present, and future applications of the auditory middle latency response. *Laryngoscope, 94*, 1545–1553.

Naulty, C.M., Weiss, I.P., and Herer, G.R. (1986). Progressive sensorineural hearing loss in survivors of persistent fetal circulation. *Ear and Hearing, 7*, 74–77.

Pappas, D.G. (1983). A study of the high-risk registry for sensorineural hearing impairment. *Otolaryngology, Head and Neck Surgery, 91*, 41–44.

Paradise, J.L., Smith, C., and Bluestone, D.D. (1976). Tympanometric detection of middle ear effusion in infants and young children. *Pediatrics, 58*, 198–206.

Plotnick, C.H. and Leppler, J.G. (1986). Infant hearing assessment: A program for identification and habilitation within four months of age. *The Hearing Journal, 39*, 23–25.

Prager, D.P., Stone, D.S., and Rose, D.N. (1987). Hearing loss screening in the neonatal intensive care unit: Auditory brain stem response versus crib-o-gram; A cost effectiveness analysis. *Ear and Hearing, 8*, 213–216.

Proctor, L.R. and Kennedy, D.W. (1990). High-risk newborns who fail hearing screening: Implications of otological problems. *Seminars in Hearing, 11*, 167–176.

Richmond, K.H., Konkle, D.F., and Potsic, W.P. (1986). ABR screening of high-risk infants: Effects of ambient noise in the neonatal nursery. *Otolaryngology-Head and Neck Surgery, 94*, 552–560.

Ruth, R.A., Dey-Sigman, S., and Mills, J.A. (1985). Neonatal ABR hearing screening. *The Hearing Journal, 38*, 39–45.

Schulman-Galambos, C. and Galambos, R. (1975). Brain stem auditory-evoked responses in premature infants. *Journal of Speech and Hearing Research, 18*, 456–465.

Schwartz, D.M., Larson, V.D., and De Chicchis, A.R. (1985). Spectral characteristics of air and bone conduction transducers used to record the auditory brain stem response. *Ear and Hearing, 6*, 274–277.

Shakno, R.J. (1984). *Physician's guide to DRGs*. Chicago, IL: Pluribus Press.

Shimizu, H., Walters, R.J., Proctor, L.R., Kennedy, D.W., Allen, M.C., and Markowitz, R.K. (1990). Identification of hearing impairment in the neonatal intensive care unit population: Outcome of a five-year project at the Johns Hopkins Hospital. *Seminars in Hearing, 11*, 150–160.

Stein, L., Clark, S., and Kraus, N. (1983). The hearing-impaired infant: Patterns of identification and habilitation. *Ear and Hearing, 4*, 232–236.

Stein, L., Jabaley, T., Spitz, R., Stoakley, D., and McGee, T. (1990). The hearing-impaired infant: Patterns of identification and habilitation revisited. *Ear and Hearing, 11*, 201–205.

Stevens, J.C., Webb, H.D., Smith, M.F., Buffin, J.T., and Ruddy, H. (1987). A comparison of oto-acoustic emissions and brain stem electric response audiometry in the normal newborn and babies admitted to a special care baby unit. *Clinical Physic and Physiological Measurement, 8*, 95–104.

Stevens, J.C., Webb, H.D., Hutchinson, J., Connell, J., Smith, M.F., and Buffin, J.T. (1990). Click evoked otoacoustic emissions in neonatal screening. *Ear and Hearing, 11*, 128–132.

Stockard, J.E., Stockard, J.J., and Coen, R.W. (1983). Auditory brain stem response variability in infants. *Ear and Hearing, 4*, 11–23.

Swigonski, N., Shallop, J., Bull, M.J., and Lemons, J.A., (1987). Hearing screening of high-risk newborns. *Ear and Hearing, 8,* 26–30.

Weber, B.A. (1982). Comparison of auditory brain stem response latency norms for premature infants. *Ear and Hearing, 3,* 257–262.

Weber, B.A. (1988) Screening of high-risk infants using auditory brainstem response audiometry. In F. H. Bess (ed.), *Hearing impairment in children*, pp. 112–132. Parkton, MD: York Press.

Wegman, M. (1987) Annual summary of vital statistics-1986. *Pediatrics, 80,* 817–827.

Yang, E.Y., Rupert, A.L., and Moushegian, G. (1987). A developmental study of bone conduction auditory brain stem response in infants. *Ear and Hearing, 8,* 244–251.

PART FOUR

NEUROTOLOGIC DISORDERS AND MANAGEMENT

AUDITORY BRAINSTEM RESPONSE MEASURES IN ACOUSTIC NERVE AND BRAINSTEM DISEASE

GARY P. JACOBSON
JOHN T. JACOBSON
NABIH RAMADAN
MARTYN HYDE

INTRODUCTION

During the past two decades, the introduction and refinement of the auditory brainstem response (ABR) test has added new clinical dimensions to the diagnosis and management of acoustic neuromas (AN). The ABR technique has been shown to be highly sensitive in assessing retrocochlear pathology to the exclusion of other audiometric tests. However, the ABR remains susceptible to several clinical shortcomings which, if not thoroughly understood, may lead to errors in test analysis and inappropriate clinical assumptions.

In an attempt to describe and clarify its use in neurotologic diagnosis, this chapter will examine the status of the ABR with regard to the identification and diagnosis of lesions that affect the cochleovestibular nerve (CN VIII) and the auditory pathways in the brainstem. Additionally, technical factors which influence the ABR, including recording, stimulus characteristics, and measurement criteria, will be detailed. This chapter also will describe the relationship of hearing loss and ABR findings and provide recommendations on the use of compensating formulae.

It is hoped that by the time the reader completes this chapter it will become apparent that there is *not any one* ABR configuration which is diagnostic for a particular disease process. For example, it is not possible on the basis of an ABR alone to diagnose an AN or multiple sclerosis (MS). In fact, patients with these two disease processes may present with identical ABR waveform characteristics. Indeed, it is the rule rather than the exception that any permutation of abnormality (e.g., delayed interpeak latencies, wave V latency differences, abnormal wave V/I amplitude ratios) can occur with any neurologic disease that can affect the proximal CN VIII nerve and brainstem. Therefore, instead of providing a complete listing of CNS diseases and a comprehensive review of reported ABR abnormalities, the authors have adopted a unique illustrative approach. In this chapter, an attempt is made to describe the pathophysiology that underlies each major classification of neural damage (e.g., compression, traction, ischemia, hemorrhage, demyelination, and neurodegeneration). This introductory material will be followed by a description of the more "classic" diseases caused by these mechanistic processes. In this manner it is hoped that the reader will be able to predict, based upon knowledge of the pathophysiology of a disease, *why* and *how* the ABR may be affected. The reader is directed to existing comprehensive reviews of neurologic diseases and their effects on the ABR (See Chiappa, 1990 and Hall, 1992).

BACKGROUND ABR IN NEUROTOLOGY AND NEUROLOGY

An exhaustive comprehension of the anatomy and physiology of the auditory pathway is essential in the evaluation and diagnosis of neurotologic disease. First and foremost, it is important to understand the fundamental concepts of sensory stimulation and physiologic response. Recall that ABR measures represent synchronized neural discharge patterns evoked by specific (transient) types of stimuli. Whereas there is ample evidence (see Møller, Chapter 2, *Neural Generator of Auditory Evoked Potentials*) that ABR waves I and II are generated from the distal and proximal regions of the CN VIII respectively, there is growing consensus that later wave peak configurations result from activity evoked from multiple, concurrently discharging neural generators located in the pons. The

complexity of these interactions has yet to be resolved (See the Section entitled *Mechanisms of Damage Identified by ABR* later in this chapter for expanded rationale). Thus, it is ill-advised to predict the pathology or location of a lesion on the basis of an abnormal wave peak configuration. Figure 16.1 illustrates a series of ABR traces recorded from patients with surgically confirmed posterior fossa lesions. Importantly, specific disease cannot be identified from any one ABR trace. The clinician often must work with pieces (clinical, audiologic, electrophysiologic, and radiologic

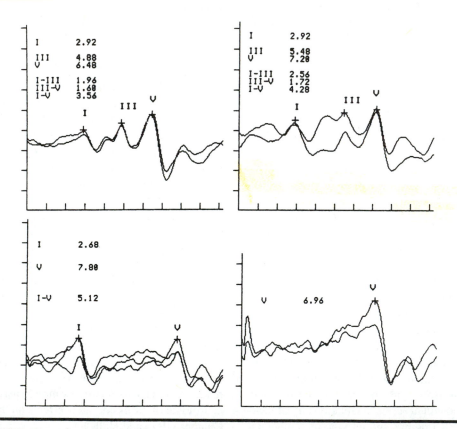

FIGURE 16.1.   A series of ABR traces obtained using standard click protocol from four patients with surgically confirmed brainstem lesions: top left, normal ABR latency and amplitude resulting in a false-negative record; top right, prolonged I–III latency in the presence of a normal I–V interwave interval; bottom left, prolonged I–V interwave interval; bottom right, absent I to IV wave peaks and prolonged wave V latency. Other records typically found in brainstem lesions but not illustrated include: 1) poor morphology; 2) nonrepeatable wave peak configurations; and 3) earlier waves only (I, II and possibly III) associated with prolonged wave V.

studies) of a puzzle (disease process) that do not simply fit into an unequivocal pattern. However, a knowledge of all the components that fit the puzzle will enhance the opportunity of a correct assessment of central auditory system dysfunction.

Despite these limitations, several auditory system disorders reveal certain electrophysiologic trends. For example, given a fixed stimulus level of 75 dB nHL the entire ABR is increased in latency and decreased in amplitude in the presence of conductive auditory pathology. Conversely, abnormally increased interpeak latencies (e.g., wave I–wave V) may be observed in central nervous system disease. In this regard, the ABR should be considered as a supplementary screening tool in the diagnosis of auditory pathology and used in conjunction with other clinical, radiologic and laboratory findings.

Anatomic Correlates of the Auditory Brainstem Response

Neuroelectric signals generated from specialized receptor cells in the cochlea are transmitted to the cerebral cortex via the acoustic nerve and brainstem auditory nervous system. This pathway includes at least four major nuclei that act as relay stations. The major elements of the pathway are duplicated on either side of the cranial midline. These neuronal connections propagate impulses and participate in the interpretation and integration of sensory stimuli. The following section briefly reviews the caudal aspects of the classic ascending auditory pathway. A more detailed account of the auditory system may be found in this book in Møller, Chapter 2, *Neural Generators of Auditory Evoked Potentials*.

CN VIII and Pontine Central Auditory Pathway. The cranial nerve VIII subserves hearing and balance function. The auditory segment consists of bipolar neurons containing cell bodies in the spiral ganglion of the modiolus situated within the central aspects of the bony shell within which the cochlea resides. The ascending axons exit the spiral ganglion to form the cochlear branch of CN VIII. At the entrance of the internal auditory canal (IAC), the cochlear branch of CN VIII is joined by the vestibular fibers. After a distance of about 5 mm, the auditory nerve enters the brainstem at the junction of

the pons and the medulla. Nerve fibers of the CN VIII exit the bony labyrinth through cribriform areas to form the main nerve trunk in the IAC. CN VIII enters the IAC in a common meningeal sheath with the facial nerve (CN VII). As they exit, both CN VII and CN VIII enter the caudal pons at the cerebellopontine angle (CPA) in close proximity to CN V (This is illustrated in Figure 16.2). Upon entering the brainstem, the nerve bifurcates, sending branches to the dorsal and ventral cochlear nuclei (Powell and Cowan, 1962). All primary fibers from the cochlea synapse with second order neurons at the cochlear nuclei. As such, auditory pathology within the IAC and more rostral sites tend to affect the later ABR wave (III–V) latency and amplitude configurations with little influence on the morphology of waves I and II.

The acoustic nerve has a twisted pattern such that fibers from the apical cochlea (low frequency) are innermost. As the nerve courses rostrally to terminate in the cochlear nuclei, the spatial arrangement originating in the cochlea (tonotopic organization) is maintained (Lorente de No, 1933; Rose et al., 1963). Second order neurons leave the cochlear nuclei in three acoustic striae: 1) The dorsal stria (Monakow's area) originates in the dorsal cochlear nucleus and passes through the reticular formation to the opposite side of the brainstem to join the medial partition of the contralateral lateral lemniscus and inferior colliculus (Osen, 1969; Bredberg, 1981). Fibers from the dorsal stria also project to the ipsilateral inferior colliculus (Warr, 1966; 1969). 2) The intermediate stria (commissure or tract of Held) arises from the posteroventral cochlear nucleus, sending fibers bilaterally to the superior olivary complex and the lateral lemniscus (Osen, 1969). As implied, the intermediate stria provides secondary avenues for decussating fibers. 3) The principle bundle, or, the ventral stria (trapezoid body) is formed by fibers from the anteroventral cochlear nucleus which decussate and terminate at the nucleus of the trapezoid body and the medial superior olivary nucleus. This activity is routed to the lateral lemniscus and inferior colliculus. Additional fibers ascend ipsilaterally to the lateral superior olive. Thus, it is apparent that such anatomical complexity makes it difficult to localize accurately pathologic lesions which affect the central auditory system.

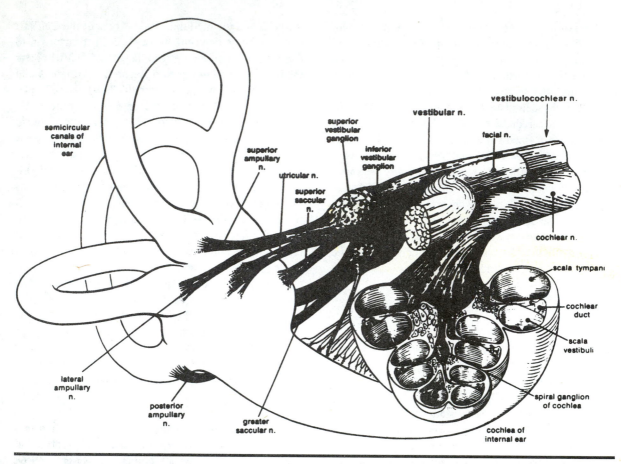

FIGURE 16.2.   Anatomical relationship between the sensory end-organ and the acoustic (CN VIII) and facial (CN VII) nerve. Reprinted with permission from *Melloni's Illustrated Medical Dictionary, 3rd ed*; The Parthenon Publishing Group, Inc., 1983.

The posterior cranial fossa is a shallow depression containing the cerebellum and the brainstem. The brainstem is comprised of the medulla, pons, midbrain, and diencephalon. It is at the junction between the pons and the cerebellum (cerebellopontine angle, CPA) that CN V, VII, VIII, IX, and X are in close proximity and, thus, CPA lesions may affect any or all of these CNs.

MECHANISMS OF DAMAGE IDENTIFIED BY ABR

Various mechanisms of neuronal/axonal damage can affect the ABR. Neurophysiologic changes that lead to an abnormal ABR may be caused by *compression* or *traction* injury of neural structures (e.g., CN VIII or brainstem), *ischemia* to the cochlea, CN VIII, or brainstem, *hemorrhage* into the auditory nerve or brainstem, and *demyelination* or *degeneration* of these same structures. It is certain that any or all of these conditions can coexist.

We are aware of the underlying mechanisms that cause changes in the neurophysiology of the auditory system because of the extensive body of research that has amassed over the years from those investigators who have conducted animal studies to determine the origins of the ABR (Wada and Starr, 1983a,b,c; Zaaroor and Starr, 1991a,b). Most of this work has involved the use of ablative permanent lesions or anesthesia-induced temporary changes in function of portions of the classical auditory pathway. These investigators have subsequently observed changes in the ABR. Additionally, some information has been derived from systematic observations of intraoperative changes in humans undergoing neurotologic and neurosurgical procedures (Møller and Jannetta, 1981, 1983, 1984).

In order to understand the effect that neurologic disease has on the ABR, it is important first to reconsider the method by which averaged evoked potentials (AEP) are recorded. In order for an evoked potential to be recorded, an electrical response must be emitted by a neural structure (or structures) following stimulus onset at an identical instant every time the stimulus is presented. If the neural response is not synchronized with the presentation of a suitable auditory stimulus (e.g., if the electrical response to the stimulus is temporally dispersed) there will be no recordable AEP. Therefore, the AEP test is an evaluation of neural synchronization. Stated another way, in the present context, the ABR examination is *not* a test of whether afferent information reaches the auditory nerve or brainstem, but instead, it *is* a test of whether auditory information passes through these structures in a synchronized manner. This being known, it is possible to predict what might cause AEP abnormalities.

Another basic consideration in the understanding of the effects of otoneurologic disease on the ABR is that each ABR component (beyond waves I and II) takes its CNS origins from multiple co-active dipole sources that are located in the pons. Accordingly, there is no point-by-point relationship between the waves of the ABR and the structures generating these responses. As stated earlier, it is well accepted that there are multiple ascending auditory pathways. For each of these pathways there may be three or more synapses from the level of the cochlear nucleus to the cortex. Therefore, once electric activity enters the brainstem the electrical responses may ascend directly and reach the cortex within approximately 15 ms. Alternately, many synapses may be interposed and this activity may reach the cortex later.

Additionally, it is known that the majority of electrical activity entering one ear crosses in the brainstem (at the level of the trapezoid body) and terminates in the contralateral auditory cortex although a small amount of this activity remains in an ipsilateral ascending pathway. Therefore, at any one moment in time during the development of the ABR (after wave II), multiple sources may be activated at varying levels of the brainstem. The non-inverted electrode on the scalp records the algebraic summation of these co-active voltage fields. Once activated, each of these sources generates an electrical field that is dipolar in shape and has a specific orientation in three-dimensional space. The unique spatial distribution of these generator sources and the temporal relationship of their activation in normal subjects is responsible for the wave shape of the normal ABR. Individual differences in the geometry of the voltage fields emanating from auditory structures in the brainstem (with respect to the recording electrode) and the temporal activation of these structures may account for some of the interindividual variation in ABR morphology (e.g., bifid wave III).

In this regard, a number of investigators have demonstrated that if single structures that are known to be part of the lemniscal system are selectively ablated or anesthetized, the effects on the ABR are quite complex (Wada and Starr, 1983a,b,c; Zaaroor and Starr, 1991a,b). For instance, unilateral lesioning of the superior olivary complex results in a modest latency change in the cat ABR component P3 (analogous to human wave IV) to ipsilateral ear stimulation. There were no changes noted in the ABR to contralateral stimulation (Zaaroor and Starr, 1991a). Therefore, the effects of brainstem disease might expectedly result in unpredictable changes in the latencies, amplitudes and (equally likely) morphology of the ABR.

Physiologic Origins of ABR Measurement Variables

Latency.   Latency refers to the time of onset or peak of an evoked potential component. When viewed in the context of single neurons, faster neuronal conduction (e.g., evoked potential with shorter latency) is associated with: 1) larger diameter axons that have decreased axoplasmic resistance, 2) neurons with membranes with lower depolarization thresholds, and, 3) higher core body temperatures (Kimura, 1984). The time required to depolarize an adjacent node of Ranvier in a single neuron is determined by the longitudinal axoplasmic resistance, and the capacitance and conductance of the internodal membrane. As these values increase (as occurs in small diameter axons), the current along the membrane decreases before electrical activity reaches the next node (Kimura, 1984). A large diameter axon is more heavily myelinated than one of small diameter. For these neurons, conduction occurs only at the nodes of Ranvier as opposed to the entire length of the axon. The internodal distance for a large diameter axon is approximately 1 mm which yields a conduction velocity of 50 m/s. Pathology can affect the axoplasmic resistance, capacitance, and conductance in a manner that decreases the speed of neuronal conduction resulting in longer than normal ABR component latencies.

Amplitude.   The amplitude of a scalp surface recorded far-field evoked response is related to the total number of neuronal events that occur at a given moment in time (e.g., at the peak latency of wave III), and the geometry of the electrical fields that are generated by these sources. Thus, it is possible for pathology to directly reduce the number of neurons that respond at any given moment in time, or, change the timing and field strengths of sets of neurons (e.g., generator sources). Both of these mechanisms would result in a reduction in ABR component amplitude (Kimura, 1984).

ABR NEURODIAGNOSTIC TEST PROTOCOL

If there were a typical, minimal, otoneurologic ABR testing approach, it would probably be as follows. The ABR is recorded using a single, differential channel, with one electrode in the midline upper forehead to vertex, from Fpz to Cz in the nomenclature of the International 10–20 System (Jasper, 1958); the other electrode is periauricular, in or near the test ear. The signal is amplified 50,000–100,000 times, filtered from 100–3000 Hz, and a data window (sweep) of 10–12 ms length is digitized. Ensemble averaging of at least

1000–2000 sweeps yields an average record, and at least two such records are required, to confirm the replicability of response waveforms. Stimuli are monaural clicks at a moderate to high intensity level, presented at about 20 per second.

Interpretation is based primarily on wave latencies, especially of the relatively prominent waves I, III and V. Absolute values and interaural differences (ILDs) of the latencies themselves or of interwave intervals (IWIs) are possible diagnostic indices, as well as wave absence.

Unfortunately, many variables relating to the stimulus and recording parameters and to the state of the subject, especially the presence of conductive or cochlear hearing loss, also affect the diagnostic indices. This section is devoted in part to a more detailed examination of those effects and how to deal with them.

Stimulation Methods

Stimulus Types.   Many types of stimuli can elicit an ABR, but most measurements involve discrete, brief, transient stimuli such as clicks or tonepips. Here, brief means having rise times (and durations) of less than about 5 ms. The stimulus must elicit a sufficient volume and synchrony of neuronal activity to generate a detectable gross response. The key evoking events appear to occur in the first few milliseconds of the stimulus (see Hecox, Squires, and Galambos, 1976; Suzuki and Horiuchi, 1981), so it must have a short rise time. The use of a longer rise time, such as with a shaped toneburst, will result in a less effective stimulus, much of which is irrelevant for response generation.

For otoneurologic ABR measurements, the click is by far the most common stimulus. It is simple to generate, using a rectangular voltage pulse, and because it has the most rapid pressure rise possible, it tends to elicit a relatively high degree of neuronal synchrony, leading (at least in a functional auditory pathway) to clear ABR waveforms with the full complement of wave components.

So-called filtered clicks have been produced by passing the rectangular pulse through an electronic bandpass filter such as an octave or a one-third-octave filter. Nowadays, the waveform would be generated digitally. The terms filtered click and tonepip are often used interchangeably, but it seems better to reserve the former term for transient waveforms that are actually derived, at least theoretically, from some well-defined filter transfer function. In any case, filtered clicks are no longer widely used, even for threshold audiometry.

Tonepips are nowadays also generated digitally, and can be viewed as amplitude modulated (windowed) sinusoids; the Blackman window (Harris, 1978) is popular because, at least acoustically, it causes less spectral energy spread than the more traditional envelope with a linear rise and flat plateau.

Clicks.   The classical click stimulus is generated by driving an earphone with a rectangular pulse of duration about 100μs. The pressure response of the earphone comprises a rapid, initial rise, followed by a brief, oscillatory return to baseline. Condensation clicks have a positive initial pressure change, and rarefaction clicks have negative initial change. The exact pressure waveform depends on many factors. It varies between transducer types and makes, with the coupling to the ear, between transducers of a given type and make (such as between different TDH-49 earphones), and over time as a given transducer ages and eventually breaks down.

In the language of systems theory (Bendat and Piersol, 1986), the rectangular voltage pulse approximates a "unit impulse" (Dirac impulse). This electrical pulse develops an impulse response from the transducer (the click stimulus) that has the widest possible spectral bandwidth of all transient stimuli.

Because the click spectrum contains energy in a wide frequency range, much of the cochlea is excited by it. This is the main reason why the click tends to elicit a large volume and high degree of synchrony of neuronal activity. However, the excitation of the primary neuronal array is not instantaneous, but is distributed in time (over about 2–3 ms in man) because of the finite propagation velocity of the cochlear traveling wave. The velocity is greatest at the cochlear base, and the innervation density also decreases from base to apex, so the effective neuronal synchrony (spike initiation per unit time) also decreases from base to apex. The result is that while an extensive cochlear region contributes to the overall gross ABR waveform, there

is a relative weighting of the response contribution from the cochlear base.

The fact that the rectangular pulse evokes the fastest possible rise (widest response bandwidth) in the pressure response of the transducer has certain disadvantages. Any change in the state of the transducer, such as wear in the diaphragm material or coil coupling, or the use of different transducers, can lead to changes in the transducer impulse response, in turn causing changes in the evoked ABRs. Also, variation of click waveform across transducers raises calibration issues; for example, the detectability and the subjective loudness of the click depend mainly on its total energy (the integral of the square of the click pressure waveform), but the evoked ABR may depend more intimately upon the details of stimulus waveshape such as the relative sizes of the initial deflection and the subsequent *ringing*. For clicks, there are no international standards analogous to those for tonal stimuli. Intensity measures such as peak or peak-equivalent SPL focus on specific features of the click waveform.

Another issue is that electromagnetic artifact picked up by the electrodes when the transducer is activated is proportional to the rate of change of current through the transducer; the shorter the stimulus rise time, the larger the artifact, so the click evoked by a rectangular pulse has the largest possible artifact. The very fast rise of the rectangular pulse is unnecessary physiologically. Also, it is probable that rectangular pulses provoke relatively rapid wear and ultimate failure of transducers, because they represent extreme response demand.

There is a case for the use of more controlled stimulus waveforms such as one period or a half-period of a sinusoid in the 2000–4000 Hz range, or a Gaussian impulse, etc., rather than the rectangular pulse. The earphone pressure response to a one-period 4000 Hz sinusoid, say, is similar to the driving voltage waveform. It also sounds like a click. Provided the stimulus contains much of its energy in the 2000–4000 Hz region, its ability to elicit clear ABR waveforms is unlikely to be compromised significantly, relative to the rectangular driving pulse. Yet, such stimuli are more easily standardized, cause less variation between and within tranducers, cause less electromagnetic artifact, and are probably less mechanically destructive than the traditional click. Nevertheless, the rectangular-pulse click remains the most widely used stimulus. Whatever the exact form of the click stimulus, contralateral noise masking is usually appropriate. Detailed pure-tone audiometry is desirable for many reasons prior to ABR testing, one reason being to establish appropriate masking conditions. However, white noise at about 50 dB nHL is generally suitable for routine use.

Stimulus Transducers.   The most common transducers for otoneurologic ABR testing are electromagnetic earphones such as the TDH-49, often with a supraaural cushion. Piezoelectric earphones are another option (Hughes and Fino, 1980). Recently, insert earphones (tubephones; Killion, 1984) have become popular, and have certain advantages: they tend to prevent ear canal collapse, a common problem with supraaural earphones especially in elderly clients laying supine; the coupling tube introduces a time delay of about 0.9 ms between electrical excitation and acoustic stimulation, and this, as well as physical separation, reduces the stimulus artifact problem; also, tubephones give better interaural attenuation. Adequate calibration data for these earphones are now widely available. Disadvantages include expense and limitations of maximum intensity.

Stimulus Level.   The simplest approach is to use a single stimulus level, but which level? The dominant factor here is whether there is pure-tone hearing loss, because even conductive or cochlear hearing loss can depress, delay, or abolish any or all of the ABR waves. This can lead to ABR test results that are false-positive, that is, they falsely indicate the presence of retrocochlear disease. Wave I is relatively vulnerable to effects of hearing loss, especially at 2000 Hz and above, but it is important to try and elicit a clear wave I, so that interwave intervals can be determined. The lower the click level, the greater the effects of hearing loss, so it seems reasonable to use a high level. The upper limit is governed by the transducer capabilities and by client discomfort and damage risk. Selections in the range from about 70 dB to 100 dB nHL are common.

If the subject has near-normal hearing, or has a cochlear hearing loss with recruitment, then 100 dB

nHL clicks are unnecessary and most unpleasant. The subject may be aroused, uncomfortable, or may find the stimulus painful, which is undesirable because even if the stimuli are tolerated, the level of electromyogenic activity will rise, degrading the signal to noise ratio (SNR) of the recording and confounding the goal of using such a high stimulus level.

With regard to possible cochlear damage, risk criteria designed for chronic noise exposure may not apply to acute exposure to intense, impulsive sounds. The cautious view is that any stimulus that can cause acute loudness discomfort, tinnitus, or temporary threshold shift is potentially hazardous and should be avoided.

One strategy is simply to use a fixed absolute click level for all subjects, such as 85 dB nHL. This is likely to elicit a clear wave I, unless sensorineural hearing loss in the 4000 Hz region is severe or profound, yet rarely causes significant discomfort. A level of 95–100 dB may cause discomfort in a significant number of subjects, but when the hearing loss is severe, the results are much clearer and easier to interpret than those at about 85 dB nHL. An adaptive protocol using, say, two levels (such as 85 and 95 dB nHL) based upon the actual clarity and interpretability of the elicited ABR waveforms, is a possibility.

Another strategy, which has been called the quasi-sensation level method, is to adjust the stimulus level according to some aspect of the puretone audiogram, such as an average threshold (Jerger and Johnson, 1988). Because hearing losses tend to delay ABR wave V, whereas increase in stimulus level tends to reduce wave latency, this strategy should, at least in principle, tend to stabilize wave V latency over a range of hearing losses. A more extreme option is to try and achieve stimulation at a constant sensation level (SL), but this involves measuring the perceptual threshold for the stimulus, which takes time. It also is based on the assumption that presenting stimuli at constant SL, if feasible, will actually reduce the intersubject variability of latency shift caused by peripheral dysfunction. This is not proven definitively; changing the stimulus level may actually increase the intersubject latency variability relative to that using a fixed level strategy, because relationships between stimulus audibility, hearing loss severity and frequency profile, and ABR latency shift are complex. Furthermore, in order to cope with subjects having severe hearing losses, low click levels must be used in subjects with near normal hearing; this can raise problem of poor detectability for wave I, and increased variability of latencies.

All three approaches have their proponents. Fixed-level methods are endorsed by, for example, Selters and Brackmann (1977), Hyde and Blair (1981), Arslan, Prosser, and Rosignoli (1988), among others. Jerger and Johnson (1988) have reported on the quasi-SL approach, but seem to favor an SL approach such as that originally reported by Prosser and Arslan (1987). However, it appears these authors have now moved towards a fixed-level approach (Arslan et al., 1988).

On balance, it seems reasonable to adapt the stimulus level according to both hearing loss and to the quality of the observed ABR, at least so far as to use two or three levels (such as 85 and 95 dB nHL). Thus, 85 dB nHL could be used initially if hearing loss at 4000 Hz or average hearing loss at 1000, 2000 and 4000 Hz were 60 dBHL or better, and 95 dB nHL otherwise or if the 85 dB records were not clear. Further investigation is required before the effects of the various possible intensity strategies on the overall diagnostic decision error rates are fully understood.

Stimulus Repetition Rate. The main concern is a choice of rate that is generally efficient in terms of SNR enhancement per unit test time. The higher the rate, the more averaging can be accomplished but the more loss of amplitude due to adaptation will occur. See Hyde and Blair (1981) and Picton, Linden, Hamel, and Maru (1983), for a more detailed discussion of rate optimization. A common error is to use rates that are inefficiently low, because of a tendency to focus upon the loss of wave amplitude with increasing rate, as opposed to the more important measure, namely the SNR. Because adaptation profiles differ for the various ABR waves, no single rate will be optimal for all waves. Wave V adapts less than wave I; whereas the average SNR-optimizing rate for wave V in adults is 50–100 stimuli per second, that for wave I is 10–30 per second. Because of the need for wave I to determine interwave intervals, and because wave I is usually more difficult to recognize, the choice of rate is usually

tailored to favor wave I. A rate of about 20 per second is usually most efficient, in adults. Of course, the actual rate will be an odd value such as 21 per second, to avoid synchronizing the averaging to a submultiple of the power line frequency.

Stimulus Polarity. Stimulus artifact pickup from electromagnetic stimulus transducers is a common problem. It is possible to shield conventional earphones in mumetal cans (Coats, 1983), to use piezo-electric transducers (Hughes and Fino, 1980) or insert tubephones (Killion, 1984). However, most ABR measurements are still performed with conventional earphones, and artifact pickup can be problematic. At very high stimulus levels, the artifact can drive the recording amplifier into overload, can cause an oscillatory response from EEG data filters and severely distort the average, especially in the area of waves I and II, and can trigger artifact rejection systems.

The most common way to "solve" the stimulus artifact problem is to alternate the stimulus polarity. While this does not protect the amplifier from overload, it essentially cancels the pickup in the average, for even numbers of sweeps. Alternating click polarity is convenient, but has drawbacks. Averaging assumes that the evoked potential is the same for all sweeps and if the ABR evoked by condensation and rarefaction clicks are not the same, then averaging may produce waveforms that are completely different from the actual underlying response evoked by either type of stimulus.

For many subjects, especially those with normal hearing, the ABRs for condensation and rarefaction clicks are almost identical. The rarefaction click tends to cause slightly shorter latencies, but the effects are small and not consistent across subjects. In most such cases, alternating click polarity causes no problem. For a small proportion of subjects, however, the differences can be substantial, even dramatic, and the averaged result can be difficult to interpret; waves can be broadened, shifted, split, or even abolished, despite the fact that the underlying ABRs to the condensation or the rarefaction stimuli may appear to be normal. The potential for misinterpretation is clear, especially false positive determination of retrocochlear lesion presence. See Figure 16.3 for an example of polarity ef-

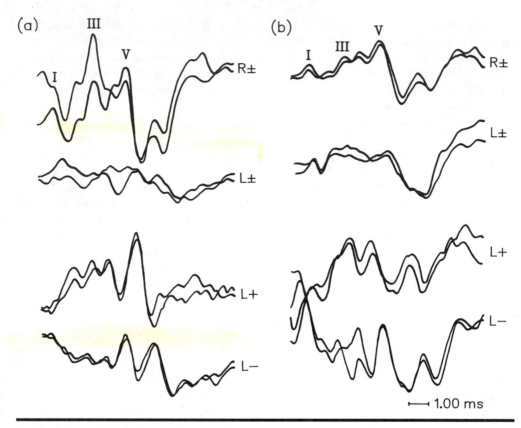

FIGURE 16.3.   Click polarity effects on the ABR, for two subjects, (a) and (b), with left moderate high-frequency cochlear hearing loss. Top: Normal ABRs to alternating(+−) clicks. Second row: ABRs to +− clicks in the suspect ears suggest retrocochlear disease. Bottom two rows: ABRs for + and − clicks show completely different morpholology, with antiphasic appearance. For the right ears, there were no such effects. One potential source of false-positive interpretation in the left alternating records is therefore identified, but the best decision rule is unclear; one view is that if either the + or − click response is normal, then retrocochlear disease is absent. Note that peak latencies to rarefaction clicks are often but not always smaller; a full intensity input-output function may be needed to confirm wave identity. ABRs to 2x2000 monaural clicks, 100 μs (TDH-49), forehead/mastoid recording, 100–3000 Hz recording bandwidth, 1 ms post-stimulus sweep delay.

fects. These large polarity effects tend to be most common and most pronounced in subjects with substantial high-frequency cochlear hearing losses.

How can this problem be handled, practically? One solution is to use a single stimulus polarity, but this can lead to a substantial artifact problem. Also, it is not clear which polarity, if any, is systematically a better choice. Another approach is to examine the condensation or rarefaction click ABRs only if the ABR elicited by alternating clicks is morphologically unusual or apparently abnormal. This is very straightforward if the ABR instrumentation being used is of the type that automatically can extract the monopolar subaverages from an alternating click average. Otherwise, additional averages are required. The goal is to determine first of all whether any apparent abnormality in the alternating average is attributable to polarity effects. If it is, then inferences from the alternating averages are suspect, and interpretation must be based on the "monopolar" averages, despite the possible difficulties with artifact (such as obscured wave I). An alternative viewpoint is that better overall decision performance will be achieved by considering the test to be normal if either the condensation or the rarefaction ABR is normal, there being no clear understanding of how an acoustic tumor can coexist with a normal ABR for either stimulus polarity.

Recording Methods

Electrode Placement. The ABR is a three-dimensional pattern of electrical potential that evolves in time, within the head and on its surface. Certain restricted features of that pattern are registered by the customary differential recording channels with electrodes pairs on the head and neck. The basic issues are how many electrodes are needed, where should they be placed, and what mathematical manipulations of the data are required, to optimize the measurement objectives.

The simplest and most parsimonious approach is to use a single differential channel with one electrode in the midline, say at Fpz or Cz, and the other in or near the ear, anywhere from the mastoid process to the middle ear promontory. The midline electrode mainly registers the later waves (III–VI) of the ABR and the ear electrode mainly registers waves I and II. The skin-negative waves I and II are inverted relative to the skin-positive later waves, to give the classical "vertex-positive" ABR wave sequence I–VI.

A single differential pair is not optimal for all waves. For example, skin-positive wave V activity is present at the midline and the ear, so some cancellation occurs due to the differential action. A neck placement registers very little wave V, so a vertex-neck montage leads to a larger wave V, but at the expense of loss of waves I and II due to the lack of an electrode close to the ear, as well as a probable increase in the level of myogenic noise. See, for example, Parker (1981); Hughes, Fino, and Gagnon, (1981); and Hall, Morgan,

Mackey-Hargadine, Aquilar, and Jahrsdoerfer (1984), for more detailed information on the topographic distribution of the ABR and the resulting effects of various differential pair sites. Overall, when the entire wave sequence is of interest, as is usually the case in otoneurologic ABR applications, the midlinear montage is a good compromise, and still the most widely used.

It is commonly believed that wave I is very important, and many maneuvers designed to increase its clarity have been proposed over the years, each with its advocates and critics. Much of the evidence is anecdotal, and the reports are inconsistent. Some believe, for example, that the earlobe is better than the mastoid, but this has not been substantiated in large-sample studies. It is also commonly believed that wave I is enhanced by using an ear-to ear recording channel, or by deriving such a record mathematically from two-channel recordings from the midline to each ear, but the results of Ruth, Hildebrand, and Cantrell (1982), for example, do not support this assertion. Certainly, the effects are not consistent across subjects.

By far the most effective approach for increasing the amplitude of wave I involves placing one of the electrodes closer to the cochlea of the test ear. Transtympanic placement of a needle electrode gives the greatest increase in wave I (Eggermont, Don, and Brackman, 1980), but is not commonly used, at least in North America. The next most effective placement is endomeatal, preferably in contact with the tympanic membrane at its annulus. A flexible wick electrode is increasingly popular for that purpose (Stypulkowski and Staller, 1987). Other placements in the external meatus are considerably less effective, but even earplug-type electrodes can give some improvement over the traditional mastoid or earlobe placements; such enhancement is very variable across subjects, however.

It should not be forgotten that even with a single, vertex-ear channel, simply choosing an efficient stimulus rate and increasing the amount of averaging and the number of averages can improve the success rate in wave I identification substantially, without the need for special techniques.

Signal Processing. The various manipulations of the recorded electrophysiologic data are described in detail in Hyde, Chapter 3, *Signal Processing and Analysis*, of this text. In routine otoneurologic ABR measurements, the most important, basic manipulations are artifact rejection, filtering, and averaging.

For EEG artifact rejection, directed primarily at high-amplitude myogenic artifacts, the most common procedural flaw is the use of insufficient artifact rejection. The rejection level should be set to achieve about five to ten percent rejection when the ongoing EEG is satisfactory.

Typical filtering at about 100–150 Hz high-pass, 1500–3000 Hz low-pass, 12 dB per octave, usually with a Butterworth design, is appropriate for most otoneurologic measurements. Stronger filtering than this runs the risk of not only loss of important waveshape information, but also the introduction of significant waveform distortion, especially phase distortion (Boston and Ainslie, 1981; Doyle and Hyde, 1981). Excessive high-pass filtering, in particular, can introduce artifactual peaks by phase distortion, as well as abolish low-frequency wave activity that has been desynchonized by retrocochlear pathology.

With regard to averaging, there are still no clear guidelines about how much averaging is needed, or how many averages. In the awake adult subject, a workable absolute minimum per stimulus condition is two averages of 1000 sweeps each, but 2000 sweeps each is preferable.

INTERPRETATION OF ABR RECORDS

This section is oriented towards screening of acoustic tumor suspects but much of it is relevant more generally. The intent is to identify principles and approaches. As yet, there is no unequivocally optimal interpretive procedure, and there is limited consensus, despite many recommendations.

ABR interpretation is a statistical decision problem. The classical approach is to categorize the client into one of two classes: retrocochlear lesion present ("disease-positive," D+) or absent ("disease-negative," D–), using observed values of one or more decision variables (such as ILD V). The decision variable (diagnostic index) will have a statistical distribution for each of the D+ and D– populations (Arslan, Prosser, and Rossignoli, 1988). If

the observed decision variable exceeds some criterion, often the 90th to 95th percentile of the D– distribution, then the test is deemed positive for disease (T+), otherwise it is negative (T–). This approach leads to the standard 2×2 decision matrix and test performance measures such as sensitivity, specificity, and positive predictive value. See, for example, Hyde, Davidson, and Alberti (1991) for a full description of this and other approaches.

The quality of any test is intimately related to overlap of its D+ and D– distributions. Less overlap yields better diagnostic performance. For any given pair of distributions, changing the criterion reveals a trading relationship between sensitivity and specificity (a Relative Operating Characteristic or ROC), and the intrinsic test quality is better expressed by "criterion-free" measures such as d-prime (d') or A (the area under the ROC; see Turner, Shepard, and Frazer, 1984; Swets, 1988; Hyde et al., 1991).

The main issues in ABR interpretive methodology are to select a decision variable that optimizes test accuracy and to select an abnormality criterion that gives appropriate sensitivity and specificity, this compromise being based on the relative costs associated with false-positive and false-negative errors. Another approach, not yet common in this field, recognizes that applying a dichotomy (T+, T–) to the diagnostic index is artificial and wastes information. For example, if ILD V is the index and 0.4 ms is the criterion, what does an observed value of 0.4 mean, and is 0.9 not more strongly indicative of retrocochlear disease than, say, 0.5? Approaches based on the likelihood ratio for the test result are more powerful than the traditional "normal-abnormal" approach, and encompass both equivocal test results and degrees of abnormality (see Hyde et al., 1991; Sackett et al., 1991).

Regardless of whether a likelihood ratio or dichotomous approach is used to express the test result, and regardless of whether the decision variable is simple (univariate) or complex (compound or multivariate), test quality depends almost entirely upon the form and overlap of the D+ and D– distributions. Variables that increase this overlap degrade test accuracy, especially in the sense of increasing the false-positive rate. For common diagnostic indices such as L V, ILD V, IWI I–

V and ILD I–V, peripheral hearing loss, age, and gender are of special interest in this regard.

Detailed Effects of Hearing Loss, Age, and Gender

The overall ABR waveform is the sum of all of the activity initiated from throughout the cochlea, so it is not unreasonable to predict that hearing loss can have complex and substantial effects on the various component waves. Because it takes several milliseconds for the traveling wave to traverse the cochlea, a complex array of simultaneous neuronal events ensues. For example, brainstem neuronal activity originally triggered from the cochlear base can occur simultaneously with primary neuronal excitation in the cochlear apex. For this and many other reasons, the click ABR is not a simple sequence of neuronal events triggered by a single cochlear event. Multiple activity sources distributed in time and space can contribute to any particular feature of the overall ABR waveform. Accordingly, it may not always be a straightforward matter to disentangle the effects of cochlear and retrocochlear function and dysfunction upon the overall ABR waveform.

Effects on Absolute Latencies and Their ILDs. Middle ear and cochlear function can affect the latencies of all ABR waves. Usually, these effects are expressed in relation to the puretone audiogram, but it must be remembered that the audiogram itself is merely one facet of the overall impact of a given anatomical or physiological abnormality. Moreover, the audiogram is a threshold descriptor, and its relationship to cochlear events at high stimulus levels is open to question. These limitations may underlie some of the intersubject variation observed in attempts to relate click ABR properties to pure-tone audiogram features. Another difficulty is that the pure-tone audiogram is actually quite a complicated, multivariate entity. Whenever an attempt is made to express the audiogram in very simple terms, such as the threshold at a single frequency, some kind of weighted average, or a slope measure, there is the potential to overlook some more subtle aspect, to lose information, and to increase variation in associations with other variables, such as ABR parameters.

Notwithstanding these caveats, hearing loss affects the ABR. Conductive and cochlear hearing losses have different effects. The simplest model of the effects of conductive loss is that of a linear attenuator, modifying the effective stimulus level reaching the cochlea. One approach is to compute the average conductive hearing loss component at the most relevant frequencies for click ABR generation (2000 and 4000 Hz, for example). The expected latency increase caused by such a loss can be calculated from the normal intensity-latency input-output function (Picton, Stapells, and Campbell, 1981; Hyde, 1985). Because the input-output function is non-linear, flattening out at high click levels, the effect of a given conductive loss will decrease with increasing click level. See van der Drift, Brocaar, and van Zanten (1988) for a detailed discussion.

The latency shift that occurs for a given click level and amount of conductive loss in a given individual can differ from the expected amount for at least three reasons: first, the input-output function in the individual is not necessarily the same as that of the population mean function, perhaps because of natural variation, or because of coexistent cochlear hearing loss. Second, the effects of different profiles of conductive loss are not fully captured in the single, average loss figure. Third, different etiologies of conductive loss may not have equivalent effects (McGee and Clemis, 1982). Conductive loss effects can at least partially be compensated by adjustment of the stimulus level to equalize the effective level of cochlear excitation. The rationale for this is stronger than it is for the case of cochlear hearing loss, because a conductive loss is more closely related to a simple change in stimulus level than is a cochlear loss. A behavioral example of this concept is the recruitment of loudness.

Cochlear hearing loss also has substantial effects on the absolute latencies of all ABR waves. Its effects are not as straightforward as those of conductive loss, and it is not in any sense equivalent to a simple change in effective stimulus level. The complexity of the effects are not unexpected, bearing in mind the physiologic mechanisms involved at the hair cell level, as well as the variety of frequency contours and etiologies.

In general, cochlear hearing loss at frequencies above about 1000 Hz increases wave latencies. Many authors have shown that these effects are nonlinear, being small at low loss values and increasing more rapidly for severe losses (Selters and Brackmann, 1977; Hyde, 1985; Elberling and Parbo, 1987; Jerger and Johnson, 1988; Bauch and Olsen, 1989). The effects are more marked for wave I than for wave V (Elberling and Parbo, 1987), but as noted earlier, wave I is not usually detectable with severe high-frequency losses when using an earlobe or mastoid electrode. Also, the effects would be expected to be smaller, the higher the stimulus level.

It should be noted that the effects of cochlear hearing loss will depend on the details of the audiometric profile, and generally in a manner that is consistent with the view of the click ABR as a weighted sum of contributions from the various regions of the cochlear partition. Differential effects on wave I and wave V are explicable by taking into account the more basal weighting of wave I initiation, and intensity effects are consistent with what is known about the cochlear traveling wave at various stimulus levels (Yamada et al., 1979; Gorga, Worthington, Reiland, Beauchaine, and Goldgar, 1985; Hyde, 1985; Keith and Greville, 1987). The results of experiments with high-pass masking noise, derived-band responses and frequency specific responses are also consistent (Keith and Greville, 1987).

For practical purposes, noteworthy points are that precipitous high-frequency hearing losses tend to produce wave delays that are independent of stimulus level, whereas the more common, gradually sloping high-frequency cochlear losses cause delays that are reduced or abolished at the highest stimulus levels.

From the above observations, it follows that cochlear hearing loss also will tend to increase the error rates for retrocochlear lesion detection with ILD V. There are at least four approaches to this problem, and they are not mutually exclusive, nor is any one of them clearly applicable universally or clearly superior. Indeed, it is possible that a combination of all four techniques would be needed to produce the best error rates. The first and most obvious approach is to use not wave V latency itself but an interwave interval, such as IWI I–V. The second approach is to manipulate the click intensity so as to reduce the impact of hearing loss as much as possible, and some intensity strategies were noted earlier. The third approach is to use a stimulus with a more restricted basilar membrane excitation pattern than the simple click, either by using ipsilateral high-pass masking noise or a mid-frequency tonepip (Telian and Kileny, 1989); this will tend to lessen the impact of high-frequency hearing loss on the elicited ABR. The fourth approach is to determine the intersubject distributions of the chosen ABR decision index, whether it is based on absolute or interwave measures, and then develop diagnostic decision criteria that are in essence conditional upon the observed hearing loss. This is sometimes referred to as the "correction factor" method.

With regard to age effects, despite contradictory reports there is a body of evidence that age increases ABR peak latencies (Jerger and Hall, 1980; Hyde, 1985: Elberling and Parbo, 1987; Jerger and Johnson, 1988). It can be difficult to unravel the effects of age and hearing loss, and to ensure sufficient sample size and diversity that all pertinent effects are represented. Age and hearing loss effects may be nonlinear and interactive (Otto and McCandless, 1982; Hyde, 1985), so age may need to be taken into account even with ILD V. A gender effect on wave latency is well established, with L III and L V being about 0.2 ms larger in males; there may be interactions among the effects of gender, age and hearing loss (Elberling and Parbo, 1988; Jerger and Johnson, 1988), so again, caution may be required even with ILD measures.

Effects on IWI I–V and its ILD.   Conductive hearing loss and sloping high-frequency cochlear loss can decrease IWI I–V (Keith and Greville, 1987); the effects are smaller than for L V, but may still be large enough to affect diagnostic error rates. Flat cochlear losses have negligible effects. Notched cochlear losses at 3000–4000 Hz increase IWI I–V, because of differential effects on waves I and V. Use of ILD I–V does not protect against these effects, if the hearing losses are not symmetrical. Reports on age effects are inconsistent, but the large sample study by Elberling and Parbo (1987) showed an increase in IWI I–V with age of 0.2–0.3 ms over the range 20–80 years. Use of ILD I–V should negate this effect.

Quantitative Decision Procedures

Diagnostic decision indices based on discriminant, factor, or multiple regression analysis are not yet well-established in clinical practice, and there are many analytic subtleties to be considered in their derivation and application. Here, the focus will be upon the more primary, classical measures.

The choice of absolute or interaural indices depends on many factors, the most important of which are the relative error rates for the disorders that are most common or most significant in the local referred population. However, these error rates will rarely be known exactly, and are time-consuming to compile. Whatever the decision index selected, the error rates will be governed by the amount of variation, mean separation, and tail overlap for the distribution of neurologically and non-neurologically impaired subjects.

Interaural measures have the advantage that they greatly reduce the need to assemble large-scale normative data; ILD V and ILD I–V are distributed with zero expectation and an SD of about 0.2 ms, regardless of many aspects of stimulus and recording technique, in non-neurologically impaired persons with at most moderate hearing losses. The objections concerning possible false-negatives due to bilateral disease can be handled by incorporating a conservative absolute L V or IWI I–V sub-rule into the decision process.

Despite widespread enthusiasm for wave I, in routine screening for CP angle lesions it is far from clear whether ILD V or ILD I–V is superior in terms of diagnostic error rates, provided the ILD V measure is handled appropriately. Also, it is not necessarily a matter of choosing one measure or the other; it is possible to develop compound decision rules that incorporate several measures. If ILD I–V were considered more desirable, then it could form the primary decision index, with ILD V as an alternative when wave I is not elicitable.

Unless transtympanic or at least tympanic recording is to be used routinely, it will be necessary to use the ILD V measure, at least for some subjects. Then, it is advisable to take certain steps to improve its properties as a decision variable. As is perfectly clear from the large-sample studies of Selters and Brackmann (1977), and Arslan, Prosser, and Rosognoli (1988), the main problem with ILD V is a high false-positive rate of retrocochlear lesion detection, if a fixed decision criterion (0.3 ms, say), is used. The cause of the problem is wave V delay due to severe, high-frequency cochlear hearing loss. The problem is aggravated by the use of low stimulus intensity levels, but even with a quasi-SL strategy that includes levels up to about 95 dB nHL, severe hearing losses will inflate the false-positive error rate of the raw ILD V (Elberling and Parbo, 1987; Jerger and Johnson, 1988).

The seminal report by Selters and Brackmann (1977) introduced the concept of making the ILD V abnormality criterion conditional upon the observed degree of hearing loss. Noting the strong correlation between wave V latency and the sensorineural hearing level at 4000 Hz, which has subsequently been verified repeatedly, they chose 4000 Hz as the audiometric basis parameter for criterion adjustment. While it is better to think of this process as one of criterion adjustment, in practice it is simpler to alter or "correct" the observed wave V latency. Without correction, the sensitivity and false positive rate were 0.98 and 0.24, respectively (d'= 2.75). Selters and Brackmann (1977) suggested subtracting 0.1 ms for every 10 dB or fraction thereof of hearing loss above 50 dB HL at 4000 Hz, and this gave sensitivity and false-positive rate values of 0.97 and 0.08 (d'=3.25). Reanalysis using a correction of 0.1 ms per 5 dB or fraction thereof above 55 dB HL at 4000 Hz improves the d' to 3.6, which is excellent performance (Hyde et al., 1991). The point is not so much the precise criterion adjustment rule, but the fact that test performance is radically improved by this maneuver. Despite this compelling large-sample evidence, there is an ongoing debate about the merits of latency correction.

One of the misconceptions that may be fueling the debate is that the correction procedure appears to be based on the population average effect of hearing loss on L V, whereas individuals may behave quite differently from the mean. It is true that individuals vary, but the arithmetical manipulation should be based not on the population mean L V but on the overlap between the D+ and D– distributions, for various degrees of hearing loss (Figure 16.4). This is why it is better to conceive of the maneuver as the use of an abnormality criterion that is a function of hearing loss, rather than the "correction" of

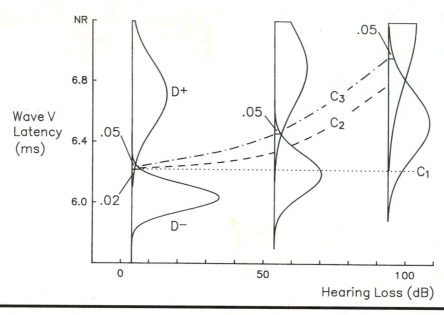

FIGURE 16.4. A model illustrating several important principles about the effect of cochlear hearing loss (2–4kHz) on ABR interpretation for acoustic tumor. For any degree of hearing loss, there will be some statistical distribution of wave V latency in clients who have cochlear (D–) or retrocochlear (D+) disease. As hearing loss increases, both the mean and the variance of the D– distribution increase. The same effects occur, but less markedly, for the D+ distribution. Note the increasing censoring of the D+ distributions at the point (NR) where the lesion abolishes wave V. CI is a binary decision criterion for tumor detection with sensitivity O.98 and specificity O.95. If C1 is applied without regard to hearing loss, the specificity will decrease dramatically; the exact net value will depend on the local population mix of hearing loss severities. C2 is an abnormality criterion function that depends upon the hearing loss. It is a shift of C1 by an amount equal to the increase in mean of the D– distribution. It is nonlinear, and more marked above 50 dB hearing loss. Use of C2 tends to keep the specificity in the 0.9–0.95 region, but the sensitivity decreases somewhat, especially for the most severe hearing losses. C1 does not take account of the D– variance increase with hearing loss. C3 is another criterion function that depends on hearing loss; it is the locus of all criterion points such that the specificity is held at 0.95, regardless of hearing loss. With this function, overall specificity is 0.95, but sensitivity is more compromised than for C2. The point is that failure to account for effects of hearing loss lowers the predictive value of a positive ABR test dramatically, and some better compromise between sensitivity and specificity than is offered by C1 seems indicated. The optimal scheme is not yet clear.

observed latency. The optimal criterion function is not yet known; it is certainly nonlinear. Furthermore, the reported interactions between age and hearing loss, and possibly between gender and hearing loss, will probably lead to the use of criterion functions that are functions of three variables, not just hearing loss. Also,

the criterion adjustment procedure will depend upon the stimulus intensity strategy that was used. Furthermore, some criterion adjustment procedure may well be appropriate for ILD I–V, not just ILD V.

This all sounds more complicated that it really is. As noted earlier, the essence of the differential diagnostic problem is to distinguish optimally between the behaviors of the diagnostic decision index for the diseased and non-diseased states, all other variables being held as constant as possible. This inevitably leads to the use of decision criteria that are functions of the variables that affect the decision index. It makes no sense, for example, to use an abnormality criterion based on normal-hearing males, when dealing with female patients who have severe sensory hearing loss. Because the variability of wave latencies increases as hearing loss increases, the absolute accuracy of the diagnostic decision may itself depend on hearing loss. This may also be true for the age and gender variables; it is certainly true for different target diseases. Thus, the concept of a single, invariant level of test accuracy for all subjects is inherently flawed.

Any attempt to reduce the variance of the diagnostic index by adjusting stimulus level on the basis of hearing loss will, of course, alter the abnormality criterion function. Changing the level on the basis of, say, an average hearing loss assumes that the same level adjustment is appropriate for all audiometric profiles that yield the same average loss. Similarly, basing criterion adjustment on single frequencies is equally suspect. One way to research this problem would be to explore latency effects of a wide variety of hearing loss severity and profile, using multiple regression analysis; the sample size requirements, however, would be formidable.

Limits of Testability by ABR

As hearing loss becomes more and more severe, wave V will tend to be the only detectable wave, and then will itself disappear. At some point that is not well defined, the accuracy of the test will become unacceptably poor. There appear to be no large-sample studies of the manner in which ABR test accuracy declines for severe and profound hearing losses. An informal opinion is that useful information can be expected in most cases provided the pure-tone threshold at 2000 Hz is about 80 dB HL or better, even if the hearing loss is profound at higher frequencies. For hearing losses that are severe or profound and extend down to 1000 Hz or below, the diagnostic information obtainable from a severely delayed wave V or an absent ABR is very limited.

PATHOPHYSIOLOGY OF COMPRESSION AND TRACTION

Compression

Neuronal structures are compressed by tumors, hematomas, and edema with resultant demyelination followed by axonal degeneration. Demyelination results in slowing of conduction velocity and increased evoked potential component latencies. Temporal dispersion of electrical activity (from compression and demyelination) produces broadened evoked potential components (decreased evoked potential component amplitudes) or absent responses. Focal compression decreases the axonal diameter which possibly could result in decreased capacitance at the internodal membrane and faster conduction. However, focal compression also results in increased axoplasmic resistance which serves to increase the delay in impulse generation at the next internode, resulting in increased evoked potential latency (Kimura, 1984). Therefore, compression of the CN VIII and/or brainstem by a mass such as a tumor or hematoma can result in delayed evoked potential components, reduced amplitude, or, absent wave components.

Traction (Stretching)

Sekiya and Møller (1987a,b) reported the effects of traction injuries on auditory nerve function. The results of their investigations indicated that extreme traction causes avulsions of the internal auditory artery (IAA) and cochlear nerve fibers. These injuries occurred in the area cribosa. In the extreme, hemorrhage resulted in an abrupt total loss of the ABR, probably due to cochlear ischemia. Histologic analysis demonstrated damage present at the fundis of the IAC at the level of the area cribosa. In another study (Møller and Sekiya, 1988) the authors associated traction injury with disintegration of the myelin sheath and petechial hemorrhages of the vasa nervorum of the cochlear nerve. In this study abrupt loss of the ABR was associated with a discontinuity of the peripheral (Schwann cell derived) and central (oligodendroglial cell derived) myelin at the Obersteiner-Redlich zone.

Clinical Correlates of Compression and Traction: Acoustic Neuroma (AN)

This section will focus on the acoustic neuroma since: 1) it is the most common (non-surgically induced) source of compression and traction injury, 2) it is the most frequently cited retrocochlear lesion, and, 3) because other lesions of the same anatomic vicinity tend to mimic its electrophysioloic outcome.

The most common tumor lesion within the CPA is the acoustic neuroma arising from the Schwann cells of the vestibular nerve. Brackmann and Bartels (1980) reported that in over 200 CPA tumor cases 92% were AN. Other CPA tumors (See Table 16.1) include: meningiomas (3%), primary cholesteatomas (2.5%) and facial nerve schwannomas (1%). Some 1.5% are caused by unusual lesions which often mimic the AN and are only correctly diagnosed at surgery.

Recent developments in radiologic and electrophysiologic techniques have improved the diagnosis of acoustic tumors that comprise about 80% to 90% of all posterior fossa lesions. ABR measures, computerized axial tomography (CT), and MRI have reportedly high operating characteristics in detecting intracanalicular AN and other CP angle tumors. Table 16.2 lists a series of studies that have reported operating characteristics

TABLE 16.1. Various types of neoplasms found in and around the posterior cranial fossa.

Arachnoid Cysts
Brainstem Gliomas
Glioma
Glomus Jugulare Tumors
Hemangioblastomas
Hemangiomas
Lipomas
Medulloblastoma
Meningiomas
Primary Cholesteatomas
Schwannomas CN VII and CN VIII

for the detection of AN. As evident, the ABR has a sensitivity rate in excess of 95% (Brackman, 1984; Selters and Brackman, 1979; Josey 1987; Josey et al., 1980, 1988; Musiek and Gollegly, 1985; Telian et al., 1989) for AN of the CPA; whereas, other lesions in the posterior fossa have demonstrated ABR detection rates of about 75% (Brackman and Forquer, 1983).

Historical Perspective. In a comprehensive review of the historical development of ANs, House (1985) reported that acoustic tumors were observed initially in the late 17th century at autopsy and later described in detail by Bell (1830). By the end of the 18th century, Sir Charles Ballance (1907) reported the successful surgical removal of an AN within the CPA. Mortality rates at that time frequently exceeded 80%, prompting Cushing (1917) to advocate subtotal intracapsular removal of tumors which reduced mortality to about 30%. Further improvements in neurosurgical techniques (e.g., hemostasis) and the use of ventriculostomy lowered the operative mortality to about 4% (Cushing, 1932). Dandy (1925, following the earlier work of Cushing) provided surgical insight into the radical removal of cranial tumors. However, this reduction in mortality often came at the expense of total hearing loss and facial paralysis.

By the 1950s, improved surgical techniques made it possible to preserve the facial nerve in about 50 to 60% of patients. It was not until the decade of the 1960s however, that otosurgical microscopic techniques were successfully introduced (House, 1961). House (1964) reported the first translabyrinthine removal of AN in 47 consecutive patients resulting in the reduction of facial nerve injury and central nervous system (CNS) complications. Today, the morbidity and mortality rates of AN surgery continue to decrease due to improved intraoperative skills, and improved microsurgical, interventional, and intraoperative monitoring techniques.

Demographics. The incidence of intracranial tumors range between 5 and 12% per 100,000 in the general population (Davis and Robertson, 1991) with about 20% occurring in childhood (Okazaki, 1983). In comparison, the incidence of ANs is about 1/100,000 or about 2500 cases per year in the US. Tos and Thomsen

TABLE 16.2. Results of past studies that have examined the efficiency of the ABR in the detection of acoustic neuroma (AN). NT: non-tumor; Hits: Hit Rate; FN: false-negative; FP: false-positive.

Investigation	Criteria	Number of Subjects				
		Tumor	NT	Hits	FN	FP
Selters & Brackmann (1977)	ILD V >.4	46	54	91%	9%	12%
Clemis & McGee (1979)	ILD V >.3	26	128	93%	7%	18%
House & Brackmann (1979)	ILD V >.2	146		98%	2%	
Glasscock et al. (1979)	I–V> 4.4 or ILD V > .2	39	511	98%	2%	6%
Josey et al. (1980)	I–V > 4.4 or ILD V > .4	52		98%	2%	
Bauch et al. (1982)	ILD V > .2 or V > 6.1	26	239	96%	4%	25%
Barrs et al. (1985)	ILD V > .2	229		98%	2%	
Musiek et al. (1986)	I–V or ILD V > .3	16		94%	25%	
Josey et al. (1988)	I–V > 4.4 or ILD V > .4	93		97%	3%	
Telian et al. (1989)	I–V > 4.4 or ILD V > .4	93		98%	2%	

(1984) have reported an incidence of 8:1,000,000 per year in Denmark, a nation with a centralized medical accounting system.

House and Hitselberger (1986) reported a series of 1667 patients with surgically treated AN. Of this sample 51% of patients were males and 0.2% were black. Tumor site was symmetrical with 48% of the cases occurring on the left side and 52% observed on the right. The average age of the sample was 47.3 years with significant differences in reported age of onset. Similar demographic findings were reported by Tos and Thomsen (1988) in a group of 400 translabyrinthine ANs removals. Their population consisted of 54% females with 44% of the total ranging between 40 and 60 years of age.

Pathophysiology

ANs, also termed neurinoma, neurilemmoma and most accurately, vestibular schwannoma, are benign encapsulated tumors arising for the most part, from the Schwann cells of the superior branch of the vestibular nerve in about two thirds of all patients. Infrequently, the acoustic portion of CN VIII or the inferior branch of the vestibular nerve are the sites of tumor origin. The tumors tend to encroach on and displace neurovascular structures without direct invasion. Their consistency varies from firm and dense to soft with large cystic spaces, commonly seen in larger tumors. They arise at the Schwann cell-oligodendroglial cell junction (at the Obersteiner-Redlich zone) near the porus acousticus.

Small intracanalicular tumors originating in the IAC are usually asymptomatic until they increase in size and apply pressure directly against the originating nerve fiber, adjacent nerves and vascular supply. As tumors grow outward into the CPA, they tend to compress nerve fiber bundles introducing auditory and vestibular symptoms and impaired function.

Clinical Profile of CN VIII Lesions

For the most part, removal of smaller acoustic tumors translates into reduced morbidity and the possibility of hearing preservation in the operated ear (see Kileny and Niparko, Chapter 18, *Neurophysiologic Intraoperative Monitoring* in this text). Thus, early diagnosis of AN significantly reduces associated morbidity and mortality rates. Early diagnosis of AN rests on complete neuroradiological or neurotologic evaluations. In this regard, *when* surgery will be performed, *what* surgical approaches will be considered, and *will* monitoring (either CN VII, CN VIII or both) be available, are determinations that depend upon the size and location of the tumor.

Signs and Symptoms. The earliest clinical manifestation of AN is unilateral hearing loss (Singh et al., 1978). Approximately 95% of patients with ANs present with unilateral sensory hearing impairment that is progressive in nature. About 10% to 15% of patients present with sudden hearing loss (Sataloff et al., 1985; Pulec and House, 1964). Cushing (1963) suggested that symptoms of unilateral hearing loss and tinnitus were warning signals of ANs and that patients should always receive a thorough neurodiagnostic evaluation for possible retrocochlear pathology.

Tinnitus and dizziness in the form of unsteadiness are also very common in patients (Singh et al., 1978; Mathew et al., 1978; Fisch and Wegmuller, 1974). Tumor size, extension, and stage affect the clinical presentation, signs, and symptoms. Since these tumors are usually slow-growing lesions, some patients may not complain of symptoms until brainstem compression starts. Occasionally, acute onset facial palsy can be an early manifestation of acoustic tumors (Ellis and Wright, 1974; Singh et al., 1978; Pulec and House, 1964; Hitselberger and House, 1966). Unilateral hearing loss also can be related to viral neronitis, neurosyphillis, autoimmune disease, perilymphatic fistula, Meniere's disease or other inner ear disorders. Such conditions should be considered in the differential diagnosis of AN.

Auditory evaluation. As indicated, tumors that compromise CN VIII function do not generate predictable audiometric patterns. As a result, there has been a proliferation of audiometric tests that have been devised to differentiate retrocochlear lesions from sensory abnormalities.

When hearing loss is measurable, it is commonly high frequency in spectrum and cochlear in origin. The degree of loss varies greatly in most patients (Johnson, 1977). Johnson (1979) found profound hearing loss in 16% of 500 patients with AN; tumor size positively correlated with the degree of peripheral hearing loss. These initial findings were later confirmed by Thomsen and Tos (1988). Patients with CPA tumors often complain of impaired communication skills, despite normal or near-normal pure-tone threshold measures (Jacobson and Reams, 1991).

The first audiometric test battery for the identification of retrocochlear pathology was not clinically available to the otologic community until the early 1960s. In retrospect, the ability of the early test battery to correctly dichotimize neural pathology from cochlear pathology occurred at the expense of a high degree of false-positive and false-negative test results. For example, it has been estimated that the sensitivity (correct identification of disease in the presence of CN VIII pathology) for the classic audiometric retrocochlear test battery is about 50% (Johnson and House, 1964; Fisch and Wegmuller, 1974). With advances in computer technology the role of electrophysiologic tests in the identification of retrocochlear disease has expanded dramatically. Suffice it to say, the use of immittance audiometry and evoked potentials have reduced our reliance on the behaviorally oriented retrocochlear test protocol. A detailed account of conventional behavioral test operating characteristics are beyond the scope of this chapter; the reader is referred to Turner et al. (1984); Schwartz (1987), and Olsen (1991).

In general, middle ear compliance is normal unless middle ear pathology coexists. Acoustic reflexes are typically elevated or absent and positive acoustic reflex decay often is demonstrated when the evoking stimulus is presented to the affected ear. However, several investigators have reported low sensitivity for acoustic reflex testing in patients with CPA tumor lesions (Palva et al., 1978; Jerger et al., 1980; Mathew et al., 1978; Hirsch and Anderson, 1980; Dauman et al., 1987). Recently, Hendrix et al. (1990) evaluated retrospectively 225 patients suffering from asymmetric sensory hearing loss; 31 had retrocochlear disease. They reported sensitivity and specificity values of 61% and

42% respectively for acoustic reflex testing. Sensitivity and specificity values for "roll-over" testing (word recognition materials were unspecified) were 25% and 88% respectively for patients with asymmetric pure-tone audiometric test scores.

Because of high false-positive and false-negative rates identified with the conventional behavioral test protocol, auditory diagnosticians increasingly have relied on the use of the ABR in the clinical confirmation of neurotologic pathology. A summary of the operating characteristics of various audiologic tests suggests that the ABR is by far the most powerful and accurate tool available for retrocochlear identification (Turner et al., 1984).

It has been estimated that approximately 5% of all patients with posterior fossa tumors will present with normal pure tone hearing (Beck et al., 1986; Musiek et al., 1986; Thomsen and Tos, 1988). According to Schuknecht (1974), normal threshold sensitivity can be measured despite a significant reduction in auditory nerve fiber activity. Jerger and Jordan (1980) and Hendley et al. (1987) have documented a series of 40 patients with neurotologic and CNS disease that all demonstrated pure-tone and "PB max" scores within normal limits. These findings, in conjunction with the fact that 2 to 5% of patients with AN have normal ABR results (Josey et al., 1980; Telian et al., 1989; also see next section) demonstrate that close clinical scrutiny is indicated when objective evidence of retrocochlear disease is equivocal. Given the earlier detection of ANs with electrophysiologic and radiologic tests (e.g., before patients become symptomatic) it is not surprising that a number of reports have appeared showing normal pure-tone audiometry in the presence of acoustic neuroma (see next sections).

Given this concern, the otolaryngologist and neurologist community often will use other neurodiagnostic tests when the clinical suspicion of retrocochlear disease is high. Jacobson and Reams (1991) reported four patients with posterior fossa tumors who presented with normal hearing as measured by conventional audiometry. All patients underwent diagnostic work-up that included immittance, PI/PB function and ABR that led to the detection of neurotologic pathology. Thus, clinical evaluation, electrophysiologic and radiologic testing are

complementary in the diagnosis of AN. Table 16.3 describes a series of criteria that have been useful in the evaluation of patient who show normal audiometric patterns but present with unequivocal neurotologic complaint. Figure 16.5 illustrates one such case.

Relationship Between Radiographic Imaging Studies and ABR Results—Acoustic Neuroma.   In the past 10 years several reports have demonstrated false negative findings in ABR testing for AN. These studies have differed in sample sizes, criteria of abnormal ABR (e.g., ILD V, I–V IPL etc.), the size of tumors studied, and the radiologic techniques used to verify the presence of the AN (at the time of this writing the MRI enhanced with Gadolinium-Gd-DTPA is considered the "gold-standard" for the identification of AN, Daniels et al. 1987; Mikhael et al. 1987). Thus, different false-negative rates for ABR in detecting AN have been reported. For instance, Bockenheimer et al. (1984) evaluated 2700 patients for possible AN. Nineteen of 85 patients evaluated with air contrast CT examination had small ANs, and 5 patients had normal ABRs (26% false negative rate). Legatt et al. (1988) reported that of 39 patients with AN or neurofibromas 4 cases had normal ABRs when click stimuli were presented at routine test levels. Telian et al. (1989) reported 2 patients of MRI diagnosed AN where the ABR was normal. One patient had an intracanalicular AN and the other had an intracanalicular AN with extension into the CP angle. Finally, Grabel et al. (1991) found that 5 of 56 patients with AN (10 intracanalicular and 46 extracanalicular) had a normal ABR (11% false negative rate). Table 16.2 summarizes the published series of investigations that have assessed the diagnostic utility of the ABR in detecting AN. In most of these studies there has been a trend for false negatives to be observed for intracanalicular tumors. Most recently, a retrospective analysis of 697 ABR examinations was conducted at Henry Ford Hospital (Gillen, Mandych, Jacobson, and Monsell, 1991, unpublished observations). The patients were referred for ABR on the basis of asymmetry of hearing (309 observations), unilateral or asymmetric tinnitus (203 observations), dysequilibrium (242 observations), and other reasons (e.g., facial numbness, facial weakness—

(A)

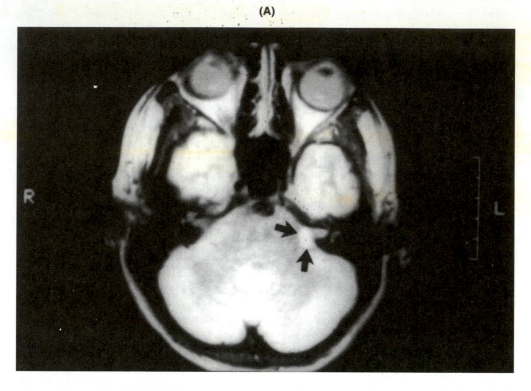

(B)

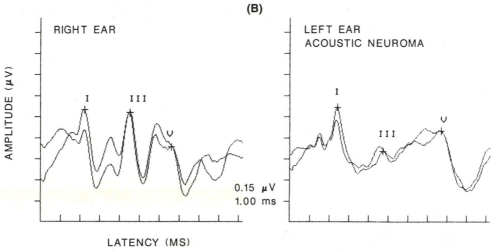

FIGURE 16.5. A 34-year-old female presented with a brief history of unsteadiness and aural fullness. Audiologic study resulted in normal audiometric and immittance findings. Both PIPB roll-over function and acoustic reflex decay were negative. (A) shows the MRI confirmation of an 1.2 cm CPA tumor from the superior branch of the vestibular nerve. (B) displays the abnormal ABR traces obtained from this patient.

TABLE 16.3.   Objective and subjective audiologic indicators of possible retrocochlear pathology.

Primary Indicators (objective)	Secondary Indicators (subjective)
asymmetric hearing loss	unilateral tinnitus
positive roll-over function	unsteadiness
positive reflex patterns	stuffy feeling
reduced vestibular response	subjective hearing loss unexplained by the audiogram

N=134 observations). There were 49 abnormal ABRs in this sample (7%) that went on to have MRI with Gd. Of this subsample there were 40 false positive ABRs. No false negative test was observed. There were 9 patients with AN, meningiomas, or neurofibromas and all were identified with ABR. More recently we have observed two patients who presented with false negative ABR findings. These patients demonstrated asymmetries on pure-tone audiometry but had excellent word recognition scores and normal immittance test results. These cases are shown in Figure 16.6A–F.

It is likely that the Gd MRI scan is identifying ANs which might never become symptomatic. Most recently, Bederson et al. (1991) studied 70 patients with AN using serial MRIs over a 26-month period. They found that the mean tumor growth was 1.6 mm at 1 year, and 1.9 mm at two years. Tumor regression was observed in 6% of patients. There was no change in tumor size in 40% of the cases. The authors suggested only repeat MRI testing for patients with incidental AN since a significant number of these individuals will demonstrate no tumor growth or regression. Recently, von Glass et al. (1991) reported 2 patients with Gd-MRI diagnosed AN. At surgery, both patients had luxuriant arachnoidal tissue suggestive of arachnoiditis instead of AN. These same patients had abnormal ABRs (Case 1 had a severe sensory hearing loss). However, caloric testing was normal in both cases. Therefore, it is highly possible that the ABR and balance function testing will be used in the future to determine which patients with AN should be considered for surgery. Those patients with a small AN and negative ABR and caloric (and rotational test) findings would be followed with serial MRIs to detect changes in tumor size and rate of tumor growth.

Clinical Correlates of Compression and Traction: Neurofibromatosis

Neurofibromatosis is a hereditary autosomal dominant disorder affecting cell growth of neural tissue. Recently, the National Institutes of Health (NIH, 1987) adopted a numbering system to identify the two known but different (peripheral versus central) entities. NF-1 (formerly von Recklinghausen's neurofibromatosis-peripheral) is the most common disorder affecting approximately 1:4,000 individuals although the incidence varies (Carey et al., 1986; Riccardi and Eichner, 1986). The NF-1 gene has been localized to chromosome 17. Although NF-1 does not appear to affect peripheral auditory sensitivity as measured by pure-tone and speech audiometry, Pensak and colleagues (1989) have reported significant ABR abnormalities (32%) in a group of 44 children and young adults ranging in age from 2 to 22 years.

NF-2 (central) is less frequently observed than NF-1 (incidence = 1:50,000) and is associated with bilateral ANs. Diagnostic evaluation for NF-2 (NIH, 1987) should include: audiometry, ABR, vestibular evaluation, and MRI. The NF-2 gene is thought to be localized on chromosome 22. Although neurofibromas and ANs originate similarly from Schwann cells, they grow differently (Baldwin and LeMaster, 1989). ANs grow as an expanding mass, pushing the remainder of the nerve

(A)

RIGHT INTRACANALICULAR
VIIIth N. ACOUSTIC TUMOR

AUDIOMETRIC DATA

	500	1000	2000	4000	8000	Hz
LT.	10	10	10	20	20	dB
RT.	10	15	25	60	55	dB

LT. WAVE V = 5.62 msec   WAVE I-WAVE V = 3.58 msec
RT. WAVE V = 5.62 msec   WAVE I-WAVE V = 3.74 msec

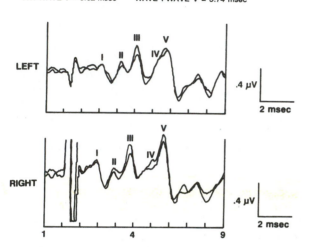

(B)

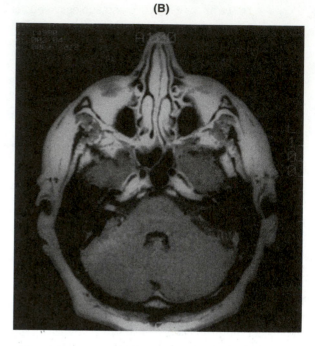

(C)

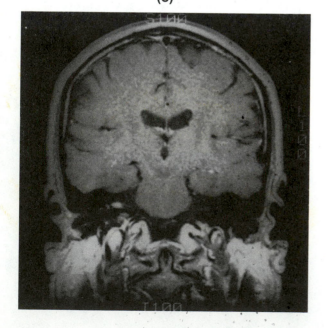

(D)

RIGHT VIIIth N. ACOUSTIC TUMOR

AUDIOMETRIC DATA

	500	1000	2000	4000	8000	Hz
LT.	10	15	20	15	20	dB
RT.	20	25	55	65	65	dB

LT. WAVE V = 5.54 msec
RT. WAVE V = 5.62 msec

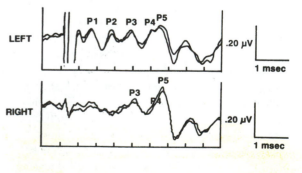

(E)   (F)

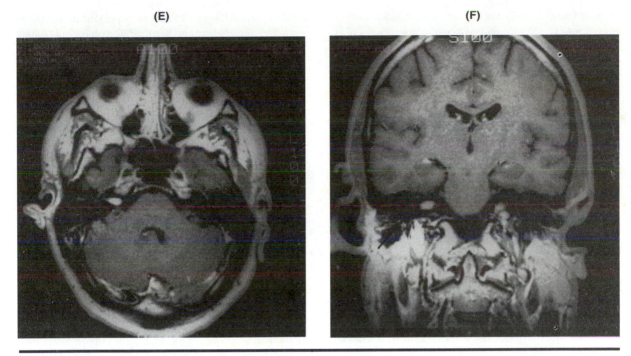

FIGURE 16.6.   Pure-tone audiometry, ABR (A and D) and MRI scans (transverse view—B and E; coronal view—C and F) for two patients (a and b) who had small ANs. In each case an asymmetry in pure-tone audiometic thresholds existed, however, word recognition ability was bilaterally excellent and immittance testing was normal. Please note that ABRs were normal in each instance. The ABR were collected using a click rate of 21.3 sec. (optimal polarity) presented at 75 dB nHL or 85 dB nHL. The filter bandpass was 100–3000 Hz. Clicks were presented through headphones.

away. The neurofibroma appears to harvest from many fascicles and ultimately involves the entire nerve. As such, the description of NF-2 is often cited as bilateral eight nerve tumors leading to deafness. Neurofibromas are found in only 5% of NF-1 patients and in more than 95% of NF-2 patients, although neurofibromas may be present in other locations intracranially and throughout the spinal cord (Hall, 1992).

Since patients with NF-2 present with bilateral pathology, the authors recommend the use of ABR interwave interval latency values of I–III and I–V for clinical analysis. A comparison of interwave latency differences (ILD-V) between ears is problematic. Obviously, there is no assurance that the presence of bilat-eral neurofibromas affect the auditory system in a similar manner. Thus, bilateral pathology limits the utility of between ear comparisons.

PATHOPHYSIOLOGY OF ISCHEMIA AND HEMORRHAGE

Cerebrovascular disease (CVD) or stroke is a common disorder in the adult population and is the commonest cause of disability in the United States (Wolf, 1990). Ischemic CVD accounts for 75%–85% of all strokes, two-thirds of those involving nervous system structures supplied by the anterior cerebral circulation (internal carotid artery-ICA territory, Mohr et al., 1978).

Hemorrhagic strokes including subarachnoid hemorrhage (SAH) and intraparenchymal hemorrhage (ICH) also are more commonly seen in the anterior circulation territories.

Abnormal ABRs have been reported in both ischemic and hemorrhagic strokes, predominantly affecting the posterior circulation (vertebrobasilar) territories. Ischemia and hemorrhage result in an abnormal ABR when the central auditory pathways extending from the upper medulla caudally to the mesencephalon are damaged by the ischemic or hemorrhagic process. Ischemia to the cochlear nerve proper, ischemic mononeuropathy, can also alter the ABR. Ischemic mononeuropathy is defined as dysfunction of a specific nerve (e.g., the cochlear nerve) when the arterial feeders of the nerve trunk (the vasa nervosa) are occluded. Ischemic mononeuropathy is encountered in conditions such as Lyme's disease, neurosyphillis, and systemic vasculitis (systemic lupus erythematosis-SLE, rheumatoid arthritis-RA, polyarteritis nodosa-PAN). In such diseases the arteries feeding the axons are directly injured. When the vasa nervosa are occluded, the axonal fibers are deprived of nutrients like oxygen and glucose, resulting in energy failure along the axon and subsequent conduction failure across the involved segments of that axon.

Brainstem strokes affect not only the central auditory structures but also cranial nerves III–XII, the ascending reticular activating system (ARAS), the ascending and descending cerebellar tracts, the descending corticospinal, corticofugal, and tectospinal tracts, the ascending spinothalamic and quintothalamic tracts and the lateral lemniscal system. Structures in the brain stem are packed so tightly such that a small lesion (hemorrhagic or ischemic) can result in major neuronal damage and subsequent disability. Common symptoms of brainstem strokes include: diplopia, perioral numbness, vertigo, dysarthria, depressed level of consciousness, unsteadiness of gait, headache (more common with ICH) and unilateral or bilateral sensorimotor dysfunction. Hearing loss as a result of ischemia or hemorrhage is observed uncommonly in patients with brainstem strokes unless the internal auditory artery, or, anterior inferior cerebellar artery are selectively involved.

In order to understand the underlying mechanisms of abnormal ABR in stroke it is important to know the sequelae of ischemia and hemorrhage on neural tissues and the microvascular anatomy of the central and peripheral auditory pathways. The brainstem is divided into the medulla oblongata, pons, mesencephalon and diencephalon. The rostral extension of the brainstem is the diencephalon which houses the thalamus, a major subcortical structure which integrates peripheral and central pathways (sensory and motor). The cochlear nerve enters the brain at the pontomedullary junction to synapse in the cochlear nuclei that are located at the same level. Central auditory structures which generate the ABR are predominantly supplied by the posterior cerebral circulation including the basilar artery (and its branches) and the posterior cerebral arteries (and their branches). The basilar artery (BA) is formed at the pontomedullary junction by the confluence of the two vertebral arteries (VA). The BA branches are divided into four groups (Caplan, 1988):

1. median branches, which supply the paramedian structure of the basis pontis and the pontine tegmentum;
2. short circumferential branches, which supply the intermediolateral portions of the pontine base and lateral tegmentum;
3. long lateral circumferential branches, which supply the lateral pontine tegmentum and midbrain tegmentum; and
4. long circumferential branches which include the:
   a. Anterior Inferior Cerebellar Artery (AICA) together with the circumferential branches supplies the lateral pontine tegmentum and the dorsal pontine structures. The internal auditory artery (IAA) branches off the AICA and supplies blood to the cochlea. In humans, the external diameter of the AICA ranges between 0.3 mm and 2.4 mm and between 0.1 mm and 0.25 mm for the IAA (mean of 1.3 mm, Sekiya and Møller, 1987b). These arteries float in the cerebrospinal fluid of the subarachnoid cisterns. Therefore, it is likely that slight compression or stretch of the AICA or IAA can decrease the luminal diameter, thus reducing cochlear perfusion.
   b. Superior Cerebellar Artery (SCA) supplies the upper portions of the cerebellar vermis and supe-

rior portions of the cerebellar hemispheres. The SCA also supplies the midbrain tegmentum.

The midline central auditory structures including the trapezoid body, the lateral lemniscus and the superior olivary nuclei in the caudal pons are supplied by the median and short circumferential branches of the basilar artery. Long lateral circumferential branches of the BA and the SCA supply the more rostral portions of the lateral lemniscus while the SCA supplies the inferior colliculus. The cochlear nucleus is supplied by the AICA while the cochlear nerve is supplied by the IAA.

The posterior cerebral arteries arise from the basilar artery at the pontomesencephalic junction. The PCA supplies the superior portions of the inferior colliculus and the medial geniculate body. The distal-most central auditory connections including the auditory association cortices, Heschl's gyrus and the auditory radiations crossing through the posterior limb of the internal capsule are supplied by branches of the middle cerebral artery which originate from the internal carotid artery.

From the above discussion, it becomes clear that the ABR can be affected at several levels in the brainstem and infarction of one arterial territory could lead (theoretically) to a specific abnormality (e.g., absent wave I when the IAA is occluded). However, ischemic strokes rarely affect only one neuropil island (unless one or two small penetrators are occluded). Furthermore, the edema which accompanies ischemia can lead to abnormalities in the ABR not expected from one particular infarcted zone. Distal Wallerian degeneration and diaschisis (e.g., electrochemically mediated neuronal dysfunction at a distance from the infarcted zone) are two other phenomena associated with strokes which could alter the ABR in a way not expected from involvement of the territory of the primary infarction.

Clinical Correlates of Ischemia and Hemorrhage-Ischemia of the CN VIII and Brainstem

Ischemia of CN VIII.   Ischemia of the nervous system can affect the nerve cell proper, the axon, or a combination of both. Often nerve cell ischemia leads to axonal damage secondarily, as part of the Wallerian degeneration phenomenon. Therefore, it is conceivable that ischemic injury of any one part of the auditory pathways (nerve cell, axon or both) can potentially alter the ABR.

Ischemic injury of neurons results first in a slowing of fast conducting, synchronized, large diameter fibers leaving slower conducting and less well-synchronized fibers to contribute to the evoked response. Ischemic injury to the central auditory pathways can be primary (e.g., brainstem stroke, discussed below) or could be related to tumors like AN, with compression of arterial structures like the IAA and subsequent ischemia. Sekiya and Møller (1987a,b) have shown in an elegant series of experiments that stretching of the auditory nerve (intraoperatively, or, due to large posterior fossa masses) may also stretch the IAA. As already mentioned, the IAA perfuses the VIIIth nerve and cochlea and has a luminal diameter of < 0.3 mm. Therefore, even modest stretch of this nerve can severely limit the effectiveness with which blood is delivered to these structures. The effect of prolonged ischemia in the cochlea is irreversible deafness. The effect of ischemia of the VIIIth nerve is associated with a slowing of VIIIth nerve conduction velocity, a decrease in the amplitude of the VIIIth nerve action potential (AP) and a broadening of the AP (e.g., due to a temporal dispersion of slower and faster conducting neurons (Sekiya and Møller, 1987a,b).

Brainstem Ischemic Stroke

Ischemic stroke is the prototype of ischemic neuronal injury. Ischemic stroke resulting from cessation of cerebral blood flow to a part of brain tissue causes a cascade of events which ultimately lead to cell death and axonal damage. Soon after cessation of blood flow to a neuron, the nerve cell swells secondary to failure of the Adenosine triphosphate (ATP)- dependent Na-K pump. Additionally, calcium enters the neuron in large amounts and causes the release of various neurotransmitters, including neuroexcitotoxins like aspartate and glutamate which act locally and at a distance by causing depolarization injury to neurons (Rothman and Olney, 1986; Albers et al., 1989). The initial phase of ischemia which leads to cytotoxic edema results in dysfunction of the nerve cell with failure of electrical conduction downstream along the terminal axon. Following this cytotoxic edema phase, a glial/endothelial injury process results in accumulation of extracellular fluid, the phenomenon of vasogenic edema. Vasogenic edema causes displacement and shift and in the severest cases causes brain herniation (Plum and Posner, 1980). Such a mass effect phenomenon results in: 1) compression injury of the white matter tracts in the nervous system with resultant focal and multifocal demyelination; 2) compression of parenchymal vascular structures with resultant ischemia of nerve tissues remote from the original injury site; 3) compression of vascular structures in the subarachnoid space (e.g., PCA or ACA) with resultant infarction in territories quite remote from the original site and frequently in totally different vascular territories than the initial ones (e.g., right anterior cerebral artery from left middle cerebral artery stroke, or, right posterior cerebral artery territory infarction from right middle cerebral artery stroke).

Furthermore, nerve dysfunction can occur remote from the infarction zone without actual ischemic injury. This phenomenon of diaschisis has been demonstrated by positron emission tomography (PET), single photon emission computerized tomography (SPECT), and Xenon-CT (Meyers et al., 1987). The diaschisis phenomenon is not well understood, nonetheless it can theoretically alter the ABR even when the structures commonly believed to generate and propagate the ABRs are not directly involved. Finally, ischemic nerve injury is not always purely ischemic. Some thrombotic strokes and a large number of embolic strokes are associated with some degree of hemorrhage (Hart and Easton, 1986). Hemorrhage can lead to neuronal and axonal injury, not only by compression, but also secondary to release of various toxic byproducts originating from the blood. These platelet-derived factors like serotonin, platelet-aggregating factors, and arachidonic acid byproducts not only directly injure tissues but also propagate the injury with accumulation of free radicals (Flamm et al., 1978; Hossman, 1988).

Studies by Branston et al. (1984) have demonstrated that cortical structures are more susceptible to the effect of ischemia than are subcortical structures. Post-synaptic components of cortical somatosensory

evoked potentials (SEP) disappear at flow levels of 15–18 ml/100gm/min whereas presynaptic components disappear at lower flow levels of 12 ml/100gm/min (Sato et al., 1984). Additionally, Branston et al. (1984) demonstrated that SEPs that emanate from the rostral medulla comparatively are more resistant to the effects of ischemia (SEP changes occur at flow levels of 10 ml/100gm/min). The changes in the SEP are initially latency prolongations. The latency prolongations were histologically correlated with cerebral edema and small effluxes of potassium into the extracellular space when the Na-K pump fails. As blood flow decreases further than this, latency prolongations become greater and finally the response disappears entirely. These phenomena were associated with infarction of brain tissue. It is reasonable to assume that the effects of brainstem ischemia are associated with the same pathophysiological processes for the auditory system as for the somesthetic system.

Brainstem Hemorrhage

Hemorrhagic injury resulting in abnormalities of the ABR is due to: 1) compression of neighboring structures by the expanding hematoma or by the associated vasogenic edema; 2) compression of neighboring vascular structures (intraparenchymal and subarachnoid) with resultant ischemic brain injury; and, 3) accumulation of toxic byproducts of blood with secondary direct damage from free radicals and neuroexcitotoxins, and indirect damage from vasoactive products which can potentiate edema, induce intraluminal vascular thrombosis, damage the blood brain barrier and induce vasospasm.

Abnormalities of the ABR in hemorrhagic strokes (ICH, SAH) are variable. Amplitude changes, prolonged latencies or both are encountered and a particular abnormality depends on the location of the hemorrhage, the extent of direct and indirect damage and the differential involvement of the nerve cell, the axon or both.

In light of the above discussion, the literature on ABRs in stroke is placed into perspective. It is generally believed that infarctions of the medulla and midbrain are not represented by abnormal ABRs since the ABR is generated by the CN VIII and pontine auditory pathways. Additionally, it is possible for the ABR to be normal in the presence of ventral pontine vascular injury. This occurs because the auditory tracts are more dorsal and lateral in the pontine tegmentum (Chiappa, 1991). This ventral pontine injury results in a phenomenon called "locked-in" syndrome wherein the patient is fully aware (because sensory pathways are intact) but unable to respond (because motor tracts contained in the ventral pons are damaged). A pure locked-in state does not result in abnormal ABR. However, many "impure" syndromes are reported where structures neighboring on the basis pontis (ventral pons) are variably involved. Such structures include the facial nucleus (causing facial paralysis), the abducens nucleus (causing horizontal gaze paralysis) in addition to the central auditory pathways (causing abnormal ABR). Thus, the patient with auditory pathway involvement in the brainstem presents with other obvious clinical signs like facial palsy or gaze palsy and the ABR is performed (by and large) for confirmatory purposes.

The earliest investigations of effects of cerebrovascular injury on the ABR were conducted by Starr and Hamilton (1976). The investigators reported their findings of a number of patients with neurological diseases, four of these patients had ischemic pontine infarcts and all of these patients demonstrated only wave I. Oh et al. (1981) reported their findings of 2 patients with lateral medullary infarctions. One had an expectedly normal ABR while the other had an abnormal ABR likely due to distant effects of the ischemic stroke as discussed above.

Several investigators have reported their findings evaluating patients with transient ischemic attacks (TIA). Ragazzoni et al. (1982) reported their findings after evaluating 26 patients with TIAs involving the vertebrobasilar system. The investigators found that over 50% of their subjects demonstrated ABR abnormalities (e.g., IWI wave I-wave V, and wave III-wave V aberrations) when tested one week following the TIA. Of 11 patients who demonstrated recovery following their TIA over 50% demonstrated persistent interwave interval aberrations. These findings were later verified by Factor and Dentinger (1987) who evaluated 8 patients with TIA in the vertebrobasilar territory. The investigators reported persistent ABR

abnormalities 1–16 days following the TIA even when the patients were normal by neurological examination. The authors subsequently followed 6 patients. The ABR was found to normalize in 83% of these cases. These findings attest to the sensitivity of the ABR to detect subclinical deficits in neuronal conduction. Lynn and Gilroy (1984) stated that the ABR is usually normal in patients with brainstem TIA unless the damage involves the auditory pathways. These findings of abnormal ABR in patients with vertebrobasilar TIA are in keeping with the concept that actual neuronal damage occurs when the cerebral blood flow to a specific brain region is interrupted by >30 minutes (Jafar and Crowell, 1987). In fact, the current definition of TIA (e.g., transient neurologic deficit lasting <24 hours—Whisnant et al. 1990) is only arbitrary. Recent natural history data (Levy, 1988; Werdelin and Juhler, 1988) showed that most TIAs last a few minutes and if magnetic resonance imaging studies are performed, a significant number of patients will have demonstrable infarctions when the classic TIA definition is used (Kinkel et al., 1986).

Stern et al. (1982) evaluated 35 patients with ischemic brainstem strokes. The authors found that the initial ABR was abnormal in 63% of the subjects. Of the sample of 35 patients, 54% had progression or remission and relapse of symptoms and the initial ABR was abnormal in 79% of these patients. Forty-four percent of those whose clinical course was stable had an abnormal initial ABR. Nine of 35 patients died and 89% of these patients demonstrated an initially abnormal ABR. The authors suggested that an abnormal initial ABR might help predicting the clinical course of brainstem strokes.

Faught and Oh (1985) recorded ABRs in 40 patients with brainstem infarction at various levels (e.g., medullary, pontine, mesencephalic). Additionally the patients were further subclassified as to whether the infarcts were medial or lateral, and whether they were unilateral or bilateral. Overall, the authors found abnormal ABRs in 70% of their cases. On closer inspection the authors failed to observe abnormal ABRs in patients with medullary infarcts. However, 87% of the patients with pontine infarcts, and 73% of the patients with mesencephalic infarcts demonstrated abnormal ABRs. Further, the authors usually found (e.g., 78% of the time) unilateral ABR abnormalities with stimulation presented to the side ipsilateral to the infarction. Unusual was the finding that patients with pontomedullary junction infarctions could have a normal wave I-wave V interwave interval, yet have an abnormal wave I-wave III interwave interval. The authors interpreted these findings as evidence that a laterally placed infarct could delay ipsilateral conduction, however, contralateral conduction (e.g., the dominant pathway) would be unimpeded. Finally, the authors reported that 90% of the patients with laterally placed infarctions demonstrated abnormal ABRs.

All previous reports have indicated that patients with evidence of pontine hemorrhage demonstrate ABR abnormalities (and grave neurological consequences). For example, Stockard and Rossiter (1977) reported their observation of one patient with pontine hemorrhage that destroyed the cochlear nuclei bilaterally. They also described three patients with hemorrhages in the pontine tegmentum. The former patient demonstrated only wave I and the latter patients demonstrated no ABR components after wave III. As described above for ischemic infarction it is possible to observe lateralized ABR abnormalities in the presence of lateralized hemorrhage. Oh et al. (1981) reported a patient with a right-sided hemorrhage at the junction of the pons and midbrain. The patient demonstrated a normal left ABR and an absent wave V following right sided stimulation.

It is noteworthy that in most if not all reports audiometric data were lacking for the patients who participated in these investigations. Additionally, laboratory upper limits of normal often were not presented. Thus, it is not possible to determine whether what one investigator called abnormal might have been within normal limits for another investigator. Also, it is not possible to determine whether hearing loss might have been responsible for what some investigators considered abnormal ABRs (e.g., delays in the absolute latencies of ABR components).

PATHOPHYSIOLOGY OF DEMYELINATION

Myelin is the protein coating of the axon in the central and peripheral nervous system. Myelination is needed for fast conduction of nerve impulses. Central nervous system myelin is generated by the oligodendroglial cells (Raine, 1984) whereas peripheral myelin is generated by Schwann cells (Raine, 1984). The mechanisms of electrical conduction through nerve terminals is described as saltatory because of the presence of the myelin sheath coating which is interrupted by the nodes of Ranvier. Saltatory conduction is a "skip-conduction" phenomenon whereby electrical charge transfer is accomplished between two subsequent nodes rather than through the axon itself. Such a process makes conduction much faster and more efficient. Therefore, it is conceivable that any injury process which involves the myelin-forming system including the oligodendroglia and Schwann cells can result in impaired conduction of electrical impulses.

The effect of demyelination is the thinning of the myelin sheath resulting in increased internodal capacitance and conductance and leakage of current through the internodal region. Additionally, current is lost to charge the capacitors along the neuronal membrane. Therefore, there is a possibility that current will dissipate before the next node of Ranvier is reached. This would result in a conduction block (conduction failure). If conduction along the affected neuron is maintained, the thinning of the myelin will result in slowed conduction in the affected neurons and temporal dispersion of electrical activity. Additionally, conduction may become continuous instead of saltatory (e.g., less efficient). Thus, it can be seen that the effects of demyelination also may vary.

Axonal demyelination and associated increases in membrane capacitance may serve to decrease the velocity of spike propagation (Waxman, 1982). The decrease in transmission velocity in remitting and relapsing multiple sclerosis (MS) also occurs as a function of the decrease in sodium channels (e.g., in comparison with the density found at the nodes of Ranvier) in the demyelinated internodal region (Ritchie and Bogart, 1977). Other investigators have suggested that abnormal neuronal transmission occurs because of synaptic blocking factors that may be present in the body as a complement-dependent factor that is associated with IgG (Schauf et al., 1981). Segmental demyelination of neurons is followed by remyelination. The remyelination is associated with a redistribution of sodium channels along the demyelinated axon. However, the internodal distance is shorter in the remyelinated axon. This results in less efficient (e.g., slower) neural conduction. Therefore, the ABR in demyelinating disease may take different forms. ABR components will be delayed in the instance where demyelination is mild and synchronization is intact. There will be reduced amplitude and delayed ABR components where demyelination is moderate and synchronization is affected. In this case the desynchronization of neural activity will lead to a loss of high amplitude, sharply peaked components. If demyelination is severe to the extent that the membrane potential requires long periods of time to equilibrate it is possible that a conduction block will occur. This will appear as absent ABR components at and above the level of damage.

Demyelinating disorders can be related to 1) loss of myelin after it has been formed, 2) production of defective myelin, or, 3) failure of myelin formation (Elias, 1987). A prototype example of failure of myelin generation might be MS (Elias, 1987). Examples of myelin destruction would be focal compressive lesions of the axons and antibodies generated against various components of myelin (e.g., myelin basic protein).

Clinical Correlates of Demyelination—Multiple Sclerosis

The prototype example of central myelin disorder is multiple sclerosis. MS is a chronic remitting and relapsing disorder of the CNS characterized by episodes of visual loss, paresthesias, unsteadiness, and various other motor dysfunctions. Those clinical manifestations are likely related to demyelination of the various pathways that subserve those neuronal functions. Accordingly, it is possible for an individual with MS to present with multiple abnormalities in nervous system function involving any level of the spinal cord, brainstem, midbrain, diencephalon, and cerebral cortex.

The reported rates of ABR abnormality in MS have ranged from 19 to 93% (Lynn et al., 1980; Stockard et al., 1977). The differences in the numbers of individuals demonstrating ABR abnormalities has occurred due to the unpredictable presentation of the disease. Additionally, it has been suggested that differences in evoked potential recording techniques (e.g., stimulus rate, polarity, intensity, electrode placement, statistical criteria for abnormality) might explain some of the

interstudy variability in reported rates of ABR abnormality in MS (Jacobson, Murray, and Deppe, 1987; Jacobson and Jacobson, 1991). Generally, higher rates of ABR abnormality have been associated with MS patients diagnosed with clinical evidence of brainstem involvement. For example, Robinson and Rudge (1977) demonstrated ABR abnormality in 79% of patients with definite evidence of brainstem lesions and in only 51% of those without clinical signs of brainstem disease. Rossiter (1977) observed ABR abnormalities in 93% of MS patients who demonstrated *definite* MS.

Several permutations of ABR abnormalities have been reported (Keith and Garza-Holquin, 1987; Keith and Jacobson, 1985), and, attempts have been made to subclassify these aberrant ABR waveforms (Jerger et al., 1986). It is generally believed that axonal demyelination and subsequent remyelination can result in several types of neural transmission deficits of graded severity. In its mildest form, the presence of demyelination is thought to cause neural transmission delays that are manifested as abnormal absolute and interpeak latencies. In these instances waveform integrity is preserved. As the disease becomes more severe, temporal dispersion of once synchronized neural activity combines with neural delays. The result is a reduction in ABR amplitude and waveform latency prolongations. Total conduction block occurs in the most severe instances. Examples of ABRs obtained from two patients with MS are shown in Figure 16.7A and B. It is interesting to note the variability in the ABR abnormalities for these two patients.

It is significant to note that a number of authors have commented upon the effects that certain stimulus and subject-related variables have on the ABR of patients with MS. Increasing body temperature in MS patients (e.g., hyperthermia) has been shown to exacerbate clinical symptoms and has been used in the past to assist in the diagnosis of this disease (Guthrie, 1951). Hyperthermia may be induced by having a patient seated in a warm bath or by placing a patient in a sauna or steam bath. Normal subjects demonstrate slightly faster (e.g., shorter latency) neuronal conduction when body core temperature increases. The opposite effect is observed in patients with MS. In fact, changes in the ABR were observed by increasing body temperature

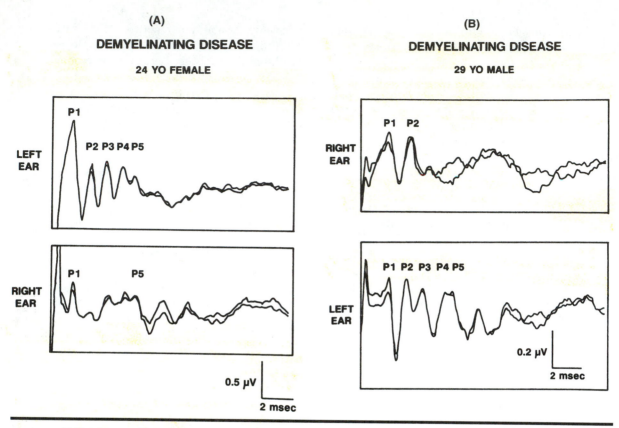

(A)

DEMYELINATING DISEASE

24 YO FEMALE

LEFT EAR

P1
P2 P3 P4 P5

RIGHT EAR

P1   P5

(B)

DEMYELINATING DISEASE

29 YO MALE

RIGHT EAR

P1   P2

LEFT EAR

P1 P2 P3 P4 P5

0.5 µV

2 msec

0.2 µV

2 msec

FIGURE 16.7.   Two patients with MS and ABR abnormalities. Please note that for the first patient (A) there was an abnormal wave V/wave I amplitude ratio with the click stimulus presented to the left ear. In the second instance (B) all components beyond wave 2 were absent. In each case the findings suggest that the ascending electrical activity has become desynchronized and/or blocked due to the demyelinating lesion.

by only .7 degrees C (Geraund et al., 1982). In the study by Geraund et al. (1982) there was no change noted in 10/18 cases whereas statistically significant increases in ABR latency were observed in the remaining 8 cases. The investigators suggested that the heating induced a slight increase in conduction velocity until a blocking point was reached after this point conduction velocity was reduced. These findings have been supported by some investigators (Phillips et al. 1983) and disputed by others (e.g., Rolak and Ashizawa, 1985). The reader is directed to Keith and Jacobson, Chapter 17, *Evoked Potentials in Multiple*

Sclerosis and Other Deymelinating Diseases, wherein the ABR in MS is discussed in great detail.

PATHOPHYSIOLOGY OF NEURODEGENERATION

CNS and peripheral nervous system (PNS) dysfunction can result from a host of disorders which damage the neuron, the axon, or both. Some of these disorders have a defined metabolic abnormality (e.g., Refsum disease), while others have unclear etiopathogenesis (e.g., olivopontocerebellar degeneration, OPCA). In addition, a specific inheritance mode has been found in some diseases (e.g., autosomal recessive inheritance in metachromatic leukodystrophy, MLD) but not in others (e.g., Parkinson's disease). A comprehensive discussion of the neurodegenerative/inherited metabolic disorders which have been reported to alter the ABR is beyond the scope of this chapter and the reader is referred to both Chiappa (1990) and Hall (1992) for this information.

Abnormalities of the ABR have been described in a vast array of neurodegenerative disorders ranging from Wilson's disease (Fujita et al., 1981) to OPCA. The abnormalities described vary depending upon the underlying degenerative process, the location of the damaged neuronal tissue and the extent of the damage. For example, diseases such as MLD which affect myelin in the nervous system and diffusely in the subcortical white matter and the brainstem can result in major amplitude reductions, latency delays, and dispersion of neuronal activity. On the other hand, Wilson's disease, or non-Wilsonian hepatolenticular degeneration, causes primarily nerve cell loss and axonal damage secondarily. Furthermore, such conditions affect the lower brainstem structures late in the course of the disease. Therefore, it would be expected that the Wilsonian and non-Wilsonian forms of CNS damage may result probably in dispersion and absence of the ABR waves before causing delays in conduction of the early waves.

Parkinson's disease (PD) and Huntington's disease (HD) rarely damage the wave-generating structures of the ABR. Although there are isolated reports of abnormal ABR in patients with PD and HD (Gawel et al., 1981), it is more likely that the mechanism of damage is indirect and secondary to dysfunction of various feedback loops in the CNS some of which are positive and excitatory while others are negative or inhibitory. Those loops function not only by altering the electrical medium of the ABR generating structures but also they participate in maintaining a "vital" environment for these structures. Therefore, damage to these loops can lead to secondary degeneration of the ABR generating structures and therein alterations of the ABR.

The more common of the neurodegenerative diseases that have been reported to affect the ABR are Friedreich's Ataxia and OPCA and these will be briefly described along with the reported ABR abnormalities.

Clinical Correlates of Neurodegeneration—Friedreich's Ataxia (FA)

FA is an autosomal recessive inherited disease that is typified by progressive ataxia. The disease usually becomes apparent before puberty and is slightly more prevalent in males. The mean life expectancy from diagnosis is 24 years (Harding, 1984). The initial presenting complaint is difficulty with ambulation. On examination the patient may be found to be ataxic only in the lower extremities. With age the patient demonstrates a progressive ataxia and dysarthria that evolves into clumsiness and staggering. It is not uncommon to observe gaze nystagmus in these patients. It is believed that the neurologic damage is limited to the brainstem and cerebellar parenchyma. However, the results of vestibular function studies (Baloh et al., 1975; Monday et al., 1978) and auditory evoked potential studies suggest that damage to both systems in FA occurs at the level of the cell body of the primary afferent neuron, or, in the neuron itself (see below).

Sensory evoked potential studies in patients with FA are almost always abnormal whereas motor evoked response studies are usually normal. For instance, sensory nerve conduction measures in electromyography generally are abnormally slowed in the upper extremities and often cannot be measured in the lower extremities. A number of investigations have been conducted evaluating the ABR in patients with FA. The most consistent general finding has been either an absent response in light of relatively good pure tone hearing sensitivity (Satya-Murti et al. 1980; Rossi et al., 1982; Cassandro et al., 1984), or, the presence of wave I and absent later responses (Rossi et al., 1982; Jabbari et al., 1983). Spoendlin (1974) evaluated the temporal bones of two patients with FA. The investigator noted that these patients demonstrated degeneration of spiral ganglion cells and primary CN VIII afferents. The cochlear end organ was normal for these subjects. In this regard, it is interesting that Satya-Murti et al. (1980) and Rossi et al. (1982) conducted extensive audiometric examinations on patients with FA and showed that patients with FA performed well on conventional audiometry but showed poor performance on "sensitized" speech tests (e.g., synthetic sentence identification with ipsilateral competing message, SSI-ICM). These findings have suggested that the neural pathology observed in FA involves only cell bodies or first order afferents. The primary disorder would be neuronal loss which would result in low amplitude or absent evoked potentials. However, other investigators have reported either delayed wave I-wave V interwave intervals (Hecox et al., 1981; Rossini and Cracco, 1987), or, normal ABRs in patients with FA (Nuwer et al., 1983; Cassandro et al., 1984). The former finding would suggest that the primary effect is one of demyelination and not cell loss. The latter finding attests to the variability of presentation of most neurologic diseases.

Clinical Correlates of Neurodegeneration— Olivopontocerebellar Atrophy (OPCA)

Patients with progressive ataxia may have degenerative changes at the level of the olivary nuclei, pons, and cerebellum. These disease entities have been grouped into what have been termed olivopontocerebellar atrophies. Konigsmark and Weiner (1970) have developed a comprehensive classification system for these disorders (Harding, 1984). This system is based upon whether the disease is inherited and whether it is inherited in a dominant or recessive manner. Accordingly, the OPCAs have been subtyped. For example, Type I (Menzel) is autosomal dominant and is typified by gait and limb ataxia, head and limb tremor, dysarthria, choreiform movements and impaired vibration, and position sense. Pathologically, atrophy of the cerebellar folia, dentate nuclei, inferior olives, substantia nigra, spinal cord and long tracts are observed. Type II (Fickler-Winkler) OPCA is autosomal recessive and is typified by gait and limb ataxia, and limb tremor. Sensation is normal in Type II OPCA and there are no choreiform movements. Atrophy of the cerebellar folia, inferior olives, substantia nigra, and spinal cord are observed in Type II OPCA (Harding, 1984).

Patients with OPCA may have normal or abnormal ABRs. Gilroy and Lynn (1978) evaluated three patients with OPCA and reported abnormal wave I-wave III interpeak intervals. Other investigators including Nuwer et al. (1982), Rossini and Cracco (1987) and Hammond and Wilder (1983) who evaluated small numbers of patients (N < 6) all reported abnormalities ranging from absent responses (Rossini and Cracco, 1987) to abnormalities in the wave V/wave I amplitude ratio (Nuwer et al., 1982) to wave I-wave V interwave interval delays (Nuwer et al., 1982; Hammond and Wilder, 1983; Rossini and Cracco, 1987). Alternately both Fujita et al. (1981, N=20) and Chokroverty et al. (1984, N=6) have reported normal ABRs in the presence of OPCA.

SUMMARY

What may be gathered from this discussion is that each of the effects of compression, traction, ischemia, hemorrhage, demyelination, and neurodegeneration, can result in the same types of changes in the ABR waveform. Each type of injury can result in identical changes in the latency and amplitude of the ABR, and therefore, ABR latency and amplitude abnormalities are not indicative of any specific disease process. Thus, although the underlying neuropathologic processes may differ, the ABR abnormalities may be quite similar.

REFERENCES

Adams, R.D. and Lyon, G. (1982). *Neurology of hereditary metabolic diseases of children*, pp. 384–408. New York: McGraw-Hill.

Albers, G.W., Goldberg, M.P., and Choi, D.W. (1989). N-methyl-D-aspartate antagonists: Read for clinical trials in brain ischemia. *Annals of Neurology, 25*, 398–403.

Arslan, E., Prosser, S., and Rosognoli, M. (1988). The behaviour of wave V latency in cochlear hearing loss. *Acta Otolaryngologica, 105*, 467–472.

Baldwin, R.L. and Lemaster, K. (1989). Neurofibromatosis-2 and bilateral acoustic neuromas: Distinctions from neurofibromatosis-1 (von Recklinghausen's disease). *American Journal of Otology, 10*, 439–442.

Ballance, C. (1907). *Some points in the surgery of the brain and its membranes*. London: Macmillan & Co.

Baloh, R.W., Konrad, H.R., and Honrubia, V. (1975). Vestibulo-ocular function in patients with cerebellar atrophy. *Neurology, 25*, 160–168.

Bauch, C.D. and Olsen, W.O. (1989). Wave V interaural latency differences as a function of asymmetry in 2000–4000 Hz hearing sensitivity. *American Journal of Otology, 10(5)*, 389–392.

Beck, H.J., Beatty, C.W., Harner, S.H., and Ilstrup, D.M. (1986). Acoustic neuromas with normal pure tone hearing levels. *Otolaryngology—Head and Neck Surgery, 94*, 96–103.

Bederson, J.B., von Ammon, K., Wichmann, W.W., and Yasargil, M.G. (1991). Conservative treatment of patients with acoustic tumors. *Neurosurgery, 28*, 646–651.

Bendat, J.S. and Piersol, A.G. (1986). Random data. *Analysis and Measurement Procedures*. New York: John Wiley and Sons.

Bockenheimer, S., Schmidt, C.L., and Zöllner, C. (1984). Neuro-otological findings in patients with small acoustic neuromas. *Archives of Otorhinolaryngology, 249*, 31–39.

Boston, J.R. and Ainslie, P.J. (1980). Effects of analog and digital filtering on brainstem auditory evoked potentials. *Electroencephalography and Clinical Neurophysiology, 48*, 361–364.

Brackman D. (1984). A review of acoustic tumors: 1979–1982. *American Journal of Otology, 5*, 233–244.

Brackmann, D.E. and Forquer, B.D. (1983). Evaluation of the auditory system: An update. *Annals of Otology, Rhinology, and Laryngology, 92*, 651–656.

Brackmann, D.E. and Bartels, L.J. (1980). Rare tumors of the cerebellopontine angle. *Otolaryngology—Head and Neck Surgery, 88*, 555–559.

Bredberg, G. (1981). Innervation of the auditory system. *Scandinavian Audiology, (Suppl.) 13*, 1–10.

Caplan, L.R. (1988). Vertebrobasilar system syndromes. In Toole, J.F. (ed.), *Handbook of clinical neurology, vascular diseases*, part I, 53, pp. 371–408. New York: Elsevier.

Carey, J.C., Baty, B.J., Johnson, J.P., Morrison, T., Skolnick, M., and Kivlin, J. (1986). The genetic aspects of neurofibromatosis. In A.E. Rubenstein, R.P. Bunge, and D.E. Housman (eds.), Neurofibromatosis, *Annals of New York Academy of Sciences, 486*, 45–46.

Cassandro, E., Mosca, F., Sequino, L., DeFalco, F.A., and Campanella, G. (1986). Otoneurological findings in Friedreich's ataxia and other inherited neuropathies. *Audiology, 25*, 84–91.

Chiappa, K.H. (1990). *Evoked potentials in clinical medicine*, pp. 223–305. New York: Raven.

Chokroverty, S., Duvoisin, R.C., Lepore, F., and Nicklas, W. (1984). Brainstem auditory and pattern-reversal visual evoked potential study in olivopontocerebellar degeneration. In R.H. Nodar and C. Barber (eds.), *Evoked potentials II: The second international evoked potentials symposium*, pp. 637–642. Butterworth: Boston, MA.

Coats, A.C. (1983). Instrumentation. In Moore, E.J.(ed.), *Bases of auditory brain-stem evoked responses*, pp. 197–220. New York: Grune & Stratton.

Cushing, H. (1917). *Tumors of the nervus acousticus and the syndrome of the cerebellopontius angle*. Philadelphia, PA: W.B. Saunders Co.

Cushing, H. (1932). *Intracranial tumors*. Springfield, IL: Charles C. Thomas.

Cushing, H. (1963). *Tumors of the Nervus Acousticus and the syndrome of the cerebellopontine angle*. New York: Hafner Publishing.

Dandy, W.E. (1925). An operation for the total removal of cerebellopontine (acoustic) tumors. *Surgical Gynecology and Obstetrics, 41*, 129–148.

Daniels, D.L., Millen, S.J., Meyer, G.A., Pojunas, K.W., Kilgore, D.P., Shaffer, K.A., Williams, A.L., and Haughton, V.M. (1987). MR detection of tumor in the internal auditory canal. *American Journal of Neuroradiology, 8*, 249–252.

Dauman, R., Aran, J.M., and Portman, M. (1987). Stapedius reflex and cerebellopontine tumors. *Clinical Otolaryngology, 12*, 119–123.

Davis, R.L. and Robertson, D.M. (eds.) (1991). *Textbook on neuropathology*, 2nd ed. Baltimore, MD: Williams & Wilkins.

Doyle, D.J. and Hyde, M.L. (1981). Analogue and digital filtering of auditory brainstem responses. *Scandinavian Audiology, 10*, 81–89.

Eggermont, J. J., Don, M., and Brackmann, D. E. (1980). Electrocochleography and auditory brainstem electric responses in patients with pontine angle tumors. *Annals of Otology, Rhinology and Laryngology, 89 (supp 75)*, 1–19.

Elberling, C. and Parbo, J. (1987). Reference data for ABRs in retrocochlear diagnosis. *Scandinavian Audiology, 16*, 49–55.

Ellis, P.D.M. and Wright, J.L.M. (1974). Acoustic neuroma. A plea for early diagnosis and treatment. *Journal of Laryngology and Otology, 88*, 1095–1100.

Factor, S.A. and Dentinger, M.P. (1987). Early brain-stem auditory evoked responses in vertebrobasilar transient ischemic attacks. *Archives of Neurology, 44*, 544–547.

Faught, E. and Oh, S. J. (1985). Brainstem auditory evoked responses in brainstem infarction. *Stroke, 16*, 701–705.

Fisch, U. and Wegmuller, A. (1974). Early diagnosis of acoustic neuromas. *ORL, 36*, 129–140.

Flamm, E.S., Demopoulos, H.B., Seligman, M.L., Poser,

R.G., and Ransohoff, J. (1978). Free radicals in cerebral ischemia. *Stroke, 9,* 445–447.

Fujita, M., Hosoki, M., and Miyazaki, M. (1981). Brainstem auditory evoked responses in spinocerebellar degeneration and Wilson disease. *Annals Neurology, 9,* 42–47.

Gawel, M.J., Das, P., Vincent, S., and Rose, F.C. (1981). Visual and auditory evoked responses in patients with Parkinson's disease. *Journal of Neurology, Neurosurgery, and Psychiatry, 44,* 227–232.

Gilman, S., Bloedel, J.R., and Lechterberg, R. (1982). *Disorders of the cerebellum,* pp. 231–262. Philadelphia, PA: F.A. Davis.

Gilroy, J. and Lynn, G.E. (1978). Computerized tomography and auditory-evoked potentials: Use in the diagnosis of olivopontocerebellar degeneration. *Archives of Neurology, 35,* 143–147.

Gorga, M.P., Worthington, D.W., Reiland, J.K., Beauchaine, K.A., and Goldgar, D.E. (1985). Some comparisons between auditory brainstem response threshold, latencies, and the pure-tone audiogram. *Ear and Hearing, 6,* 105–112.

Grabel, J.C., Zappulla, R.A., Ryder, J., Wang, W., and Malis, L.I. (1991). Brain-stem auditory evoked responses in 56 patients with acoustic neuroma. *Journal of Neurosurgery, 74,* 749–753.

Hall, J.W. (1992). *Handbook of auditory evoked responses,* pp. 419–472. Boston, MA: Allyn and Bacon.

Hall, J.W., Morgan, S., Mackey-Hargadine, J., Aguilar, E., and Jahrsdoerfer, R. (1984). Neuro-otologic application of simultaneous multi-channel auditory evoked response recordings. *Laryngoscope, 94,* 883–889.

Hammond, E.J. and Wilder, B.J. (1983). Evoked potentials in olivopontocerebellar atrophy. *Archives Neurology, 40,* 366–369.

Harding, A.E. (1984).*The hereditary ataxias and related disorders,* pp. 57–96. New York: Churchill Livingstone.

Harris, F.J. (1978). On the use of windows for harmonic analysis with the discrete Fourier transform. *Proceedings of the IEEE, 66,* 51–83.

Hart, R.G. and Easton, J.D. (1986). Hemorrhagic infarcts. *Stroke, 17,* 586–589.

Hecox, K., Cone, B., and Blaw, M.E. (1981). Brainstem auditory evoked responses in the diagnosis of pediatric neurological disease. *Neurology, 31,* 832–840.

Hecox, K., Squires, N., and Galambos, R. (1976). Brainstem evoked responses in man: I. Effect of stimulus rise-fall time and duration. *Journal of the Acoustical Society of America, 60,* 1187–1192.

Hedley, A.J., Jerger, J.F., and Stach, B.A. (1987). Normal audiometric findings revisited. (Abstract). *ASHA, 29,* 125.

Hendrix, R.A., DeDio, R.M., and Sclafani, A.P. (1990). The use of diagnostic testing in asymmetric sensorineural hearing loss. *Otolaryngology—Head and Neck Surgery, 103,* 593–598.

Hirsch, A. and Anderson, H. (1980). Audiologic test results in 96 patients with tumors affecting the eighth nerve. *Acta Otolaryngologica (Suppl), 369,* 1–26.

Hitselberger, W.E. and House, W.F. (1966). Acoustic neuroma diagnosis. *Archives of Otolaryngology, 83,* 219–221.

Hossmann, K.A. (1988). Pathophysiology of cerebral infarction. In Toole, J.F. (ed.), *Handbook of clinical neurology, Vascular Diseases,* pp. 107–153. New York: Elsevier.

House, W.F. and Hitselberger, W.E. (1986). The neuro-otologist's view of the surgical management of acoustic neuromas. *Clinical Neurosurgery, 32,* 214–222.

House, W.F. (1961). Report of cases, Monograph. Transtemporal bone microsurgical removal of acoustic neruomas, *Archives of Otolaryngology, 80,* 617.

House, W.F. (1964). Transtemporal bone microsurgical removal of acoustic neuromas. *Archives of Otolaryngology, 80,* 599–756.

House, W.F. (1985). A history of acoustic tumor surgery. In House, W.F. and Luetje, C.M., (eds.), *Acoustic Tumors. Vol. 1: Diagnosis,* pp. 1–32. Los Angeles, CA: House Ear Institute.

Hughes, J.R. and Fino, J.J. (1980). Usefulness of piezoelectric earphones in recording the brain stem auditory evoked potentials: A new early deflection. *Electroencephalography and Clinical Neurophysiology, 48,* 357–360.

Hughes, J.R., Fino, J.J., and Gagnon, L. (1981). The importance of phase of stimulus and the reference recording electrode in brain stem auditory evoked potentials. *Electroencephalography and Clinical Neurophysiology, 51,* 611–623.

Hyde, M.L. and Blair, R.L. (1981). The auditory brainstem response in neuro-otology: Perspectives and problems. *Journal of Otolaryngology, 10,* 117–125.

Hyde, M.L. (1985). The effect of cochlear lesions on the ABR. In Jacobson, J.T. (ed.), *The auditory brainstem response,* pp. 133–146. San Diego, CA: College-Hill.

Hyde, M.L., Davidson, M.J., and Alberti, P.W. (1991). Auditory test strategy. In Jacobson, J.T. and Northern, J.L. (eds.), *Diagnostic Audiology,* pp. 295–322. Austin, TX: Pro-ed.

Jabbari, B., Schwartz, D.M., MacNeil, D.M., and Coker, S.B. (1983). Early abnormalities of brainstem auditory evoked potentials in Friedreich's ataxia: Evidence of primary brainstem dysfunction. *Neurology, 33,* 1071–1074.

Jacobson, J. and Jacobson, G.P. (1990). Auditory brainstem responses in multiple sclerosis. *Seminars in Hearing, 11,* 248–264.

Jacobson, J. and Reams, C. (1991). Neurotologic disease in four patients with normal audiometric findings. *American Journal of Otology, 12,* 114–118.

Jacobson, J.T., Murray, T.J., and Deppe, U. (1987). The effects of ABR stimulus repetition rate in multiple sclerosis. *Ear and Hearing, 8,* 115–120.

Jacobson, G.P. and Newman, C.W. (1989). Absence of rate-dependent BAEP P5 latency changes in patients with definite multiple sclerosis: Possible physiological mechanisms. *Electroencephalography and Clinical Neurophysiology, 74,* 19–23.

Jafar, J.J. and Crowell, R.M. (1987). Focal ischemic thresholds. In Wood, J.H. (ed.), *Cerebral blood flow-physiologic and clinical aspects,* pp. 449–457. New York: McGraw-Hill.

Jasper, H.H. (1958). The ten twenty electrode system of the international federation. *Electroencephalography and Clinical Neurophysiology, 10,* 371–375.

Jerger, J., Neeley, G., and Jerger, S. (1980). Speech, impedance and auditory brainstem response audiometry in brainstem tumors. Importance of a multiple test strategy. *Archives of Otolaryngology, 106,* 218–223.

Jerger, J. and Jordan, C. (1980). Normal audiometric findings. *American Journal of Otology, 1,* 157–159.

Jerger, J. and Johnson, K. (1988). Interactions of age, gender, and sensorineural hearing loss on ABR latency. *Ear and Hearing, 9,* 168–176.

Johnson, E.V. (1977). Auditory test results 500 cases of acoustic neuroma. *Archives of Otolarynology, 103,* 153–158.

Johnson, E.V. (1979). Results of auditory tests in acoustic neuroma patients. In House, W.F. and Luetje, C.M. (eds.), *Acoustic tumors: Vol. 1. Diagnosis,* pp. 209–224. Baltimore, MD: University Park Press.

Johnson, E.W. and House, W.F. (1964). Auditory findings in 53 cases of acoustic neuromas. *Archives of Otolaryngology, 80,* 667–677.

Josey, A.F. (1987). Audiologic manifestations of tumors of the VIIth nerve. *Ear and Hearing (Suppl.), 8,* 195–215.

Josey, A.F., Glasscock, M.E., and Musiek, F.E. (1988). Correlation of ABR and medical imaging in patients with cerebellopontine angle tumors. *American Journal of Otology, 9,* 12–16.

Josey, A.F., Jackson, C.G., and Glasscock, M.E. (1980). Brainstem evoked response audiometry in confirmed

eighth nerve tumors. *American Journal of Otolaryngology, 1,* 285–289.

Keith, R.W. and Jacobson, J.T. (1985). Physiological responses in multiple sclerosis and other demyelinating diseases. In Jacobson, J.T. (ed.), *The auditory brainstem response,* pp. 219–235. San Diego, CA: College-Hill.

Keith, R.W. and Garza-Holquin, Y. (1987). Acoustic reflex dynamics and auditory brainstem responses in multiple sclerosis. *American Journal of Otology, 8,* 406–413.

Keith, W.J. and Greville, K.A. (1987). Effects of audiometric configuration on the auditory brain stem response. *Ear and Hearing, 8,* 49–55.

Killion, M. (1984). New insert earphones for audiometry. *Hearing Instruments, 35,* 28–29.

Kimura, J. (1984). *Electrodiagnosis in diseases of nerve and muscle: Principles and practice,* pp. 59–81. Philadelphia, PA: F.A. Davis.

Kinkel, P.R., Kinkel, W.R., and Jacobs, L. (1986). Nuclear magnetic resonance imaging in patients with stroke. *Seminars in Neurology, 6,* 43–52.

Konigsmark, B.W. and Weiner, L.P. (1970). The olivopontocerebellar atrophies: A review. *Medicine, 49,* 227, 1970.

Legatt, A.D., Pedley, T.A., Emerson, R.G., Stein, B.M., and Abramson, M. (1988). Normal brain-stem auditory evoked potentials with abnormal latency-intensity studies in patients with acoustic neuromas. *Archives of Neurology, 45,* 1326–1330.

Levy, D.E. (1988). How transient are transient ischemic attacks? *Neurology, 38,* 674–677.

Lorente de No, R. (1933). Anatomy of the eighth nerve. I. The central projection of the nerve endings of the internal ear. *Laryngoscope, 43,* 1–8.

Mathew, G.D., Facer, G.W., Suh, K.W., et al. (1978). Symptoms, findings, and methods of diagnosis in patients with acoustic neuroma. *Laryngoscope, 88,* 1893–1903.

McGee, T. and Clemis, J. (1982). Effects of conductive hearing loss on the auditory brainstem response. *Annals of Otology, Rhinology, and Laryngology, 91,* 304–309.

Meyer, J.S., Hata, T., and Imai, A. (1987). Clinical and experimental studies of diaschisis. In Wood, J.H. (ed.), *Cerebral blood flow—physiologic and clinical aspects,* pp. 481–502. New York: McGraw-Hill.

Mikhael, M.A., Wolff, A.P., and Ciric, I.S. (1987). Current concepts in neuroradiological diagnosis of acoustic neuromas. *Laryngoscope, 97,* 471–476.

Mohr, J.P., Caplan, L.R., Lelski, J.W., Goldstein, R.J., Duncan, G.W., Kistler, J.P., Pessin, M.S., and Bleich, H.L. (1978). The Harvard cooperative stroke registry: A prospective registry. *Neurology, 28,* 754–762.

Monday, L.A., Lemieux, B., St-Vincent, H., and Barbeau, A. (1978). Clinical and electronystagmographic findings in Friedreich's ataxia. *Canadian Journal of Neurological Science, 5*, 71–73.

Musiek, F.E. and Gollegly, K.M. (1985). ABR in eighth nerve and low brainstem lesions. In Jacobson, J., (ed.), *The auditory brainstem response*, pp. 181–202. San Diego, CA: College Hill Press.

Musiek, F.E., Kibble-Michal, K., and Geurkink, N.A. (1986). ABR results in patients with posterior fossa tumors and normal pure tone hearing. *Otolaryngology—Head Neck Surgery, 94*, 568–573.

Møller, A.R. and Jannetta, P.J. (1981). Compound action potentials recorded intracranially from the auditory nerve in man. *Journal of Experimental Neurology, 74*, 862–874.

Møller, A.R. and Jannetta, P.J. (1983). Monitoring auditory functions during cranial microvascular decompression operations by direct recording from the eighth nerve. *Journal of Neurosurgery, 59*, 493–499.

Møller, A.R. and Jannetta, P.J. (1984). Monitoring auditory nerve potentials during operations in the cerebellopontine angle. *Otolaryngology—Head and Neck Surgery, 92*, 434–439.

Møller, A.R. and Sekiya, T. (1988). Injuries to the auditory nerve: A study in monkeys. *Electroencephalography and Clinical Neurophysiology, 70*, 248–255.

National Institutes of Health (NIH). (1987). Neurofibromatosis. *National Institutes of Health Consensus Development Conference Statement, 6*, No. 12.

National Institutes of Health (NIH). (1988). Conference of neurofibromatosis. *Archives of Neurology, 45*, 575–578.

Nuwer, M. R., Perlman, S.L., Packwood, J.W., and Kark, R.A.P. (1982). Evoked potential abnormalities in the various inherited ataxias. *Annals of Neurology, 13*, 20–27.

Oh, S.J., Kuba, T., Soyer, A., Choi, I.S., Bonikowski, F.P., and Vitek, J. (1981). Lateralization of brainstem lesions by brainstem auditory evoked potentials. *Neurology, 31*, 14–18.

Okazaki, H. (1983). *Fundamentals of Neuropathology.* New York: Igaku-Shoin.

Olsen, W.O. (1991). Special auditory tests: A historical perspective. In Jacobson, J. and Northern, J. (eds.), *Diagnostic audiology*, pp. 19–52. Austin, TX: Pro-ed.

Osen, K.K. (1969). The intrinsic organization of the cochlear nuclei in the cat. *Acta Otolaryngologica, 657*, 352–359.

Palva, T., Jauhiainen, C., Sjoblom, G., et al. (1978). Diagnosis and surgery of acoustic tumors. *Acta Otolaryngologica, 86*, 233–240.

Parker, D.J. (1981). Dependence of the auditory brain stem response on electrode location. *Archives of Otolaryngology, 107*.

Pensak, M.L., Keith, R.W., Dignan, P.S., Stowens, D.W. Towin, R.B., and Kathamna, B. (1989). Neuroaudiologic abnormalities in patients with type 1 neurofibromatosis. *Laryngoscope, 99*, 702–706.

Picton, T.W., Linden, R.D., Hamel, G., and Maru, J. (1983). Aspects of averaging. *Seminars in Hearing, 4*, 327–342.

Picton, T.W., Stapells, D.R., and Campbell, K.B. (1981). Auditory evoked potentials from the human cochlea and brainstem. *Journal of Otolaryngology, 10*, 1–14.

Plum, F. and Posner, J.B. (1980) *The diagnosis of stupor and coma*, pp. 87–151. Philadelphia, PA: F.A. Davis.

Powell, T.P. and Cowan, W.M. (1962). An experimental study of the projection of the cochlea. *Journal of Anatomy, 96*, 269–284.

Prosser, S. and Arslan, E. (1987). Prediction of auditory brainstem wave V latency as a diagnostic tool of sensorineural hearing loss. *Audiology, 26*, 179–187.

Pulec, J., House, W.F., and Huges, R.I. (1964). Vestibular involvement and testing in acoustic neuromas. *Archives of Otolaryngology, 80*, 677–681.

Ragazzoni, A., Amatini, A., Rossi, L., Pagnini, P., Arnetoli, G., Marini, P., Nencioni, C., Versari, A., and Zappoli, R. (1982). Brainstem auditory evoked potentials and vertebral-basilar reversible ischemic attacks. In Courjon, J., Mauguiere, F., and Revol, M. (eds.), *Clinical applications of evoked potentials in neurology*, pp. 187–194. New York: Raven Press.

Raine, C.S. (1984). Morphology of myelin. In Morrell, P. (ed.), *Myelin*, pp. 1–50. New York: Plenum.

Riccardi, V.M. and Eichner, J.E, (1986). *Neurofibromatosis phenotype, natural history, and pathogenesis.* Baltimore, MD: Johns Hopkins University Press.

Rose, J.E., Greenwood, D.D., Goldberg, J.M., and Hind, J.E. (1963). Some discharge characteristics of single neurons in the inferior colliculus of the cat. *Journal of Neurophysiology, 26*, 294–320.

Rossi, L., Amantini, A., Bindi, A., de Scisciolo, G., Pagnini, P., Ronchi, O., Papini, M,. Pasquinelli, A., and Bigozzi, M. (1982). Brainstem auditory evoked potentials and electronystagmography findings in Friedreich's ataxia. In Chiarenza, G.A. and Papakostopoulos, D. (eds.), *Clinical application of cerebral evoked potentials in pediatric medicine*, pp. 385–396. Amsterdam: Excerpta Medica.

Rossini, P.M. and Cracco, J.B. (1987). Somatosensory and brainstem auditory evoked potentials in neurodegenerative system disorders. *European Neurology, 26*, 176–188.

Rothman, S.M. and Olney, J.W. (1986). Glutamate and the pathophysiology of hypoxic-ischemic brain damage. *Annals of Neurology, 19*, 105–111.

Ruth, R.A., Hildebrand, D.L., and Cantrell, R.W. (1982). A study of methods used to enhance wave I in the auditory brain stem response. *Otolaryngology—Head and Neck Surgery, 90*, 635–640.

Sataloff, R.T., Davies, B., and Myers, D.L. (1985). Acoustic neuromas presenting as sudden deafness. *American Journal of Otology, 6*, 349–352.

Satya-Murti, S., Cacace, A., and Hanson, P. (1980). Auditory dysfunction in Friedreich's ataxia: Result of spiral ganglion degeneration. *Neurology, 30*, 1047–1053.

Schauf, C.L., Ptacek, T.L., Davis, F.A., and Rooney, M.W. (1981). Physiological basis for neuroelectric blocking activity in multiple sclerosis. *Neurology, 31*, 1337–1340.

Schunknecht, H.F. (1974). *Pathology of the Ear*. Cambridge, MA: Harvard University Press.

Schwartz, D. (1987). Neurodiangotic audiology: Contemporary perspectives. *Ear and Hearing, 8*, 43–48.

Sekiya, T. and Møller, A.R. (1987*a*). Cochlear nerve injuries caused by cerebellopontine angle manipulations: An electrophysiological and morphological study in dogs. *Journal of Neurosurgery, 67*, 244–249.

Sekiya, T. and Møller, A.R. (1987*b*). Avulsion-rupture of the internal auditory artery during operations in the cerebellopontine angle: A study in monkeys. *Neurosurgery, 21*, 631–637.

Selters, W.A. and Brackman, D.E. (1979). Brainstem electric response audiometry in acoustic tumor detection. In House, W. and Leutje, C., (eds.), *Acoustic tumors, vol I: diagnosis*, pp. 225–235. Baltimore, MD: University Park Press.

Selters, W.A. and Brackmann, D.E. (1977). Acoustic tumor detection with brain stem electric response audiometry. *Archives of Otolaryngology, 103*, 181–187.

Singh, K.P., Smyth, G.D.L., and Gordon, D.S. (1978). The diagnosis of acoustic neuroma, A retrospective study. *Journal of Laryngology and Otology, 92*, 1–7.

Spoendlin, H. (1974). Optic and cochleovestibular degenerations in the hereditary ataxias. II. Temporal bone pathology in 2 cases of Friedreich's ataxia with vestibulo-cochlear disorders. *Brain, 97*, 41–48.

Stapells, D.R. and Picton, T.W. (1981). Technical aspects of brainstem evoked potential audiometry using tones. *Ear and Hearing, 2*, 20–29.

Starr, A. and Hamilton, A.E. (1976). Correlation between confirmed sites of neurologic lesions and abnormalities of far-field auditory brainstem responses. *Electroencephalography and Clinical Neurophysiology, 41*, 595–608.

Stern, B.J., Krumholz, A., Weiss, H.D., Goldstein, P., and Harris, K.C. (1982). Evaluation of brainstem stroke using brainstem auditory evoked responses. *Stroke, 13*, 705–711.

Stockard, J.J. and Rossiter, V.S. (1977). Clinical and pathologic correlates of brain stem auditory response abnormalities. *Neurology, 27*, 316–325.

Stypulkowski, P. and Staller, S. (1987). Clinical evaluation of a new ECochG recording electrode. *Ear and Hearing, 8*, 304–310.

Suzuki, T. and Horiuchi, K. (1981). Rise time of pure-tone stimuli in brain stem response audiometry. *Audiology, 20*, 101–112.

Telian, S.A. and Kileny, P.R. (1988). Pitfalls in neurotologic diagnosis. *Ear and Hearing, 9*, 86–91.

Telian, S.A., Kileny, P.R., Niparko, J.K., Kemink, J.L., and Graham, M.D. (1989). Normal auditory brainstem response in patients with acoustic neuroma. *Laryngoscope, 99*, 10–14.

Telian, S.A. and Kileny, P.R. (1989). Usefulness of 1000 Hz toneburst-evoked responses in the diagnosis of acoustic neuroma. *Otolaryngology—Head and Neck Surgery, 101*, 466–471.

Thomsen, J. and Toss, M. (1988). Diagnostic strategies in search for acoustic neuromas. *Acta Otolaryngolgica (Suppl.) 452*, 16–25.

Tos, M. and Thomsen, J. (1984). Epidemiology of acoustic neuromas. *Journal of Laryngology and Otology, 98*, 685–692.

Turner, R.G., Shepard. N.T., and Frazier, G.J. (1984). Clinical performance of audiological and related diagnostic tests. *Ear and Hearing, 5*, 187–194.

van der Drift, J.F., Brocaar, P., and van Zanten, G.A. (1988). Brainstem response audiometry: I. Its use in distinguishing between conductive and cochlear hearing loss. *Audiology, 27*, 260–270.

von Glass, W., Haid, C.-T., Cidlinsky, K., Stenglein, C., and Christ, P. (1991). False-positive MR imaging in the diagnosis of acoustic neuromas. *Otolaryngology—Head and Neck Surgery, 104*, 863–867.

Wada, S.-I. and Starr, A. (1983). Generation of auditory brain stem responses (ABRs). I. Effects of injection of a local anesthetic (Procaine HCL) into the trapezoid body of guinea pigs and cat. *Electroencephalography and Clinical Neurophysiology, 56*, 326–339.

Wada, S.-I. and Starr, A. (1983). Generation of auditory brain stem responses (ABRs). II. Effects of surgical section of the trapezoid body on the ABR in guinea pigs and cat. *Electroencephalography and Clinical Neurophysiology, 56*, 340–351.

Wada, S.-I. and Starr, A. (1983). Generation of auditory brain stem responses (ABRs). III. Effects of lesions of the superior olive, lateral lemniscus and inferior colliculus on the ABR in guinea pig. *Electroencephalography and Clinical Neurophysiology, 56*, 352–366.

Warr, W.B. (1966). Fiber degeneration following lesions in the anterior ventral cochlear nucleus of the cat. *Experimental Neurology, 14*, 453–474.

Warr, W.B. (1969). Fiber degeneration following lesions in the posteriorventral cochlear of the cat. *Experimental Neurology, 23*, 140–155.

Waxman, S.G. (1982). Membranes, myelin, and the pathophysiology of multiple sclerosis. *New England Journal of Medicine, 306*, 1529–1532.

Werdelin, L. and Juhler, M. (1988). The course of transient ischemic attacks. *Neurology, 38*, 677–680.

Whisnant, J.P., Basford, J.R., Bernstein, E.F. et al. (1990). Special report from the National Institutes of Neurologic Disorders and Stroke Committee: Classification of cerebrovascular diseases III. *Stroke, 21*, 637–676.

Wolf, P.A. (1990). An overview of the epidemiology of stroke. *Stroke, 21 (Suppl.)*, 4–6.

Yamada, O., Kodera, K., and Yagi, T. (1979). Cochlear processes affecting wave V latency of the auditory evoked brain stem response: A study of patients with sensory hearing loss. *Scandinavian Audiology, 8*, 67–70.

Zaaroor, M. and Starr, A. (1991). Auditory brain-stem evoked potentials in cad after kainic acid induced neuronal loss. I. Superior olivary complex. *Electroencephalography and Clinical Neurophysiology, 80*, 422–435.

Zaaroor, M. and Starr, A. (1991). Auditory brain-stem evoked potentials in cad after kainic acid induced neuronal loss. II. Cochlear nucleus. *Electroencephalography and Clinical Neurophysiology, 80*, 436–445.

CHAPTER 17

EVOKED POTENTIALS IN MULTIPLE SCLEROSIS AND OTHER DEMYELINATING DISEASES

ROBERT W. KEITH

JOHN T. JACOBSON

INTRODUCTION

The use of sensory evoked potentials has played a prominent role in the detection and diagnosis of neurologic disorders. Neurodegenerative diseases, including multiple sclerosis, are usually diagnosed according to clinical symptomology and the time course of the disease process. Because multiple sclerosis frequently presents with subclinical "silent" plaque formations that are difficult to demonstrate, confirmation is often evasive. Therefore, it is important to recognize the pathophysiology and clinical manifestation of the disease under investigation.

A consensus of evoked potential literature suggests that multimodality (auditory, visual, and somatosensory) evoked potentials (EP) have demonstrated a comprehensive and preferred method of clinical evaluation in demyelinating disease study. This chapter unit focuses on one aspect of the battery; that of auditory evoked potentials (AEPs) and in particular, the auditory brainstem response (ABR). Additional electrophysiologic measures and audiologic test protocol will be described to illustrate the effects of demyelinating diseases in the auditory pathway.

The auditory brainstem response has emerged as the AEP of choice in identifying demyelinating lesions of the central nervous system (CNS). The purpose of ABR testing in the detection of multiple sclerosis is twofold: 1) to substantiate objectively CNS disease in the presence of clinical symptomology; and 2) to identify "silent" subclinical disease in the absence of patient complaint (Jacobson and Jacobson, 1990). The value of the brainstem response measure lies in its ability to monitor neural conduction within the auditory system. Further, the ABR wave components show minimal subject variability, are easily replicated, and appear insensitive to attention, sleep, sedation, or general anesthesia. Specific response parameters such as the relative latency difference between peak components and the amplitude ratio have proven invaluable as measures of neuropathology. Therefore, this chapter will examine the relevant clinical applications of ABR and other physiologic responses in the assessment of demyelinating lesions.

BACKGROUND

Demyelinating Disease

The term "demyelinating disease" refers to a group of related neurologic disorders characterized by concentrations of plaque demyelination. Criteria used to delineate demyelinating disease normally include destruction of the nerve fiber myelin sheath, the relative sparing of associated axons, nerve cells, and supporting structures, and perivenous distribution of lesions throughout the brain and spinal cord (Adams and Kubik, 1952). Redefining the criteria limits, Posner (1969) recommends that any definition of demyelinating disease be considered not in terms of myelin as an isolated tissue, but rather as a complex, integrated functional system comprising the neuron, axon, myelin formation, and the spiral wrapping of the myelin sheath.

Myelin diseases may be divided into two major categories: 1) those that disrupt the normal formation of myelin; and 2) those disorders, known as leukodystrophies, that result in abnormally formed myelin as a result of oligodendrocyte destruction (Pryse-Phillips and Murray, 1982).

Though speculative, etiologic agents implicated in myelin destruction include those immune (allergic), virally induced, and inherited (leukodystrophies) diseases, toxic diseases, and those associated with physical and traumatic demyelination. Regardless of the inferred cause, demyelination adversely affects nerve transmission by total conduction block, a reduction in conduction velocity, and/or an impairment in the ability to transmit trains of impulses (Sears, Bostock, and Sherratt, 1978).

Neural Conduction

To appreciate the complexity and impact of demyelinating diseases on neural conduction, a brief review of neural properties and function follows. Nerve cells are encapsulated by a semipermeable membrane that regulates the exchange of potassium and organic anions found in relatively high concentrations within the axoplasmic cell interior with surrounding interstitial fluid rich in sodium and chloride. Transmembrane ionic concentration differences maintain the cell interior at about −70mV at rest. During excitation, the cell membrane experiences a transient electrochemical disturbance whereby an influx of positive sodium ions enters the cell cytoplasm. This transient voltage reversal is known as a spike or action potential.

Depolarization is immediately followed by a reversal in membrane permeability in which the cell returns to its resting state following a spontaneous disruption in the sodium current and a delayed outward flow of potassium, a process called repolarization. During repolarization, regardless of excitation intensity, a second action potential cannot be evoked, and the neuron is said to be in an absolute refractory state. This period is followed by a relative refractory period during

which the initiation of an impulse results from sodium ions flowing down their electrochemical gradient, exciting adjacent areas of resting cell membrane.

In the CNS, myelin, which serves as an electrical insulator, is manufactured and maintained by specialized glial cells (oligodendroglia). As illustrated in Figure 17.1, the myelin sheath consists of a lamellar structure of protein and lipids that concentrically wraps the axon. At regular intervals, the sheath is interrupted by gaps known as the nodes of Ranvier. These sites are characteristically devoid of myelin and as such exhibit a pronounced decrease in electrical resistance. During neural propagation, impulses tend to jump between these internodes, an activity called saltatory conduction. This process increases the speed of neural conduction in myelin fibers to an extent predicated on axon diameter, internode length, and myelin efficiency. As indicated, myelin destruction will either reduce the speed of or block signal transmission, resulting in abnormal electrophysiologic measures.

Multiple Sclerosis

Multiple sclerosis is the primary human demyelinating disease of the CNS, characterized by exacerbations and remissions of symptoms in about one-quarter of all patients, with remitting and progressive symptoms occurring in 40% (Rivera, 1990). Although a test battery is usually required to support the neurologic examination, no pathognomonic laboratory tests have been found to confirm the disease process. Epidemiologic findings suggest that multiple sclerosis is acquired early in life, with a peak risk age in the teens, but onset of symptoms is usually in the third or fourth decade. During the early stages of the disease, clinical diagnosis is sometimes difficult since it requires the objective demonstration and involvement of at least two distinct sights within the CNS over a long duration or on a number of occasions.

The clinical diagnosis of multiple sclerosis normally requires evidence of fluctuations in the course of the disease and symptoms and signs indicating scattered lesions in the white matter of the CNS (Schumacher, 1971) although other focal lesions have been identified (Lammaglia et al., 1989). While symp-

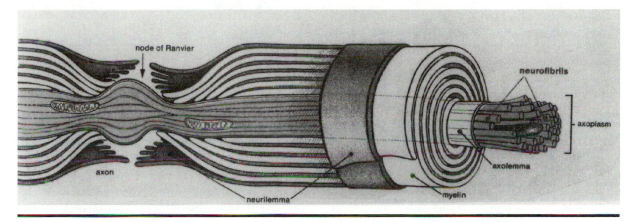

FIGURE 17.1.   Anatomical structure of a nerve showing myelin sheath and nodes of Ranvier. Plaque formation as observed in demyelinating disease will tend to reduce or block neural conduction thereby reducing impulse velocity. Reprinted with permission from *Melloni's Illustrated Medical Dictionary, 3rd ed.*; The Parthenon Publishing Group, Inc., 1983.

toms vary in degree, duration, and character, they usually involve, in isolation or combination, impairment of the sensory and motor systems. For example, Jerger and colleagues (1986a) have observed auditory system abnormality in 90% of confirmed multiple sclerosis patients.

Pathophysiology.   In demyelination, plaque formation usually begins with perivenular infiltration of lymphocytes and monocytes, most often in the optic tract, the lateral and posterior columns of the spinal cord, the brainstem, and the cerebellum. The loss of myelin is characterized by glial cell proliferation, perivascular edema, inflammation, and gliosis (scarring). As the disease progresses, plaques increase in number and size, depending on the manifestation of pathologic interstitial space. Plaques frequently remit; and while segmented remyelination is predictable, in the CNS it is usually restricted to a few layers of new myelin. Thus, normal function in the fiber tract is rare and conduction is slower.

The causative agent for multiple sclerosis remains elusive. There is growing support, however, that the pathogenesis of demyelination is likely found in alterations of the autoimmune regulation system. This theory is supported by the presence of increased concentrations of myelin basic protein in the cerebrospinal fluid (CSF) and has led to a possible immunologic basis for multiple sclerosis (Cohen et al., 1976). About two-thirds of all active, clinically diagnosed multiple sclerosis patients have increased immunoglobulin G (IgG) in the CSF, whereas 90% of all cases show the presence of oligoclonal IgG bands on CSF immunoelectrophoresis (Johnson and Nelson, 1977). In addition, CSF analysis has been useful in the reclassification of multiple sclerosis patients with subclinical lesions of the CNS (Cosi et al., 1987). Myelin basic protein has also been found in patients with metachromatic leukodystrophy in central pontine myelinolysis (Cohen et al., 1980). Thus, the excessive synthesis of immunoglobulin may produce antibodies responsible for destruction of myelin in multiple sclerosis and other demyelinating diseases.

Another possible etiologic source has been attributed to a slow-virus infection that may explain the unusual dormant period between the early risk age and the later symptoms onset. The finding of increased levels of measles virus antibody in the serum and CSF in multiple sclerosis patients has placed the measles virus under suspicion, although many viruses can produce the same disorder (Hankins and Black, 1986).

Classification.   Through the years, there have been several criteria proposed for the classification of multiple sclerosis (Schumacher et al., 1968). Bauer (1980) reported the results of a survey that established four categories into which all multiple sclerosis patients could be clinically diagnosed. They were 1) multiple sclerosis proven by autopsy, 2) "definite", 3) "probable", and 4) "possible" multiple sclerosis. While specific criteria varied among the later three categories, those listed in the diagnosis of "definite" multiple sclerosis include a relapsing and remitting course, a slow or stepwise progression, documented neurologic signs of predominately CNS white matter pathology, characteristic CSF findings, symptom onset between 10 and 50 years, and "no better" neurologic explanation.

Epidemiology.   Numerous epidemiologic studies have been undertaken in an attempt to uncover possible eti-

ologies, risk factors, and the pathogenesis of multiple sclerosis (Alter, 1980). The results of such investigations indicate a unique geographic distribution as displayed in Figure 17.2. The prevalence of multiple sclerosis is substantially greater at higher latitudes in both hemispheres. For example, in North America, the prevalence is approximately 50/100,000 between 40 and 50 degrees latitude compared to 6 to 14/100,000 between 25 and 30 degrees latitude (Kurkland and Reed, 1964; Rivera, 1986; Waksman and Reynolds, 1982). In comparison, geographic regions with the highest reported prevalence rate per 100,000 are the Orkney and Shetland Islands with 258 and 152/100,000, respectively (Poskanzer et al., 1976).

Although no direct link exists between latitude and etiology, epidemiologic evidence indicates that genetic factors may be active in multiple sclerosis susceptibility. Residence in low-prevalence areas during

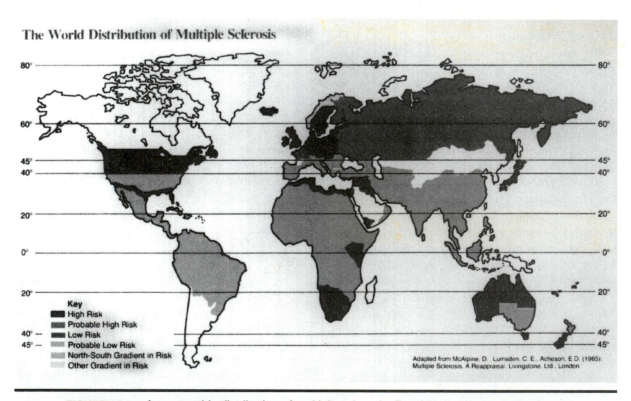

FIGURE 17.2.   A geographic distribution of multiple sclerosis. Reprinted with permission from U.S. Department of Health, Education, and Welfare.

early life ensures long-term immunity, and migration to a low-prevalence area may modify the risks of clinical multiple sclerosis (Detels et al., 1974).

Further inspection of epidemiologic evidence shows that multiple sclerosis is more common in females, approximating a two-to-one ratio (Waksman and Reynolds, 1982; McAlpine, Lumsden, and Acheson, 1972). Approximately two-thirds of all multiple sclerosis patients experience initial onset in their early thirties (Leibowitz, Alter, and Halper, 1964), and familial incidence is higher than that in the general public (McAlpine et al., 1972). According to Pryse-Phillips and Murray (1982), about 10% of all multiple sclerosis patients have a positive family history suggesting inherited immune factors. Other genetic influences have been described from twin series with elevated concordance rates among monozygotic twins (Kinnunen et al., 1988). In part, epidemiologic studies have accounted for the unique effects of environmental, genetic, and infectious conditions associated with geographic distribution.

AUDIOLOGIC FINDINGS

The reported prevalence and degree of peripheral auditory impairment varies widely in multiple sclerosis patients. In a comprehensive review, Noffsinger et al. (1972) found the incidence of pure-tone deficits to range from 1 to 86%. Fischer et al. (1985) considered hearing loss to be an infrequent symptom in multiple sclerosis and estimated it to be no more than 3%. Although the most frequently observed peripheral abnormality is a mild high-frequency cochlear hearing loss, a diversity of audiometric configurations have been described (Dayal and Swisher, 1967; LeZak and Selhub, 1966; Rose and Daly, 1964; Simpkins, 1961). Recent literature has documented varying degrees of sudden hearing loss associated with multiple sclerosis. Acute onset of hearing loss has been, for the most part, restricted to the high frequency regions of the cochlea with prolonged abnormal ABR results and auditory sensitivity recovery (Hansen and Christiansen, 1985; Shea and Brackmann, 1989; Schweitzer and Shepard, 1989; Barratt, Miller, and Rudge, 1988; Furnman, Durrant, and Hirsch, 1989; Franklin, Coker, and Jenkins, 1989).

Special Tests for Site of Lesion

In general, conventional site-of-lesion tests are insensitive to demonstrate clinical severity in multiple sclerosis patients. Abnormal adaptation has been reported (Daughtery et al., 1983; Noffsinger et al., 1972) with some evidence of fluctuation and a return to normal status during remission (Rose and Daly, 1964). The presence of recruitment is not common (Dix, 1965; Noffsinger et al., 1972), nor has any conclusive diagnosis resulted from the Short Increment Sensitivity Index test (LeZak and Selhub, 1966; Noffsinger et al., 1972). Thus, any relationship between multiple sclerosis and hearing loss is ill-defined without correlating neurologic evidence (Antonelli and Demitri, 1963; Citron et al., 1963; Parker, Decker, and Richards, 1968; Rose and Daly, 1964).

Sensitized Speech Tests

Acoustically modified linguistic stimuli have gained a prominent role in the diagnosis of central auditory nervous system dysfunction. Unfortunately, sensitized speech materials have been infrequently employed in multiple sclerosis patients (Antonelli and DeMitri, 1963; Noffsinger et al., 1972; Stephens and Thornton, 1976). The results of sensitized speech tests appear to be related to the degree of extrinsic redundancy found in the speech material, the intrinsic redundancy of the auditory system, and the nature, site, and size of the neurologic lesion. In multiple sclerosis, test results vary depending on the specific test and the status (classification, remission, exacerbation, etc.) of the patient. Conventional speech recognition thresholds and word recognition scores are usually normal and in good agreement with pure tone sensitivity (Parker et al., 1968), although reduced word recognition scores have been reported in the presence of competing noise (Daughtery et al., 1983; Dayal, Tarantino, and Swisher, 1966).

In comparison to conventional speech material, sensitized speech has shown diagnostic promise in multiple sclerosis patients. Jacobson, Deppe, and Murray, (1983), compared dichotic speech paradigms in a group of 20 "definite" multiple sclerosis patients. The results suggested that dichotic consonant-vowel nonsense-syllables and Synthetic Sentence Identification (SSI) tests proved clinically useful in the overall diagnosis of central auditory deficits in multiple sclerosis patients. The SSI results have been confirmed in other test observations (Hannley, Jerger, and Rivera, 1983; Russolo and Poli, 1983). Jerger et al. (1986b) found that 55% of 62 subjects with "definite" multiple sclerosis showed some abnormality in word recognition using either the PAL PB-50 words or the SSI with ipsilateral competing messages. Binaural fusion, dichotic digit and sentence tests, and low-pass filtered speech have also demonstrated abnormal findings in varying classifications of multiple sclerosis patients (Daugherty et al., 1983; Musiek et al., 1989).

Recently van der Poel, Jones, and Miller (1988) found that discrimination of alternating monaural clicks and interaural time difference (IATD) discrimination of binaural clicks were abnormal in 53% and 82% respectively in patients with "definite" multiple sclerosis. These results were thought to be caused by disruption of the auditory pathway peripheral to the superior olivary complex, where binaurally responsive units are sensitive to IATD (Matathias, Sohmer, and Biton, 1985). With advances in electrophysiologic techniques there has been little recent research in behavioral testing of patients with multiple sclerosis. Behavioral and psychoacoustic research still has relevance, however, because it investigates functional disorders of hearing as they relate to counseling for communication deficits. This notion is different than the administration of tests of physiologic responses to sound that are useful for diagnostic purposes.

PHYSIOLOGICAL RESPONSES

Acoustic Reflex (AR)

Several physiologic responses have been used successfully in the evaluation of patients with possible multiple sclerosis. The acoustic reflex measure is one such response that, due to its ease of application, has been used frequently in multiple sclerosis diagnosis. The acoustic reflex refers to the involuntary contraction of the stapedius muscle in response to a sufficiently intense auditory stimulus. Measurements of the acoustic reflex response can include response threshold, latency of onset, rise time, time to maximum contraction, am-

plitude of response, offset, and adaptation to sustained stimulus presentation. Acoustic reflex testing has been shown to be useful in detecting retrocochlear pathology with common findings that include elevated or absent reflexes, and/or abnormal adaptation to sustained tones.

Similarly, abnormalities in the acoustic reflex response have been observed in patients with multiple sclerosis and have been reported to range from 21 (Grenman et al., 1984) to 60% (Kofler, Oberascher, and Pommer, 1984). Acoustic reflex abnormalities in this disease include prolongation of reflex onset latency (Bosatra, 1977; Hess, 1979) and increases in the rise time (Colletti, 1975; Hess, 1979). In addition, patients with multiple sclerosis have aberrations in acoustic response amplitude, with many patients showing reduced amplitude (Bosatra, Russola, and Poli, 1976; Colletti, 1975), whereas others show opposite amplitude effects (Bosatra et al., 1976).

Keith and Garza-Holquin (1987) reported that five of 23 normal hearing subjects with "definite" or "probable" multiple sclerosis had absent acoustic reflexes. Responses of the other 18 subjects were characterized as showing normal onset latencies followed by increased rise times and normal responses amplitude. Jerger et al. (1986a) reported that 75% of 122 patients with "definite" multiple sclerosis showed some abnormality of the acoustic reflex including elevation or absent reflex thresholds, or some abnormality in either absolute amplitude, latency, or relative amplitude indices. In contrast, Wiegand and Poch (1988), comparing a group of normal and sensory hearing-impaired and multiple sclerosis patients, found that acoustic reflex rise time and onset latency was not a sensitive measure to screen for the presence of otherwise asymptomatic multiple sclerosis. Despite this study, the majority of evidence supports abnormal reflex activity in multiple sclerosis patients.

Evaluation of studies of acoustic reflex dynamics completed on multiple sclerosis subjects indicates that abnormalities occur in a substantial number, although not a majority of persons. When acoustic reflex abnormalities occur in the presence of normal peripheral hearing, they are a sensitive measure of a lesion involving the brainstem reflex arc. In this regard, acoustic reflex testing continues to be an important and integral part of the diagnostic evaluation of patients with possible neurologic disorders.

Electronystagmography (ENG)

Approximately 50% of patients with multiple sclerosis report vertigo at some time during the course of the disease. Pathologic nystagmus has been observed at one time or another in approximately 90% of multiple sclerosis patients (Baloh and Honrubia, 1979). According to these authors, ENG recordings of patients suspected of having multiple sclerosis are valuable in detecting smooth pursuit, saccadic, and optokinetic nystagmus abnormalities that are not apparent on visual inspection of eye movements. In a study of 53 patients by Pitt and Rawles (1989), 40% had subclinical abnormalities of saccadic eye movement supporting a diagnosis of "probable" multiple sclerosis. These authors state that abnormal detection rates by saccadic eye movement recording was equal to that of visual evoked responses but greater than ABR. Prolonged latency of gaze was the most common saccadic abnormality detected. Similarly, Tedeshi et al. (1989) reported that saccadic eye movements were as sensitive as visual and auditory EPs in diagnosing multiple sclerosis as the most sensitive saccadic eye movement parameter.

Multiple sclerosis produces every other variety of vestibular abnormality, including gaze and positional nystagmus, unilateral or bilateral caloric weakness, and directional preponderance. These ENG findings are found with both CNS and peripheral abnormalities as a result of plaques within the nerve root where peripheral nerves contain CNS myelin (Baloh and Honrubia, 1979). Whereas a high percentage of multiple sclerosis patients present with vestibular abnormality at one point or another, the ENG is not however particularly helpful in differentiating multiple sclerosis from other neurologic disease processes.

ROLE OF THE ABR IN NEUROLOGIC DIAGNOSIS

The application of sensory evoked potentials (SEP) continues to play an important role in the diagnosis of patients who present with symptoms suggesting possible multiple sclerosis. According to Maurer and Lowitzsch (1982), the diagnosis of multiple sclerosis is based on the clinical course of the disease, the dissemination of the demyelinating process, and characteristic changes in the CSF. The notion of dissemination of lesions in the CNS means that the diagnosis of multiple sclerosis is dependent upon fulfilling a diagnostic requirement of a second nervous system lesion. In patients with suspected multiple sclerosis but clinical evidence of only a single lesion, electrophysiologic studies may provide evidence for subclinical involvement elsewhere in the CNS, thereby helping to establish the diagnosis with greater confidence. They may also provide objective evidence of neurologic dysfunction in patients with nonspecific symptoms whose true nature is not otherwise apparent. Normal recordings may also be valuable in reassuring patients with uncharacteristic symptoms that they may not be suffering from multiple sclerosis. For example, Nuwer et al. (1985) found that relatives of patients with multiple sclerosis tended to have prolonged visual and somatosensory evoked potential results, but were not considered likely to have future appearance of clinical multiple sclerosis. Nuwer et al. cautioned that clinicians should be aware not to overinterpret small EP changes in relatives of multiple sclerosis patients. In view of the fact that Nuwer et al. did not study the ABR, it is not known whether similar prolonged findings would occur in this modality.

While earlier optimism predicted that EPs may be useful in monitoring the effectiveness of treatment of multiple sclerosis, recent evidence fails to confirm that hypothesis. Milanese et al. (1989) found that electrophysiologic test results were not affected by treatment of ACTH, dexamethasone, or methylprednisolone. Anderson et al. (1987) also found multimodality EPs to have limited use in studying the effectiveness of hyperbaric oxygen treatment of chronic multiple sclerosis. Smith, Zeeberg, and Sjo (1986) found that EPs did not change in parallel to the clinical effect of high-dose methylprednisolone infusion therapy. In his definitive text on electrodiagnosis, Kimura (1989) states that evoked potential studies may not provide information for monitoring progression of disease, and there may be frequent disparity between clinical and electrophysiologic courses. Nevertheless, the ease of such non-invasive procedures will continue to be used and helpful within clinical limits.

Somatosensory and Visual Evoked Potentials

Although the focus of this chapter and text deal with auditory evoked responses, we would be remiss if somatosensory and visual EPs were not acknowledged, since their application has proven significant in multimodality assessment of multiple sclerosis patients. Somatosensory evoked potentials can be elicited from multiple peripheral nerve sites. Clinical studies often stimulate mixed nerves containing both sensory and motor fibers because the motor response assures proper electrode placement and adequate stimulus levels. Nerves that are commonly stimulated include the median nerve at the wrist, the posterior tibial nerve at the ankle, and the peroneal nerve at the knee. A constant current stimulus is applied at these sites using durations of 0.1 to 0.5 ms at presentation rates of one to five per second.

A response can theoretically be recorded from any place along the nerve pathway, although some sites offer such a low-voltage response that they offer little clinical utility (e.g., the cervical spine). Cortical EPs are larger voltage, and are usually easy to record in a cooperative, unanesthetized patient. The cortical response is best recorded from the midparietal scalp over the posterior portion of the fissure of Rolando. Filter settings of 1 to 250 Hz optimize SEP response using an analysis time window of approximately 40 ms for the median nerve and 100 ms for posterior tibial nerve stimulation. The cortical evoked potential consists of a biphasic wave with Pa, Pb response at 16 and 24 ms for median nerve stimulation and 40 and 60 ms for the posterior tibial nerve, respectively.

Similarly, visual evoked potentials (VEP) can be recorded from the visual cortex in response to the flash of a strobe light or a pattern reversing checkerboard design on a television screen. The VEP response of primary interest occurs at approximately P 100 ms. According to Chiappa and Ropper (1982) both the absolute latency of P 100 and the difference in latency between the two eyes are very sensitive indicators of disease. Amplitude measurements are more variable than latency and have less clinical utility.

In the evaluation of patients suspected of having demyelinating disease, Matthews, Wattam-Bell, and Pountney (1982) comment that VEPs have "the greatest predictive value" over other EP measurements. That finding has been confirmed repeatedly by many investigators. For example, Baumhefner et al. (1990) found VEPs to be abnormal in 85% of 62 patients with "definite" multiple sclerosis, whereas ABRs were abnormal in 46% and SEPs in 19%. Similar findings are reported by Javidan, McLean, and Warren (1986). Kjaer (1980) identified clinically silent lesions by VEPs in 50% of subjects evaluated, with ABRs abnormal in 38% and somatosensory EPs in 13%. Clearly, the finding of CNS abnormalities is determined primarily by the focus of the demyelinating process and the tests are more or less interdependent. Since they are noninvasive they can be done in a relatively short time with little discomfort to the patient. They provide supplemental information and increase the certainty of the diagnosis.

Auditory Brainstem Responses

Prevalence of Abnormalities.   The development of techniques used to record and measure short-latency electric events generated along the auditory pathway of the brainstem resulted in a dramatic change in the approach to differential diagnosis in patients with various eighth nerve and brainstem lesions, including multiple sclerosis.

Early studies by Robinson and Rudge (1975, 1977), Shanon et al. (1979), Starr and Achor (1975), and Lynn, Taylor, and Gilroy (1980) indicated that a substantial number of patients with multiple sclerosis showed ABR abnormalities. Estimates of abnormalities ranged from 34% (Chiappa and Norwood, 1977) to 73% (Robinson and Rudge, 1975) of all patients tested. The overall percentage of abnormalities is the summation of patient subgroups classified as "definite," "probable," or "possible" multiple sclerosis. Lynn et al. (1980), for example, found 75% of "definite," 33% of "probable," and 29% of "possible" multiple sclerosis patients with ABR abnormalities. Similarly, patients with clinical evidence of brainstem involvement show a higher rate of ABR abnormalities than patients who show no evidence of brainstem disorder. For example, 79% of Robinson and Rudge's (1977) patients with positive evidence of brainstem lesion and 51% of those without clinical sign of brainstem involvement had ABR abnormalities. Further, Antonelli et al. (1988) observed 81% ABR abnormality in 21 patients with positive neurologic evidence of brainstem involvement.

Manifestations of brainstem abnormalities include internuclear ophthalmoplegia, sixth or seventh nerve palsy, horizontal or vertical gaze nystagmus (Robinson and Rudge, 1977), dizziness, gait disturbance, cerebellar signs, and sensory or motor abnormalities (Chiappa et al., 1980). Other studies have shown evidence of ABR abnormalities in an even higher percentage of patients with "definite" clinical brainstem involvement with estimates as high as 88% (Paludetti et al., 1985) and 93% (Stockard and Rossiter, 1977). It should be noted that some results are reported in the absence of symptomatic hearing impairment, although many investigators are vague about procedures used in assessing peripheral hearing levels. Since ABR results are dependent upon middle ear and cochlear function, the technique should be used in conjunction with standard audiometry.

Types of ABR Abnormalities. There is considerable variability in ABR abnormalities observed in multiple sclerosis patients. The findings include abnormality of symmetry, delay in latency, fragmented response, decreased amplitude or absence of peaks, poor response reliability, abnormal responses to changes in rate, and latency-intensity function. Jerger et al. (1986b) observed a series of patterns in 62 patients diagnosed with "definite" multiple sclerosis. These authors classified these into four abnormal conditions: 1) delayed interwave intervals; 2) degraded waveforms; 3) loss of late waves; and, 4) wave I only. From our experience, we add two additional classification patterns. They include: 5) non-replicable traces; and, 6) wave I prolongation with normal peripheral hearing. As discussed, plaque formations may result in normal conduction delay or blockage, thus modifying the synchronization of the neural discharge patterns. The consequence is a dispersion pattern of neural activity and an absent array of ABR traces based on severity and status.

Figure 17.3 illustrates some of the ABR abnormalities previously described. These results were obtained from patients with "definite" multiple sclerosis who

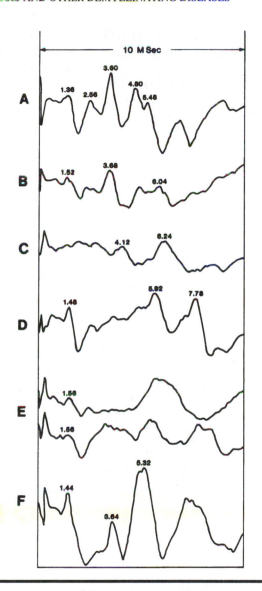

FIGURE 17.3. ABR traces obtained from a normal subject (A) and several (B–F) multiple sclerosis patients. See text for a description of morphology.

were in a state of remission. All persons had normal hearing sensitivity. The responses were obtained using alternating click polarity presented monaurally at 80 dB nHL at a rate of 21.1 per second. The data were obtained (Garza, 1981) and presented in part by Garza, Keith, and Barajas (1982).

Tracing A is a response obtained from a normal subject; tracing B has a normal wave I and III with delayed wave V, resulting in a prolonged III–V interval. Tracing C has an absent wave I and delayed latency to wave III with a normal III–V interval. Tracing D has waves I and V present at normal latencies with an absent wave III. In fact, it is not possible to determine if the response at 5.92 ms is wave V or a delayed wave III with normal III–V conduction between the responses at 5.92 and 7.98 ms. Tracing E shows two trials from the same subject with a normal wave I response and nonrepeatable waves III and V. Tracing F has responses with normal latencies but abnormally large amplitude of waves I and V.

Latency and Amplitude. Chiappa, Young, and Goldie (1979) report that 13% of 202 patients had abnormal I–V separation, 55% had only wave V amplitude abnormalities, and 33% had both abnormalities. Stockard and Rossiter (1977) reported that 69% of abnormalities were related to latency, while 31% were amplitude related. Robinson and Rudge (1977) also reported that latency was a more reliable discriminator than amplitude, with wave V the single most important component. For example, wave V was the only abnormality in 71% of patients reported by Robinson and Rudge (1977). These authors and others (Hausler and Levine, 1980) report normal wave I responses in all of their subjects.

The most common interwave interval (IWI) latency abnormality appears to occur in the III–V separation (Chiappa, 1980; Lynn et al., 1980; Shanon, Gold, and Himmelfarb, 1981), although Shanon et al. (1981) found significant I–III interval prolongation. Similarly, Barajas (1982) reported 25% of ABR abnormalities were related to IWI alone, 45% to wave V amplitude, and 30% had both abnormalities.

Whereas absolute and relative latency has been shown to be a sensitive indicator of brainstem dysfunction associated with multiple sclerosis, Robinson and Rudge (1975) found that in patients with normal brainstem latencies, 50% showed a decrease in response amplitude. Starr and Achor (1975) report that with the exception of wave I, all multiple sclerosis patients showed reduced amplitude. Chiappa et al. (1980) found 87% of multiple sclerosis patients show absent or abnormally low wave V amplitude. Finally, clinical evidence suggests that the diagnosis of multiple sclerosis increases when the combined amplitudes of waves III, IV, and V were compared between ears (Javidan et al., 1986).

Peripheral Nerve Involvement.   Until recently, the effects of multiple sclerosis were thought to be restricted to the CNS. However, evidence has shown segmental demyelination (Pollack, Calder, and Allpress, 1977) and abnormal refractory periods (Hopf and Eysholdt, 1978) in the peripheral nerves of multiple sclerosis patients. Using ABR and electrocochleography to confirm wave I presence, Hopf and Maurer (1983) tested 71 multiple sclerosis patients. Eight (11%) exhibited prolonged wave I latencies (>3 SD). They attributed peripheral involvement to segmental demyelination of the distal part of the acoustic nerve. Further clinical findings have been reported that support peripheral involvement as reflected in ABR measures. Fischer et al. (1985) observed 25% wave I abnormality in 12 multiple sclerosis patients with acute hearing loss. Verma and Lynn (1985) reported 22% abnormality in 29 "definite" multiple sclerosis patients with normal auditory and otologic findings and Jacobson, Murray, and Deppe (1987) identified 40% latency prolongation or wave I absence in multiple sclerosis patients with confirmed brainstem lesions. There appears to be anatomical support for their conclusions. The neuroglial-neurilemmal junction of the acoustic nerve is located 7 to 13 mm distal to the brainstem near the fundus of the internal meatus (Nager, 1969). This junction may be the functional site of peripheral demyelination. Recently, Furnman et al. (1989) observed an acute high-frequency hearing loss in a multiple sclerosis patient who demonstrated an abnormal ABR trace (wave I only) on initial evaluation. Axial magnetic resonance imaging supported the hypothesis of an eighth nerve root-entry lesion.

Repeatability.   Test-retest repeatability in normal subjects is excellent with highly reproducible waveform morphology and latency. In contrast, a common finding in multiple sclerosis patients is poor repeatability of ABR results. The absence test-retest reliability has been reported in as many as 80% of multiple sclerosis patients (Garza et al., 1982; Nodar, 1978; Prasher and Gibson, 1980; Robinson and Rudge, 1980). Figure 17.4 demonstrates this common finding in one patient disguised with multiple sclerosis. Lacquaniti et al. (1979) report that response variability is independent of stimulus intensity and support the common clinical practice of repeated measurements at each stimulus intensity and repetition rate.

Polarity Effects.   In a group of 95 multiple sclerosis patients, Tackman and Vogel (1987) found that rarefaction and condensation clicks could independently elicit ABR abnormalities with increased latencies of one or more peaks, whereas clicks of alternating polarity failed to detect abnormalities in greater number. Hammond, Yiannikas, and Chan (1986), in contrast, found that ABR latency and amplitude measures were independent of click polarity. Additional study is warranted to confirm these conflicting findings.

Rate Effects.   The effects of increased repetition rate on the ABR have been documented in normal (Don, Allen, and Starr, 1977; Hyde, Stephens, and Thornton, 1976; Pratt and Sohmer, 1976; Weber and Fujikawa, 1977) and neurologic impaired human subjects (Hecox, Cone, and Blaw, 1981; Pratt et al., 1981; Stockard and

Rossiter, 1977; Yagi and Kaga, 1979). Generally, an increase in repetition rate will differentially prolong wave latency while decreasing amplitude. The more rostral the response, the greater the latency shift. A number of investigators have shown small but consistent wave I latency increases (Terkildsen, Osterhammel, and Huis in't Veld, 1975; Thornton and Coleman, 1975; Yagi and Kaga, 1979; Zollner, Karnahl, and Stange, 1976).

Despite the evidence that rate effects are clinically useful in the identification of neurologic disorders, little information exists with regard to demyelinating diseases and those results are conflicting. Chiappa et al. (1980) confirmed earlier work (Chiappa and Norwood, 1977) that rate effects did not alter the incidence of multiple sclerosis abnormality. Using a constant click stimulus polarity and an abnormality criterion of 3 SD above the normal mean, they found no significant difference in relative latency values in 57 multiple sclerosis patients tested at 10 and 70/s. In comparison, Shanon et al. (1981) employed alternating click polarity at three rates of 10, 50, and 100/s in 10 multiple sclerosis patients. Brainstem results produced greater wave variability, amplitude alterations, and increases in latency (N1-P4) of 0.66 ms between rates of 10 and 100/s. Increases in the identification of multiple sclerosis abnormality associated with higher rates have been reported by Robinson and Rudge (1977), Stockard and Rossiter (1977), and Stockard et al. (1978). Finally, Jacobson and colleagues (1987) reported the results of rate effects on 20 multiple sclerosis patients diagnosed with "definite" multiple sclerosis. Patients exhibited normal peripheral hearing sensitivity and positive neurologic evidence of brainstem abnormality. The results indicated that the incidence of abnormality was dependent on the rate of presentation. Abnormal IWI (I–V) increased from 52.5% at 10/s to 65% at 67 and 80/s. Figure 17.5 illustrates a series of ABR traces from one patient with multiple sclerosis. The left ear is well with normal absolute and relative latencies at slower presentation rates, but abnormal for both resources as the "system" is stressed at higher rates. Latency shifts have been attributed to adaptation or fatigue (Don et al., 1977), reduced refractory period, and decreased synaptic efficiency (Pratt and Sohmer, 1976). Jacobson and Newman

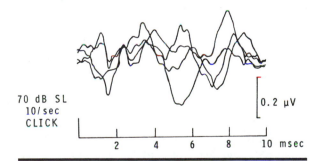

70 dB SL
10/sec
CLICK

0.2 µV

2   4   6   8   10 msec

FIGURE 17.4.   ABR traces recorded consecutively form the same ear of one patient diagnosed with "definite" M.S. A 70 dB SL alternating click polarity was presented monaurally at a rate of 10/sec. Conventional ABR protocol was used throughout this single channel recording.

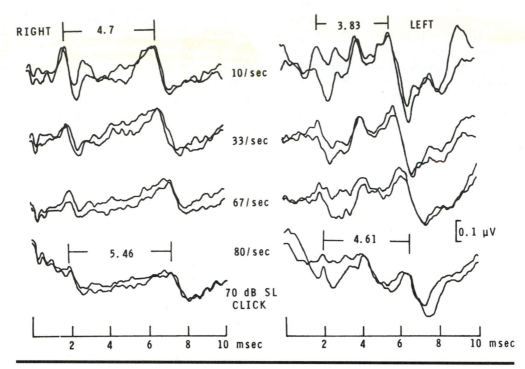

FIGURE 17.5.   Abnormal increases in I–V central conduction time (left ear) observed from the same ear of one patient with multiple sclerosis as a function of four repetition rates. Abnormal interwave intervals are present in the right ear of the same M.S. patient at all presentation rates. Note the early identical latency shift for the left (0.78 ms) and the right (0.76 ms) ears.

(1989) found that certain patients with clinically "definite" multiple sclerosis failed to demonstrate a significant enhancement of rate abnormality following rapid click presentation rates. They hypothesize that it may be possible to subclassify patients with evidence of brainstem demyelination based on the presence or absence of ABR rate-dependent abnormalities.

It is well known that response variability increases with rate; the multiple sclerosis population is no exception. Brainstem responses may alter wave morphology, amplitude, and response replicability on consecutive runs. Figure 17.6 illustrates wave aberrations from one multiple sclerosis patient as a function of rate increase.

Latency-Intensity Effects.   Parving, Elberling, and Smith, (1981) studied 15 patients with "definite" multiple sclerosis using electrocochleography and ABR.

Stimulus intensities of 35–115 dB peSPL were used to obtain latency-intensity functions. Although absolute wave I and the I–V latency results were normal, the latency-intensity function was abnormal for both latency and amplitude at low stimulus intensities despite normal hearing sensitivity at 2000 Hz. Parving et al. interpret the difference between their results and others as: 1) difficulties in the ability to assign values to ABR components; 2) influences on the ABR from cochlear dysfunction; and, 3) data interpretation. It would appear that based on the results of the latency-intensity function on multiple sclerosis patients further research is required before it can be used with diagnostic confidence.

Ipsilateral versus Contralateral Stimulation.   Initially, binaural stimulus presentation was used in obtaining ABR in multiple sclerosis patients (Robinson and Rudge,

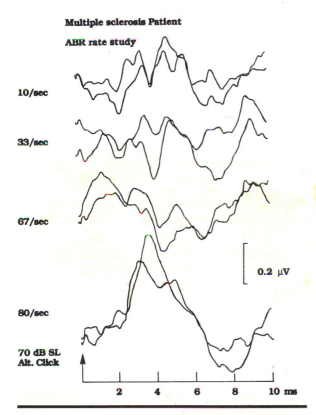

Multiple sclerosis Patient

ABR rate study

10/sec

33/sec

67/sec

80/sec

70 dB SL
Alt. Click

0.2 μV

2   4   6   8   10 ms

FIGURE 17.6.   ABR traces obtained from the same ear of one multiple sclerosis patient. Alternating click stimulus rates from 10 to 80/s were presented monaurally. Substantial changes in wave morphology are noted as rate is increased. See text for explanation.

1977). This technique obscured a lateralized abnormality because of the normal response from the contralateral site. Several investigators have since documented the need for using monaural stimulation to identify patients with lateralized lesions (Barajas, 1982; Prasher and Gibson, 1980; Rowe, 1981).

Two publications (Barajas, 1982; Prasher and Gibson, 1980) suggest that occasionally only contralateral stimulation results in an abnormally late response in multiple sclerosis. Their data are vague regarding specific abnormalities. Quaranta, Mininni, and Longo (1986) found that detection of abnormality using contralateral derivation increased detectability from 74% to

89% in patients with confirmed multiple sclerosis and from 9% to 21% in cases of undefined multiple sclerosis. Hammond and Yiannikas (1987) found that the contralateral responses generally mirrored the ipsilateral responses and did not contribute significantly to the sensitivity of lesion detection. However, contralateral recordings did aid in the recognition of waves when they were not clearly seen in the ipsilateral channel.

ABR Related to Psychophysical Data.   There is presently a lack of sufficient published information relating ABR findings to results of psychoacoustic studies. Clinically, investigators have observed patients for whom no repeatable ABR could be recorded who had normal hearing sensitivity and 100% word recognition scores in quiet. One study (Hausler and Levine, 1980) attempted to relate estimates of the just-noticeable difference (JND) for intra-aural time and intensity in multiple sclerosis patients. In general, their results showed that patients with abnormal time JNDs had abnormal ABRs on at least one side, while those with normal time JNDs tended to yield normal ABRs. The authors suggest that these results indicate that the same auditory structure of the brainstem subserves intra-aural time discrimination and short-latency, click-evoked potentials. While the data available on relationship between psychophysical testing and EPs are scant, the study by Hausler and Levine suggests further avenues of exploration to understand auditory function better in normal and disordered populations.

Hyperthermia on ABR.   An increase in body temperature can provoke a transitory worsening of clinical symptoms of multiple sclerosis, and has been used in the past to help diagnose multiple sclerosis (Guthrie, 1951). Geraund et al. (1982) have reported on ABR changes observed following warming multiple sclerosis subjects by an average of 0.7 degree C. Of 18 multiple sclerosis subjects studied, there was no change of wave V latency or amplitude in 10 cases, whereas eight patients showed a significant alteration in the response. The result is due to a slight increase in conduction velocity with increased temperature until a blocking temperature is reached, at which time conduction velocity slows (Geraund et al., 1982). Although these authors indicated that ABR testing after warming has possible clinical advantages, induced hyperthermia has shown only slight diagnostic value.

Occult Lesions of the Auditory System

Acoustic neuromas are often identified with neurofibromatosis Type II, known as von Recklinghausen's disease. Type I neurofibromatosis is not usually associated with acoustic tumors. In a study of 44 children diagnosed as having Type I neurofibromatosis, Pensak et al. (1989) found that 32% had significant abnormalities on ABR test results, even though most were asymptomatic for auditory disorders. Twenty-eight percent of children also had abnormal acoustic reflex test results. Only one of the children had an identifiable mass lesion. These findings were interpreted as indicating delays in neural conduction resulting from myelin dysfunction in this population. Whether the findings predict later degenerative changes or the presence of mass lesions was not know, indicating the need for following children with Type I neurofibromatosis who have abnormal EP studies.

Other degenerative diseases have been shown to have similar effects on ABR results. They include, for example, Charcot-Marie-Tooth disease (Musiek, Weider, and Mueller, 1982; Triantafyllou et al., 1989); multiple system degeneration (Kawahara et al., 1988); Pelizaeus-Merzbacher disease (Feldman et al., 1990); sarcoidosis, Jamaican neuropathy, and vascular disease (Robinson and Rudge, 1980). During the past few years a number of investigators have reported abnormal EP results in patients with leukodystrophy, a disease of degeneration of the white matter of the brain characterized by demyelination and glial reaction, probably related to defects of lipid metabolism (De-Meirleir, Taylor, and Logan, 1988;

Kurokawa et al., 1987; Krevit et al., 1987; Goto et al., 1986). In general, due to the nature of the degenerative process, diseases that manifest demyelination properties, mimic those EP results found in multiple sclerosis patients and therefore any attempt to differentiation between demyelinating lesion using EPs must be approached cautiously.

Comment. There is a great disparity of ABR results demonstrated in multiple sclerosis patients. Wave V responses are likely to be prolonged since the area between the superior olivary complex and the inferior colliculus is "the longest tract of white matter in the CNS, and therefore the most susceptible to the effects of demyelinating disease" (Shanon et al., 1979). Wave I results are more complex due to the anatomical composition and functional structure of the auditory nerve where the myelin sheath is formed. Demyelination results in increased refraction period of transmission of the axons with reduced conduction velocity along the central auditory pathways, yielding delays in latency of progressive waves of the AEP. (Lacquaniti et al., 1979; Thornton and Hawkes, 1976).

In the final analysis, clinicians should not expect to find a homogeneous pattern of test results in the described patient population. Further, it is worthy of repeating that ABR abnormalities are not specific to the identification of multiple sclerosis. Robinson and Rudge (1980) note that the ABR is similar to many tests of the CNS in that it merely indicates dysfunctional abnormality of the system. Nevertheless, ABR testing is a cost-effective method of assessing the integrity of the auditory system, and provides important information that is used in the diagnosis of degenerative and space occupying lesions of the auditory nervous system.

REFERENCES

Adams, R. and Kubik, C. (1952). Morbid anatomy of the demyelinative diseases. *American Journal of Medicine, 12*, 510.

Alter, M. (1980). The geographic distribution of multiple sclerosis: New concepts. In H.J. Bauer, S. Poser, and G. Ritter (eds.), *Progress in multiple sclerosis research*, pp. 495–502. Berlin: Springer-Verlag.

Anderson, D.C., Slater, G.E., Sherman, R., and Ettinger, M.G. (1987). Evoked potentials to test a treatment of chronic multiple sclerosis. *Archives of Neurology, 44*, 1232–1236.

Antonelli, A. and DeMitri, T. (1963). Reperti audiometrici nella sclerosi a placche. *Sistema Nervosa, 15*, 138–145.

Antonelli, A.R., Bonfioli, F., Cappiello, J., Peretti, G., Zanetti,

D., and Capra, R. (1988). Auditory evoked potentials test battery related to magnetic resonance imaging for multiple sclerosis patients. *Scandinavian Audiology Supplement, 30,* 191–196.

Baloh, R. and Honrubia, V. (1979). *Clinical neurophysiology of the vestibular system.* Philadephia, PA: Davis.

Barajas, J.J. (1982). Evaluation of ipsilateral and contralateral brainstem auditory evoked potentials in multiple sclerosis patients. *Journal of Neurological Sciences, 54,* 69–78.

Barratt, H.J., Miller, D., and Rudge, P. (1988). The site of lesion causing deafness in multiple sclerosis. *Scandinavian Audiology, 17,* 67–71.

Bauer, H.J. (1980). IMAB-enquete concerning the diagnostic criteria for MS. In H.J. Bauer, S. Poser, and G. Ritter (eds.) *Progress in multiple sclerosis research,* pp. 555–563. Berlin: Springer-Verlag.

Baumhefner, R.W., Tourtellotte, W.W., Syndulko, K., Waluch, V., Ellison, G.W., Myers, L.W., Cohen, S.N., Osborne, M., and Shapshak, P. (1990). Quantitative multiple sclerosis plaque assessment with magnetic potentials, and intra-blood-brain barrier IgG synthesis. *Archives of Neurology, 47(1),* 19–26.

Bosatra, A. (1977). Pathology of the nervous arc of the acoustic reflexes. *Audiology, 16,* 307–315.

Bosatra, A., Russola, M., and Poli, P. (1976). Oscilloscopic analysis of the stapedius muscle reflex in brain stem lesions. *Archives of Otolaryngology, 102,* 284–285.

Chiappa, K.H. (1980). Pattern shift visual, brainstem auditory, and short-latency somatosensory evoked potentials in multiple sclerosis. *Neurology, 30,* 110–123.

Chiappa, K.H., Harrison, J.L., Brooks, E.B., and Young, R.R. (1980). Brainstem auditory evoked responses in 200 patients with multiple sclerosis. *Annals of Neurology, 7,* 135–143.

Chiappa, K.H. and Norwood, A.E. (1977). Brainstem auditory evoked responses in clinical neurology: Utility and neuropathological correlates. *Electroencephalography and Clinical Neurophysiology, 43,* 518–527.

Chiappa, K.H. and Ropper, A.H. (1982). Evoked potentials in clinical medicine: Part I. *New England Journal of Medicine, 30,* 1140–1210.

Chiappa, K.H., Young, R.R., and Goldie, W.D. (1979). Origins of the components of human short latency somatosensory evoked responses. *Neurology, 29,* 598–604.

Citron, L., Dix, M.R., Hallpike, C.S., and Hood, J.D. (1963). A recent clinicopathological study of cochlear nerve degeneration resulting from tumor pressure and disseminated sclerosis with particular reference to the finding of

normal threshold sensitivity for pure tones. *Acta Oto-Laryngologica (Stockholm), 97,* 291–295.

Cohen, S.R., Brune, M.J., Herndon, R.M., and McKhann, G.M. (1980). Diagnostic value of myelin basic protein in cerebrospinal fluid. In H.J. Bauer, S. Poser, and G. Ritter, (eds.), *Progress in multiple sclerosis research,* pp. 161–168. Berlin: Springer-Verlag.

Cohen, S.R., Herndon, R.M., and McKhann, G.M. (1976). Radioimmunoassay of myelin basic protein in spinal fluid: An index of active demyelination. *New England Journal of Medicine, 295,* 1455–1457.

Colletti, V. (1975). Stapedius reflex abnormalities in multiple sclerosis. *Audiology, 14,* 63–71.

Cosi, V., Citterio, A., Battelli, G., Bergamaschi, R., Grampa, G., and Callieco, R. (1987). Multimodal evoked potentials in multiple sclerosis: A contribution to diagnosis and classification. *Italian Journal of Neurological Science, 6,* 109–112.

Daugherty, W.T., Lederman, R.J., Nodar, R.H., and Conomy, J.P. (1983). Hearing loss in multiple sclerosis. *Archives of Neurology, 40,* 33–35.

Dayal, V. and Swisher, L. (1967). Pure tone thresholds in multiple sclerosis. *Laryngoscope, 77,* 2169–2177.

Dayal, V.S., Tarantino, L., and Swisher, L.P. (1966). Neuro-otologic studies in multiple sclerosis. *Laryngoscope, 76,* 1798–1809.

De-Meirleir, L.J., Taylor, M.J., and Logan, W.J. (1988). Multimodal evoked potential studies in leukodystrophies of children. *Canadian Journal of Neurological Science, 15,* 26–31.

Detels, R., Visscher, B., Coulson, A., Malmgren, R., and Dudley, J. (1974). Multiple sclerosis in Japanese-Americans. A preliminary report. *International Journal of Epidemiology, 3,* 341–45.

Dix, M.R. (1965). Observations upon the nerve fibre deafness of multiple sclerosis, with particular reference to the phenomenon of loudness recruitment. *Journal of Laryngology and Otology, 79,* 695–706.

Don, M., Allen, A.R., and Starr, A. (1977). The effect of click rate on the latency of auditory brainstem responses in humans. *Annals of Otology, Rhinology, and Laryngology, 86,* 186–196.

Feldman, J.I., Kearns, D.B., Seid, A.B., Pransky, S.M., and Jones, M.C. (1990). The otolaryngologic manifestations of Pelizaeus-Merzbacher disease. *Archives of Otolaryngology—Head and Neck Surgery, 116,* 613–616.

Fischer, C., Mauguiere, F., Ibanez, V., Confavreux, C., and Chazot, G. (1985). The acute deafness of definite multiple sclerosis: BAEP patterns. *Electroencephalography and Clinical Neurophysiology, 61,* 7–15.

Franklin, D.J., Coker, N.J., and Jenkins, H.A. (1989). Sudden sensorineural hearing loss as a presentation of multiple sclerosis. *Archives of Otolaryngology—Head and Neck Surgery, 115*, 41–45.

Furnman, J.M., Durrant, J.D., and Hirsch, W.L. (1989). Eighth nerve signs in a case of multiple sclerosis. *American Journal of Otolaryngology, 10(6)*, 376–81.

Garza, Y.A. (1981). Acoustic reflex dynamics and auditory brainstem responses in normal and multiple sclerosis subjects. Unpublished master's thesis. University of Cincinnati, Cincinnati.

Garza, Y.A., Keith, R.W., and Barajas, J. (1982). Acoustic reflex latency and auditory brainstem, response in multiple sclerosis. Presented at the International Symposium on Evoked Potentials, Cleveland, Ohio.

Geraund, G., Coll, J., Arne-Bes, C., Arbus, L., Lacomme, Y., and Bes, A. (1982). Brainstem auditory evoked potentials in multiple sclerosis: Influence of body temperature increase. *Advances in Neurology, 32*, 501–505.

Goto, I., Kobayashi, T., Antoku, et al., (1986). Adrenoleukodystrophy and variants. *Journal of Neurological Science, 72*, 103–112

Grenman, R., Lang, H., Panelius, M., et al. (1982). Stapedius reflex and brainstem auditory evoked responses in multiple sclerosis patients. *Scandinavian Audiology, 13*, 109–113.

Guthrie, T.C. (1951). Visual and motor changes in patients with multiple sclerosis. *Archives of Neurology and Psychiatry, 64*, 437–451.

Hammond, S.R. and Yiannikas, C. (1987). The relevance of contralateral recordings and patient disability to assessment of brainstem auditory evoked potential abnormalities in multiple sclerosis. *Archives of Neurology, 44*, 382–387.

Hammond, S.R., Yiannikas, C., and Chan, Y.W. (1986). A comparison of brainstem auditory evoked responses evoked by rarefaction and condensation stimulation in control subjects and in patients with Wenicke-Korsakoff syndrome and multiple. *Journal of Neurological Science, 74(2–3)*, 177–90.

Hankins, R.W. and Black, F.L. (1986). Western blot analyses of measles virus antibody in normal persons and in patients with multiple sclerosis, subacute sclerosing panencephalitis, or atypical measles. *Journal of Clinical Microbiology, 24(3)*, 324–329.

Hannley, M., Jerger, J.F., and Rivera, V. (1983). Relationships among auditory brain stem responses, masking level differences and the acoustic reflex in multiple sclerosis. *Audiology, 22*, 20–33.

Hansen, P.H. and Christiansen, C.B. (1985). Sudden deafness in multiple sclerosis. *Ugeskr Laeger, 147*, 711–712

Hausler, R. and Levine, R. (1980). Brainstem auditory evoked potentials are related to interaural time discrimination in patients with multiple sclerosis. *Brain Research, 191*, 589–594.

Hecox, K., Cone, B., and Blaw, M.E. (1981). Brainstem auditory evoked response in the diagnosis of pediatric neurological disease. *Neurology, 31*, 832–839.

Hess, K. (1979). Stapedius reflex in multiple sclerosis. *Journal of Neurology, Neurosurgery, and Psychiatry, 42*, 331–337.

Hopf, H.C. and Eysholdt, M. (1978). Impaired refractory periods of peripheral sensory nerves in multiple sclerosis. *Annals of Neurology, 4*, 499–501.

Hopf, H.C. and Maurer, K. (1983). Wave I of early auditory evoked potentials in multiple sclerosis. *Electroencephalography and Clinical Neurophysiology, 56*, 31–37.

Hyde, M.L., Stephens, S.D.G., and Thornton, A.R.D. (1976). Stimulus repetition rate and the early brainstem responses. *British Journal of Audiology, 10*, 41–50.

Jacobson, G. and Newman, C. (1989). Absence of rate-dependent BAEP P5 latency changes in patients with definite multiple sclerosis: Possible physiological mechanisms. *Electroencephalography and Clinical Neurophysiology, 74*, 19–23.

Jacobson, J.T., Deppe, U., and Murray, T.J. (1983). Dichotic paradigms in multiple sclerosis. *Ear and Hearing, 4*, 311–317.

Jacobson, J.T. and Jacobson, G.P. (1990). The auditory brainstem response in multiple sclerosis. *Seminars in Hearing, 11(3)*, 248–264.

Jacobson, J.T., Murray, T.J., and Deppe, U. (1987). The effects of ABR stimulus repetition rate in multiple sclerosis. *Ear and Hearing, 8*, 115–120.

Javidan, M., McLean, D.R., and Warren, K.G. (1986). Cerebral evoked potentials in multiple sclerosis. *Canadian Journal of Neurological Science, 13*, 240–244.

Jerger, J., Oliver, T., Chimiel, R., and Rivera, V. (1986b). Patterns of auditory abnormality in multiple sclerosis. *Audiology, 25*, 193–209.

Jerger J, Oliver, T.A, Rivera, V., and Stach B.A. (1986a). Abnormalities of the acoustic reflex in multiple sclerosis. *American Journal of Otolaryngology, 7*, 163–176.

Johnson, K.P. and Nelson, B.J. (1977). Multiple sclerosis: Diagnostic usefulness of cerebrospinal fluid. *Annals of Neurology, 2*, 425–501.

Kawahara, H., Tomita, Y., Takashima, S., Nishimura, S., and Takeshita, K. (1988). Neurophysiological and neuropathological studies in two children with unusual form of multiple system degeneration. *Brain Development, 10,* 312–318.

Keith, R.W. and Garza-Holquin, Y. (1987). Acoustic reflex dynamics and auditory brainstem responses in multiple sclerosis. *American Journal of Otology, 8,* 406–413.

Kimura, J. (1989). *Electrodiagnosis in diseases of nerve and muscle: Principles and practice,* Edition 2. Philadephia, PA: F.A. Davis Company.

Kinnunen, E., Juntunen, J. Ketonen, L., Koskimies, S., Konttinen, Y.T., Salmi, T., Koskenvuo, M., and Kaprio, J. (1988). Genetic susceptibility to multiple sclerosis. A co-twin study of a nationwide series. *Archives of Neurology, 45(10),* 1108–1111.

Kjaer, M. (1980). Variations of brain stem auditory evoked potentials correlated to duration and severity of multiple sclerosis. *Acta Neurologica Scandinavia, 61,* 157–166.

Kofler, F., Oberascher, G., and Pommer, B. (1984). Brain-stem involvement in multiple sclerosis: A comparison between brain-stem auditory evoked potentials and the acoustic stapedius reflex. *Journal of Neurology, 231,* 145–147.

Krevit, W., Lipton, M.E., Lockman, L.A., et al. (1987). Prevention of deterioration in metachromatic leukodystrophy by bone marrow transplantation. *American Journal of Medical Science, 294,* 80–85.

Kurkland, L. and Reed, D. (1964). Geographic and climatic aspects of multiple sclerosis: A review of current hypotheses. *American Journal of Public Health, 54,* 588–597.

Kurokawa, T., Chaen, Y.J., Nagata, M., Hasuo, K., et al. (1987). Late infantile Krabbe leukodystrophy. *Neuropediatrics, 18,* 182–183.

Lacquaniti, F., Benna, P., Gillis, M., Trone, W., and Bergamasco, B. (1979). Brainstem auditory evoked potentials and blink reflexes in quiescent multiple sclerosis. *Electroencephalography and Clinical Neurophysiology, 47,* 607–610.

Lammoglia, F.J., Short, S.R., Sweet, D.E., Pay, N., and Abay, E.A. (1989). Multiple sclerosis presenting as an intramedullary cervical cord tumor. *Kansas Medicine, 90(7),* 219–221.

Leibowitz, V., Alter, M., and Halper, L. (1964). Clinical studies of multiple sclerosis in Israel: III. Clinical course and prognosis related to age of onset. *Neurology, 14,* 926.

LeZak, R.J. and Selhub, S. (1966). On hearing in multiple sclerosis. *Annals of Otology, Rhinology, and Laryngology, 75,* 1102–1110.

Lynn, G., Taylor, P., and Gilroy, J. (1980). Auditory evoked potentials in multiple sclerosis. *Electroencephalography and Clinical Neurophysiology, 50,* 167 (Abstract).

Matathias, O., Sohmer, H., and Biton, V. (1985). Central auditory tests and auditory nerve-brainstem evoked responses in multiple sclerosis. *Acta Oto-Laryngologica (Stockholm), 99,* 369–376.

Matthews, W.B., Wattam-Bell, J.R.R., and Pountney, E. (1982). Evoked potentials in the diagnosis of multiple sclerosis. A follow-up study. *Journal of Neurology, Neurosurgery, and Psychiatry, 45,* 303–307.

Maurer, K. and Lowitzsch, L. (1982). Brainstem auditory evoked potentials in reclassification of 143 multiple sclerosis patients. *Advances in Neurology, 32,* 481–486.

McAlpine, D., Lumsden, C.E., and Acheson, E.D. (eds.) (1972). *Multiple sclerosis: A reappraisal.* Baltimore, MD: Williams and Wilkins.

Milanese, C., La-mantia, L., Salmaggi, A., et al. (1989). Double blind randomized trial of ACTH versus dexamethasone versus methylprednisolone in multiple sclerosis bouts. *European Neurology, 29,* 10–4.

Musiek, F., Gollegly, K.M., Kibbe, K.S., and Reeves, A.G. (1989). Electrophysiologic and behavioral auditory findings in multiple sclerosis. *The American Journal of Otology, 10,* 343–350.

Musiek, F.E., Weider, D.J., and Mueller, R.J. (1982). Audiologic findings in Charcot-Maria-Tooth disease. *Archives of Otolaryngology, 108,* 595–599.

Nager, G.T. (1969). Acoustic neurinomas. *Archives of Otolaryngology, 89,* 252–280.

Nodar, R.H. (1978). The effects of MS on brainstem auditory evoked potentials. Presented at the Annual Convention of the American Speech-Language-Hearing Association, San Francisco, California.

Noffsinger, D., Olsen, W.O., Carhart, R., Hart, C.W., and Sahgal, V. (1972). Auditory and vestibular aberrations in multiple sclerosis. *Acta Otolaryngologica, 303, Suppl.,* 1–63.

Nuwer, M.R., Visscher, B.R., Packwood, J.W., and Namerow, N.S. (1985). Evoked potential testing in relatives of multiple sclerosis patients. *Annals of Neurology, 18,* 30–34.

Paludetti, G., Ottaviani, F., Fallai, V., Tassoni, A., and Maurizi, M. (1985). Auditory brainstem responses (ABR) in multiple sclerosis. *Scandinavian Audiology, 14(1),* 27–34.

Parker, W., Decker, R., and Richards, N. (1968). Auditory function and lesions on the pons. *Archives of Otolaryngology, 87,* 26–38.

Parving, A., Elberling, C., and Smith, T. (1981). Auditory electrophysiology: Findings in multiple sclerosis. *Audiology, 20,* 123–142.

Pensak, M.L., Keith, R.W., Dignan, P., Stowens, D.W., Towbin, M.D., and Katbamna, B. (1989). Neuroaudiologic abnormalities in patients with Type I neurofibromatosis. *Laryngoscope, 99*, 702–706.

Pitt, M.C. and Rawles, J.M. (1989). The value of measuring saccadic eye movement in the investigation of non-compressive myelopathy. *Journal of Neurology, Neurosurgery, and Psychiatry, 52*, 1157–1161.

Pollack, M., Calder, C., and Allpress, S. (1977). Peripheral nerve abnormalities in multiple sclerosis. *Annals of Neurology, 2*, 41–48.

Poskanzer, D.C., Walker, A.M., Yokondz, J., and Sheridan, J.L. (1976). Studies in the epidemiology of multiple sclerosis in the Orkney and Shetland Islands. *Neurology, 26*, 14–17.

Posner, C.M. (1969). Disseminated vasculomyelinopathy: A review of the clinical pathologic reactions of the nervous system in hypergic diseases. *Acta Neurologica Scandinavica, 45, Suppl. 37*, 3–44.

Prasher, D.K. and Gibson, W. (1980). Brainstem auditory evoked potentials: A comparative study of monaural vs. binaural stimulation in the detection of multiple sclerosis. *Electroencephalography and Clinical Neurophysiology, 50*, 247–253.

Pratt, H. and Sohmer, H. (1976). Intensity and rate functions of cochlear and brainstem evoked responses to click stimuli in man. *Archives of Otology, Rhinology, and Laryngology, 212*, 85–92.

Pratt, H., Ben-David, Y., Reled, R., Podoshin, L., and Sharf, B. (1981). Auditory brain stem evoked potentials: Clinical promise of increasing stimulus rate. *Electroencephalography and Clinical Neurophysiology, 51*, 80–90.

Pryse-Phillips, W. and Murray, T.J. (1982). *Essential neurology.* Garden City, NY: Medical Examination Publishing Co.

Quaranta, A., Mininni, F., and Longo, G. (1986). ABR in multiple sclerosis. Ipsi versus contralateral derivation. *Scandinavian Audiology, 15*, 125–128.

Rivera, V.M. (1986). Multiple sclerosis: Is the mystery beginning to unfold? *Postgraduate Medicine, 79*, 217–232.

Rivera, V.M. (1990). The nature of multiple sclerosis. *Seminars in Hearing, 11(9)*, 207–220.

Robinson, K.H. and Rudge, P. (1977). Abnormalities of the auditory evoked potentials in patients with multiple sclerosis. *Brain, 100*, 19–40.

Robinson, K.H. and Rudge, P. (1975). Auditory evoked responses in mulitple sclerosis. *Lancet, 24*, 1164–1166.

Robinson, K.H. and Rudge, P. (1980). The use of the auditory evoked potential in the diagnosis of multiple sclerosis. *Journal of Neurological Science, 45*, 235–244.

Rose, R.M. and Daly, J.F. (1964). Reversible temporary threshold shift in multiple sclerosis. *Laryngoscope, 74*, 424–432.

Rowe, J. (1981). The brainstem auditory evoked response in neurologic disease. A review. *Ear and Hearing, 2*, 41–49.

Russolo, M. and Poli, P. (1983). Lateralization, impedance, auditory brainstem response, and synthetic sentence audiometry in brainstem disorders. *Audiology, 22*, 50–62.

Schumacher, G.A. (1971). Demyelinating diseases. In A.G. Baker and L.H. Baker (eds). *Clinical Neurology*, pp. 1–92. New York: Harper & Row.

Schumacher, G.A., Beebe, G., Kibler, R.F., Kurkland, L.T., et al. (1968). Problems of experimental trials of therapy in multiple sclerosis: Report by the panel on the evaluation of experimental trial of therapy in multiple sclerosis. *Annals of the New York Academy of Science, 122*, 552–568.

Schweitzer, V.G. and Shepard, N. (1989). Sudden hearing loss: an uncommon manifestation of multiple sclerosis. *Otolaryngology—Head and Neck Surgery, 100(4)*, 327–32.

Sears, T.A., Bostock, H., and Sherratt, M. (1978). The pathophysiology of myelination and its implication for the symptomatic treatment of multiple sclerosis. *Neurology, 28*, 21–26.

Shanon, E., Gold, S., and Himmelfarb, M. (1981). Assessment of functional integrity of brainstem auditory pathways of stimulus stress. *Audiology, 20*, 65–71.

Shanon, E., Gold, S., Himmelfarb, M., and Carasso, R. (1979). Auditory potentials of cochlear nerve and brainstem in multiple sclerosis. *Archives of Otolaryngology, 105*, 505–508.

Shea, J.J. and Brackmann, D.E. (1989). Multiple sclerosis manifesting as a sudden hearing loss. *Otolaryngology—Head and Neck Surgery, 97*, 335–338.

Simpkins, W.T. (1961). An audiometric profile in multiple sclerosis. *Archives of Otolaryngology, 73*, 557–563.

Smith, T., Zeeberg, I., and Sjo, O. (1986). Evoked potentials in multiple sclerosis before and after high-dose methylprednisolone infusion. *European Neurology, 25*, 67–73.

Starr, A. and Achor, J. (1975). Auditory brainstem responses in neurological disease. *Archives of Neurology, 32*, 761–768.

Stephens, S. and Thornton, A. (1976). Subjective and eletrophysiologic tests in brainstem lesions, *Archives of Otolaryngology, 102*, 608–613.

Stockard, J.J. and Rossiter, V.S. (1977). Clinical and pathological correlates of brainstem auditory response abnormalities. *Neurology, 27*, 316–325.

Stockard, J.J., Sharbrough, J.W., and Tinker, J.A. (1978). Effects of hypothermia on the human brainstem auditory response. *Annals of Neurology, 3*, 368–370.

Tackmann, W. and Vogel, P. (1987). Brainstem auditory evoked potentials evoked by clicks of different polarity in multiple sclerosis patients. *European Neurology, 26,* 193–198.

Tedeshi, G., Allocca, S., Di-Constanzo, A., et al. (1989). The contribution of saccadic eye movements analysis, visual and auditory evoked responses to the diagnosis of multiple sclerosis. *Clinical Neurology and Neurosurgery, 91,* 123–128.

Terkildsen, K., Osterhammel, P., and Huis in't Veld. (1975). Far-field electrocochleography adaptation. *Scandinavian Audiology, 4,* 215–220.

Thornton, A.R.D. and Coleman, M.J. (1975). The adaptation of cochlear brainstem auditory evoked potentials in humans. *Electroencephalography and Clinical Neurophysiology, 39,* 399–406.

Thornton, A.R.D. and Hawkes, C.H. (1976). Cochlear and brainstem evoked responses in multiple sclerosis. Read before the 13th International Congress of Audiology, Jerusalem, August.

Triantafyllou, N., Rombos, A., Athanasopoulou, H., and Siafakas, A. (1989). Electrophysiological study in patients with Charcot-Marie-Tooth disease. *Electromyography and Clinical Neurophysiology, 29,* 259–63.

van der Poel, J.C., Jones, S.J., and Miller, D.H. (1988). Sound lateralization, brainstem auditory evoked potentials and magnetic resonance imaging in multiple sclerosis. *Brain, 111,* 1453–1474.

Verma, N.P. and Lynn, G.E. (1985). Auditory evoked responses in multiple sclerosis: Wave I abnormality. *Archives of Otolaryngology, 111,* 22–24.

Waksman, B.H. and Reynold, W.E. (1982). *Research on multiple sclerosis.* New York: National Multiple Sclerosis Society.

Weber, B.A. and Fujikawa, S.M. (1977). Brainstem evoked response (BER) audiology at various stimulus presentation rates. *Journal of American Audiology Society, 3,* 59–62.

Wiegand, D.A. and Poch, N.E. (1988). The acoustic reflex in patients with asymptomatic multiple sclerosis. *American Journal of Otolaryngology, 9,* 210–216.

Yagi, T. and Kaga, K. (1979). The effect of the click repetition rate on the latency of the auditory evoked brain stem response and its clinical use for neurological diagnosis. *Archives of Otolaryngology, 222,* 91–97.

Zollner, C., Karnahl, T., and Stange, G. (1976). Input-output functions and adaptation behavior on the five early potentials registered with the earlobe-vertex pickup. *Archives of Otology, Rhinology, and Laryngology, 212,* 23–33.

NEUROPHYSIOLOGIC INTRAOPERATIVE MONITORING

PAUL R. KILENY
JOHN K. NIPARKO

INTRODUCTION

The medical literature of the 20th century, and in particular of the last three decades, documents a remarkable evolution in surgical techniques performed in proximity to the central and peripheral nervous systems. Early in this century, for example, acoustic neuroma removal was performed with little regard for the preservation of cranial nerve function. This practice reflected the formidable operative task of safely separating cranial nerves from tumor, as well as the complex surgical anatomy of the posterior fossa. Subsequent understanding of the anatomical relationships of cranial nerves, as well as advances in surgical instrumentation, greatly improved operative management of such tumors. In otology and neuro-otology in particular, the advent of refinements in operative techniques of temporal bone surgery has fostered a stronger emphasis on preservation of auditory and facial functions.

Along with the increased complexity of neuro-otologic and neurosurgical procedures, the sophistication of diagnostic tests based on electroneurophysiologic principles has also increased. This has contributed to the earlier diagnosis of neuro-otologic and neurologic problems, leading to the availability of earlier surgical intervention. One of the important contributions to this field was made by Jewett and his colleagues (1970) by discovering the auditory brain stem response (ABR). Subsequent early efforts by Starr and Achor (1975) and by Selters and Brackmann (1977, 1979) have contributed to the establishment of the ABR as a valuable neurodiagnostic tool. Today, the ABR is a universally accepted clinical neurophysiologic measure used, among other things, for the early detection of mass lesions of the cerebellopontine angle (CPA). Electromyography of facial muscles is also rapidly gaining acceptance as a neurophysiologic tool contributing to the diagnosis and management of facial nerve pathology.

Concern about preservation of neural function has provided the motivation for the development of neurophysiologic techniques applicable to providing feedback about the neurophysiologic status of neural structures during surgery. These intervention neurophysiology techniques complement the increasingly sophisticated microsurgical techniques, and in combination, have achieved improved preservation of facial and auditory function following acoustic neuroma resection, retrolabyrinthine vestibular nerve section, microvascular decompression of cranial nerves VII or VIII, and others. The emergence of intraoperative monitoring (IOM) as a legitimate adjunct in the surgical armamentarium of neurotologists and neurosurgeons has further enhanced the ability to perform surgical tasks in the posterior fossa, while averting neural injury.

What is IOM? What exactly does it involve? How does it differ from an outpatient neurodiagnostic procedure? How does a clinician performing IOM function in the operating room? We hope to provide answers to most of these questions on the subsequent pages of this chapter.

Several statements about the principles of IOM and our philosophy are in order at this point. In an editorial statement, Luetje (1989) warned that while facial and auditory nerve monitoring in neuro-otologic surgery may minimize intraoperative complications, it cannot replace the skill, experience, and clinical judgment of the surgeon. In addition to the potential for instilling a false sense of security in a novice surgeon, another potentially serious pitfall of IOM is to instill a sense of insecurity if monitored activity is not properly interpreted. IOM is a dynamic process involving positive interactive feedback and collaboration between the surgeon and the clinician responsible for IOM. Skill and experience play an important role in the surgery and an equally important role in determining the quality of IOM. The individual responsible for monitoring must have extensive experience in clinical neurophysiology, must understand the pathology of the lesion to be treated by surgery, and must be familiar with the surgical anatomy and technique. In addition, this must be an individual who appreciates the pace and flow of the surgical procedure. Intraoperative monitoring performed by such skilled individuals must be distinguished from non-attended IOM consisting solely of acoustical or other types of warning signals indicating possible contact or inadvertent stimulation of a neural structure. Surgery in the posterior fossa is sufficiently intricate to require more than bells and whistles, signals that distract rather than help the surgeon. The specific experience needed to become proficient in IOM will depend on an individual's background, motivation, and talents. Clearly, solid footing in the principles of neural stimulation and recording, electrophysiology, and surgical anatomy are all critical attributes of a training program. Precept or apprentice-type teaching may provide a valuable method of obtaining practical experience in the operative room. Although these educational activities cannot guarantee quality, they can serve as guidelines in developing a training program.

INTRAOPERATIVE MONITORING OF AUDITORY FUNCTION

The ABR is uniquely well-suited for neurophysiologic monitoring of surgical procedures in the posterior cranial fossa. Studies by Møller and Jannetta (1985) indicate that the neural generator sources of ABR peaks I through V extend from the cochlear nerve to the nucleus of the lateral lemniscus. The first two scalp-positive components, waves I and II, are generated by the distal and proximal segments of the cochlear nerve, respectively. The presence of two compound action potentials (CAP) originating from the same cranial nerve is attributed to the transition from neuroglial to Schwann's cell covering, just lateral to the porus acusticus. This transition is thought to be responsible for changes in neural conduction properties. Waves III and IV are associated with activity in the cochlear nucleus and the superior olivary complex, respectively. Wave V is associated with neural activity in the area of the nucleus of the lateral lemniscus.

Electrophysiologic Recording of Auditory Function

In most cases, the monitoring of the scalp-recorded ABR can reasonably assure the detection of intraoperative changes associated with auditory nerve or brain stem manipulation. However, other options also exist. Real-time feedback on the status of the auditory nerve can be obtained by monitoring the CAP of the cochlear nerve between porus acusticus and the brain stem, using a cotton wick or other type of electrode. Direct nerve monitoring necessitates an exposed cochlear nerve, and in acoustic neuroma surgery, can only be carried out after the resection of the extracanalicular portion of the neoplasm and the exposure of the cochlear nerve. The advantage of direct nerve monitoring is in its capacity to provide real-time moment-to-moment feedback obtained from the proximal segment of the auditory nerve. One inherent disadvantage is that this method, if not used in conjunction with simultaneous ABR recording, would not provide feedback about the condition of the auditory brain stem.

A third option is to monitor auditory function using one of the many variants of electrocochleographic recording, using a transtympanic needle electrode or some type of ear canal or tympanic membrane electrode. This technique enhances the first action potential of the cochlear nerve (wave I of the ABR), but necessitates some averaging, although somewhat less than that required for surface-recorded ABR. A combination of ABR, electrocochleography, and direct proximal nerve recording could be used alternately or simultaneously as the type and course of the surgery warrants.

ABR recording remains the most popular method for monitoring auditory function. With the use of a stimulus repetition rate of approximately 30 per second, a well-defined response may be obtained in an anesthetized patient after 256 to 512 sweeps. This results in an averaged response every 10 to 20 seconds. In addition, the observation of the buildup of the averaged response can provide some real-time information as well. We have often observed that during surgery, especially acoustic neuroma resection, desynchronization or deterioration of the averaged response occurs with surgical manipulation. In other words, instead of improving with averaging, the response actually deteriorates. This underscores the importance of monitoring the ongoing as well as the final averaged product.

Non-surgical Factors Affecting the ABR

Physiologic Factors. The purpose of neurophysiologic IOM is to help protect neural structures that may be at risk due to the nature of the surgical procedure by detecting and reporting changes in the monitored neurophysiologic response. However, neurophysiologic responses may also be adversely affected by nonsurgical physiologic and pharmacologic factors. Therefore, prior to associating an observed change in the neurophysiologic response with specific intraoperative events, one must be able to rule out possible physiologic and pharmacologic effects. The patient's altered state or environmental conditions in the operating room (relatively cold, contributing to localized hypothermia of the exposed surgical field) may alter the monitored neurophysiologic response (i.e., delay in response latency) similarly to intraoperative manipulation (i.e., retraction or compression).

Systemic physiologic changes may affect evoked potentials by interfering with normal metabolic and biochemical environments of neural structures. These changes may be manifested as a reduction or cessation of electrical activity, especially in areas with the highest metabolic needs. Oxygen supply, a basic metabolic component, may be impaired during surgery by way of

hypoxemia as a result of inadequate ventilation or due to excessive hemodilution. Systemic hypotension or regional ischemia may also bring about hypoxia by reducing perfusion. A specific phenomenon associated with the auditory receptor is the reduction of the endocochlear potential (thought to be generated by the stria vascularis) caused by anoxia. Konishi (1979) demonstrated that this coincides with a decrease in K+ concentration and an increase in Na+ concentration in the endolymph. A diminished endocochlear potential may in turn cause a decrease in the cochlear neural output and may affect all subsequent auditory electrophysiologic events. While hypoxia and hypercapnia adversely affect both the EEG and cortical evoked potentials, Sohmer and associates (1982) have shown that the ABR was resistant to both hypoxia and hypercapnia at levels that depressed both the EEG and cortical evoked potentials. The ABR also proved more resistant to the effects of systemic hypotension than the auditory middle latency response (MLR) when both were monitored during open heart surgery (Kileny et al., 1983).

Another important factor to consider during neurophysiologic IOM is hypothermia, which is known to interfere with synaptic transmission and neural conduction velocity as a result of a reduction of the enzymatic reactions necessary for neural activation. With progressive reductions in core body temperature, latencies of both auditory MLR and ABR become progressively prolonged (Kileny et al., 1983; Kaga et al., 1979; and Stockard et al., 1978). At 20–23°C measured in the nasopharynx, both the MLR and the ABR disappeared. Temperature reduction brings about delays in all three major ABR components, waves I, III, and V. The effect is cumulative, as the later components are delayed to a greater extent than the earlier ones. For instances, a reduction in body temperature of 2–4°C would bring about a I–III interpeak latency prolongation of up to 0.5 ms and a I.V. interpeak latency of up to 0.75 ms. In addition to a reduction in core body temperature, local hypothermia of the VIIIth or VIIth cranial nerves may occur as a result of exposure to the relatively colder operating room temperature or the introduction of cold irrigating solutions. This would not necessarily be associated with a reduction in temperature measured rectally or in the nasopharynx. Effective neurophysiologic monitoring involves, therefore, constant vigilance of the patient's vital signs, such as core body temperature, mean arterial pressure, or systolic and diastolic pressures, end-tidal carbon dioxide concentration, intracranial pressure, if available, as well as oxygen saturation hematocrit (Schwartz et al., 1988).

Pharmacologic Effects.   An unavoidable component of intraoperative neurophysiologic monitoring is the consideration needed to be given to the effects of anesthetic and other pharmacologic agents on the monitored bioelectric activity. The understanding of the physiologic events associated with the anesthetic state is incomplete. As a result, the effects of anesthetic agents on various evoked potentials or other bioelectric event cannot be predicted with certainty, since exact mechanism and site of action have yet to be precisely determined (Koblin and Eger, 1981). It is considered that anesthetics exert their effects by interacting with neural membranes and disrupt transmission in many parts of the central nervous system (CNS). The activity of excitatory synapses is depressed by reducing the magnitude of the post-synaptic depolarization caused by the release of acetylcholine. At higher doses, anesthetics may also block axonal conduction. Some anesthetics potentiate inhibitory synapses. For instance, barbiturates potentiate gamma-aminobutyric acid-mediated post-synaptic inhibition (Gage and Hamill, 1981).

The ABR is generally considered to be quite resistant to pharmacologic effects. Although mild to moderate changes in ABR amplitude and latency associated with certain pharmacologic agents have been documented, to date there is no documentation of a complete pharmacologic agent-related blockade of the ABR. Table 18.1 divides anesthetics and other pharmacologic agents that may be used during surgery into those that do not affect the ABR whatsoever and those that do have mild to moderate effects. For instance, fentanyl (an artificial narcotic agent), nitrous oxide (an inhalational anesthetic), and pentobarbital (a barbiturate) have no significant effects on the ABR. On the other hand, volatile anesthetics such as halothane or isoflurane may affect wave V latency or I-V interpeak latency. These volatile anesthetics depress neuronal activity and cerebral metabolic rate.

Those anesthetic agents that do affect the ABR usu-

TABLE 18.1.   Effects of Pharmacologic Agents on the ABR

No Effect	Adverse Effects
Althesin	Enflurane: Up to 1 ms wave V latency change
Anticholinergics	Halothane: Up to 0.5 ms delay in wave V latency
Etomidate	
Fentanyl	Isoflurane: Beyond 15% end-tidal concentration over 0.5 ms increase in I∠V interpeak latency
Ketamine	
Nitrous oxide	Lidocaine: Reduction of the amplitude and delay in the latency of wave V
Pentobarbital	Sodium thiopental: At very high doses (77.5 mg/1 kg), a 0.5 ms increase in wave V latency was documented

From Kileny, P.R. and Niparko, J.K. (1988). Interoperative monitoring of auditory and facial functions in neurotologic surgery. *Advances in Otolaryngology—Head and Neck Surgery, 1*, 55–88. Reprinted with permission

ally prolong interpeak latencies or predominantly the latencies of the later components of the response. At an end-tidal concentration of 3% of enflurane, the latency of wave V may be delayed by up to 1.0 ms (Thornton et al., 1984). Halothane may delay the absolute latency of wave V by up to 0.5 ms at end-tidal concentrations of up to 1.5%. Beyond 1.5% end-tidal concentration, isoflurane can prolong the I-V interpeak latency by 0.5 ms (Manninen et al., 1985). Lidocaine is sometimes administered intravenously to control myocardial irritability. Ruth et al. (1985) have studied the effects of lidocaine infusion in humans on the latency and amplitudes of the ABR components. While waves I and III remain unaffected, significant reductions in the amplitude and delays in the latency of wave V were documented by these investigators. At very high doses (77.5 mg/kg), sodium thiopental has been documented to introduce a 0.5 ms increase in wave V latency (Drummond et al., 1985).

In summary, while the ABR is in general very resistant to anesthetic and non-anesthetic pharmacologic agents, it is not totally immune to these effects. Therefore, during IOM with the ABR, careful note must be taken of pharmacologic agents administered to the patient, in order to be able to rule out surgical effects on changes in latency or amplitude.

IOM with the ABR and CN VIII AP: Technical Factors

The Operating Room Environment.   Involvement in IOM thrusts audiologists/neurophysiologists into a working environment that is very likely unfamiliar to most. It is therefore important to first become acquainted with the operating room environment, including the concepts of sterile fields and procedures, and with the roles of the various professionals working in this environment. It is also important to become acquainted with the general working conditions, priorities, and typical work pace in an operating room. In addition to the surgical team, usually consisting of a staff surgeon assisted by one or more resident surgeons or a physician's assistant, there are usually at least two operating room nurses (one who is circulating, the other the scrub nurse assisting the surgical team) and the anesthesia team, consisting of an anesthesiologist, a certified registered nurse anesthetist or both. Equally important to becoming acquainted with the various functions these professionals fulfill in the operating room is communicating effectively the role of the audiologist (or neurophysiologist) who will perform IOM, in order to become integrated into the operating room team. Since neurophysiologic IOM is the latest addition to the operating room team, prior to initiating a monitoring program, its roles, limitations, and physical needs must be discussed with all of the operating room staff. Operating rooms often provide limited space for all of the new technology that has been introduced during the past decade; therefore, the introduction of yet another piece of equipment may be problematic. However, it has been the authors' experience that effective interaction with the operating room team leads to a collegial and cooperative willingness to accommodate these new needs. In moving about the operating room, one needs to be extremely cautious to avoid violating sterile fields, which include instrument tables, the surgical team, and the patient. Prior to first entering the operating room, it makes good sense to enlist the help of an experienced colleague to learn about adequate attire, placement of the surgical mask, shoe covers, etc. In addition, it is also important to learn the functions of all electronic instrumentation used in the operating room, including electrocoagulators, various anesthesia monitors, and surgical instruments, such as ultrasonic dissectors and lasers. Last but not least, it is necessary to become familiar with universal precautions for the avoidance of contact with body fluids and to know the measures to be taken if such contact occurs (Center for Disease Control, 1988; American Speech-Language Hearing Association, 1990).

Patient Preparation.   It is the audiologist's (or neurophysiologist's) responsibility to prepare the patient for monitoring prior to the preparation of the surgical field and subsequent placement of surgical drapes. It is important to remember that beyond this point, access to the patient for the purpose of adjustments of equipment is virtually impossible. Therefore, extreme care needs to be taken in securing electrodes and transducers. For the purpose of auditory stimulation, we recommend the use of insert transducers. Coupling to the ear canal is achieved by means of a soft, approximately 10 cm polyethylene (Wilber et al., 1988) tube ending with a disposable foam plug coupled to the tube by means of its own rigid polyethylene tube and a nipple. Extreme care needs to be taken with the placement of the foam plug and the routing of the polyethylene tube to avoid extruding the plug or compressing the tube during surgery. Therefore, the plug needs to be placed deep into the ear canal—if possible, far medially, into the bony portion of the canal. The polyethylene tube needs to be routed in such a way as to avoid compression during surgery or even prior to surgery, when the pinna is often reflected anteriorly to accommodate a postauricular incision. If the rigid polyethylene coupler belonging to the foam plug protrudes from the ear canal, this maneuver can kink this tube and cut off the delivery of the acoustic stimuli. Therefore, we often cut off half or more of this tube in order to avoid this problem. The placement of the foam plug too laterally may result in the extrusion of the foam plug following a postauricular incision with the placement of a self-retaining retractor to keep the incision open. This self-retaining retractor often rests against the cartilaginous portion of the canal, and with pressure can expel the foam plug. In order to avoid the seepage into the ear canal of disinfectant solutions used to prepare the surgical area, following the placement of the foam plug, it is also helpful to pack the ear canal with bone wax and a cotton ball. The cotton ball may soak up some of the excess solution and may be removed at the completion of the preparation.

Secure and appropriate placement of recording electrodes is equally important. It is recommended that until an individual becomes comfortable and competent with preoperative patient preparation, each electrode have a double available to connect to the recording equipment, in case the other fails for any reason. The use of subdermal needle electrodes is recommended for both evoked potential monitoring and electromyographic muscle function monitoring. Unless they come pre-sterilized, these electrodes must be cleaned and sterilized prior to use. For patient and clinical staff safety, it is recommended that pre-sterilized single-use disposable needle electrodes be used for this purpose. At the completion of the procedure, these electrodes are removed and appropriately discarded into the "sharps" disposal container. The electrodes need to be adequately secured with waterproof plastic tape with a strong adhesive. Prior to electrode placement, electrode sites need to be cleaned with alcohol or other disinfectant solution. Care must be taken to place these electrodes in such a way as to avoid any possible injury during surgery due to dislocation of an electrode or pressure exerted on an electrode. Therefore, prior to establishing a protocol, the surgical team needs to be consulted on their preferences and limitations. For patient safety, placement of a ground electrode in such a manner that its lead will cross the heart should be avoided. While this is usually the responsibility of the nursing or medical staff in the operating room, the individual responsible for neurophysiologic monitoring needs to ascertain that the ground electrode on the monopolar electrocoagulator has been properly placed, secured, and connected. Failure of this may result in

electrode burns caused by current being shunted by the needle electrodes used for monitoring.

Artifacts.   In spite of careful patient preparation, electrical artifacts obscuring and distorting the intended response are not altogether avoidable. Electrical artifacts specific to the operating room environment may be divided into two general groups:

1. First, there are transient but unavoidable artifacts, such as those associated with the use of a specific powered surgical instrument (such as a monopolar or bipolar electrocoagulator or cutter or an ultrasonic dissecting device). These instruments are used from time to time for various lengths of time by the surgeon for tumor resection or hemostasis purposes. It is important that everyone concerned, the surgical and the monitoring team, be aware that during the use of such instrumentation, electrophysiologic responses may be non-interpretable. If it is necessary to use these instruments for relatively prolonged periods of time, an agreement needs to be made with the surgical team a priori to provide periodic breaks in order to allow effective neurophysiologic monitoring.

2. The other type of artifact is a constant electrical interference that may originate from poorly grounded equipment, electrical radiation from other monitoring equipment such as the equipment used by the anesthesiologist, or other electrical sources. This type of artifact is more troublesome because of its constant nature and because its source is not always identifiable. Not all constant electrical artifacts take the form of 60-cycle interference. High-frequency interference may originate, for instance, from cathode ray tubes, which may be part of the IOM equipment or the anesthesia monitoring equipment. Proximity to cables attached to the EKG electrodes may result in an EKG artifact. These types of artifacts need to be dealt with in a systematic manner. First, the monitoring team needs to be aware of the various types of artifacts produced by the various types of instrumentation in a specific operating room. This, in our experience, changes from one room to the next. Therefore, familiarity with one specific operating room may not help to solve problems next door. Moving electrode cables, patient interface connectors, and preamplifiers often solve many of these problems. It is important to remember to avoid sharing an electrical outlet with other electronic monitoring or dissecting equipment. At times, the best attempts fail to completely obliterate these constant artifacts. That is when the knowledge of general electrophysiology takes over. Recording parameters may need to be changed, especially the cutoff settings of the band-pass filter. It is important to have a good understanding of the general effects of filter cutoff settings on the specifically recorded response in order to facilitate continued interpretation of the response.

Intraoperative ABR Protocol

Prior to initiating an IOM program, it is necessary to establish a fixed protocol designed to assist in the various procedures. At times, different protocols need to be developed for the same EP modality, depending on the specific application. Other times, the same protocol may serve a variety of applications. In general, an intraoperative protocol should maximize efficacy, reliability, and flexibility.

The intraoperative ABR protocol begins outside the operating room during preoperative outpatient testing. Even when the diagnosis is known and the patient has had previous diagnostic ABR tests, it is imperative to establish a preoperative baseline outside the operating room. This is in order to provide the clinician with information about the status of the response. For instance, the ABR of patients with acoustic neuroma may change rather rapidly. A preoperative absence of an ABR may negate its use in the operating room in a hearing preservation attempt. On the other hand, if the patient presents preoperatively with a poor click-evoked response and a reasonable and replicable tone-pip response, that may be the choice for IOM. Once in the operating room, it is desirable to re-establish a pre-anesthesia baseline response, which may differ from the response obtained in the outpatient clinic because of the electronic environment, patient positioning, or the often reduced body temperature of the patient. It is also important to establish a pre-anesthesia response in order to check the equipment, electrode and transducer reliability, and other factors. This may also be the time

that some troubleshooting may be necessary to manage electrical artifacts. A new baseline needs to be established following the induction of anesthesia, as some anesthetics may affect the ABR to some extent. It is important to monitor the ABR prior to opening the dura mater, primarily for the purpose of determining equipment reliability. The true preoperative baseline is established following opening of the dura and prior to the positioning of the retractors. This will serve as the intraoperative reference regarding changes associated with retractor placement, dissection, irrigation, and the administration of additional pharmacologic agents by the anesthesiologist. Throughout this period, the clinician responsible for IOM needs to remain vigilant regarding any changes in the patient's vital signs. Constant communication with the anesthesia staff is therefore of paramount importance.

Monitoring continues throughout the procedure, with the role of the clinical neurophysiologist now being to correlate changes in the electrophysiologic response with the surgical procedure (retractor placement, surgical dissection, etc.) referenced to changes in the anesthesia regimen, body temperature, etc. In addition to serial evoked response recording and the measurement of latencies and amplitudes, monitoring the ongoing continuous electrophysiologic activity (essentially the EEG) is also very important. One can often see changes in ongoing baseline activity related to surgical manipulations. Furthermore, the buildup of the averaged response also needs to be monitored at the same time. For instance, it is important to note a sudden deterioration of the averaged response associated with an intraoperative event after it had been building up predictably with averaging. This deterioration in configuration may also coincide with a sudden increase in baseline activity. Depending upon previously established criteria, changes in response status need to be communicated to the surgical team. The surgical team then will have the option of taking corrective action if possible. For instance, if the maximum wave V latency prolongation established for a certain procedure is 3.0 ms, the surgical team needs to be informed about gradual changes in wave V latency associated with the procedure. Thus, if wave V latency prolongation reaches 1.5 ms, based on the previously established protocol, the surgeon may remove or reposition the retractors for the time needed for wave V to return to baseline value or for the prolongation to be reduced by 0.5 ms. The overall principle of such intraoperative protocols is to avoid warnings with extreme changes when it may be too late to take corrective action.

Clinical Applications

As indicated in the previous section, the principle of IOM of auditory function is an interactive process consisting of on-line interpretation of changes in consecutively obtained electrophysiological responses, their correlation with surgical events, and the communication of significant changes to the surgical team. This provides the surgical team with the opportunity to take corrective action whenever possible in an effort to maximize preservation of hearing.

Any surgical procedure involving the posterior cranial fossa and cerebellar retraction for the purpose of access to the CPA can benefit from auditory function monitoring. The purpose is to avoid irreversible changes associated with direct or indirect manipulation of the auditory nerve and the brain stem. The following procedures can benefit from auditory function monitoring: 1) acoustic neuroma resection with planned hearing preservation (suboccipital or transtemporal approach); 2) vestibular nerve section; 3) microvascular decompression of cranial nerves V–IX; 4) resection of meningiomas in the CPA; 5) the resection of schwannomas of cranial nerves V, VII, and IX; 6) skull base tumors and others. Most of these procedures involve cerebellar retraction, resulting in a lateral to medial traction of the VIIIth cranial nerve (Sekiya et al., 1986). In addition to this particular risk factor, acoustic neuroma resection involves an increase risk associated with the intent to remove tumor and leave the VIIIth cranial nerve intact.

Although some of the intraoperative risk factors differ between the various surgical procedures in the vicinity of the cerebello-pontine angle and the VIII cranial nerve, the principles are similar. For instance, in both vestibular nerve section and microvascular decompression of nerves VII, VIII or IX one of the risk factors is cerebellar retraction. The specific risk factor in vestibular nerve section is the separation of the cochlear and vestibular branches of the VIIIth cranial nerve and the division of the vestibular branch. In microvascular decompression, the specific risk factor is the placement of the Teflon sponge to separate the vascular loop creating symptoms from the affected cranial nerve. The concept of attempting to maintain the integrity of the auditory brainstem response or the action potential of the VIIIth cranial nerve is the same. This can be achieved through continuous monitoring and the initiation of corrective action, such as retractor relaxation, until the response recovers or a change of the angle of retraction. At times however, due to the nature of the pathology, irreversible changes may be unavoidable.

Suboccipital Resection of Acoustic Neuroma. The following case illustrates the application of intraoperative ABR monitoring in the resection of an acoustic neuroma with planned hearing preservation.

A 42-year old male patient was diagnosed with a 1 cm intracanalicular acoustic neuroma. Preoperatively his pure-tone audiogram indicated hearing within normal limits in the affected ear with excellent speech recognition scores, as shown in Figure 18.1. Tumor size, pure-tone thresholds, and speech recognition scores all fulfilled our criteria for planned hearing preservation via the suboccipital approach (Kemink et al., 1990). His preoperative ABR was grossly intact with waves I, III and V, replicable and easily identified. The I–III interpeak latency was prolonged (2.57 ms) and fulfilled our diagnostic criteria for retrocochlear involvement (I–III > 2.30 ms; Kileny et al., 1991a).

Following anesthesia, the patient was placed in the lateral decubitus position and his head was fixed in a Mayfield head holder. Once in position, subdermal needle electrodes were placed for ABR monitoring and for facial EMG monitoring. The ABR electrodes were placed at FP_Z, anterior to the tragus of the right, operated ear and the right shoulder (ground). The foam plug of the ER3A acoustic transducer was placed in the external ear canal as described earlier, and the lateral end of the ear canal was packed with bone wax to avoid the infiltration of the liquid surgical disinfectant used to scrub the surgical site. Figure 18.2 illustrates the intraoperative ABR sequence obtained during the re-

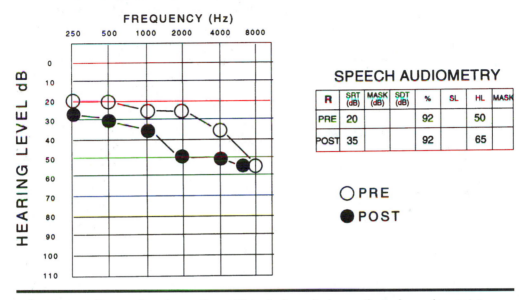

RIGHT EAR
1 cm AN: PRE & POSTOP AUDIOGRAM

SPEECH AUDIOMETRY

R	SRT (dB)	MASK (dB)	SDT (dB)	%	SL	HL	MASK
PRE	20			92		50	
POST	35			92		65	

○ PRE
● POST

FIGURE 18.1.   Pre- and postoperative audiological results in a patient who underwent a suboccipital resection of an acoustic neuroma with hearing preservation.

section of this patient's acoustic neuroma. The top trace is the preoperative diagnostic ABR obtained a few days prior to surgery. The second trace was obtained following the establishment of anesthesia and upon completing the preoperative preparation but prior to draping in order to allow for any adjustments that may be necessary. Note the stability of wave I and the mild delay of waves III and V that may be attributed to the isoflurane used as the main anesthetic agent in this case. The opening of the dura and the beginning of cerebellar retraction to allow access to the cerebello-pontine angle affected the ABR peak latencies minimally however, there is an overall reduction of amplitude probably due to moderate desynchronization. An increase in retraction further delayed waves III and V (0.76 ms for wave III and 0.65 ms for wave V with respect to the post-anesthesia baseline). Nevertheless, the retractors were relaxed momentarily to allow for some recovery and an excellent ABR was obtained at this point with a wave V latency nearly identical to

baseline and an increased amplitude. Retraction was increased again to allow the exposure of the petrous apex and drilling was started to expose the IAC and the acoustic neuroma within. Recording ABR during drilling is not very informative due to the masking effect of the drill, therefore, it is recommended that the surgeon take occasional breaks and a sample can then be obtained during that time. The third trace illustrates the effect of tumor dissection in the IAC following its exposure. At this point, wave V was further delayed. The next trace was obtained immediately following the successful resection of the tumor which left the cochlear nerve intact and was characterized by a reduction of wave V latency. The last trace illustrates the effects of completely removing the retractors just prior to closing. The ABR is well defined: wave V latency is prolonged by less than 0.5 ms with respect to the post-anesthesia baseline; wave III latency is, in fact at this point, reduced when compared to the post-anesthesia baseline by 0.3 ms. One can speculate that the comple-

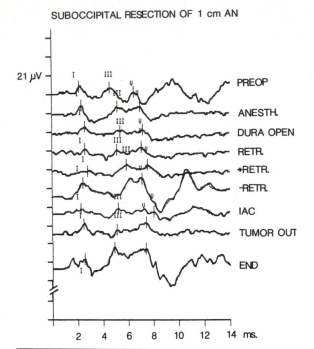

SUBOCCIPITAL RESECTION OF 1 cm AN

FIGURE 18.2.   Intraoperative ABR sequence during the suboccipital resection of an acoustic neuroma with hearing preservation in the patient illustrated in Figure 18.1.

tion of tumor resection and the cessation of compression of the cochlear nerve may have contributed to this. The patient's postoperative audiogram is illustrated in Figure 18.1; hearing and speech recognition scores remained within normal limits with minimal postoperative change.

We recently reviewed the IOM records of 29 patients who underwent suboccipital acoustic neuroma resection with planned hearing preservation (Kileny et al., 1992). Mean tumor size in this group was 1.69 cm (standard deviation, 0.84 cm). Wave V, at least, was identifiable in all preoperative ABRs from these patients. Table 18.2 summarizes postoperative outcome and intraoperative ABR changes in these cases. Hearing preservation was successful in 15 of these cases (52%). The criteria for successful postoperative hearing preservation was discussed in detail by Kemink et al. (1990) and involved a less than 20 dB elevation of

SRT and a less than 15% reduction in speech recognition scores. At no time during the course of surgery was wave V of the ABR lost in these 15 cases. The mean maximal wave V latency shift for this group was 1.17 ms (standard deviation, 0.86 ms). Figure 18.3 charts changes in wave I and V latency during the suboccipital resection of 1.0 cm acoustic neuromas in two different patients. In the first case (Figure 18.3A), hearing was successfully preserved. The latency of wave I remained stable throughout the various intraoperative manipulations but there were more appreciative changes in wave V latency. These latency changes culminated during tumor dissection in the IAC. At the end of the procedure, wave V latency was only slightly delayed with respect to its baseline value.

In the second case (Figure 18.3B), the latency of wave I also remained stable throughout the procedure, however, wave V latency increased progressively, was lost during tumor dissection in the IAC, and returned with substantially delayed with respect to baseline toward the end of the operation. Post-operatively, this patient presented with measurable but nonfunctional hearing characterized by an 80 dB elevation of the average pure-tone threshold and an absence of appreciable speech recognition.

In our experience, the strongest prognostic indicator in auditory function monitoring in acoustic neuroma surgery is the preservation of an intact ABR. Since wave V is the most robust ABR component, it is often necessary to rely on its configuration and latency in neurophysiologic IOM. The preservation and stability of wave I alone is not a good prognostic indicator in hearing preservation. It appears that even the temporary loss of wave V constitutes a poor prognosis. While one of the main concerns in acoustic neuroma surgery with hearing preservation is the onset of a vascular insult affecting the cochlea (Sekiya et al., 1986), the loss of wave V or waves III and V while wave I remains intact would indicate a destruction of the more proximal components of the auditory pathway.

The following case presentation illustrates the interactive decision-making process leading to acoustic neuroma resection with planned hearing preservation. Furthermore, it illustrates the role that IOM can play in determining the final outcome.

TABLE 18.2. Intraoperative ABR monitoring in suboccipital acoustic neuroma surgery (*n*=29; tumor size: 1.69/0.84 cm)

	Successful result	*Poor result*	*No measurable hearing*
Number	15 (52%)	5 (17%)	9 (31%)
Tumor size	1.73/1.01 cm	1.5/2.0 cm	1.74/0.71 cm
Wave V	+1.17/0.86 ms	V lost (*n*=2)	V lost
		V delayed: 2.70–4.30 ms	

A 64-year-old female patient with a profound hearing loss in her left ear since early childhood was referred to us with a history of progressive, sensorineural hearing loss in her right ear. She had first noted a hearing impairment in her right ear approximately six years prior to being referred to our clinic and has had amplification for the past four years. Her main complaint was that she no longer benefited from amplification and that she had increasing difficulty to communicate. Pure-tone audiometry (Figure 18.4) indicated a profound hearing loss in the left ear and a mild-to-severe high-frequency sensorineural hearing loss in her right ear. Speech recognition was extremely reduced at 28%. Auditory brainstem response evaluation was car-

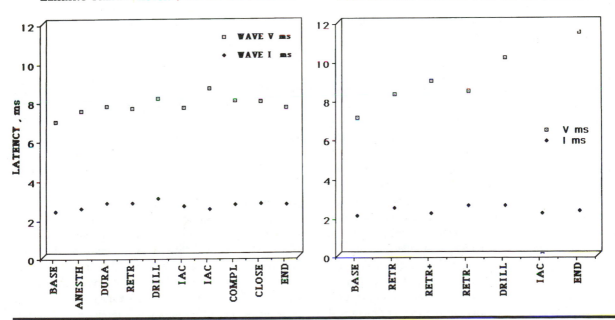

FIGURE 18.3. Graphs charting wave I and V latency changes during suboccipital resections of 1 cm acoustic neuromas in two patients.

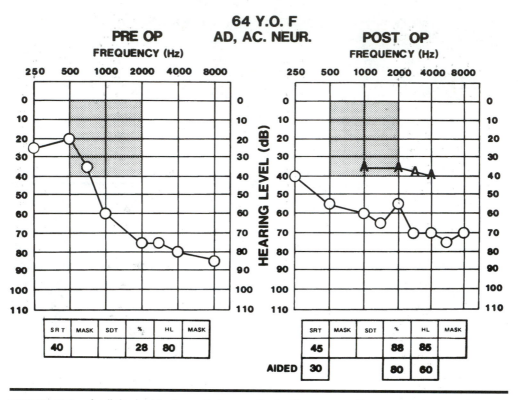

FIGURE 18.4. Audiological test results in a patient with an acoustic neuroma in an only hearing ear planned for subtotal resection with hearing preservation.

ried out and reasonably well replicated responses were obtained following right ear stimulation with 95 dB clicks. The response was characterized by poor morphology and an extended I–V innerpeak latency at 6.91 ms. A CT scan with contrast demonstrated a 3.5 cm right-sided acoustic neuroma. Since tumor size and preoperative hearing were outside the range considered as rule for hearing preservation at our institution (SRT 30 dB or less; speech recognition 70% or more; tumor size 1.5 cm or less) a translabyrinthine resection was considered. In order to provide the patient with auditory input, a cochlear implant was considered for the left ear following the resection of the right sided acoustic neuroma. Following the routine at our institution, the left ear was evaluated by means of electrical stimulation (promontory testing). Several attempts, however, failed to elicit any auditory sensations at the

limits of our equipment. Since an absence of response to electrical stimulation is a contra-indication for implantation in our program, that plan had to be abandoned. Instead, a suboccipital approach was planned for a subtotal resection with hearing preservation and careful intraoperative monitoring. Based on our experience, a decision was made to avoid exceeding the preoperative latency of wave V by more than 2.5 ms. Figure 18.5 illustrates the intraoperative ABR sequence in this case. It is interesting to note a reduction in wave V latency following the opening of the dura. The latency of wave V reached 13.05 ms during the debulking of the tumor by means of cavitron (an ultrasonic dissection instrument). After the cessation of the cavitron use, wave V latency was reduced by approximately 1.5 ms however, its morphology was poor and the amplitude reduced. At this point in time, approxi-

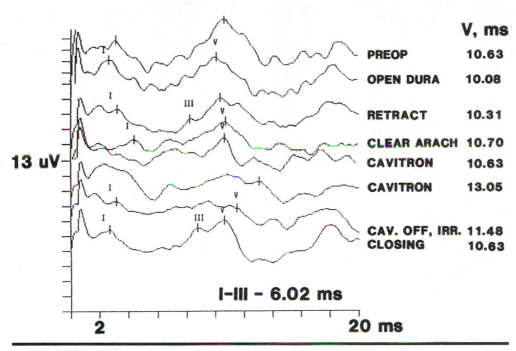

FIGURE 18.5.   Intraoperative ABR sequence during the suboccipital subtotal resection of an acoustic neuroma in the patient whose audiological results are illustrated in Figure 18.4.

mately 70% of the tumor had been resected and in view of the changes in morphology and the previous latency delay, it was decided to end the procedure. The last trace in Figure 18.5 illustrates the ABR following closing. It is characterized by a better morphology with wave III identifiable and wave V with a latency identical to the preoperative latency. Figure 18.6 illustrates the preoperative and postoperative CT scan. Postoperatively, the patient's hearing improved in the mid and high frequency range and threshold was elevated in the lower frequencies. Speech discrimination improved significantly to 88% and with proper amplification her speech reception threshold was 30 dB. The patient is being followed with periodic magnetic resonance imaging scans and audiological testing. At the writing of this chapter she is three years postoperative, her hearing is unchanged and there has been no significant growth of

her tumor. It is possible that she will have to undergo another operative procedure sometime in the future and she may lose her hearing as a result of tumor growth or the surgical procedure; however, in the mean time the quality of her life has been greatly improved.

Retrolabyrinthine Vestibular Nerve Section.   The following example illustrates auditory brainstem response monitoring in retrolabyrinthine vestibular nerve section. This is a last resort surgical procedure in patients with intractable vertigo with intact or near intact hearing on the affected side. Therefore, in this case the surgeons operate on and near structurally and functionally intact auditory neural structures and auditory function is not inherently at risk, as is the case with acoustic neuroma. Therefore, hearing preservation becomes perhaps an even more important goal than in

(A)   (B)

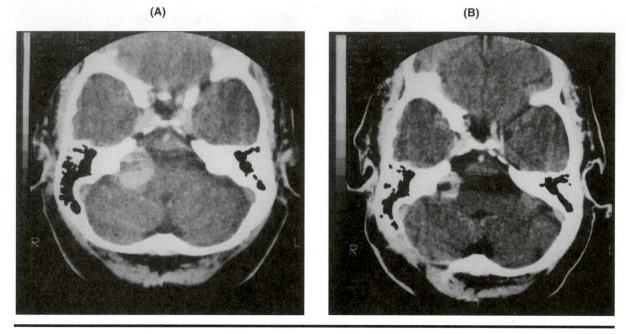

FIGURE 18.6.   Pre- and postoperative CT scans in a patient with a suboccipital subtotal resection of an acoustic neuroma with hearing preservation (also illustrated in Figures 18.4 and 18.5).

acoustic neuroma surgery. The intraoperative changes in ABR latency and morphology tend to be less drastic than in acoustic neuroma surgery and auditory function is at substantial risk during the separation of the cochlear and vestibular branches of the VIIIth cranial nerve and during the division (section) of the vestibular branch. Figure 18.7 illustrates a sequence of ABRs during a retrolabyrinthine vestibular nerve section. Retraction following the opening of the dura resulted in a slight delay of waves III and V (wave I remained stable). During the separation of the vestibular and cochlear branches, there was further delay in waves III and V and the overall amplitude and definition of the response became reduced. While wave I latency remained fairly stable, its amplitude diminished significantly. The removal of the retractor following the completion of the vestibular nerve section contributed to a reversal of the previous effect, however—the latency values were still prolonged in comparison of baseline values.

PEDIATRIC APPLICATIONS OF THE ELECTRICALLY EVOKED ABR (EABR)

The preoperative establishment of electrical stimulability is an important contribution to a successful outcome following cochlear implant surgery. Wherever possible, the psychophysical determination of promontory electric thresholds is an excellent indicator of postoperative stimulability. In our experience, accurate promontory thresholds can be established by means of behavioral testing in most children 10 years of age or older. In the younger age group, particularly the three to six years age range, we have relied exclusively on the EABR.

Children selected for cochlear implantation are taken to the operating room on the day scheduled for surgery, anesthetized and paralyzed, but not prepared otherwise for surgery. In the operation room, a needle electrode is placed on the promontory in the usual fashion, and subdermal needle electrodes are placed anterior to the tragus (to serve as an indifferent electrode

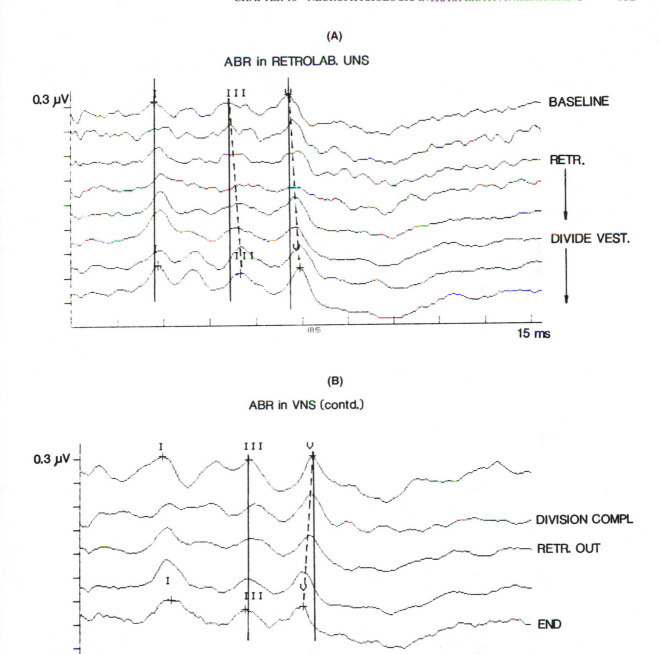

FIGURE 18.7.   ABR sequence during retrolabyrinthine vestibular nerve section.

for promontory stimulation), at the vertex, the contralateral earlobe, or the nape of the neck (EABR recording electrodes), and at the forehead (ground electrode). Biphasic balanced rectangular current pulses with phase durations of either 400 or 800 μs, generated by a modified Cochlear Corporation promontory stimulator, or a custom-made stimulator are delivered at a rate of 10 per second. Responses are recorded by means of a Bio-logic Traveler or a Bio-logic Navigator electrodiagnostic system triggered by the amplified and rectified "monitor" output of the Cochlear Corporation promontory stimulator. The custom made stimulator is triggered by a sync (TTL) pulse generated by the electrodiagnostic system. Responses are amplified (x 100,000 to 150,000), filtered (10 Hz or 30 Hz to 1500 Hz), and stored on floppy diskettes. To avoid overloading the digital-to-analog converters and scaling problems, the stimulus artifact is blocked digitally during response averaging. The recorded waveform may be further filtered digitally (30 or 100 Hz high pass, zero phase) to improve response appearance. Typically, we begin delivering stimuli at current levels of 400–500 μA and either descend or ascend from there up to a maximum of 1 mA. Following the completion of the evaluation of one ear, the contralateral ear is usually evaluated in like fashion.

The following is an example of pediatric perioperative application of the EABR. B.A. is an 11-year-old girl with profound bilateral congenital sensory hearing impairment. She was evaluated at our center for cochlear implant candidacy. Our preoperative protocol includes promontory testing carried out behaviorally in adults and older children (Kileny et al., 1991*b*) and electrophysiologically (ABR or MLR) in younger children and in adults in whom the psychophysical results are unreliable (i.e., pre-lingually deaf) (Kileny and Kemink, 1987; Kileny, 1991). In B.A.'s case it was decided to asses the electrical excitability of the auditory system by means of perioperative EABR. The left ear was stimulated first. EABR's to 400 μs biphasic pulses ranging in level from 650 μA to 400 μA are illustrated in Figure 18.8. These responses are characterized by well-defined wave V components with latencies of 3.79–4.18 ms. Threshold was estimated to be 400 μA or possibly lower (no attempt was made to

obtain responses at lower levels). In our experience, a threshold of 400 μA or less as a rule translates into adequate postoperative electrical thresholds and functional gain from a cochlear implant (subject to other variables such as language development, age at implantation, duration of preoperative auditory deprivation, etc.). Right ear stimulation resulted in atypical waveform configuration possibly due to contamination by facial nerve stimulation. Because of the satisfactory nature of the responses obtained with left ear stimulation, there were no further attempts to validate the excitability of the right ear and the left ear was recommended for implantation. Had this not been the case, several options were available: increase the amount of neuromuscular blocking agent administered to the patient; reposition the stimulating transtympanic needle electrode; retest the ear. Figure 18.9 illustrates B.A.'s preoperative and three months postoperative pure-tone audiogram with a Cochlear Corporation multichannel implant in her left ear. Her postoperative thresholds are in the typical 30–40 dB HL range. Three

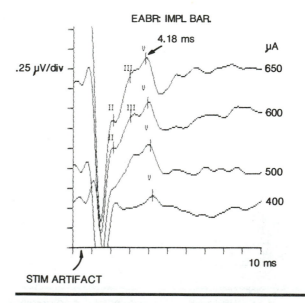

FIGURE 18.8. Perioperative electric ABR elicited by 400 μs biphasic current pulses in an 11-year-old patient prior to cochlear implant surgery.

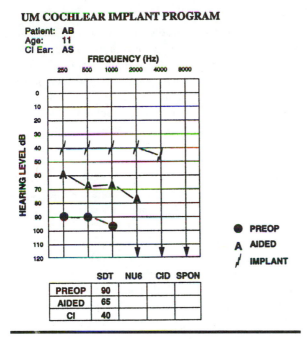

UM COCHLEAR IMPLANT PROGRAM

Patient: **AB**
Age: **11**
CI Ear: **AS**

FIGURE 18.9. Pre- and postoperative pure-tone audiogram in an 11-year-old cochlear implant patient.

months post activation she responds consistently to her name and correctly identifies several environmental sounds. She can also discriminate second formant (i.e., "bee" vs "boo") differences consistently.

FACIAL NERVE MONITORING

Postoperative facial paralysis imposes cosmetic and function deficits that carry a heavy psychological impact. Functionally, facial paralysis places the eye at risk for exposure and drying, and incapacitates perioral musculature, thereby interfering with speech and mastication. The inability to control facial expression is quite conspicuous and creates a communication barrier that frustrates the patient. Because most paralyses are unilateral, the asymmetry is more apparent when the contralateral muscles are used.

Once incurred, the rehabilitation of a complete facial paralysis presents a difficult challenge. Although surgical approaches have been developed to reanimate the paralyzed face, each of the currently available techniques has significant limitations underscoring the need for prevention.

Anatomy of the Facial Nerve

The facial nerve courses through the posterior cranial fossa and temporal bone to the peripheral facial musculature via a circuitous route. The intracranial segment of the facial nerve is comprised of fibers from the facial motor and superior salivatory nuclei and emerges from the brain stem at the pontomedullary junction. The nerve trunk crosses the subarachnoid space of the CPA and then passes into the internal auditory canal. The intracranial segment of the nerve is at risk for surgical injury because it lacks an epineural sheath, the fibrous sheath that enhances surface integrity of more peripheral segments of the nerve. After traversing the internal auditory canal, the facial nerve enters the fallopian canal of the temporal bone at the site of the canal's smallest diameter, the meatal foramen. The nerve then passes distally to form the labyrinthine, geniculate, tympanic, and mastoid portions of the fallopian canal to exit from the skull base through the stylomastoid foramen. The extratemporal segment of the nerve enters the parotid gland where it branches before finally terminating on the motor-end plates of the sixteen muscles of facial expression on each side.

Electrophysiologic Recording of Facial Muscle Activity

The ultimate goal of facial nerve IOM is to help maximize the postoperative preservation of the facial nerve in procedures that place the facial nerve at risk. The achievement of this goal depends on the ability to: 1) indicate direct or indirect mechanical manipulation of the facial nerve; 2) detect conditions that may lead to the injury of the facial nerve; and 3) assist in the localization, identification, and mapping of the facial nerve. Direct electrophysiological recordings of facial nerve responses and activity may be the ideal way to achieve these goals. However, due in a large part to its anatomy, this method is impractical for the time being. While the facial nerve is the source of taste sensation to the anterior two-thirds of the tongue (chorda tympani) and provides sensory innervation to the mucous membrane of the soft palate (greater superficial petrosal nerve) the main part of the nerve originates from the motor root arising from the motor nucleus located deep in the pons. It is responsible for the supply of motor innervation to the many muscles of facial expression as it branches out after its exit from the stylomastoid foramen. Therefore, electromyographic recording of facial muscle activity is another electrophysiologic method for the determination of facial nerve status and activation.

As a rule, facial muscle activity as a means of facial nerve monitoring is recorded intraoperatively by means of intramuscular needle electrodes. Depending upon limitations imposed by the monitoring equipment, EMG activity can be sampled from any number of facial muscles. Beyond activity immediately following electrode insertion (insertional activity) normal muscle at rest is quiet. Muscle contraction resulting from the recruitment of motor units within the recording range of the electrodes is manifested as the appearance of one to several, to numerous motor unit potentials. The synchronized recruitment of a substantial number of motor unit such as may result from electrical stimulation of a motor nerve results in the mass contraction of the target muscles and is recorded as a biphasic compound muscle (or myogenic) action potential. These two electromyographic phenomena serve as the basis for neurophysiologic IOM of any motor nerve function including the facial nerve. Both phenomena are, as a rule, recorded in real time as they do not require signal averaging for definition.

Recording Techniques

Electromyographic activity may be recorded using a variety of electrodes: monopolar and bipolar hooked wire electrodes, monopolar needle electrodes, bipolar concentric needle electrodes, surface electrodes, and others. We recommend the use of short (1 cm or less) non-insulated needle electrodes commonly known as subdermal electrodes. These can be used for intramuscular recording. They are extremely stable over long durations with impedances ranging from less than 3 kohm to about 6 kohm and because they are not insu-

lated, can sample electromyographic activity from a relatively wide area, thus contributing to the sensitivity of monitoring. For monitoring purposes, we usually utilize two channels: differential recording from frontalis and orbicularis oculi ("upper face") and orbicularis oris and mentalis ("lower face") as shown in Figure 18.10. This recording montage provides us with sufficient sensitivity and versatility. For instance, if one of the electrodes malfunctions during surgery this montage can be quickly converted to a single-channel recording by eliminating one of the three remaining electrodes or, the malfunctioning facial muscle electrode can be replaced with an electrode placed away from the face (thigh) providing us with one channel of monopolar facial muscle monitoring. It is important to set the high pass filter relatively low (5–10 Hz) to avoid significant ringing induced by the electric stimulus artifact. Low-pass filter may be set anywhere between 3000 and 10,000 Hz. This two-channel recording may also help observe restricted discharges of facial muscles particularly with dissection around the extratemporal portion of the nerve. If necessary, and the appropriate equipment is available, electrodes can be inserted into several individual facial muscles for more detailed monitoring. The recorded output may be visually displayed on the cathode ray tube of the electrophysiologic equipment and an acoustic analog of the myogenic activity is also routed

INTRAOPERATIVE CN VII MONITORING FACIAL EMG

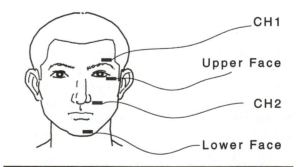

FIGURE 18.10. Subdermal needle electrode placement for intraoperative facial EMG monitoring.

to a speaker to provide a simultaneous acoustic signal. The acoustic signal offers immediate feedback to the operating surgeon who is unable to view the visual display of the evoked activity. The use of devices consisting solely of an acoustic output (raw EMG or tonal alarm) is not recommended as stimulus artifacts or contact between operating instruments within the field can mimic the sound of EMG and/or trigger the alarm. Video monitoring of the operative procedure is also recommended to enable the clinician responsible for monitoring to determine the relationship between surgical and neurophysiologic events. For instance, it is not necessary to warn the surgical team about EMG activity elicited by irrigation. Failure to observe the surgical procedure can result in unnecessary and confusing warnings and would greatly detract from the value of monitoring.

Stimulus Source and Stimulating Electrodes

Surgery of the medial temporal bone and CPA entails dissection through an array of tissues and fluid media of varying resistivities. Tumor removal from the posterior fossa, for instance, is performed in a field intermittently bathed with cerebrospinal fluid. Møller and Jannetta (1984) described the potential for current diversion to this fluid-filled medium. Under these circumstances, stimulus delivery to the nerve reduced by the fluid shunt might produce a false-negative stimulation. To correct for this dynamic shunt, they recommended a constant voltage stimulus source. This source varies current according to the degree of stimulus shunting, as determined by the impedance encountered at the electrode terminal. Depolarization, however, is a function of electric current therefore, in most applications constant current stimulation is used. This type of source varies voltage as a function of impedance to maintain a constant current at the tip of the stimulating electrode.

Prass and Luders (1985) demonstrated the effect of various stimulus electrode designs on preventing shunt-related inaccuracies. Under "worst-case" shunting conditions—a cerebrospinal fluid-filled environment—neural stimulation was inefficient with either constant current or constant voltage when a large area of the stimulus probe was not insulated. In contrast,

probes insulated so that only the tip was exposed consistently—a flush tip design—gave accurate excitation, regardless of shunt conditions. Similar results were obtained with these probes with both constant current and constant voltage stimulus-generating sources.

In contrast to monopolar stimulation in which response amplitude does not vary with changes in electrode probe orientation, bipolar stimulation is optimized by orienting the probe tips longitudinally along the axis of nerve fibers (Møller and Janetta, 1984). In the setting where the course of the nerve is obscured by tumor effacement, and is not immediately appreciable, a monopolar stimulus probe effectively maps regions of the tumor remote from the nerve. In contrast, bipolar probe design can provide a means of differentiating nerves, particularly when they lie in close proximity to one another, as in the internal auditory canal. The greater specificity of bipolar stimulation reflects confinement of current to the electrode terminals and less tendency for stimulus shunting and can therefore be of value in distinguishing the facial nerve from other regional cranial nerves.

Safety of Direct Nerve Stimulation

Few studies have critically evaluated the safety of electrical stimulation of surgically exposed cranial nerves. Concern for the safety of such stimulation is underscored by the lack of epineural covering of the nerve in its intradural segment. Love and Marchbanks (1978) described a case of facial paralysis after acoustic neuroma removal, possibly related to the use of a disposable nerve stimulator. The site of nerve stimulation demonstrated a blanched area and "bubbling" of the surface fluids under microscopic visualization. This observation suggested that a cautery-like effect may have been exerted by the nerve stimulator. Further experimental studies carried out by these investigators in the rabbit model suggested that direct-current nerve stimulation may produce neural damage by inducing thermal or iontophoretic injury.

Hughes and co-workers (1984) demonstrated that repetitive, prolonged direct-current stimulation produced significant myelin and axonal degeneration in the rodent model. Pulsed-current stimulation was not associated with these neuropathic changes. In a follow-up investigation, Chase et al. (1984) demonstrated that damaging effects of direct-current stimulation were absent if the nerve and stimulator were in contact for periods lasting less than one second.

Studies of chronic stimulation of the CNS suggests that neural injury induced by current injection is most closely correlated with current density and coulombs per phase of stimulation. In order to maximize control of these parameters, constant current stimulation is recommended.

These investigations suggest that limiting the density of injected current and limiting the time of exposure of the nerve to unbalanced current are important factors in minimizing morbidity associated with direct stimulation of the surgically exposed nerve.

PHARMACOLOGIC EFFECTS

Excitation of the facial nerve resulting in muscle contraction involves a sequence of physiologic events. A change in the ion permeability of the nerve fiber to elevate the membrane potential beyond threshold elicits an action potential. Propagation of the potential to the neuromuscular junction results in acetylcholine release. This elicits depolarization of the post-junctional membrane, which produces contraction of muscle fibers.

Several drugs used clinically in the operative setting may interfere with the propagation of potentials along nerve and muscle membranes (DeJong, 1977; Koelle, 1980). Most notably, drugs of the local anesthetic and neuromuscular blocking agent groups may interfere with the accuracy of intraoperative nerve monitoring by virtue of their interference with the propagation of potentials. Local anesthetic agents, including those of the amide group (e.g., lidocaine and bupivacaine) and the ester group (e.g., cocaine and tetracaine), act to interfere with ionic exchange at the nerve cell membrane by stabilizing the membrane to prevent the generation of action potentials. The duration of the anesthetic effect of these agents varies with the amount of drug reaching the tissue membrane. The maximal duration of activity of these agents is three to four hours.

Neuromuscular blocking agents may be classified as either competitive (stabilizing) agents such as d-tubocurarine, gallamine, and pancuronium, or depolarization agents, such as succinylcholine (Koelle, 1980). These agents vary markedly in their duration of activity. For example, although the paralyzing effect of a single moderate dose of d-tubocurarine begins to abate in 20 minutes, the residual effect is still discernible after 4 hours or more. The long duration of this agent is attributable to its elimination via renal excretion. In contrast, the duration of activity of succinylcholine is extremely brief—two to three minutes. This is due to its rapid hydrolysis by pseudocholinesterase of the plasma and liver.

Local anesthetics and neuromuscular blocking agents affecting neuromuscular transmission can influence monitored activity, and their use should be strictly regulated by the anesthesiologist and surgeon. Past studies have suggested the possibility that facial motor activation may be differentially responsive to neuromuscular blockade, perhaps as a reflection of different densities of cholinergic receptors between cranial and peripheral neuromuscular junctions. The major question is whether peripheral neuromuscular blockade can be achieved while leaving the facial and other cranial neuromuscular axes responsive to electrical and mechanical stimulation. This could potentially prove helpful in maintaining an adequate level of anesthesia with less dependence on sedatives, hypnotics, and inhalation agents.

Response Characteristics—Electrically Evoked Activity

Effective nerve stimulation produces a single compound MAP synchronized to the delivered electrical stimulus. The amplitude of this response is often biphasic or triphasic in configuration and is typically larger in amplitude than typical motor unit potentials. It is easily separated from surrounding artifact and does not require averaging techniques.

Direct electrical stimulation of the facial nerve can be used to identify, localize, and map the course of the nerve. In addition, direct facial nerve stimulation can provide information about the functional status of the nerve. To obtain this information, the nerve is alternately stimulated distal and proximal to the site or segment of the nerve previously dissected. The two sites of stimulation therefore bracket the segment of the nerve from which the tumor was removed or otherwise manipulated. Symmetry of these responses reflects the integrity of the facial motor axons crossing the operative site either during or at the completion of the procedure. The prognostic utility of this technique is described below under applications of intraoperative nerve stimulation during acoustic neuroma removal. Because electrical stimulation of the surgically exposed nerve provides only a "snapshot" of its functional capacity to conduct an action potential, ongoing tracking of nerve activity is required to detect changes in its status on a continuous basis.

Response Characteristics—Spontaneous and Mechanically Evoked Activity

It is necessary to establish that surgical maneuvers bear an appropriate temporal relationship to motor unit activity, while accounting for non-pathologic factors. Interpreting such activity therefore requires correlation with the patient's baseline and ongoing physiologic status, delivered pharmacologic agents as well as ongoing surgical events.

"Burst" activity, consisting of brief bursts of two or more motor unit potentials, is the most frequently observed pattern with direct manipulation of the facial nerve intraoperatively. Blunt dissection, brief traction, and fluid irrigation in the vicinity of the nerve are known inducers of burst activity. Bursts occasionally follows monopolar or bipolar cauterization in proximity to the facial nerve, representing an after discharge depolarization of the electrical field. The tendency for facial nerve manipulation to elicit burst activity varies significantly between cases. The same intraoperative event may evoked very different activity patterns in the same patient as well. Burst activity indicates local mechanical stimulation of the facial nerve and is often inevitable during tumor separation from the nerve. When direct nerve manipulation occurs in the course

of a surgical procedure, evoked burst activity can serve as an index of the status of the facial nerve. A decline in burst activity with continued mechanical stimulation may be interpreted as evidence of evolving neural injury or fatigue and the surgical strategy should be adjusted accordingly.

The association between specific surgical events and monitored responses can vary heavily depending on the preoperative status of the nerve. In cases where a tumor involves the facial nerve, monitored activity may vary with tumor-induced ischemia and compression of the nerve. Kugelberg (1946) assessed the effects of ischemia and compression on electrical responses to mechanical stimulation of limb nerves. With compression, regional irritation of the median nerve resulted in heightened sensitivity to mechano-stimulation and early generation of spontaneous activity. Bergmans (1983) has summarized data indicating that chronic demyelinating neuropathies are associated with heightened levels of spontaneous firing and mechano-sensitivity of motor nerves. This abnormal activity is attributed to heightened activity of sodium-potassium channels that occur in demyelinated nerve fibers (Bostack and Sears, 1978). A potential gradient may develop between normal and demyelinated nerve segments and can serve to trigger action potentials. Once initiated, this postulated mechanism may act in an autoregenerative fashion to elicit repetitive neural excitation.

Asynchronous, autoregenerative discharges are commonly known as train activity. They consist of prolonged "trains" of motor unit activity temporally unrelated to surgical manipulation and may also be referred to as "spasms." The presence of train activity should be interpreted as a sign of increased sensitivity of the facial nerve resulting in prolonged high-frequency activation and facial spasm. Train activity can follow prolonged or repetitive lateral to medial traction of the facial nerve during tumor removal. Laser and cavitron tumor dissection as well as irrigation of the surgical field can also produce varying periods of train activity.

Artifacts.   Effective IOM of facial function depends to a great extent on the ability to distinguish artifacts from electromyogenic events. Because facial function monitoring consists mostly of the observation of the continuous activity sampled by the recording electrodes, it is particularly prone to artifacts. Motor unit potentials are predominantly biphasic events with a duration of 1–2 ms. With the differential recording technique described earlier, their configuration may change depending upon the relationship between the activities sampled by each of the two electrodes. For instance, if the motor unit potential activity sampled by the two electrodes is identical in temporal and polarity configuration, there is a risk of complete cancellation. In addition, for the same reason, the configuration of the motor unit potentials recorded may not always have the typical biphasic configuration. Therefore, it is extremely important to monitor the video display of the surgical procedure simultaneously. Depending upon the nature of the intraoperative manipulation of the facial nerve motor unit activity may be observed on both "upper face" and "lower face" channels. Seldom if ever are these activities completely identical. One common source of artifact is created by contact between surgical instruments within the operative field. Acoustically, these events are indistinguishable from motor unit activity. Visually however, these artifacts tend to be displayed as monopolar events synchronized in time between the two recording channels and 180°

out of phase as illustrated in Figure 18.11. Only a qualified observer can distinguish these from true motor unit activity. Non-attended acoustic monitoring can not make this distinction.

Another source of more obvious artifact is created by the use of electrocautery instrumentation or at times by ultrasonic dissection instrumentation. These events are distinguished by their large amplitude overwhelming any other activity. Some types of equipment used in intraoperative monitoring are equipment with sensors that can pick up the considerable electric field generated by such instrumentation and activate a muting switch.

Other artifacts may be associated with electrical stimulation used to identify and map the course of the facial nerve. An erroneous interpretation due to such artifacts can have very serious negative consequences. These artifacts usually derive from the electric stimulus artifact. If the high-pass filter is set too high, the electrical stimulus can generate a ringing artifact that may bear both configuration and latency resemblance to a compound muscle action potential (CMAP). This would result in a false positive identification that in turn may lead to the inadvertent sacrifice of an unidentified facial nerve. As with the previous artifacts, acoustic monitoring is incapable of distinguishing this type of event from a true CMAP.

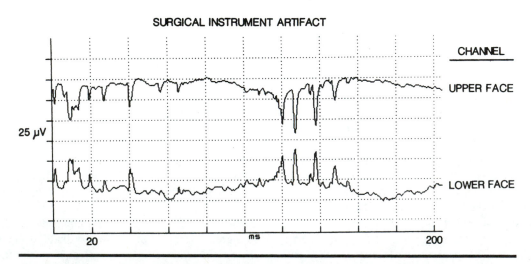

FIGURE 18.11. Example of artifacts recorded during intraoperative facial EMG monitoring.

Applications of Intraoperative Monitoring

Posterior Cranial Fossa Tumors.   Neurophysiologic recording techniques have found extensive use in assisting with the management of the facial nerve in removing tumors from the CPA of the posterior fossa and internal auditory canal. IOM represents another stride in the development of safe surgical approaches to lesions of this area, particularly acoustic tumors. Glasscock et al. (1984) have presented an historical perspective and summarized approaches currently utilized for the exposure and removal of tumors of this region. Six modified or combined techniques are based on three principal approaches: suboccipital, translabyrinthine and middle fossa (Figure 18.12).

The suboccipital, or posterior route, has been utilized throughout this century for exposing posterior fossa lesions. This approach utilizes a posterior craniectomy between the sigmoid and lateral sinuses and the foramen magnum. The dura is reflected from the posterior aspect of the temporal bone and the cerebellum is retracted to expose the CPA. In cases of tumor removal, the tumor must often be debulked before essential neural structures anterior and medial to the tumor can be identified. Identification of the nerve medial to the tumor may re-

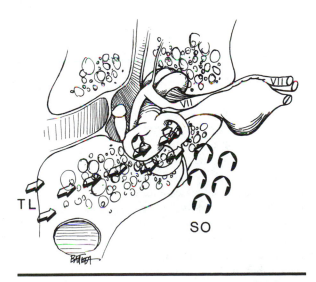

FIGURE 18.12.   Surgical approaches to the posterior fossa.

quire reliance upon brain stem landmarks that are often obscured by tumors that efface the brain stem surface.

House (1964) described modification of transtemporal bone removal that greatly enhanced the exposure, and hence the safety and utility of the translabyrinthine approach. This approach provides direct access to the CPA and internal auditory canal through removal of the mastoid air cells and vestibular portion of the otic capsule—a labyrinthectomy—and drill-out of bone between the jugular bulb inferiorly and middle fossa dura superiorly. The internal auditory canal is thus opened from a posterior orientation. The neural elements contained by the internal canal are identified in relation to vertically and horizontally positioned bony landmarks in the lateral extent of the canal.

House (1964) is also credited with the development of a technique to expose the internal auditory canal via the middle cranial fossa. A lateral craniectomy is created by removal of a 2.0 × 3.0 cm rectangle of squamous laterally, followed by superior retraction of the temporal lobe. This exposes the floor of the middle cranial fossa. Guided by landmarks of the middle cranial fossa floor, the roof of the internal canal is surgically removed exposing its dura. Opening of the dura provides access to the neural contents of the internal canal. Limited exposure of the CPA is provided with this approach.

Acoustic tumors comprise the largest group of neoplasms proximate to the facial nerve in the CPA. Meningiomas, primary cholesteatomas, gliomas, glomus and matastatic tumors occur in the CPA less frequently and may secondarily involve the facial nerve (Brackmann and Bartells, 1980)

The great majority of tumors in this region are histologically benign. In contrast to direct nerve infiltration, which often occurs with malignancies, involvement of the facial nerve with benign neoplasms produces a well-recognized pattern of compression. Compressional involvement with benign tumors can make identification and preservation of the facial nerve exceedingly difficult. Patterns of involvement of the facial nerve with acoustic neuromas have been detailed by House (1974) and Brackmann and Horn (1986). By virtue of reflecting the arachnoid sheath covering acoustic neuromas, adherence of the tumor to the nerve, particularly at the medial extent of the internal auditory canal, may be considerable. Attenuation of the nerve by tumor may be so pronounced that the nerve resembles a transparent membrane on the tumor surface. Usually the facial nerve will be displaced anterior and superior to the tumor. Less commonly, the nerve may course directly superior or even inferior to the tumor. Occasionally the facial nerve will be interposed between lobes of larger tumors.

Adherence, attenuation and displacement of the facial nerve by tumor is best managed by the experienced surgeon who is able to identify visually the variable involvement of the nerve with tumor. The difficulties imposed by such variable involvement of the nerve however, underscore the need for methods of improving the accuracy of nerve identification and detection of impending nerve compromise.

Several fundamental principles are commonly followed in removing posterior cranial fossa tumors after their exposure. Tumors are commonly debulked from within their capsule to reduce the volume of the tumor. This allows progressively better visibility about the tumor's periphery. Tumor dissection is kept within the capsule to maintain anatomic orientation to regional neural structures. Vessels on the tumor surface are coagulated and devascularized portions of the tumor are removed, further reducing tumor volume. Once the tumor is adequately reduced in volume to allow viewing the facial nerve both proximal and distal to the site of tumor involvement, the capsular attachment to the facial nerve is divided. Separation of tumor from nerve is most intricate at the most medial extent of the internal auditory canal (porus acusticus). This often requires sharp division of fine adhesions to complete removal of the tumor and its surrounding capsule.

As mentioned previously, two distinct patterns of responses to mechanical stimulation of the facial nerve during acoustic neuroma removal are recognized: bursts and trains. The more frequently encountered pattern is burst activity which may occur in association with direct nerve manipulation such as that occurring with blunt dissection of tumor capsule from the nerve, brief periods of traction, or with fluid irrigation in the vicinity of the facial nerve. Asynchronous, repetitive train activity often occurs with traction of the facial

nerve produced by manipulation of a tumor that is adherent to the nerve.

Figure 18.13 demonstrates the effects of traction of the facial nerve during resection of an acoustic neuroma. The traction resulted in burst-type activity consisting of polyphasic potentials separated by approximately 10–20 ms. Cessation of traction produced a return to baseline activity. However, in some instances, such mechanically-induced activity may persist for several minutes after cessation of the triggering activity and may progress to recurring train activity. Should this occur, a break in the surgical procedure is recommended until cessation of the bursts and/or train activity occurs.

Figure 18.14 illustrates the use of electrically evoked facial responses during the course of resecting an acoustic neuroma. The traces represent activity recorded with monopolar, constant current electrical stimulation of the nerve at sites proximal and distal to the point of tumor removal. As mentioned previously, this technique detects conducting axons crossing the site of tumor removal.

Although a number of reports have suggested that intraoperative facial nerve monitoring facilitates its identification, delineation of contour, and preservation, few comparative trials of postoperative results of monitored and unmonitored acoustic tumor surgery exist. In two separate studies, Harner and colleagues (1986, 1987) compared postoperative functional results obtained with unmonitored acoustic neuroma removal with those obtained with the use of monitoring through the suboccipital approach. In an initial series of 21 matched cases, monitoring did not appear to confer a significant advantage in facial nerve function preservation. In a subsequent study of 48 matched cases of acoustic tumors removed through the suboccipital approach, monitoring substantially improved the rate of facial nerve preservation with large, greater than 4.0 cm acoustic tumors. The incidence of immediate postoperative incomplete facial palsy and complete paralysis was similar in monitored and unmonitored cases. However, after three months, the degree of improvement in the monitored group exceeded that of the unmonitored group, particularly in patients with medium (greater than 2 cm) and large (greater than 4 cm) tumors.

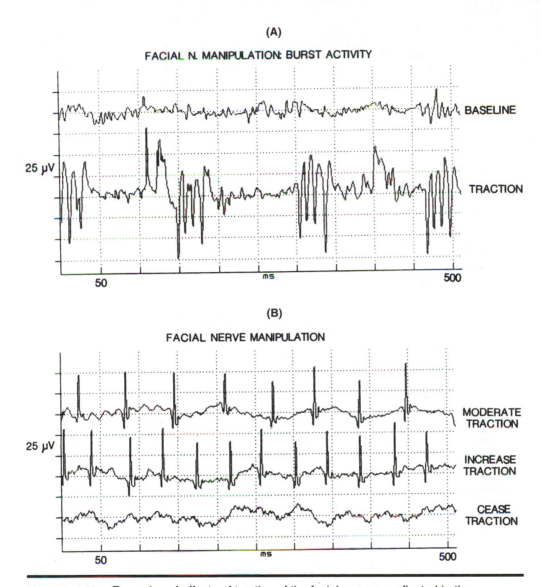

FIGURE 18.13.   Examples of effects of traction of the facial nerve as reflected in the intraoperative facial EMG. (A) Burst activity, with bursts of several motor unit potentials separate by about 100 ms; (B) Train activity with motor unit potentials separated by about 50 ms.

Historic controls do not serve as a satisfactory comparative population for evaluating the potential benefits of monitoring posterior fossa surgery. This study design flaw notwithstanding, the results suggest that facial nerve monitoring during translabyrinthine re-

moval of large acoustic neuroma may limit operative neural injury, enhancing the potential for recovery of satisfactory facial function.

In a previous study (Niparko et al., 1989), we compared facial function outcome in 29 patients who had

(A)

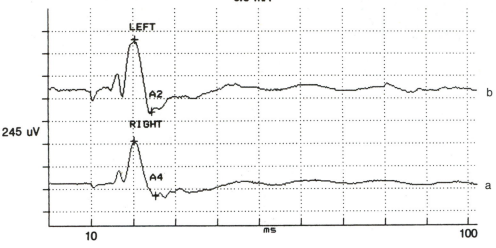

(B)

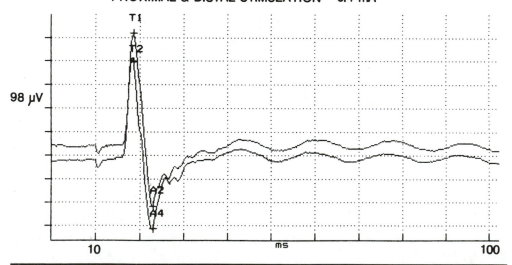

FIGURE 18.14.   The use of electrically evoked facial muscle compound action potentials in intraoperative monitoring. (A) Proximally evoked responses before (b) and after (a) the resection of an acoustic neuroma; (B) Identical proximal and distally evoked compound facial action potentials at the completion of acoustic neuroma resection.

undergone translabyrinthine resections of acoustic neuroma with facial nerve monitoring to 75 patients who had undergone translabyrinthine resections prior to the introduction of IOM. The mean patient age in the control group was 54.5 years and the mean tumor size was 2.14 cm. One year postoperative, in the unmonitored group, 43 of the 75 patients (57%) demonstrated satisfactory facial function. In the monitored group, one year postoperative facial function was satisfactory in 25 of 29 patients (86%). The association of satisfactory facial function one year postoperatively with monitoring was statistically significant ($p < 0.05$). This effect was stronger when comparing subgroups with larger tumors.

In order to determine the relationship between specific intraoperative neurophysiologic events and facial function outcome, we reviewed 71 additional acoustic neuroma cases operated on during 1989–1990 at the University of Michigan Medical Center (Kileny et al., 1992). In 32 patients the surgical approach was suboccipital; in 39 cases the surgical approach was translabyrinthine. One year following surgery, 66 of the 71 patients (93.8%) presented with normal facial function (two had some moderate residual mass action). In 42 of these patients (59%), facial function was normal immediately postoperatively and remained normal. In 38 of these 42 patients (90%), the amplitude of the proximally evoked CMAP differed from the distally evoked CMAP by 20% or less (proximal equals distal). In 27 of these patient (65%), the IOM course was characterized by frequent mechanically induced motor unit activity.

In 22 of the 71 patients (31%) with normal postoperative facial function, facial weakness occurred with a postoperative delay of from a few hours to a few days. In 16 of these patients (72%), the proximal and distal responses obtained prior to closing were equal. Frequent mechanical or spontaneous EMG activity was present in nine of 22 patients (41%). In seven of the 71 patients (10%), there was immediate postoperative facial paralysis. In two of these patients, the proximal and distal evoked CMAP were considered to be equal. In these two patients, the facial nerve was anatomically intact at the end of the procedure and both recovered to normal/near normal facial function within one year after surgery.

The following may be concluded from these data. The strongest prognostic indicator is the comparison between the proximally and distally evoked compound facial MAP. Mechanical and spontaneous activity was more common in the more normal and delayed weakness groups. The degree of tumor adherence to the nerve was not documented. The normal final outcome may have been facilitated by an increase in the vigilance of the surgical and monitoring team as a result of the frequent, neurophysiologic events.

Vestibular Nerve Section

Retrolabyrinthine vestibular nerve section is one of several surgical options available for controlling disabling vertigo experienced by patients with Meniere's disease who fail medical management (Kemink et al., 1991). This procedure selectively denervates the vestibular portion of the offending inner ear while sparing function of the auditory portion of the VIIIth cranial nerve. This procedure commonly utilizes a transmastoid approach, working posterior to the semicircular canals in order to preserve function of the auditory portion of the labyrinth. Exposure of the VIIIth cranial nerve for vestibular nerve section may also be obtained through middle fossa, retrosigmoid, combined retrosigmoid-retrolabyrinthine and suboccipital approaches.

The VIIIth cranial nerve is identified in the CPA. The facial nerve is identified by gently retracting the VIIIth cranial nerve inferiorly. Direct electrical stimulation of the facial nerve provides for definitive identification. A septum commonly divides the cochlear and vestibular divisions of the VIIIth cranial nerve and is often delineated by an arteriole on the posterior aspect of the nerve. In some cases, the retrolabyrinthine approach may not permit as precise a separation of the vestibular from the cochlear fibers of the VIIIth cranial nerve. In such cases, direct nerve recordings with acoustic stimulation can enhance this determination (Kileny et al., 1988)

Facial Nerve Decompression

Bell's palsy is a common disorder than produces unilateral facial paresis or paralysis. The diagnosis of

Bell's palsy is made only after clinical and radiological assessment fail to reveal a metabolic, infectious, traumatic or neoplastic etiology for the facial paralysis. It is hypothesized that the loss of facial nerve function in Bell's palsy is secondary to nerve inflammation and compression within the unyielding perineurium of the fallopian canal. Electrical mapping in patients with Bell's palsy who have undergone nerve exploration and decompression suggests that critical nerve entrapment exists at discrete sites (Niparko et al., 1989; Fisch and Esslen, 1972; Gantz et al., 1982). Direct facial nerve stimulation at the time of middle cranial fossa nerve exposure frequently localizes the site of conduction blockade to the segment of the nerve within the narrowest portion of the fallopian canal—the meatal foramen. Figure 18.15 demonstrates that nerve stimulation, moving in a distal to proximal direction, evokes responses of diminished amplitude at the site of conduction block, and presumably nerve compression is approached. This supports the utility of intraoperative stimulation of the exposed facial nerve at the meatal segment in a patient undergoing decompression for Bell's paralysis.

Mastoid and Reconstructive Surgery

A wide range of pathologies involving the middle ear and mastoid required transtemporal bone and other tissue removal in proximity to the facial nerve. IOM can assist the surgeon in identifying and isolating the facial nerve when chronic inflammatory changes obscure its visualization. This may result in the presence of cholesteatoma, granulation tissue or thickened, infected mucosa. Irreversibly diseased tissue can be removed from sites directly adjacent to the facial nerve expeditiously by monitoring mechanically evoked activity and identifying the nerve with certainty using electrical stimulation. The utility of IOM of chronic otitis media surgery is emphasized by the common occurrence of facial nerve canal deficiencies due to either the pattern of temporal bone development or through bony erosion caused by chronic inflammation.

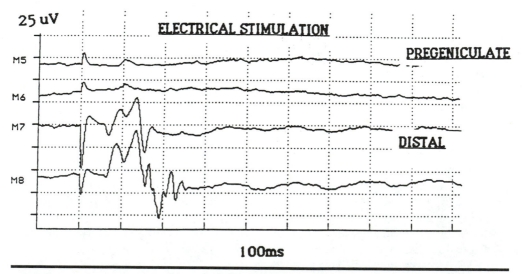

FIGURE 18.15. Proximal to distal electrical stimulation of the facial nerve demonstrating diminished compound muscle action potential amplitude at the site of the conduction block during a decompression surgery in a patient with Bell's Palsy.

REFERENCES

American Speech-Language Hearing Association. Report Update. (1990). Aids/HIV: Implications for Speech-Language Pathologists and Audiologists. *ASHA, 32,* 46–48.

Bergmans, J. (1983). Neurophysiological features of experimental and human neuropathies. In Battistin, L., Hashim, G., and Lajtha, A. (eds.), *Clinical and Biological Aspects of Peripheral Nerve Diseases,* pp. 73–100. New York: A.R. Liss.

Bostack, H. and Sears, T. (1978). The intermodel axon membrane: Electrical excitability and continuous conduction in segmental demyelination. *Journal of Physiology (London), 280,* 273–281.

Brackmann, D.E. and Bartels, W. (1980). Rare tumors of the cerebellopontine angle. *Otolaryngology—Head and Neck Surgery, 88,* 555–559.

Brackmann, D.E. and Horn, W. (1986). Surgery for acoustic neuroma. In Wiet, R.J. and Causse, J.B. (eds.), *Complications in otolaryngology—Head and neck surgery—Ear and skull base,* pp. 47–56. Toronto: B.C. Dekker.

Centers for Disease Control. (1988). Morbidity and Mortality Weekly Report: Perspectives in Disease Prevention and Health Promotion. *CDC, 37,* 377–388.

Chase, S.G., Hughes, G.N., and Dudley, A.W. (1984). Neuropathologic changes following direct-current stimulation of the rat sciatic nerve. *Otolaryngology—Head and Neck Surgery, 92,* 615–617.

De Jong, R.H. (1977). Neural blockade by local anesthetics. *Journal of the American Medical Association, 238,* 1383–1385.

Drummond, J.C., Todd, M.M., and Sang, U.H. (1985). The effect of high dose sodium thiopental on brainstem auditory and median nerve somatosensory evoked responses in humans. *Anesthesiology, 63,* 249–254.

Fisch, U. and Esslen, E. (1972). Total intratemporal exposure of the facial nerve. *Archives of Otolaryngology, 95,* 335–341.

Gage, P.W. and Hamill, O.P. (1981). Effects of anesthetics on ion channels in synapses. In R. Porter (ed.), *International Review of Physiology, Vol. 25, Neurophysiology,* Baltimore, MD: University Park Press.

Gantz, B., Gmur, A., and Fisch, U. (1982). Intraoperative evoked electromyography in Bell's palsy. *American Journal of Otolaryngology, 3,* 273–278.

Glasscock, M., Gulya, A., and Pensak, M. (1984). Surgery of the posterior fossae. *Otolaryngological Clinics of North America, 17,* 483–497.

Harner, S., Daube, J., and Ebersold, M. (1986). Electrophysiologic monitoring of the facial nerve during temporal bone surgery. *Laryngoscope, 96,* 65–69.

Harner, S.G., Daube, T.R., and Ebersold, M.J. (1987). Improved preservation of facial nerve function with use of electrical monitoring during removal of acoustic neuromas. *Mayo Clinic Proc., 62,* 92–102.

House, W. (1964). Evolution of transtemporal bone removal of acoustic tumors. *Archives of Otolaryngology, 80,* 731–742.

House, W.F. (1974). Management of the facial nerve in acoustic tumor surgery. *Otolaryngological Clinics of North America, 7,* 457–460.

Hughes, G.B., Bottomy, M.B., Jackson, C.G., et al. (1984). Myelin and axon degeneration following direct current peripheral nerve stimulation: A prospective controlled experimental study. *Otolaryngology—Head and Neck Surgery, 92,* 615–617. (not in text of manuscript)

Jewett, D.L., Romano, M.N., and Williamston, J.S. (1970). Human auditory evoked potentials: Possible brain stem components detected on the scalp. *Science, 167,* 1517–1518.

Kaga, K., Takiguchi, T., Myokai, K., et al. (1979). Effects of deep hypothermia and circulatory arrest on the auditory brain stem response. *Archives of Otolaryngology, Rhinology, and Laryngology, 225,* 199–205.

Kemink, J.L., LaRouere, M.J., Kileny, P.R., et al. (1990). Hearing preservation following suboccipital removal of acoustic neuromas. *Laryngoscope, 100(6),* 597–602.

Kemink, J.L., Telian, S.A., El-Kashlan, H., and Langman, A.W. (1991). Retrolabyrinthine vestibular nerve section: Efficacy in disorders other than Meniere's disease. *Laryngoscope, 101,* 523–528.

Kileny, P.R. (1991). Use of electrophysiologic measures in the management of children with cochlear implants: Brainstem, middle latency and cognitive (P300) responses. *American Journal of Otology, 12(Suppl),* 37–42.

Kileny, P., Dobson, D., and Gelfand, E.T. (1983). Middle latency auditory evoked responses during open-heart surgery with hypothermia. *Electroencephalography and Clinical Neurophysiology, 55,* 268–276.

Kileny, P.R. and Kemink, J.L. (1987). Electrically evoked middle-latency auditory potentials in cochlear implant candidates. *Archives of Otolaryngology, 113,* 1072–1077.

Kileny, P.R., Niparko, J.K., Shepard, N.T., and Kemink, J.T. (1988). Neurophysiologic intraoperative monitoring: I. Auditory function. *American Journal of Otology, 9,* 17–24.

Kileny, P.R., Telian, S.A., and Kemink, J.L. (1991*a*). Acoustic neuroma: Diagnosis and management. In Jacobson, J.T. and Northern, J.L. (eds.), *Diagnostic audiology,* pp. 217–233. Austin, TX: Pro-ed.

Kileny, P.R., Kemink, J.L., Zimmerman-Phillips, S., and Schmaltz, S.P. (1991*b*). Effects of preoperative electrical stimulatibility and historical factors on performance with multichannel cochlear implant. *Annals of Otology, Rhinology, and Laryngology, 100(7),* 563–568.

Kileny, P.K., Kemink, J.L., Tucci, D.L., and Hoff, J.T. (1992). Neurophysiologic intraoperative facial and auditory function monitoring in acoustic neuroma surgery. In: Tos, M. and Thomsen, J. (eds.), *Acoustic Neuroma,* pp. 569–574. Amsterdam/New York: Kugler Publications.

Koblin, D.D. and Eger E. (1981). How anesthetics work. In R.A. Miller (ed.), *Anesthesia,* New York: Churchill, Livingstone.

Koelle, G.B. (1980). Neuromuscular blocking agents. In Goodman, A.F., Gilman, C.S. (eds.), *The pharmacologic basis of therapeutics,* 6th Edition, pp. 575–588. New York: Macmillan.

Konishi, T. (1979). Some observations on the negative endocochlear potential during anoxia. *Acta Otolaryngologica, 87,* 506–516.

Kugelberg, E. (1946). "Injury activity" and "trigger zones" in human nerves. *Brain, 69,* 310–324.

Love, J. and Marchbanks, J. (1978). Injury to the facial nerve associated with the use of a disposable nerve stimulator. *Otorhinolaryngology, 86,* 61–64.

Luetje, C.M. (1989). Intraoperative monitoring: Hardware addiction is no substitute for clinical judgement. *American Journal of Otology, 10 (Editorial).*

Manninen, P., Lam, A.M., and Nicholas, J.F. (1985). The effects of isoflurane-nitrous oxide anesthesia on brainstem auditory evoked potentials in humans. *Anesth. Anal., 64,* 43–47.

Møller, A.R. and Jannetta, P.J. (1984). Preservation of facial function during removal of acoustic neuromas. *Journal of Neurosurgery, 61,* 757–760.

Møller, A.R. and Jannetta, P.J. (1985). Neurogenerators of the auditory brain stem response. In J.T. Jacobson (ed.), *The auditory brainstem response,* pp. 13–31. Boston, MA: College Hill Press.

Niparko, J.K., Kileny, P.R., Kemink, J.L., Lee, H.M., and Graham, M.D. (1989). Neurophysiologic intraoperative monitoring: II. Facial nerve function. *American Journal of Otology, 10,* 55–61.

Prass, R. and Luders, H. (1985). Constant current versus constant voltage stimulation. *Journal of Neurosurgery, 62,* 622–623.

Ruth, R.A., Gal, P.J., DiFazio, C.A., et al. (1985). Brain stem auditory evoked potentials during lidocaine infusion in humans. *Archives of Otolaryngology, 111,* 799–802.

Schwartz, B.M., Bloom, M.J., Pratt, R.E., and Costello, J.A. (1988). Anesthetic effects on neuroelectric events. *Seminars on Hearing, 9,* 99–112.

Sekiya, T., Møller, A.R., and Jannetta, P.J. (1986). Pathophysiological mechanisms of intraoperative and postoperative hearing deficits in cerebellopontine angle surgery. *Acta Neurochir. (Wien), 81,* 142–151.

Selters, W.A. and Brackmann, D.E. (1977). Acoustic tumor detection with brain stem electric response audiometry. *Archives of Otolaryngology, 103,* 181–187.

Selters, W.A. and Brackmann, D.E. (1979). Brain stem electric response audiometry in acoustic tumor detection. In House, W.F. and Luetje, C.M. (eds.), *Acoustic tumor, Vol. 1. Diagnosis,* pp. 225–236. Baltimore, MD: University Park Press.

Sohmer, H., Gafni, M., and Chisin, R. (1982). Auditory nerve brainstem potentials in man and cat under hypoxic and hypercapnic conditions. *Electroencephalography and Clinical Neurophysiology, 53,* 506–512.

Starr, A. and Achor, L.J. (1975). Auditory brainstem responses in neurological disease. *Archives of Neurology, 32,* 761–768.

Stockard, J.J., Sharbrough, F.W., and Tinker, J.A. (1978). Effects of hypothermia on the human auditory brainstem response. *Annals of Neurology, 3,* 368–370.

Thornton, C., Heneghan, C., James, M., et al. (1984). Effects of halothane or enflurane with controlled ventilation on auditory evoked potentials. *British Journal of Anesthesiology, 56,* 315–323.

Wilber, L.A., Kruger, B., and Killion, M.C. (1988). Reference thresholds for the ER-3A insert earphone. *Journal of the Acoustical Society of America, 83,* 669–676.

CHAPTER 19

AUDITORY EVOKED RESPONSES IN ACUTE BRAIN INJURY AND REHABILITATION

JAMES W. HALL III
DANIEL P. HARRIS

INTRODUCTION

Severe brain injury at any age requires intensive care and systematic monitoring to minimize the effects of the primary injury and prevent, whenever possible, secondary CNS pathophysiology. Monitoring is especially critical during the acute period following hospital admission. Auditory evoked responses (AERs) have features which are essential for reliable and valid neuromonitoring. In addition, AERs offer unique advantages for prompt and thorough assessment of otologic and audiologic status in both intensive care unit (ICU) and rehabilitation settings.

Greenberg and colleagues first applied AERs in the evaluation and management of acute brain injury, along with visual and somatosensory evoked responses (Greenberg et al., 1977). The emphasis in these early studies was prediction of long-term neurologic outcome, largely in adults, from the pattern of evoked response findings recorded during the acute period after the injury. Since then, the role of AERs in the intensive care unit (ICU) setting has expanded dramatically, and been described for both adults and children. AERs have unique value in early detection and evaluation of peripheral auditory dysfunction, which is not uncommon in patients with both traumatic and non-traumatic acute brain injury. AERs can be applied in evaluating and monitoring CNS status during the acute period following a severe brain injury, much the same as they are

used in neurophysiologic intraoperative monitoring. One of the most exciting new monitoring developments is the application of computer-controlled automated evoked response techniques in acute brain injured patients. In addition, the use of event related AERs in brain injury rehabilitation has recently been described. In this chapter we will review the various applications of AERs in both acute brain injury and during subsequent rehabilitation. We begin with a review of the rationale for monitoring, protocols for AER assessment, and factors influencing AER findings. The chapter concludes with an introduction to computed evoked response topographic assessment (brain mapping) in the brain injured population.

RATIONALE FOR NEUROLOGIC MONITORING IN ACUTE BRAIN INJURY

Measures of Structure versus Function

Management of brain injury involves medical and surgical treatment for primary traumatic or non-traumatic lesions, and prevention of secondary neuronal damage in the acute period following injury. AERs, and sensory evoked responses in general, fulfill a rather unique clinical role during this critical period. Although *structural* CNS damage can be detected by neuroradiologic techniques, principally computerized tomography (CT) or magnetic resonance imaging

Data and clinical experiences reported in this paper were in part acquired while the first author was affiliated with the Department of Otolaryngology—Head and Neck Surgery at the University of Texas Medical School in Houston.

(MRI), neither CT scanning nor MRI can be conducted at bedside and, consequently, neither offers a feasible neuromonitoring alternative. Another neuroradiologic technique, ultrasonography, has the advantage of mobility. While ultrasound imaging in the ICU is now available for management of acute brain injury as an adjunct to CT or MRI, it does not provide the necessary spatial resolution for precise evaluation of sites and extent of brain injury. In short, one limitation of CNS monitoring with neuroradiologic imaging techniques is the lack of information on the *functional* integrity of neurons. A secondary practical drawback for repeated CNS assessment with these procedures is the high cost of the service to the patient.

General Physiologic Monitoring

Constant monitoring of systemic physiologic parameters, such as blood pressure, body temperature, and cardiac output, along with periodic assessment of blood gases such as PaO_2 (arterial pressure for oxygen) and $PaCO_2$ (arterial pressure of carbon dioxide) is an essential feature of intensive care of the acute brain-injured patient. A general monitor of CNS functional status is intracranial pressure (ICP). Within days after a severe insult to the brain, there is increased risk for cerebral edema and, as a result, elevated ICP. ICP is monitored with pressure-sensitive transducers that are inserted through the skull and located either below the dura covering the brain, within the subarachnoid space, or in the CSF within the intraventricular space (via a catheter). One of the most important relationships among these parameters is the difference between mean arterial blood pressure (MAP) and ICP:

MAP – ICP = cerebral perfusion pressure (CPP).

CPP must be adequate to assure delivery of blood to brain tissue. Control of ICP is a basic and ongoing objective in intensive care of brain injury. Normally, ICP is close to 0 mmHg and increases slightly with exercise or straining. The accepted upper limit for normal ICP is 15 mmHg (1 mmHg = 1 torr = 1.36 mm H_2O). Uncontrolled increases in ICP will produce a decrease in CPP. With CPP values of less than 50 mmHg, blood flow is usually inadequate. In addition, elevated ICP

eventually may result in transtentorial (downward) herniation of the cerebrum with compression of vital structures in the brainstem and, subsequently, death. Cerebral spinal fluid is contiguous with cochlear fluids, in particular the perilymph via the cochlear aqueduct which forms the link between scala tympani and subarachnoid space. Changes in ICP may also be reflected in sensorineural status via as changes occur in fluid pressure in perineural spaces and within the endolymphatic duct (Reid, Marchbanks, Burge, Martin, Bateman, Pickard, and Brightwell, 1990; Tandon, Sinha, Kacker, Saxena, and Sing, 1973; Klockhoff, Anggard, and Anggard, 1966). The relevance of this relation for audiologists is that increased ICP can, conceivably, produce sensorineural hearing deficits. This point was illustrated by case reports in several recent publications (Hall, 1988, 1991).

The combination of these general physiologic monitoring techniques provide regular information on the CNS environment. The overall objective is to create the optimal metabolic conditions for CNS function and recovery and thus prevent secondary CNS damage due to hypoxia, hypotension, and ischemia. Neuronal hypoxia usually is a factor of reduced delivery of oxygen to the brain, either because of lowered oxygen levels within an adequate blood supply, perhaps secondary to respiratory dysfunction, or because of decreased blood flow (which results in less oxygen reaching the brain). Ischemia is the brain tissue dysfunction or damage resulting from an inadequate blood supply. It can be a product of lowered blood pressure, increased ICP, or a combination of these two factors. These general physiologic data are supplemented by the clinical neurologic examination which, in the ICU, is typically limited to the assessment of brainstem reflexes (corneal, gag, oculocephalic, pupillary response to light) and the Glasgow Coma Scale (GCS). The neurologic examination is traditionally the primary monitor of CNS function in the ICU patient.

Each of these physiologic monitoring approaches has clinical drawbacks. The general physiologic measures do not reflect status of specific regions of the CNS. Blood gas data are typically not available continuously. As usually monitored, ICP data only applies to the CNS region near the site of the transducer, and almost always the cerebral region. Brainstem ICP may differ significantly. Mechanical obstruction of the device can produce incorrectly low or high ICP readings. Furthermore, in the injured brain, ischemia may develop at variable ICP and CPP values, some of which would be adequate for normal brain functioning. Finally, the validity of the neurologic examination of a comatose patient, which mainly consists of brainstem reflexes and motor responses to crude sensory stimulation, often is compromised or completely eliminated by common therapy modalities. Intensive therapy for the acute brain-injured patient may include hyperventilation to reduce blood flow, CSF drainage, osmotic diuretics to reduce brain water content, and head elevation (all of these maneuvers in part are designed to control ICP), and maintenance of adequate MAP. Three other medical therapies are neuromuscular blockade, sedatives, and barbiturates. These medications can profoundly influence the neurologic examination.

AERs, as detailed below, can be recorded in patients treated with these drugs. This is a practical advantage of AERs in neuromonitoring. The major rationale for neuromonitoring, however, is the sensitivity of AERs to the development of brain pathophysiology. There is recent clinical and experimental evidence that alterations of AER latency, amplitude and/or threshold are associated with hypoxia (Sohmer, Freeman, and Schmuel, 1989), increased ICP and, especially, early stages of brain ischemia (Baik, Branston, Bentivoglio, and Symon, 1990; Billet, Thorne, and Gavin, 1989; Lesnick et al., 1984). With developing ischemia, evoked response abnormalities occur during disruption of metabolic processes, at the cellular level, prior to the development of irreversible structural cell damage. Thus, timing is a critical factor in neuromonitoring. Evoked responses must be recorded as ischemia develops in order to provide an early warning that aggressive medical or surgical therapy is imperative. For this reason, continuous monitoring in the ICU is optimal. Although not feasible with conventional evoked response measurement techniques, computer controlled automatic evoked response instrumentation may soon make continuous monitoring a reality, as described in the concluding section of this chapter.

FACTORS IN AER MEASUREMENT IN ACUTE BRAIN INJURY

Effect of Coma on AERs

A commonly used clinical grading scale for severity of injury is the Glasgow Coma Scale, or GCS (Jennett and Teasdale, 1981). As displayed in Figure 19.1, the GCS incorporates an eye opening, verbal and motor response to sensory stimulation. Patients with the highest possible score are generally intact neurologically. A patient with a GCS score of 3 or 4, in contrast, has minimal neurologic responsiveness to even painful stimulation. An accepted definition for severe head injury is a GCS of 8 or less. The severely injured patient, therefore, typically does not open his/her eyes to any form of stimulus, does not vocalize (most are intubated so this component of the scale is not tallied), and has abnormal motor responses to sensory stimulation (e.g. flexion or extension posturing).

In patients without primary or secondary brainstem damage, GCS is not correlated to ABR. That is, patients with the lowest possible coma score (the "deepest" coma) often, in fact usually, have a normal ABR, at least initially. This important point will be reiterated with group data and case reports which follow. Conversely, ABR abnormalities are occasionally found among patients with relatively high GCS scores (above 8) and moderate or minor head injury. The insensitivity of ABR to level of coma is probably due to the inherent difference in neurophysiologic substrate for the two CNS measures. The ABR is a sensory response with well-appreciated resistance to the effects of CNS suppressants and state of arousal, whereas the GCS is predominantly a measure of motor response and consciousness.

Can comatose patients hear? Clinicians routinely involved in AER measurement in the ICU are asked this question periodically, especially from the family members of comatose patients. For comatose patients with normal appearing AERs, especially responses presumably arising at least in part from auditory cortex (e.g. auditory middle latency, auditory late, and P300 responses), the answer is not clearcut. Auditory stimulation clearly can alter heart rate, respiratory rate, and ICP (McGraw and Cindall, 1974). This latter finding has direct implications for AER monitoring in the ICU.

GLASGOW COMA SCALE

Eye Opening	Spontaneous	4	Total
	To Voice	3	Glasgow Coma
	To Pain	2	Scale Points
	None	1	14 - 15 = 5
			11 - 13 = 4
			8 - 10 = 3
			5 - 7 = 2
Verbal Response	Oriented	5	3 - 4 = 1
	Confused	4	
	Inappropriate Words	3	
	Incomprehensible Words	2	
	None	1	
Motor Response	Obeys Command	6	
	Localizes Pain	5	
	Withdraw (pain)	4	
	Flexion (pain)	3	
	Extension (pain)	2	
	None	1	
TOTAL TRAUMA SCORE			**1-15**

FIGURE 19.1. Glasgow Coma Scale used to grade severity of brain injury and depth of coma.

High-intensity auditory stimulation in AER measurement may, in comatose patients with "tight brains," cause elevations in ICP. There is, conversely, some evidence that nonnoxious environmental stimulation may reduce length of coma and be therapeutic.

In a thought provoking and compassionate article, La Puma, Schiedermayer, Gulyas, and Siegler (1988) frankly address the issue of talking to comatose patients. They conclude by affirming that: "When caring for a comatose patient, we should identify ourselves, recognize the patient by name, tell the patient the reason for our visit, and briefly explain any procedures that are planned. We should say words that might be comforting. We should talk to comatose patients because they may hear, because some comatose patients get better, and because we are caring professionals" (La Puma et al., 1988, p. 22). This is sound advice for those clinicians who record AERs in the ICU.

Influence of Therapeutic Drugs on AERs

Drugs used therapeutically in acute management of brain injury differentially influence AERs. Four general categories of drugs which may influence AER outcome in the ICU are neuromuscular blockers (chemical paralyzers), sedatives, barbiturates, and potentially ototoxic medications. Neuromuscular blockers (e.g., Metocurine or Pavulon) chemically paralyze the patient and facilitate acceptance of intubation. These drugs also limit movement and exertion, both of which can elevate intracranial pressure. The effect of chemical paralyzers on AERs is beneficial, namely, reduction or elimination of muscle-related artifact. The rather conspicuously smooth appearance of many of the AER recordings displayed in this chapter is testimony to the positive effects of chemical paralysis.

Sedatives are also frequently administered in the ICU in an attempt to keep the patient relaxed and physically inactive. Two sedatives used for this purpose are morphine and haldol. While the effects of these sedatives on AERs have not been systematically investigated, there is no apparent change of ECochG or ABR. Some reduction of AMLR amplitude would be expected on the basis of known influences of other sedatives (e.g., chloral hydrate) and also sleep, but as illustrated in Figure 19.2, a robust AMLR can be ob-

served from patients receiving therapeutic doses of morphine, as well as haldol. The later-latency AERs are suppressed by sedatives.

Among the drugs that are sometimes administered in the ICU, barbiturates have the most profound influence on AERs. Barbiturates (specifically pentobarbital) are usually reserved as a last-resort therapy modality in management of elevated intracranial pressure (ICP). A therapeutic blood level of barbiturates is 30 μg/ml, which is defined by suppression of the EEG and is in effect a drug-induced coma. The barbiturates are thought by some investigators to contribute to lowered ICP and to offer protection from brain ischemia by reducing brain metabolism and, therefore, the brain's demand for blood, in general, and glucose and oxygen in particular. However, this theory is not universally endorsed and the effectiveness of barbiturates in management of acute brain injury has not be documented (Piatt and Schiff, 1984). The effect of barbiturates on AERs and other sensory evoked responses,

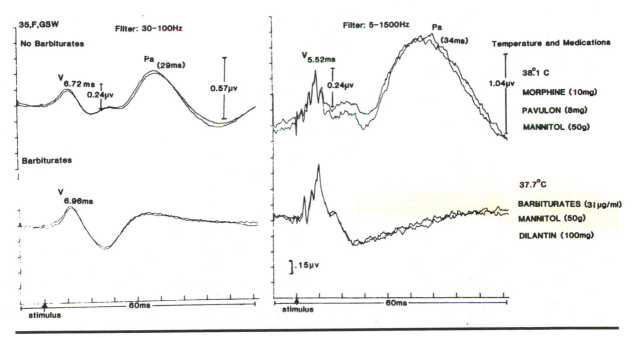

FIGURE 19.2.   Example of ABR and AMLR waveforms recorded in the ICU from a comatose patient managed with several medical therapies.

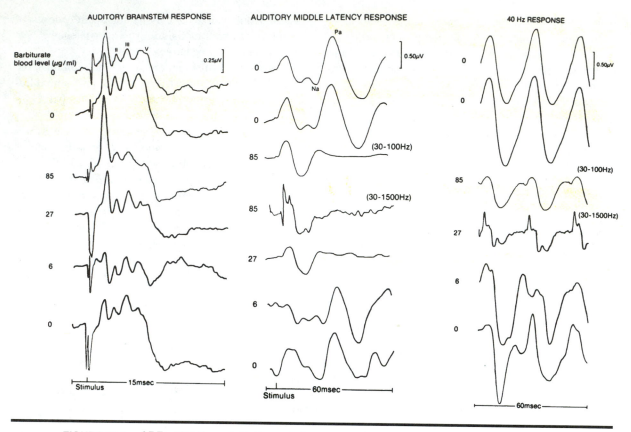

FIGURE 19.3.   ABR, AMLR, and 40 Hz waveforms recorded from an adult patient with traumatic head injury before, during, and after therapeutic barbiturate induced coma.

and also acoustic reflexes, has been described in detail (Hall, 1985), and is illustrated in Figure 19.3.

The ABR is remarkably resistant to barbiturates, even at blood levels of well over 100 μg/ml, although high dose barbiturates will produce increased ABR interwave latencies (e.g., I–V). The mechanism underlying this change in increased synaptic transmission time, rather than a reduction in the speed of axonal propagation (Sohmer and Goitein, 1988). The AMLR Pa component and the auditory 40 Hz response, in contrast, is totally suppressed by blood levels as low as 10 to 20 μg/ml (Hall, Hargadine, and Allen, 1985, Hall, 1985, 1991). It is important to keep in mind that body temperature may be reduced in barbiturate coma. The

possible effects of lowered temperature on AERs must be taken into account when monitoring a patient who is receiving high dose barbiturates. Deep hypothermia may also be employed therapeutically in management of acute brain injury.

Each of these four therapy modalities—neuromuscular blockers, sedatives, barbiturates, and hypothermia—seriously limit or totally eliminate the effectiveness of the clinical neurologic examination as a means of monitoring CNS status in the acute brain-injured patient. The neuromuscular blockers preclude assessment of motor response to stimulation. The sedatives reduce responsiveness in general. Barbiturates at therapeutic doses, and extreme hypothermia, can render the patient flaccid, with no apparent brainstem reflexes, and even fixed and dilated pupils. A major rationale for neuromonitoring in the ICU with AERs is the compromising effect of commonly used drugs on neurologic findings. However, because AERs are not entirely independent of these medications, each therapy modality must be carefully documented at the time of the assessment.

The possible effects on AERs of other therapy modalities often used in management of acute brain injury, such as osmotic diuretics (e.g., mannitol), steroids (e.g., decadron), and anticonvulsants (e.g., dilantin) are not known. Although major effects are unlikely, particularly for the earlier latency AERs, there is some recent experimental evidence (in an rat animal model) suggesting that high doses of certain anticonvulsants (phenytoin, carbamazepine, phenobarbital, clonazepam) increased the latencies for later ABR waves (Hirose, Chujo, Kataoka, Kawada, and Yoshioki, 1990). In fact, these investigators found that very high doses (maximum nonlethal) of phenytoin totally suppressed the ABR. The authors warn that high doses of anticonvulsants should be taken into account when ABR is applied in the diagnosis of brain death.

Potentially ototoxic drugs are administered to many comatose brain-injured patients in the treatment of infection or to maintain physiologic stability. Among these drugs are the aminoglycosides (e.g., gentamycin, tobramycin), other antibiotics (e.g., vancomycin, amphotericin B), and loop diuretics, such as furosemide (lasix). Prolonged administration of one or more of these ototoxic drugs during intensive care can lead to cochlear hearing impairment, initially for the higher frequencies. This possibility has two direct implications for AER test protocol in the ICU. First, AER assessment should be carried out soon after the injury to establish a pre-drug audiometric baseline. This testing would, of course, include threshold seeking for each ear. Without this test strategy, it will probably be impossible to determine later whether a patient's sensorineural hearing deficit was pre-existing, due to otologic trauma, or a result of ototoxicity or infection. For those patients who do receive an extensive course of ototoxic drugs, a follow up audiologic assessment after medical stabilization but prior to hospital discharge is advisable. This is especially important for pediatric ICU patients.

Effect of Body Temperature

Evaluating a patient with a low body temperature is a condition frequently encountered in the operating room (OR) and ICU. In the ICU, hypothermia can be seen in patients who have suffered a cardiac arrest. Additionally, patients with brainstem pathology often demonstrate an inability to regulate their body temperature. Acute care therapies, such as barbiturate coma, may also lower temperature. Temperature, both hyper- and hypothermia, has a profound effect on evoked response testing (Hall, Bull, and Cronau, 1988; Jacobson, Hall, Bull, and Mackey-Hargadine, 1991; Sohmer, Gold, Cahani, and Attias, 1989; Ahmed, 1991). In general, ABR latencies are inversely related to temperature. As temperature decreases (hypothermia), ABR latencies increase. The temperature effect is especially prominent for interwave latency values. With increased temperature (hyperthermia), ABR latency values progressively decrease. Hall (Hall, Bull, Cronau, 1988; Hall, 1991) recommends a conservative correction factor of 0.2 ms for the wave I–V latency interval for every degree of body temperature change. As an example, for a patient whose body temperature drops by two degrees during the course of monitoring, we would assume that the wave I–V latency interval would increase by about 0.4 ms strictly due to the change in temperature. Before interpreting the wave I–V latency interval, therefore, we would first correct the wave I–V latency interval (subtract 0.4 ms). Body temperature must always be documented in ICU neuromonitoring.

Effect of Environmental Artifact on AER Measurement

Environmental electrical artifact is probably the most troublesome and commonly encountered obstacle to obtaining reliable and meaningful evoked response data in an ICU environment. There are many sources of electrical artifact, including 60 Hz line noise and a spectrum of airborne electromagnetic energy. Even though an ICU is potentially a hostile environment for evoked response recording, it is possible to measure evoked responses routinely for auditory, somatosensory and visual stimulus modalities from acute, severely brain injured children and adults with commercially available equipment. Precautions for minimizing the deleterious effects of electrical artifact include reliance on well grounded evoked response measurement instrumentation, quality electrodes, low interelectrode resistance (less than 5000 ohms), and especially a very good electrical contact for the ground electrode. Guidelines for optimizing evoked response recording in general, and trouble shooting techniques for OR and ICU recordings, were recently presented in detail (Hall, 1992). As a last resort, attempt to reduce artifact contamination by restricting filter settings, e.g., from 30 to 3000 Hz to 150 to 1500 Hz for the ABR and, if that technique fails, return to the patient's bedside at another time, perhaps in the evening.

Neuromuscular artifact is a less serious problem in the acute period following brain injury. As noted later in the chapter, the patient is typically sedated, often paralyzed chemically, and sometimes in a deep barbiturate induced coma. During recovery from injury, however, increasing movement can contribute to muscular artifact that contaminates or even precludes evoked response recording. Muscle artifact is a more significant factor for the AMLR and SSERs than for the ABR. Sometimes it is necessary to request mild sedation in patients recovering from brain injury in order to successfully carry out testing.

Effect of Peripheral Otologic Pathology

Approximately two-thirds of acute severely head-injured patients have otologic pathology by physical examination (Aquilar et al., 1986). Among these, the most common pathologies are relatively minor and typically transient, such as hemotympanum, blood in the external ear canal, and serous otitis media. Conductive hearing impairment, which can seriously affect AER measurement, may be a direct result of trauma, e.g., hemotympanum, or a function of prolonged intensive care requiring intubation, mechanical ventilation,

supine positioning, or infection. Non-injury related sensorineural hearing deficits in acute brain injury may develop secondarily to necessary but potentially ototoxic drug therapy with aminoglycosides, other antibiotics (e.g., vancomycin), and the loop diuretic furosemide (lasix). For patients with any of these etiologies, AERs are a feasible means of promptly identifying hearing impairment and describing type and degree. The point at which the hearing deficit occurs may range from pre-existing impairment, to injury-related damage to post-injury secondary causes. Baseline AERs soon after the injury, and then periodically during hospital course, may assist in clarification of the onset of the deficit. This effort can yield dividends in both patient otologic management and medico-legal documentation.

Traditionally, temporal bone fractures have been categorized as either longitudinal (which are most common) or transverse (usually accounting for less than 20%), or even less frequently, mixed. Serious hearing impairment is generally considered an invariable component of most temporal bone fractures. This final point would seem to limit the value of AERs in patients with radiographically confirmed temporal bone fractures. That is, if there is radiographic evidence of temporal bone fracture conventionally one could presume a serious hearing impairment which would, in turn, preclude recording a detectable AER.

Studies within the past few years challenge these traditional viewpoints. First, acute radiologic study with high resolution CT scanning of head-injured patients with temporal bone fractures suspected by clinical criteria shows that a high percentage (68%) have fractures that are best classified as "mixed," rather than purely longitudinal or transverse (Ghorayeb, Yeakley, Hall, and Jones, 1987). Routine CT scanning of the CNS is usually inadequate for description of the status of temporal bone structures. In addition, patients with CT-confirmed temporal bone fractures may present with a wide variety of audiologic patterns, ranging from normal hearing to profound hearing impairment. Audiologic data obtained during the sub-acute period for 78 ears of 68 patients with CT-confirmed temporal bone fractures (fractures were bilateral for 10 patients), summarized in Table 19.5 (below), highlight this point. Normal hearing threshold levels (20 dB or better) were found in approximately one-third of the ears, with only a mild hearing sensitivity impairment in another 33%. The next largest percentage of patients was in the profound hearing impairment region. Although the majority of the ears (58%) showed a type A tympanogram, 46% of these also had hearing losses with a definite conductive component, implying middle ear pathology (i.e., ossicular chain disruption). Severe restriction of middle ear mobility (evidenced by a type B tympanogram) characterized almost one-half of the ears. When pure-tone audiometry and tympanometry were evaluated in combination, conductive hearing impairment was most common (57%) in this series of patients, while normal hearing, and sensorineural or mixed deficits were relatively evenly distributed. AERs can be detected, with high stimulus intensity levels, in patients with hearing thresholds as poor as 60 to 65 dB, even when the type of impairment is conductive (Hall, 1991). An AER will be present in up to three-fourths of patients with CT-confirmed temporal bone fracture, at least at the time of outpatient follow-up (Hall, 1988). Coordinated application of AERs, pure-tone audiometry and immittance measurement is an effective approach for defining functional otologic status following temporal bone fracture.

DEMOGRAPHICS OF ICU PATIENTS WITH SEVERE BRAIN INJURY

Pediatric Head Injury

Trauma is the leading cause of injury and death in children aged 1 to 14 (Walker et al., 1985; Raimondi and Hirschauer, 1984). Head injury is usually a component of life-threatening trauma. Each year head injury kills five times as many children as the second-ranking lethal disease, leukemia, and kills or causes permanent disability in more children than all other neurologic diseases combined (Division of Injury Control, 1990). Head injury is the most common CNS pathologic entity in many pediatric ICUs. The mode of injury for the majority of children is generally a motor vehicle, auto-pedestrian, or auto-bicyclist accident (Argan, Castillo, Winn, 1990). Other causes of injury are falls, child abuse, and gunshot wounds. Protocol for AER mea-

surement in pediatric brain injury is similar to that described for adults. Detailed discussions are also presented in recent publications by the author and colleagues (Hall and Mackey-Hargadine, 1984; Hall, Mackey-Hargadine, and Allen, 1985; Hall and Tucker, 1985, 1986; Hall, Winkler, and Fletcher, 1987; Hall, Tucker, Fletcher, and Habersang, 1989; Hall, 1992).

As seen in Table 19.1, the ages of traumatically head-injured children evaluated with AERs by the first author ranged from 1 month to 16 years (the arbitrary upper age limit). Mean age was 7.3 years. Approximately two-thirds were male. As with the adult population, the majority were severely injured, as defined by the GCS. Although head trauma was the mechanism of injury for more than half of the children, there were a mixture of other etiologies for patients evaluated in the pediatric ICU including meningitis, hydrocephalus, and ischemic/hypoxic insults (e.g., near drowning).

Adult Head Injury

In a regional CNS trauma center located within a private hospital, the majority of patients, usually more than three-fourths, will be injured in motor vehicle accidents (MVAs). Statistics gathered by the first author support this general finding. Most victims of MVAs (66%) were drivers or passengers in automobiles, whereas the remainder in the group were pedestrians struck by an motor vehicle (9%) or were victims of motorcycle accidents, gunshot wounds, falls, or assault. Following the injury, 89% of this series of patients was transported to the emergency center by LifeFlight helicopter. The average time elapsed from helicopter patient pickup to emergency center arrival was 41 minutes. Of all adult patients undergoing AER assessment in the ICU setting, 92% (the population just described) were traumatically head injured. The additional 8% suffered acute cerebral vascular accidents (i.e., intracranial bleeds of varying etiologies). Elderly stroke victims were not referred for AER assessment in the surgical ICU.

General characteristics of 114 consecutive adult patients evaluated with ABR are shown in Table 19.2. Three-fourths were male. CT revealed mass lesions more often than diffuse lesions. Most (80%) required

TABLE 19.1. Summary of Characteristics of a Series of Acutely Head-Injured Children (N = 102) who Underwent AER Assessment in the Pediatric ICU.

Characteristic	Number	%
Gender		
Male	66	65
Female	36	35
Initial Glasgow Coma Score *		Cumulative %
3–4	36	36
5–6	24	60
7–8	16	76
9–12	11	87
13–15	13	100

* mean = 6.4

TABLE 19.2. Summary of Characteristics of a Series of Acutely Head-Injured Adults (N = 114) who Underwent AER Assessment in the Surgical ICU.

Characteristic	Number	%
Gender		
Male	85	75
Female	29	25
Computerized tomography		
Mass lesions	66	58
Diffuse lesion	48	42
ICP		
Monitored	91	80
Not monitored	23	20
Surgery		
Neurologic *	28	24
Other	25	22
Disposition		
Died	67	59
Nursing home	9	8
Rehabilitation	25	22
Home	13	11

* Surgical intervention in addition to placement of ICP monitor prior to initial AER assessment.

ICP monitoring during intensive care, and among those not monitored were patients with a presumably fatal injury which did not warrant ICP an monitor. Less than one-quarter of the patients underwent neurological surgery, other than placement of an ICP monitor, implying that intensive care (medical) therapy was the usual management approach. The mortality rate for this series was 59%, yet one-third of the patients were discharged from the hospital to their home or to a rehabilitation facility. Relatively few patients were sufficiently impaired to require nursing home care. The distribution of GCS for the 114 patients was as follows: GCS 3, 20%; GCS 4, 23%; GCS 5, 12%; GCS 6, 14%; GCS 7, 17%; GCS 8–15, 14%. Therefore, 86% of this patient group undergoing AER assessment had GCS scores of 7 or less. By definition, therefore, they were severely brain injured.

CORRELATION OF AERS WITH CLINICAL FINDINGS

Relation between ABR and Pupillary Response and CT Findings in Adults

CT is the principal method for evaluating site and extent of CNS acute brain damage, and the pupillary response is the major neurologic sign monitored during the acute period after injury. If ABR findings were invariably correlated with each of these valuable and time-tested techniques for neuroassessment and monitoring, there would be little rationale for adding ABR to the list of sophisticated procedures applied in intensive care and management of acute brain injury. In fact, as displayed in Tables 19.3 and 19.4, there are clearcut discrepancies among ABR outcome, pupillary response, and CT findings in adults with acute traumatic brain injury. ABR and pupillary response, are both mediated in the brainstem, yet 7 of 45 patients with a normal (reactive) pupillary response showed abnormal ABRs and, conversely, over half (58%) of those patients with clearly abnormal (unreactive) pupil findings yielded a normal ABR (Table 19.3). This latter pattern is especially important for clinical management of brain injury since unreactive pupils are often viewed as a sign of irre-

TABLE 19.3.   Correlation between Initial ABR Findings and Pupillary Response Data as Recorded in the Surgical ICU and Patient Disposition at or prior to Hospital Discharge for a Series of Head-Injured Adults (N = 85).

	Pupils	
	Reactive	Nonreactive
ABR		
Normal	38	23
Abnormal *	7	17
Disposition		
Died	14	31
Nursing home	3	3
Rehabilitation	18	5
Home	10	1

* Interwave latency delay of more than 2.5 standard deviations above mean normal value, absent wave III or V, or no response.

TABLE 19.4.   Comparison of ABR Findings and CT Evidence of Transtentorial Herniation (TH) for a Series of Head Injured Adults (N = 114). *

	ABR	
	Normal	Abnormal
Mass lesion		
no transtentorial herniation	33	19
transtentorial herniation	5	9
Diffuse lesion		
no transtentorial herniation	9	14
transtentorial herniation	6	19

* CT scanning at hospital admission; ABR data collected within 25 hours after hospital admission in the surgical ICU.

versible brain dysfunction. The value of ABR in defining CNS status in conjunction with pupillary response is suggested by data on patient disposition at hospital discharge, displayed in the lower portion of Table 19.3. Among the patients with reactive pupils, 14 died, including all 7 patients with an abnormal ABR. Pupil unreactivity was not invariably associated with subsequent death, as 9 of these 40 patients survived and 6 were discharged to either home or a rehabilitation facility. Each of these 6 patients were among the group of 23 patients with normal ABRs. Thus, ABR and pupillary findings that are in agreement (i.e., both normal or both abnormal) appear to offer strong evidence of CNS integrity or dysfunction, at least on the brainstem level. However, when ABR does not confirm the pupillary finding there is the possibility of an unexpected outcome and, perhaps, reason for reconsidering the strategy for medical management.

A similar theme is found in the relationship between emergency CT scans at hospital admission and initial ABR findings, usually 24 to 48 hours later (Table 19.4). CTs were interpreted by a neuroradiologist without knowledge that ABRs had been assessed, and the ABRs were interpreted by the author without information on CT results. The neuroradiologist differentiated in his report between those patients with versus without CT evidence of transtentorial herniation (i.e., effacement of the cisterns surrounding the brainstem and/or evidence of compression of the brainstem). This judgment was made for patients with mass lesions and diffuse lesions. The expectation was that patients with evidence of brainstem compression would have abnormal ABRs and vice versa. In both groups of CT lesions, there were patients who met this expectation, but in addition, there was also a substantial proportion of patients with discrepant findings for the two procedures. For example, 5 patients with mass lesions and 6 with diffuse lesions had CT evidence of transtentorial herniation yet normal ABRs. CT interpretation appeared to overestimate the extent of CNS dysfunction. CT evidence of transtentorial herniation carries the same dire implication as unreactive pupils, namely, the likelihood of a severe, irreversible, fatal brain injury. This discrepancy would imply that the CT can provide structural evidence of brainstem compression when, in fact, brainstem function remains reasonably intact (Zuccarello et al., 1983; Toutan et al., 1984). An even greater number of patients presented the converse discrepancy between CT and ABR. The majority of patients with abnormal ABRs actually failed to show CT evidence of transtentorial herniation (Table 19.4). That is, the ABR indicated brainstem dysfunction that would not have been predicted on the basis of CT. Virtually all of these patients with abnormal ABRs went on to either die or remained severely impaired neurologically. Several possible explanations come to mind for this latter difference between ABR versus CT findings. Patients may develop brainstem hypoxic/ischemic injury (and ABR abnormalities) secondary to events other than increased ICP and transtentorial herniation. Overall, these data suggest a complimentary relationship among ABR, pupillary response, and CT findings. One measure may provide information not immediately available from the other. It is also possible the brain status changed between the time of CT scanning at hospital admission and ABR measurement within 24 hours later.

ABR and Physiologic Findings in Head-Injured Children

The pattern of ABR and pupillary findings described above for adult head-injured patients characterized data for 157 tests in the group of 102 children. For example, in 39 of the 109 tests yielding an abnormal ABR the pupillary response was normal. Conversely, in 8 tests when the pupils were totally unreactive there was a normal wave I–V latency interval. On none of these test

dates was the patient receiving a drug which is known to affect pupillary response (e.g., atropine). CT data were not available for the pediatric head injury group.

Correlations among ABR latency values and selected physiologic parameters for 129 test sessions are summarized in Table 19.5. All patients were normothermic (37 ± 1 degree Centigrade) at the time of assessment. There was a significant correlation between ICP, CPP and ABR absolute latency of waves III and V and major interwave latencies (I–III, III–V, and I–V). MAP was not associated with ABR latency according to group data analysis, perhaps because the average MAP in this series was 86 mmHg, and few patients had MAP values below 65 to 70 mmHg. ICP seemed to be the critical variable that was directly related to ABR latency, even for wave I which is a measure of peripheral (sensorineural) auditory function. This latter observation may offer some support for the relationship between elevated ICP and sensorineural impairment that was discussed above. The lack of a correlation between blood gas values and ABR latency is not unexpected, as blood for the oxygen and carbon dioxide analysis was drawn every 4 to 6 hours, and not usually within the timeframe of the AER assessment, and blood gases rarely deviated dramatically from an acceptable region for these mechanically ventilated children. Furthermore, basic research suggests a weak relationship between ABR and hypoxia. These data confirm the usefulness of ABR in detection of the pathophysiologic events that result in brain ischemia, namely, increased ICP and decreased CPP.

TABLE 19.5. Relation among ABR Latency and Physiologic Parameters in a Series of Children (N = 102; total of 129 test sessions). *

Physiologic parameter**	ABR components					
	I	III	V	I–III	III–V	I–V
MAP	–	–	–	+	–	–
ICP	+	++	++	++	++	++
CPP	+	++	++	++	++	++
PaO$_2$	–	+	–	+	–	+
PaCO$_2$	–	+	+	–	–	–

* all children had normal body temperature
** MAP = mean arterial blood pressure; ICP = intracranial pressure; CPP = cerebral perfusion pressure
 – = p > 0.05; + = p < 0.05; ++ = p < 0.01

AER TEST PROTOCOLS IN BRAIN INJURY

Measurement Parameters

The test protocol employed in AER measurement of brain injured patients in the ICU is summarized in Table 19.6. Most stimulus and acquisition parameters are comparable to those used in other clinical AER applications and described in greater detail elsewhere (Hall, 1992). Several features of the test protocol, however, warrant comment. Insert earphones (e.g., Etymotic ER-3A) are especially handy with the ICU population for at least six reasons. First, for many

TABLE 19.6. Auditory Brainstem Response (ABR) and Auditory Middle Latency Response (AMLR) Test Protocols Used in the Intensive Care Unit Setting.

Parameters	ABR	AMLR
Stimulus		
transducer	. . . . ER-3A (air conduction)	
	. . . . B-70 (bone conduction)	
type	click	tone bursts
frequency	not applicable	500, 1K, or 2K Hz
duration	0.1 ms	2-1-2 cycles
polarity	rarefaction	alternating
rate	21.1/sec	7.1/sec (or slower)
intensity	80 to 95 dB nHL	70 dB nHL
masking	occasional	never
presentation	monaural	monaural
Acquisition		
electrode arrays *		
Ch 1:	Fz-A1	C_5-linked ears
Ch 2:	Fz-A2	C_6-linked ears
Ch 3:	Fz-noncephalic	Fz-linked ears
	(optional)	
	. . . . Fpz ground	
filter	30–3000 Hz	10–500 Hz
notch filter	. . . . none	
amplification	× 100,000	× 75,000
sensitivity	±25 µv	±50 µV
analysis time	15 ms	100 ms
prestimulus time	1 ms	10 ms
sample points	512	256
sweeps	500 to 4000	250 to 500

*Noninverting-inverting electrode according to International 10–20 Electrode System. (Adapted from Hall, 1992.)

head-injured patients dressings partially cover the pinna and preclude a tight supraaural earphone coupling. The insert cushion can generally be placed under the bandage or the bandage can be cut to permit insertion. Second, some patients will have lacerations of the external ear which contraindicate supraaural earphone placement. Third, the pressure of conventional head-bands and TDH earphones against the head and ears may act as noxious tactile stimulation and actually elevate ICP. Fourth, ICP monitors, scalp lacerations, and head dressings may interfere with the typical placement of the traditional head band. Fifth, aural hygiene is enhanced because the insert cushions are disposable after use. This is particularly important in the ICU population since patients often have blood or debris in the ear canal. Before inserting the foam cushion, the clinician should of course ensure that the ear canal does not contain excessive blood or debris. Finally, a TIPtrode electrode can be used with insert earphones. TIPtrodes enhance ABR wave I (Hall, 1992). This is especially useful in the ICU population because ABR analysis is largely based on interwave latency values, yet patients often have peripheral auditory dysfunction (discussed earlier) that minimizes ABR wave I. In addition to these somewhat unique features in the ICU, insert earphones offer the usual clinical advantages, including prevention of ear canal collapse, precision in earphone placement, and minimal stimulus artifact (Hall, 1992).

As in neurodiagnostic applications of ABR, the test protocol in the ICU is generally selected to optimize detection of all waves, from wave I through wave V. Thus, the stimulus intensity is high (often maximum) to overcome any potential peripheral auditory deficit, bone conduction stimulation is whenever a conductive ABR pattern is observed, whenever possible filter settings are relatively wide to encompass maximal response energy, and multiple electrode arrays are often employed to clarify identification of specific waves. The rationale for these ABR measurement manipulations is reviewed in detail by Hall (1992). Conventional disk-type electrodes are typically adequate for ABR recordings in the ICU. Subdermal needle electrodes are also appropriate, and recommended when the response is monitored periodically over the course of a day or more. The needle electrodes can be left in place throughout the course of monitoring. After monitoring is discontinued and the needle electrodes are removed, they require sterilization before reuse. In some institutions, needle electrodes are considered disposable. Clinicians should consult with hospital policy on the use of needle electrodes.

AMLR measurement in the ICU can yield valuable information on the status of higher level auditory CNS regions. As indicated in selected figures throughout this chapter, a reliable AMLR can be consistently recorded from comatose patients. Several components of the test protocol (Table 19.6) should be highlighted. High stimulus intensities (greater than 70 to 75 dB

nHL) should generally be avoided to minimize postauricular muscle artifact (PAM). PAM, which appears as a sharp, large, peak in the 13 to 17 ms region of the AMLR waveform, may occur in comatose brain-injured patients, even if they are medically sedated. As a rule, the clinician should be very suspicious of PAM whenever an apparent AMLR Pa component is recorded at a latency of less than 23 to 25 ms (Hall, 1992). It is very important to avoid high-pass filter settings of 30 Hz in AMLR measurement. Filter-related artifacts in the AMLR waveform may be mistaken for the Pa component when restricted filter settings (e.g., 30 to 100 Hz) are used. This point was illustrated in Figures 19.2 and 19.3, and discussed in considerable detail by Hall (1992). Multiple channel recordings are essential for neurodiagnosis and neuromonitoring applications of AMLR in the ICU. Minimally, there should be a noninverting electrode located over each parietal-temporal region (e.g., C5 and C6), plus a midline electrode (Fz). There is now ample evidence that AMLR arises from cortical and subcortical (perhaps acoustic radiation and thalamic) generators (Jacobson, Newman, Privitera, and Grayson, 1991; Kraus et al., 1988; Scherg and von Cramon, 1988; Kileny et al., 1987). The hemispheric electrodes are more likely to detect activity generated in the auditory cortex or acoustic radiations, whereas the midline electrode may detect mostly subcortical activity.

Steps in ICU Neuromonitoring with AERs

Preparation.   Successful AER monitoring in the ICU begins with adequate instrumentation and preparation. Minimal requirements for the evoked response system are two- (preferably four-) channel capacity, insert earphones, sterilized subdermal needle electrodes, computer storage for AER data, and the ability to print out finished reports. Other desirable equipment features would be somatosensory and visual evoked response capacity, automatic documentation of measurement parameters, and a feature which permits the user to set up the equipment to collect AER data automatically on a periodic basis.

Before beginning AER monitoring, the clinician

should: 1) have a written order for the service, 2) appreciate the rationale for why monitoring is being done, 3) review the patient's medical history and physical findings, with special attention to possible otologic trauma and neurologic status, and 4) verify with the patient's nurse that AER measurement will not interfere with ongoing care, other neurodiagnostic procedures (e.g., travel to the CT scanner), or patient visitations. At the time of AER assessment, and throughout monitoring, it is important to document physiologic parameters (blood gases, blood pressure, ICP, body temperature), relevant medications (sedatives, chemical paralyzers, barbiturates, potentially ototoxic drugs), and clinical evidence of neurologic status, such as the GCS. With modern computer-based evoked response systems, this information can be documented within the patient's evoked response data files, much as intraoperative events are noted throughout surgery. Otherwise, pertinent patient data should be documented manually, as illustrated in Figure 19.4. The possible effects of medical therapies are a critical factor for interpretation of AMLR findings in the ICU setting. As noted above, AMLR can be totally suppressed by therapeutic dosages of barbiturates (Hall, 1985). Other anesthetic agents, and sedatives, may reduce AMLR amplitude values but do not appear to abolish the response. In the ICU, as in the OR setting, medications should always be documented before AERs are interpreted.

SPECIFIC APPLICATIONS OF AERs IN THE ICU

Monitoring Neurologic Status

Therapy modalities employed in the management of acute brain injury, as emphasized already, may invalidate the clinical neurologic examination. Sensory evoked responses (SERs), including AERs, provide a noninvasive means of objectively evaluating CNS functional status over time without contamination by necessary treatment regimens. We have focused much of our efforts on serially evaluating CNS function over time with SERs, rather than attempting to rely on data collected from a single test session 3 or 4 days after the injury, as other researchers have done (Anderson,

Bundlie, and Rockswold, 1984; Rappaport et al., 1978; Karnaze et al., 1982; Narayan et al., 1981; Lindsay et al., 1981; Rosenberg, Wogensen, and Starr, 1984; Seales, Rossiter, and Weinstein, 1979). Serial evoked response data have varied applications in the acute period following severe brain injury. Maximum exploitation of evoked responses is achieved when recordings are initially made within 24 hours of the injury and then repeated during the period of neurologic instability. One point requires emphasis at this juncture. An abnormal ABR almost always implies poor outcome, or death, whereas a normal acute ABR (within 24 to 76 hours post injury) has little predictive value, and is followed by patient death within the acute stage (Hall and Mackey-Hargadine, 1984; Hall et al., 1985; Hall and Tucker, 1985; Hall, 1992). This unfortunate sequence of events is witnessed all too often with severely brain-injured patients in the ICU.

The following case report serves to illustrate the use of AERs in monitoring neurologic status. A series of such cases were also recently presented by the first author (Hall, 1992). A 22-year-old male suffered a head injury in a MVA (case 1). At the scene, pupils were sluggishly reactive and respirations were labored. There was a decorticate motor response. GCS was 5. Following helicopter transport to the emergency room, and emergency therapy en route, pupils were equal and briskly reactive to light. Motor responses were purposeful to deep painful stimuli, but there was still no eye opening or verbal response. Emergency CT showed a right intraventricular bleed and a small left subdural hematoma. He was taken to the OR for a ventriculostomy (opening pressure of 12 cm water) and then to the ICU.

For the initial three days after injury, ICP was controlled with frequent doses of hyperosmolar (mannitol) drugs, as well as hyperventilation and CSF drainage. By one week, however, ICP was increasing to the 40s (mmHg), and barbiturate therapy was instituted. The major medical problem during barbiturate coma was a series of episodes of hypotension, which was treated with Dopamine. Follow-up CT scans indicated resolution of the intraventricular hemorrhage and neurologic status began to improve. Then, over the course of the

Test # ___1___

Patient Name: _J.C._____

Test date: _6/6/85_

Age _51_   Sex _M_____

Test time: _10:15 A.M._

PHYSIOLOGIC DATA:

P. _1_

BP _98 mm Hg_   ICP _20 - 22 mmHg_   PUPILLARY RESPONSE

T _99.6°F_   MEDS _DILANTIN_____

O_2 _172 mmHg_   _DECADRON_

LEFT   RIGHT   GCS = 6

CO_2 _23 mmHg_   _MORPHINE_____

4mm/+   4mm/+

METACURINE

DISKETTE#: _176_____

MANNITOL   ABR COMPONENTS

Note: Reactivity/size
+ = Brisk; - = sluggish;
0 = nonreactive

FILE #	MEM.	INTENSITY (RE: NORM)		I	III	V	I-III	III-V	I-V	V/I	ICP	TIME	COMMENTS
5	H_1	RIGHT	ms	1.62	3.66	5.88	2.04	2.22	4.26		21		30 - 3000 Hz
	H_2	85dB	uv	.24		.36							25 µV SENS. $\leq$ 1.1/sec N = 2000
6	Q_1	RE 85	ms										150 - 3000 Hz
		IPSILAT	uv										
	Q_2		ms										
		NONCEPH.	uv										
	Q_3		ms										
		CONTRAL.	uv										
	Q_4		ms										
		HORIZ.	uv										
			ms										
			uv										

AUDITORY MIDDLE-LATENCY/40 Hz								
FILE #	MEM.	INTENSITY (dial)	Na (ms)	Pa (ms)	Na - Pa (uv)	FILTER	AMR/40 Hz	COMMENTS
7	Q_1 Q_2	RE 75dB IPSILAT.	13	30	0.65	5-1500	AMR	Post-auricular artifact
	Q_3 Q_4	CONTRAL.	14	28	0.57	5-1500	AMR	
8	H_1 H_2	RE 75dB	—	—	0.80	5-1500	40Hz	

FIGURE 19.4.   Form used for documenting test time, physiologic data, medications, and ABR findings in the ICU setting.

next two weeks, the patient developed adult respiratory distress syndrome, at one point requiring CPR. He arrested and died one month after the injury.

Serial AER measures in this patient are illustrated in Figure 19.5. There were repeated instances of abnor-malities in interwave latency values, persisting for almost a week at one period, which were reversed, apparently with medically elevated mean arterial pressure. On day 19, a wave V component was not observed with the standard electrode array (Figure 19.6), but evaluation of

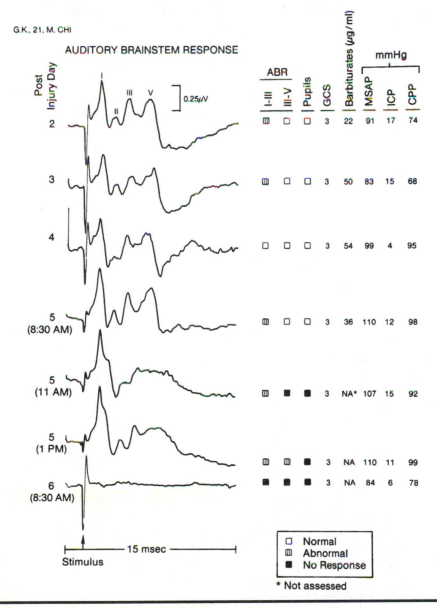

FIGURE 19.5.   Serial ABR and AMLR waveforms recorded in the ICU from a 22-year-old comatose, severely head-injured male during prolonged intensive care (case 1).

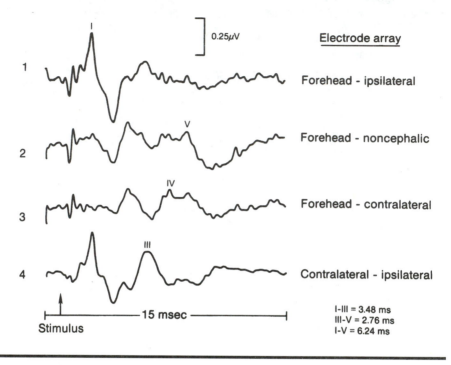

G.K., 21, M, CHI

AUDITORY BRAINSTEM RESPONSE
(Right ear stimulus, 95dB)

0.25μV

Electrode array

1   Forehead - ipsilateral

2   Forehead - noncephalic

3   Forehead - contralateral

4   Contralateral - ipsilateral

Stimulus   ————— 15 msec —————

I-III = 3.48 ms
III-V = 2.76 ms
I-V = 6.24 ms

FIGURE 19.6.   Multichannel ABR waveforms recorded in the ICU from case 1 illustrating the value of alternative electrode arrays in enhancing wave components.

the ABR with a four-channel recording array revealed a repeatable wave V. The AMLR, in contrast, was relatively stable, although suppressed of course in barbiturate coma. Finally, within 24 hours of the patient's death, ABR abnormalities were again recorded, this time in conjunction with no apparent AMLR.

In this case, the pathophysiologic feature associated temporally with the ABR changes was reduced CPP resulting not from elevated ICP but, rather, from decreased MAP. On the basis of the ABR findings, it would appear that CPPs in the 60s (mmHg) were inadequate for maintaining normal brainstem function of an already damaged CNS. An additional factor to consider, at least on day 14, was hypoxia. Repeated hypoxic episodes toward the end of the patient's hospital

course may have also contributed to the terminal ABR abnormalities.

Definition of Brain Death

Diagnosis of brain death is based on evidence of cerebral, cerebellar, and brainstem neuronal inactivity (Korein, 1984; Guidelines for the Determination of Death, 1981; Determination of Brain Death, 1987). There are numerous criteria for definition of brain death, and considerable medical, legal, and ethical discussion of the topic (Beresford, 1984; Guidelines for the Determination of Death, 1981). The primary mode of assessment in the determination of brain death has been, and will be, the physical examination. Current therapy modalities in acute severe brain injury, as we have pointed out already, may compromise the validity of the neurologic examination. Also, in the era of organ transplantation, some of the criteria requiring an established time period of physiologic inactivity before brain death can be declared are simply not feasible, since they preclude obtaining viable organs. SERs have, for these reasons, been applied as ancillary procedures in the diagnosis of brain death.

The first author and colleagues have reported group data and case reports in support of this application of SERs. These studies have been limited to adult populations with, mostly, traumatic head injury (Hall and Mackey-Hargadine, 1985; Hall, Mackey-Hargadine, Kim, 1985; Hall and Tucker, 1985). A strong correlation between the ABR and nuclear cerebral blood flow (CBF) measures (Goodman and Heck, 1977; Goodman, Heck, and Moore, 1985; Coker and Dillehay, 1986) was found for over 80 adults with acute severe brain injury (Hall, Hargadine, and Kim, 1985). The majority of these patients were chemically paralyzed or in barbiturate coma at the time of assessment, and some were assessed with the first 6 hours after injury with recreational drugs in the blood. A normal ABR or an ABR characterized by reliable waves III and/or V, either unilaterally or bilaterally (top waveforms in Figure 19.7), was invariably associated with the presence of CBF, whereas no detectable CBF was consistently reported in patients with bilateral absence of ABR components, except for waves I and II (lower waveforms in Figure 19.7). We are, therefore, in agreement with published guidelines on determinations of brain death that "a flat auditory brainstem response in the presence of viable peripheral conduction (cochlear wave) is considered unequivocal evidence of cerebral death because of the proximity of auditory nuclei to vital centers . . . Brainstem sensory evoked potentials. . . . effectively complement the information derived from spontaneous electrical cortical activity when cerebral death is suspected on clinical grounds (Determination of Brain Death, 1987, p. 18)."

One point cannot be overemphasized at this juncture. We are offering data in support of the use of ABR in diagnosis of brain death only in adult patients with traumatic head injury. The same guidelines do not ap-

AUDITORY BRAINSTEM RESPONSE

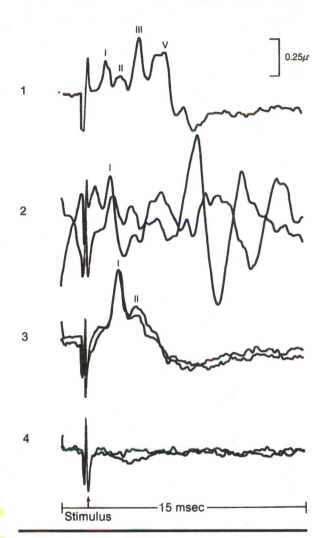

FIGURE 19.7. ABR waveforms recorded from selected patients undergoing evaluation for suspected brain death. All patients were deeply comatose and unresponsive to physical stimulation. The presence of ABR waves (after waves I and II) is not compatible with brain death.

ply to adults with other forms of brain injury, such as acute cerebrovascular insults, nor for infants and young children, regardless of the etiology for brain injury. Our clinical experience, and other published findings (Celesia, 1989; Dear and Godfrey, 1985; Toffol et al., 1987; Kohrman and Spivack, 1990), confirm that absence of an ABR is not necessarily incompatible with survival in these latter patient populations.

The application of ABR in diagnosis of brain death in adult traumatic head injury is highlighted by the following case report. A 24-year-old male sustained a gunshot wound to the right temporal region (case 2). The patient was transferred to the emergency room with normal vital signs but minimal neurologic func-

tion. Pupils were in midposition and unreactive. GCS was 5. Blood alcohol level was 158 mg/dl. He was taken to CT scanning which showed a right subdural hematoma, and then directly to the OR for a right temporal craniotomy and evacuation of the hematoma, with ventriculostomy. Marked brain swelling was noted intraoperatively. This was treated with hyperventilation, diuretics, and barbiturates, with little success. After surgery, the patient did poorly, and required Dopamine for support of blood pressure. By the

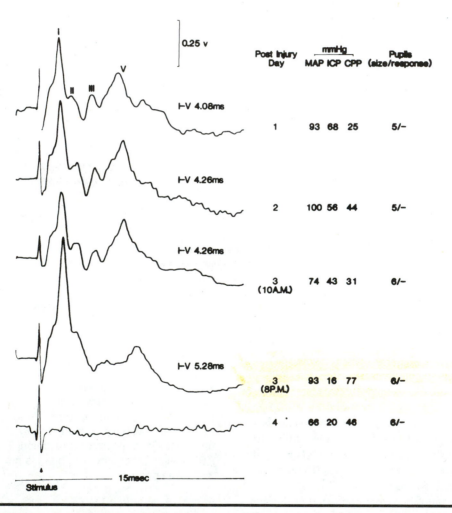

FIGURE 19.8.   Serial ABR and AMLR waveforms recorded in the ICU from a 24-year-old comatose male with gunshot wound during intensive care (case 2). Patient was in therapeutic barbiturate coma at the time of AER assessments.

evening of the injury, there was no evidence of cerebral activity by clinical examination. There was no movement to deep pain. Pupils were fixed in midposition. Brainstem reflexes were not observed. Apnea response was not assessed.

Initial AER assessment was carried out at this time. As illustrated in Figure 19.8, a well formed ABR was recorded from the left. No response could be generated with right ear stimulation at maximum intensity levels. There was no AMLR bilaterally, but this finding was considered equivocal due the barbiturate therapy.

Nuclear CBF studies were requested. The image on the left portion of Figure 19.9 indicates that flow was present. On the following morning, ABR assessment was again carried out. Neurologic status, examined after chemical paralysis was medically reversed, showed no brainstem or cerebral signs except for minimal right corneal reflex. Again, a normal ABR was recorded. ICP continued to increase into the mid 30s (mmHg) in spite of maximum medical therapy. Repeat ABRs later on day 1 after the injury yielded no response. A second nuclear CBF study failed to document flow, and the

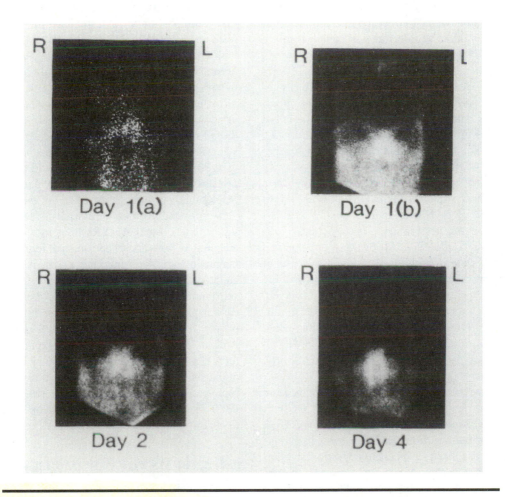

FIGURE 19.9. Nuclear cerebral blood flow studies for case 2 used in determination of brain death.

patient was declared brain dead. The patient was promptly taken to the OR for a donor nephrectomy and splenectomy. Two normal kidneys were donated.

Predicting Short Term Cognitive and Communicative Outcome

As noted in the introduction of this chapter, estimation of long term outcome was the objective of the earliest studies of SERs in severe head injury (Greenberg and Becker, 1976; Greenberg et al., 1977). These important clinical reports provided the motivation for our research and applications of AERs in this challenging population, and have led to ongoing interest and clinical research by others (Anderson et al., 1984; Karnaze et al., 1982; Narayan et al., 1981; Rappaport et al., 1978; Rosenberg, Wogensen, and Starr, 1984; Seales et al., 1979). Without exception, these previously reported studies have based estimates on long term outcome on SER data acquired, typically, on a single test session on the third day post injury, or later.

The first author has studied the relationship between serial AER data obtained within the first week after injury and cognitive and communicative outcome at 6 months as described with the Rancho Los Amigos Hospital Scale (RLAHS) (Hagen et al., 1979) in 74 survivors of severe head injury. The Rancho Scale is summarized in Table 19.7. All of these patients had ABRs. None were in barbiturate coma at the time of testing. Mean GCS was 5.7. Data for patients dying within the first post injury week were not analyzed. ABR was, as expected, not related to long-term outcome (Hall, Hargadine, and Allen, 1985; Hall, Hargadine, Kim, 1985; Hall and Tucker, 1986; Hall et al., 1983; Hall, 1988, 1992; Papanicoulaou, Loring, Eisenberg, Raz, Contreras, 1986).

AMLR was, therefore, selected as the AER measure for estimating cognitive/communicative status. One reason for this decision was the possibility that the AMLR receives contributions from auditory cortical regions that are closely related to speech recognition and language function (Lee et al., 1984; Jacobson and Newman, 1990; Liegeois-Chauvel, Musolino, and Chauvel, 1991; Kileny et al., 1987). To simplify data analysis and this potential clinical application of AMLR, cognitive/communicative outcome as assessed with the Rancho Scale was reduced to four categories, as described below. AMLR was categorized as shown in Figure 19.10. AMLR waveforms were defined as follows: Normal. A reliable Pa component bilaterally with amplitude (Pa-Nb) equal to or greater than 0.30 μv; Abnormal. A reliable Pa component unilaterally or bilaterally with amplitude of less than 0.30 μv or only a unilateral AMLR Pa component (regardless of amplitude); No response. No reliable Pa component on either side.

The results of this study were quite encouraging. Patients with excellent recovery (RLAHS level VIII) invariably had a consistently normal AMLR during the first week post injury. All but 5% of the patients with good recovery (RLAHS level VII) and 19% of those with fair recovery (RLAHS levels IV–V) also yielded normal AMLRs in the acute period. Among the patients with poor recovery (RLAHS levels I–IV) a majority had either an abnormal response (low amplitude) or no AMLR within the first week after injury. While these findings are only preliminary, they do appear to suggest that a complete recovery depends on integrity of the neuroanatomic region generating the AMLR, perhaps in part the primary auditory cortex.

Not unexpectedly, some (32%) of the patients with very unfavorable outcome, at least at 3 months after the injury, had normal AMLRs bilaterally. Other neuroanatomic regions are, of course, vital for normal speech/language/cognitive functioning than just the primary auditory cortex, and these regions may have sustained substantial damage. In addition, it is likely that in many cases significant further cognitive/communicative improvement occurred after the month limit of this study. A promising new area for research on predicting long-term cognitive outcome in head injury is exploitation of the auditory P300 (3) response, a true cognitive neurophysiologic event (Levin, 1985). The application of P300 in assessment of recovering brain-injured patients in rehabilitation is discussed next.

AERs IN BRAIN INJURY REHABILITATION

As just noted, AERs have clinical value in monitoring neurologic status in the acute stage of brain injury, and estimating short-term prognosis. It is likely that

TABLE 19.7.   Summary of Levels of Cognitive Functioning in Rancho Los Amigos Hospital Scale (RLAHS).

Level	Category	Description
I	No response	comatose; unresponsive to all sensory stimuli
II	Generalized response	inconsistent, nonpurposeful, and limited responses to stimuli; responses consist of physiologic changes, gross body movements, and vocalization.
III	Localized response	inconsistent reaction related directly to the type of stimulus; patient may withdraw extremity or vocalize to painful stimulus; may follow simple commands inconsistently and in a delayed manner; may show bias to certain people in responses
IV	Confused, agitated	disoriented, heightened state of activity, unaware of present events; behavior may be bizarre; incoherent verbalization; short attention span; unable to perform self care activities; may attempt to crawl out of bed or show aggressive behavior
V	Confused, inappropriate	appears alert; able to respond to nonagitated simple but not complex commands; gross attention to environment but cannot focus attention on specific task; can converse on social/automatic level for brief periods; verbalization may be inappropriate; severe memory impairment; difficulty learning new information; can perform self care activities with assistance
VI	Confused, appropriate	shows goal-directed behavior; follows simple commands consistently; new learning still difficult; appropriate but delayed responses; reduced ability to process information; inconsistently oriented to time and place
VII	Automatic and appropriate	appears appropriate and oriented in hospital or home setting; daily routine carried out in robot-like fashion; some carry over for new learning; increased awareness of self, family, foods, etc.; decreased judgment and impaired problem solving still prominent; independent in self care activities; needs supervision for personal safety; can start prevocational evaluation and counseling
VIII	Purposeful and appropriate	alert and oriented; can recall and integrate past; carry over for new learning; independent in physical functioning and activities; driving and vocational recommendations are indicated; may be residual decrease in intellectual functioning and tolerance for stress, judgment, and social and emotional capacities

Adapted from Hagen, Malkmus, and Durham, 1979; Harris and Hall, 1990; Hall, 1992.

AERs will eventually assume importance in the management of brain injury rehabilitation patients, after the acute phase of treatment. Before this role of AERs is secure, however, additional information is needed. Answers to four general questions are required:

1. Can AERs provide diagnostic information on the patient's post-acute neurologic status?
2. How can AERs contribute to the estimation of prognosis beyond survival and emergence from coma?
3. Are AERs of value in assessing the effects of rehabilitation treatments electrophysiologically?

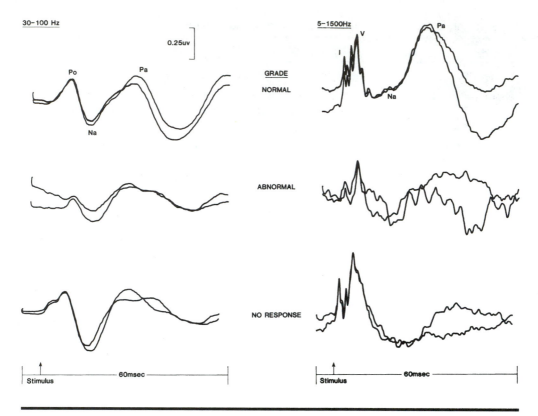

FIGURE 19.10. Categorization of AMLR findings for correlation with cognitive/communicative outcome as assessed by the RLAH scale. AMLR waveforms were recorded during the acute period following severe head injury.

4. Are AERs useful tools for clinical research of auditory cognitive deficits following brain injury?

Answers to these questions are currently lacking, perhaps due to the difficulty of performing systematic research among the very heterogeneous population of individuals that survive brain injury. Oken and Chiappa (1985) and Levin, Benton, and Grossman (1982) list six reasons why comparison of the results of evoked response studies across groups of brain injury patients is problematic. First, technical evoked response recording methods vary from study to study. Second, criteria for judging abnormalities are not consistent across studies. Third, often control groups used to develop normative data have too few subjects, are under different conditions than patient groups, and/or differ from patients in age, gender, and other important subject characteristics. Fourth, patient groups selected for study are not always controlled for pre-existing medical conditions, type of injury, severity of injury, test time post-onset, and possible medication effects. Fifth, information on the pre-injury cognitive abilities of the patients is rarely available. Finally, injury-to-test intervals vary widely, and serial tests investigating the time-course of recovery are too seldom used. To this list, we would add one more problem; namely, that there is no current consensus as to which disability and outcome measures may be most effective in the process of validating AERs as clinical tools for post-acute brain injury rehabilitation.

AERs AND BRAIN INJURY OUTCOME

Although several studies have included analysis of the relationship between AERs and long-term recovery indicators (Anderson, Bundlie, and Rockswold, 1984; Greenberg et al., 1977; Lindsay et al., 1981; Newlon and Greenberg, 1983; Rappaport et al., 1977, 1982; Shin et al., 1989), the outcome indicators used in the studies did not address any specific aspects of auditory-cognitive functioning in brain injury patients. Typically, the focus of such research was to determine the relationship between general categories of physical and cognitive recovery and multimodal evoked potential abnormalities including AERs, visual evoked responses (VERs), and somatosensory evoked potentials (SSERs). For example, Rappaport and colleagues (1977, 1982) developed the Disability Rating Scale (DRS) and then investigated the relationship among DRS scores and AER, VER, and SSER abnormalities for 88 patients admitted to a head trauma rehabilitation program. The DRS provides ratings in four categories of patient function (awareness, self-care activities, dependence on others, and psychosocial adaptability). Eight criteria items addressing basic motor responses, toileting, feeding, grooming, independence, and employability are used to assign numerical scores in the four categories. Rappaport et al. (1982) found that the correlation between DRS scores and AER abnormalities was 0.35 for ABR and 0.62 for longer latency AERs. The correlation between DRS scores and combined multimodal evoked response abnormalities (AERs, VERs, and SSERs) was 0.78. Furthermore, the correlation was 0.53 between DRS scores obtained at admission and one year later for the same patients. Because all these correlations were statistically significant (at p <0.01), the authors concluded that the evoked response measures of abnormal brain activity supported the clinical validity of the DRS.

More recently, Shin and his colleagues (1989) studied the relationship between ABR and short latency SSERs (0–50 ms), and ratings on the Rancho Los Amigos Hospital Scale of Cognitive Recovery (Hagen, Malkmus, and Durham, 1979) for 29 head trauma patients who were in rehabilitation for at least 18 months. As noted above, the Rancho Los Amigos Hospital

Scale (RLAHS) is comprised of eight scale levels (including comatose, confused, and appropriate cognitive functional states) and is widely used among rehabilitation professionals to rate recovery in brain injury patients along dimensions of response specificity and consistency, orientation, memory, and intellectual capacity. Shin et al. (1989) found that neither ABR nor short latency SSERs were significantly correlated with cognitive level on the RLAHS at one year after injury for the 29 head trauma patients studied. At 18 months after injury, ABR and short latency SSERs, in combination, accounted for only 15% of the variance in RLAHS ratings. The authors concluded that the best predictor of outcome on the RLAHS was the combination of RLAHS rating at 12 months post-injury, patient age, and SSER. These variables together accounted for 72% of the variance in RLAHS ratings at 18 months post-injury. Shin et al. (1989) theorized that ABR and short latency SSERs may be insensitive outcome predictors because they reflect only fixed neuronal damage resulting from brain injury. Therefore, measurements of these potentials cannot represent cognitive adaptations and behavioral modifications that patients make, even though there is little change in brain structure during rehabilitation (Shin et al., 1989).

Measurements of auditory event related potentials (ERPs), in brain-injury rehabilitation patients may overcome the previously described limitation of evoked responses that do not directly reflect neurophysiologic activity related to cognitive functions (Shin et al., 1989). In normal individuals, ERPs, which fall into the general category of endogenous potentials (see Chapter 9) can be elicited when a subject attempts to discriminate between nontarget and target sensory stimuli, for example tone bursts presented at two different frequencies (Goodin, Aminoff, and Mantle, 1986) or clicks presented at two different intensity levels (Snyder and Hillyard, 1976). The nontarget stimulus elicits an N1-P2 complex which represents the late auditory vertex potential, whereas the target stimulus elicits an N1-P2-N2-P3 complex (Figure 19.11) which presumably reflects cognitive processes associated with attention, evaluation, discrimination, and memory (Goodin and Aminoff, 1984; Hansen and Hillyard, 1980; Hillyard, Hink, Schwent, and Picton, 1974; Michalewski,

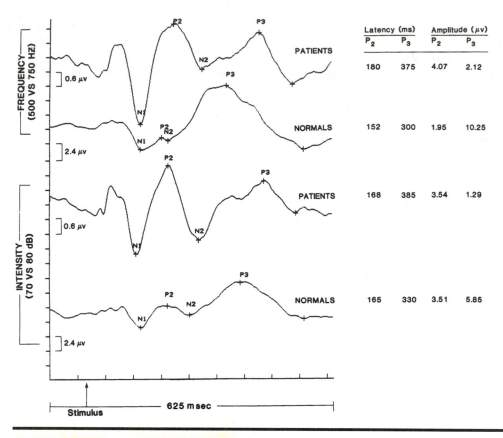

FIGURE 19.11.   Composite P300 ERP waveforms for normal subjects and brain-injured patients in a rehabilitation facility.

Prasher, and Starr, 1986; Polich, 1986; Pritchard, 1981; Sklare and Lynn, 1984). Therefore, auditory ERPs might be better indicators of cognitive function and prognosis than brainstem and other stimulus-related (exogenous) AERs.

Campbell, Deacon, and colleagues have recently investigated auditory ERPs in the recovering head injured patient (Campbell, Houle, Lorrain, Deacon-Elliott, and Proulx, 1986; Campbell, Suffield, and Deacon, 1990; Deacon and Campbell, 1991). Their studies have focused on relations among auditory ERPs and impairment of specific cognitive abilities, such as attention, memory, and speed of cognitive processing (reaction time). Yingling, Hosobuchi, and Harrington (1990) applied a passive P300 response paradigm (Hall, 1992) in the prediction of recovery from coma. They concluded that P300 can be used to assess cognitive function of unconscious patients and, ultimately, contribute to prognosis of communicative and cognitive outcome. In a similar line of research, Reuter and Linke (1989) argue that topographic mapping of P300 is important for description of "elementary forms of cognition" in coma due to head injury. Based on these collective findings, auditory ERPs appear to offer a promising approach for learning more about higher level CNS functioning in brain injury.

This literature on the use of evoked responses in brain injury rehabilitation was reviewed to illustrate the current level of knowledge on the relationship between AERs and general indicators of outcome. Even from this limited sample of papers, it is apparent that ABR is typically a poor predictor of cognitive outcome (Hall, 1988, 1992; Rappaport et al., 1977; 1982; Shin et al., 1989), and longer latency AERs may be only moderate predictors of cognitive outcome (Rappaport et al., 1977; 1982), when correlated with recovery scale measures presently in use (Hagen, Malkmus, and Durham, 1979; Rappaport et al., 1982). But, as pointed out by Shin et al., (1989), these disappointing levels of prognostic power may have stemmed from the use of AERs that do not directly represent neurophysiologic activity related to cognitive functions. Another reason may be that the DRS and RLAHS do not address any specific dimensions of auditory processing. Under such conditions it seems logical that AERs and these outcome scales should show modest agreement at best.

FEASIBILITY OF MEASURING AUDITORY ERPs FROM BRAIN-INJURY PATIENTS

Introduction

Little information has been published on the measurement of auditory ERPs in brain injury rehabilitation. Most studies involve patients at relatively high levels of cognitive recovery. Levin (1985) reported that the appearance of the auditory ERP (P3 response) coincided with the resolution of post-traumatic amnesia in head-injured patients. As orientation and memory improved, the latency of P3 approximated the normal region. Campbell et al. (1986) measured auditory ERPs from a group of 8 head-injured outpatients at least one year after injury and found that P3 latencies were delayed, and amplitudes reduced, when compared to a control group. However, auditory ERPs for these outpatients appeared to be less abnormal than those reported by Curry (1980), who studied head trauma patients only a few months after injury.

We recently conducted a detailed study of the feasibility of measuring auditory ERPs in brain injury rehabilitation inpatients at stages of cognitive recovery ranging from coma to near premorbid function (Harris and Hall, 1990). Our objective was to add to the literature on auditory ERPs recorded from patients at higher cognitive levels (Campbell et al., 1986; Curry, 1980;

Levin, 1985) and, in addition, to provide preliminary data on auditory ERPs in patients at lower cognitive levels. The criteria for evaluating the feasibility of AERP measurement in our patient sample were developed according to two main considerations.

Auditory ERP Analysis Criteria

For any particular response to be considered an auditory ERP, a replicable graphic tracing with N1, P2, N2, and P3 components was required for the waveform elicited by the target stimulus. Acceptable peak latency ranges for each major components were as follows: N1 (75 to 175 msec), P2 (125 to 225 msec), N2 (150 to 350 msec), and P3 (250 to 500 msec). We also required P2 and P3 peak amplitude values of at least 1 µV. These criteria were derived from previously reported data (Campbell et al., 1986; Curry, 1980; Levin, 1985) and our pilot work which showed that auditory ERP component latencies and amplitudes fell within these ranges for brain injury patients who were able to follow directions for AERP measurement tasks.

In addition, the feasibility of auditory ERP measurement was evaluated with the assumption that certain similarities might be observed in auditory ERP waveforms within groups of patients who were at similar stages of cognitive function. This approach represented a preliminary attempt to gain information on the sensitivity and specificity of AERPs as indicators of cognitive status in brain injury rehabilitation patients.

Characteristics of Brain-Injury Patients

Our investigation was described in detail in a recent publication (Harris and Hall, 1990). Briefly, auditory ERPs were recorded from 50 brain injury patients consecutively admitted to a 150-bed rehabilitation hospital. Ages ranged from 11 to 54 years (average of 24 years). Thirty-six of the patients (72%) were male. Etiologies included motor vehicle accidents, falls, anoxia, encephalitis, tumors, and aneurysms. Time post-injury ranged from 1 to 126 months. Patients were ranked from levels II through VII on the RLAHS according to a consensus of therapy team professionals (Table 19.7).

Test Procedures

To the degree permitted by cognitive status, each patient underwent otoscopic inspection, acoustic immittance testing, behavioral audiometry, central auditory processing assessment, as well as ABR, 40 Hertz, and AMLR measurement, before auditory ERP measurements were attempted. All AERs were recorded with commercially available equipment, including insert earphone transducers. Parameters used to record exogenous AERs are displayed in Table 19.8. The parameters used to record AERPs are not listed in the table because they were not held constant across our patient sample. For the majority of patients, audiometric tests and auditory evoked potential recordings were performed in an acoustically shielded booth. For medical reasons some comatose patients were evaluated in their hospital rooms. Insert earphones were then routinely used to reduce ambient noise.

Behavioral audiometry consisted of testing pure-tone audiometry at octave frequencies from 250 to 8000 Hz, speech recognition thresholds, and word recognition scores at 35 dB SL RE: the SRT for each ear. Tape recorded spondee words and phonetically balanced word lists (NU 6) were always used. The central auditory assessment consisted of the staggered spondaic word (SSW) test (Katz, 1962) and the competing sentences test (CST) (Willeford, 1977). The CST was administered according to a "threshold-of-interference" procedure similar to that recently described by Bergman et al. (1987). We used this procedure because some brain injury patients could not accurately repeat any words of message sentences when the message-to-competition ratio was maintained at −15 dB, as specified in the original description of the CST (Willeford, 1977).

Auditory ERP measurement paradigms were based upon intensity (loudness) or frequency (pitch) differences between nontarget (80% occurrence) and target (20% occurrence) stimuli. The type of stimuli and the degree of difference between stimuli were adjusted according to the cognitive status of the patient. That is, for those (RLAHS level VII) who could consistently count target stimuli, the loudness discrimination task employed unfiltered clicks presented at intensities of 60 dB nHL for nontarget stimuli and 70 dB nHL for target stimuli and the pitch discrimination task consisted of tone bursts presented at frequencies of 500 Hz for nontarget stimuli and 750 Hz for target stimuli. Stimulus intensity was 60 dB nHL for nontarget and target tone bursts. For patients (RLAHS levels II–VI) who could not consistently count target stimuli, we used a loudness discrimination paradigm with unfil-

TABLE 19.8. Recording Parameters for Auditory Brainstem, 40 Hertz, and Auditory Middle Latency Evoked Potentials.

Recording Parameter	Auditory Brainstem	40 Hertz	Middle Latency
Artifact Reject	25 μv	50 μv	50 μv
High Pass Filter	100 Hz	10 Hz	5 Hz
Low Pass Filter	3000 Hz	100 Hz	1500 Hz
Time Window	10 ms	100 ms	60 ms
Sweeps	2000	1000	1000
Positive Electrode	Fz	Cz	Fz
Negative Electrode	Ipsi. Ear	Ipsi. Ear	Ipsi. Ear
Com. Electrode	Nasion	Nasion	Nasion
Stimulus Type	Click	Click	Click
Stimulus Polarity	Alt.	Alt.	Alt.
Stimulus Rate	21.1/sec	39.1/sec	11.1/sec
Stimulus Intensity	80 dB nHL	70 dB nHL	70 dB nHL

tered clicks presented at intensities of 60 dB nHL for nontarget stimuli and 90 dB nHL for target stimuli.

This strategy of adjusting stimulus differences according to patient cognitive status was taken because we found that patients at RLAHS level VII may become inattentive if a discrimination task is too easy. On the other hand, patients at lower RLAHS levels were not always able to detect relatively small differences between stimuli. Also, since it was difficult to document attention in patients below level VII, relatively large differences between nontarget and target stimuli were used. A pitch discrimination paradigm was not employed for all patients at lower cognitive levels because waveforms recorded with auditory ERP test parameters, including stimulus frequency differences as great as two and one-half octaves (500 Hz nontarget versus 3000 Hz target tone bursts), did not show any P3 peaks for individual patients at RLAHS levels II, III, and V. These same patients had shown waveforms with P3 peaks for the loudness discrimination paradigm involving 60 dB nontarget and 90 dB target click stimuli.

Results

Our present sample size of nine comatose patients was too small to lead to definite conclusions about the value of auditory ERPs as indicators of prognosis. Although the limited data in this study do not seem promising, it must be recognized that severe brain injury often is associated with sequelae that are too complex for any single indicator to consistently predict outcome (Levin, 1985; Newlon et al., 1982; Oken and Chiappa, 1985; Rappaport et al., 1977; 1982). For example, one patient (at RLAHS level II) who showed a waveform with high-amplitude P2, N2, and P3 components, recovered cognitively over an 18-month period to RLAHS level VI (Figure 19.12, Patient IId). Another patient at level III (age 11 years) underwent auditory ERP measurement upon admission to the rehabilitation center (Figure 19.12, Patient IIIc) and 30 days later. During the 30-day period between auditory ERP measurements, the patient progressed rapidly from RLAHS level III to level VI. For the second AERP test she was able to raise her finger consistently to coincide with the presentation of each 90 dB click, yet auditory

ERP wave morphology did not improve greatly in correspondence with the patient's remarkable cognitive recovery. Behavioral audiometrics at the time of the AERP retest showed normal pure-tone thresholds and speech discrimination percentages bilaterally. Central auditory evaluation revealed mildly abnormal SSW test results, and a marked deficit in left ear CST performance. Finally, yet another patient (at RLAHS level III) who showed a waveform resembling a normal AERP (Figure 19.12, Patient IIIe), did not improve in his cognitive status, and eventually expired of kidney failure. The main point illustrated by these selected cases is that auditory ERP findings, viewed in isolation, may not be sensitive indicators of cognitive recovery in brain injury patients emerging from coma. We also note that waveforms recorded within each of the two RLAHS levels (II–III) bear relatively little resemblance to each other. Nor did these waveforms show peak components similar to those recorded from other patients at RLAHS levels II and III who did not suffer diffuse traumatic brain injuries. It may be that severe head trauma has greater effects than other forms of brain injury on the neural generation of auditory evoked potentials in the latency domain of auditory ERPs. However, our data are based on too small a sample of comatose patients to verify this possibility.

All patients at RLAHS level VI could demonstrate discrimination between target and non-target stimuli, whereas none of the patients at level V could consistently demonstrate signal discrimination. In normal individuals P3 amplitude is greater than P2 (Michalewski, Prasher, and Starr, 1986; Polich, 1986; Sklare and Lynn, 1984), but in our sample of brain injury patients who could follow directions to selectively attend to the target stimulus (RLAHS levels VI and VII) the amplitude of P3 was nearly always less than P2. This inversion of the normal P2/P3 amplitude relationship may indicate some degree of plasticity or compensatory activity in the neural mechanisms underlying selective auditory attention in brain injury patients at higher cognitive recovery levels. Additional patients at RLAHS levels V or VI yielded waveforms without any identifiable N1, P2, N2, or P3 components. This result is compatible with the variability of waveforms observed among our patients at RLAHS levels II and III, and could be preliminary evi-

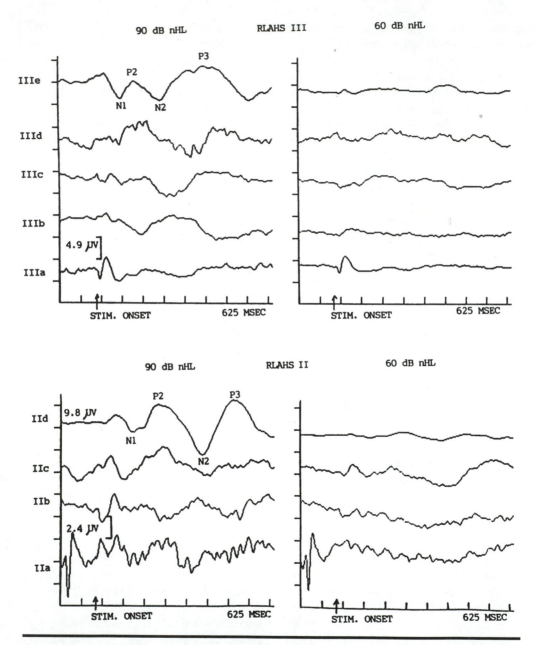

FIGURE 19.12.   Example of P300 ERP waveforms for a brain-injured patient at RLAHS level II (IId bottom portion) and two patients at RLAHS level III (IIIc, IIIe, top portion). AERs were recorded in a rehabilitation facility.

dence that auditory ERP measurement lacks sensitivity as indicators of cognitive status in confused-amnesic patients. Since none of the patients at level IV, V, or VI progressed to higher RLAHS levels during their stay at the rehabilitation hospital, information on the prognostic value of AERP measurements for confused-amnesic individuals was not available.

In our sample of 30 patients at RLAHS level VII, P3 latency was longer and P3 amplitude was lower for the automatic-appropriate patient group in pitch and loudness discrimination auditory ERP tasks. Auditory ERP data for the pitch discrimination task were compared for 30 head trauma patients at RLAHS level VII versus 10 normal-hearing young adults with no history of head injury as described above. In one analysis, means were compared between the entire group of 30 patients and the normal group. In another analysis, means were compared between the normals and a subgroup of 17 patients who all had normal results for hearing evaluations and exogenous AERs (ABR, 40 Hz, MLR) (Figure 19.11). The results showed significant overall differences between mean auditory ERP components for both patient groups compared to means for the normals. Significant univariate differences were also found when means for N2 latency, P3 latency, and P3 amplitude for both patient groups were compared to corresponding means for the normals. This outcome confirmed previous data on auditory ERPs in chronic head injury patients (Campbell et al., 1986; Curry, 1980; Levin, 1985). Further, statistical analyses indicated that latencies and amplitudes of auditory ERP P3 peaks in the 30 brain injury patients at RLAHS level VII were not significantly related to measures of hearing sensitivity, speech discrimination, central auditory processing, or other AERs.

Conclusions

Our experiences thus far indicate that it is feasible to use auditory ERP measurement paradigms for clinical study of brain injury rehabilitation patients in diverse cognitive states. Waveforms showing N1, P2, N2, and P3 components were recorded from individual patients at each of the RLAHS levels we studied (II–VII), except level IV where only 1 patient was tested. How-

ever, considerable variability in waveforms for individual patients was also observed at each scale level. Because the number of patients at RLAHS levels II–VI was small, it was difficult to draw conclusions about possible relationships between cognitive function and waveforms elicited by the AERP measurement paradigm we used for comatose or confused-amnesic patients. Also, it was not possible to resolve questions about the prognostic value of AERP measurements from these individuals, because relatively few patients advanced one or more RLAHS levels during their treatment at the rehabilitation hospital.

Earlier in this chapter we noted that the RLAHS does not address specific dimensions of auditory-cognitive functioning. Therefore, any lack of sensitivity between auditory ERP measurements from patients in this study and cognitive status as determined by the RLAHS may stem from the insensitivity of the RLAHS scale to factors involved in neural generation of auditory ERPs. Our finding of no statistically significant relationship among auditory ERP components, other AERs, and peripheral and central auditory measures for the 30 patients at RLAHS level VII indicates the need for research focused on electrophysiologic and behavioral measures that better describe auditory function and prognosis in brain injury patients. It would appear that a recovery scale which specifically addresses auditory-cognitive disabilities would be a step in the right direction.

COMPUTERIZED TOPOGRAPHIC BRAIN MAPPING OF AUDITORY ERPs AND EEG

Topographic brain mapping of auditory ERPs and the EEG has been made possible by recent advances in computer technology that permit digital representation of brain electrical activity as color maps displaying frequency, amplitude, and spatial distribution on the scalp (see Chapter 20). This technology can also be used to produce spectral maps of the VERs and SSERs. We hasten to point out, however, that at this time there is controversy as to the appropriateness of brain mapping as a routine clinical neurodiagnostic procedure (Baran et al., 1988; Musiek, 1989; Nuwer, 1989; Oken and Chiappa, 1986; Finitzo and Pool, 1987). The main areas of concern include difficulties in recognizing artifact, uncertainty regarding sensitivity and specificity for detecting abnormalities, and the general lack of knowledge about the relationship between statistical probability maps of brain activity and the functional status of any particular individual (Nuwer, 1989). However, our experiences indicate that with properly trained personnel, and knowledge of the pitfalls associated with converting analog signals of brain activity into purely digital representations, computerized evoked response topographic mapping can be a valuable tool for investigating brain function.

Recently, the second author presented preliminary results of an ongoing investigation of the relationship between central auditory test results and topographic brain maps of auditory ERPs and EEG in brain injury rehabilitation patients (Harris, 1989). The purpose of this line of research is to gain knowledge on the sensi-

tivity and specificity of central auditory testing and topographic brain mapping as complimentary techniques for assessing central auditory processing in such patients. Preliminary data were reported for five commercially available central auditory tests, including binaural fusion (Matzker, 1959), synthetic sentence identification with an ipsilateral competing message (Speaks and Jerger, 1965), the competing sentences test (Willeford, 1977), the dichotic digits test (Musiek, 1983), and the SSW test (Katz, 1962). These procedures were administered as a battery to patients with etiologies including head injury, anoxia, encephalitis, tumor, and CVA. The same patients also underwent brain mapping of auditory ERPs and EEG as part of the admission diagnostic process.

Two types of data analysis were attempted. First, auditory ERP and EEG brain maps for 1 normal non-

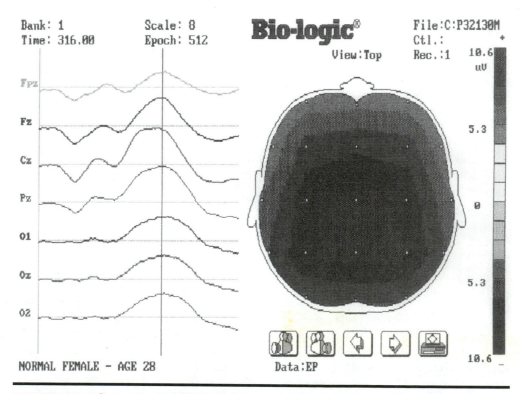

FIGURE 19.13.   Computer evoked response topographic map of the auditory P300 ERP recorded from a normal 28-year-old female.

patient and 10 consecutively admitted patients were ranked according to scores on the central auditory battery. Second, auditory ERP and EEG brain maps were compared within groups of selected patients who demonstrated consistent left ear or right ear score advantages for the five central auditory tests. Figure 19.13 shows auditory ERP topographic maps for the normal individual whose data was included in the first type of analysis. When auditory ERP and EEG topographic maps for the 10 brain injury patients and 1 normal individual were ordered according to rankings for central auditory test scores, certain patterns were observed. Patients who ranked higher generally had auditory ERP and EEG maps that were similar to the normal individual (who ranked first). These similarities included scalp distribution of auditory ERP voltages, and relative power of EEG activity in the four traditional

frequency band widths: delta (0.0–3.5 Hz), theta (4.0–7.5 Hz), alpha (8.0–11.5 Hz), and beta (12.0–15.5 Hz). Patients with lower central auditory test score rankings often demonstrated shifts in maximum auditory ERP voltages away from the midline central-parietal region, and also tended to show relatively greater EEG activity in the delta and theta bands.

We are conducting ongoing research comparing central auditory findings and brain mapping. An illustrative case is a 22-year-old female who suffered a left middle cerebral artery hemorrhage during the birth of her child. Her central auditory test scores were consistently much lower in the right ear than the left, indicating left hemispheric dysfunction. Her topographic brain map made at 10 months post-injury (Figure 19.14) showed greater auditory ERP voltage (P3 at 336 ms) over her left central region. This pattern of audi-

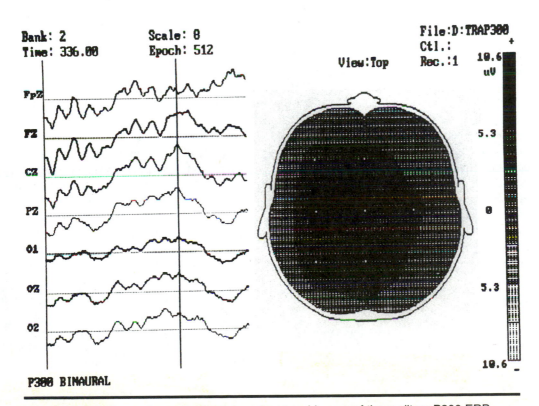

FIGURE 19.14.   Computer evoked response topographic map of the auditory P300 ERP recorded from a 22-year-old female who suffered a left middle cerebral artery hemorrhage.

tory ERP voltage distribution may have been due to encephalomacia in the left central cerebral area (as documented by CT scan), which led to increased cerebrospinal fluid volume in the region of cortical atrophy. Such a focal increase in CSF could have led to volume conduction of the auditory ERP, which would account for the area of higher voltage around the site of lesion. A topographic brain map of EEG for this patient showed a focus of high amplitude delta waves over the left temporal lobe. This pattern of EEG abnormality strongly indicates focal left temporal lobe pathology consistent with her history of left middle cerebral artery hemorrhage. Overall, comparisons between this patient's central auditory test results and auditory ERP and EEG brain maps are consistent with the effects of focal lesions of left hemispheric CNS structures known to be important to auditory processing (Baran et al., 1988; Musiek, 1989; Finitzo and Pool, 1987).

Admittedly, other patients with consistent left or right ear central auditory test score advantages have not shown such obvious correspondence between central auditory test results and topographic brain maps. Possible reasons for this lack of sensitivity and specificity are numerous. General considerations must include the current imperfect state of knowledge about the anatomy and physiology of central auditory processing. Also, the central auditory test battery employed in this investigation probably does not sample all dimensions of auditory processing. Finally, topographic maps cannot represent all the brain activity that may be involved in normal or disordered auditory processing. Continuing investigation will be necessary to improve the sensitivity and specificity of central auditory testing and topographic brain mapping as complimentary techniques for evaluating central auditory processing.

CONCLUSIONS

Although literally hundreds of papers have described applications of AERs in the ICU setting, mostly with adult populations, a better understanding of AER neuroanatomy and neurophysiology and more precise correlation of AERs with brain pathophysiology is needed before AERs can be fully exploited as an assessment and monitoring tool. Within recent years, papers describing experimental and clinical correlations among AER findings and pathophysiologic processes have begun to appear regularly. More information on the effect of pharmacologic agents employed therapeutically on AERs is essential for confident interpretation of findings in ICU patients. It is likely that much of the knowledge of pharmacologic effects on evoked responses gained in the OR will be applicable to ICU neuromonitoring as well. Nonetheless, the full potential of AERs in acute brain injury will not be realized until increased sophistication and automation in response recording and, at least to some extent, waveform analysis is commercially available. Automation in evoked response monitoring, in general, has been described for over six years (Boston and Denault, 1984; Boston, 1985). In several recent comprehensive papers, Bertrand and colleagues (Bertrand, Garcia-Larrea, Artru, Mauguiere, and Pernier, 1987; Bertrand, Bohorquez, and Pernier, 1990), have specifically addressed the issue of automated evoked response monitoring in the ICU. These authors provide a detailed review of the technical requirements for a monitoring system, among them adaptive filtering techniques, automatic peak detection and wave component amplitude measurement, and strategies for computer assisted trend curve analysis. This latter system feature includes the capacity to detect patient changes "on-line" (as they are occurring) and then to produce an alarm for the intensive care medical team. These investigations are a major step toward the future of AER monitoring of brain-injured patients in the ICU. Finally, an exciting new line of research is the clinical investigation of auditory ERPs (cognitive evoked responses) in brain injury. With the growing interest in P300 and other ERPS, and increasing availability of sophisticated techniques such as computed evoked response topography or "brain mapping" (see Chapter 20), we predict renewed interest in the application of evoked responses in brain injury.

Pending the routine application of these advances in knowledge and technology, the auditory neurophysiologist still may be a valued member of the ICU team. However, successful application of AERs in acute brain injury requires a basic understanding of CNS pathophysiology and acute management strategies and technical expertise in AER recording and interpretation. There are, from a practical standpoint, both advantages and disadvantages to implementing an ICU evoked response monitoring service. On the positive side, evoked responses can, as reviewed in this paper, contribute uniquely to decisions on surgical/medical management of patients. ICU monitoring leads to multidisciplinary professional contacts and heightened visibility in the hospital, which has a beneficial impact on other neuroaudiologic services and provides a new and potentially substantial source of revenue. There is also the possibility for clinical research on correlations among AERs and neuropathology and neuropathophysiology.

Disadvantages must nonetheless be considered. Among these are the sometimes long work hours and occasional weekend duty. As with intraoperative monitoring with evoked responses, there is usually more stress and time pressure involved in the ICU than for more traditional AER applications. The time demands of ICU monitoring may preclude other important clinical services. Finally, the auditory neurophysiologist may necessarily become involved in recording non-auditory responses (e.g., somatosensory and visual). Each clinician must weigh these advantages and disadvantages before deciding to implement an ICU monitoring service.

REFERENCES

Adamovich, B.B., Henderson, J.A., and Auerbach, S. (1985). *Cognitive rehabilitation of closed head injured patients*, pp. 15–26. San Diego, CA: College Hill Press.

Ahmed, B. (1991). Brain stem auditory evoked potentials as non-invasive measures of regional temperature and functional state during hyperthermia. *International Journal of Hyperthermia, 7*, 93–102.

Anderson, D., Bundlie, S., and Rockswold, G.L. (1984). Multimodal evoked potentials in closed head trauma. *Archives of Neurology, 41*, 369–374.

Aquilar, E.A. III, Hall, J.W. III, and Mackey-Hargadine, J. (1986). Neuro-otologic evaluation of the acute severely head-injured patient: Correlation among physical findings, auditory evoked responses and computerized tomography. *Otolaryngology—Head and Neck Surgery, 94*, 211–219.

Argan, P., Castillo, D., and Winn, D. (1990). Childhood motor vehicle occupant injuries. *American Journal of Diseases in Children, 144*, 653–662.

Baik, M.W., Branston, N.M., Bentivoglio, P., and Symon, L. (1990). The effects of experimental brain-stem ischaemia on brain-stem auditory evoked potentials in primates. *Electroencephalography and Clinical Neurophysiology, 75*, 433–443.

Baran, J.A., Long, R.R., Musiek, F.E., and Alexander, O. (1988). Topographic mapping of brain electrical activity in the assessment of central auditory nervous system pathology. *American Journal of Otology, 9, Suppl*, 72–76.

Baxter, R., Cohen, S.B., and Ylvisaker, M. (1985). Comprehensive cognitive assessment. In Ylvisaker, M. (ed.)

Head injury rehabilitation: Children and adolescents, pp. 247–274. San Diego, CA: College Hill Press.

Ben-Yishay, Y. and Diller, L. (1983). Cognitive deficits. In Rosenthal, M., Griffith, E.R., Bond, M.R., and Miller, J.D. (eds.), *Head injury rehabilitation: Children and adolescents*, pp. 167–184. Philadelphia, PA: F.A. Davis.

Beresford, H.R. (1984). Legal aspects of terminating care. *Seminars in Neurology, 4*, 23–29.

Bergman, M., Hirsch, S., Solzi, P., and Mankowitz, Z. (1987). The threshold-of-interference test: A new test of interhemispheric suppression in brain injury. *Ear and Hearing, 8*, 147–150.

Bertrand, O., Bohorquez, J., and Pernier, J. (1990). Technical requirements for evoked potential monitoring in the intensive care unit. Rossini, P.M. and Mauguiere, F. (eds.), *New trends and advanced techniques in clinical neurophysiology (EEG Supplement 41)*, pp. 51–70. New York: Elsevier.

Bertrand, O., Garcia-Larrea, L., Artru, F., Mauguiere, F., and Pernier, J. (1987). Brain-stem monitoring. I. A system for high-rate sequential BAEP recording and feature extraction. *Electroencephalography and Clinical Neurophysiology, 68*, 433–445.

Billett, T.E., Thorne, P.R., and Gavin, J.B. (1989). The nature and progression of injury in the organ of Corti during ischemia. *Hearing Research, 41*, 189–198.

Boston, J.R. (1985). An algorithm for monitoring sensory evoked potentials. *Journal of Clinical Monitoring, 1*, 201–206.

Boston, J.R. and Deneault, L.G. (1984). Sensory evoked potentials: A system for clinical testing and patient monitoring. *International Journal of Clinical Monitoring Computers, 1*, 13–19.

Campbell, K., Houle, S., Lorrain, D., Deacon-Elliot, D., and Proulx, G. (1986). Event-related potentials as an index of cognitive functioning in head-injured outpatients. In McCallum, W.C., Zappoli, R., and Denoth, F., (eds.), *Cerebral psychophysiology: Studies in event-related potentials* (EEG suppl. 38), pp. 486–488. Amsterdam: Elsevier.

Campbell, K.B., Suffield, J.B., and Deacon, D.L. (1990). Electrophysiological assessment of cognitive disorder in closed head-injured outpatients. In Rossini, P.M. and Mauguiere, F. (eds.), *New trends and advanced techniques in clinical neurophysiology* (EEG Supplement 41), pp. 202–215. New York: Elsevier.

Celesia, G.G. (1989). Brain death in children: Editorial comment. *Electroencephalography and Clinical Neurophysiology, 73*, 271.

Coker, S.B. and Dillehay, G.L. (1986). Radionuclide cerebral imaging for confirmation of brain death in children: The significance of dural sinus activity. *Pediatric Neurology, 2*, 43–46.

Curry, S.H. (1980). Event-related potentials as indicants of structural and functional damage in closed head injury. In Kornhuber, H.H. and Deecke, L. (eds.), *Progress in brain research, vol. 54, Motivation, motor and sensory processes of the brain: Electric potentials, behavior and clinical use*, pp. 507–515. Amsterdam: Elsevier.

Deacon, D. and Campbell, K.B. (1991). Effects of performance feedback on P300 and reaction time in closed head-injured outpatients. *Electroencephalography and Clinical Neurophysiology, 78*, 133–141.

Dear, P.R.F. and Godfrey, D.J. (1985). Neonatal auditory brainstem response cannot reliably diagnose brainstem death. *Archives of Disease in Childhood, 60*, 17–19.

Determination of brain death. (1987). From the Ad Hoc Committee on Brain Death. *The Journal of Pediatrics, 110*, 15–19.

Division of Injury Control. (1990). Childhood injuries in the United States. *American Journal of Diseases of Children, 144*, 627–646.

Finitzo, T. and Pool, K.D. (1987). Brain electrical activity mapping—a future for audiologists or simply a future conflict? *ASHA, 29(6)*, 21–25.

Ghorayeb, B.Y., Yeakley, J.W., Hall, J.W. III, and Jones, E.B. (1987). Unusual complications of temporal bone fractures. *Archives of Otolaryngology—Head and Neck Surgery, 113*, 749–753.

Goodin, D.P. (1986). Event-related (endogenous) potentials. In Aminoff, M. (ed.), *Electrodiagnosis in clinical neurology*, pp. 575–595. New York: Churchill Livingstone.

Goodin, D.P. and Aminoff, M.J. (1984). The relationship between the evoked potential and brain events in sensory discrimination and motor response. *Brain, 107*, 241–251.

Goodin, D.P., Aminoff, M.J., and Mantle, M.M. (1986). Subclasses of event-related potentials: Response-locked and stimulus-locked components. *Annals of Neurology, 20*, 603–609.

Goodman, J.M. and Heck, L.L. (1977). Confirmation of brain death at bedside by isotope angiography. *Journal of the American Medical Association, 238*, 966–968.

Goodman, J.M., Heck, L.L., and Moore, B.D. (1985). Confirmation of brain death with portable isotope angiography: A review of 204 consecutive cases. *Neurosurgery, 16*, 492–497.

Greenberg, R.P. and Becker, D.P. (1976). Clinical applications and results of evoked potential data in patients with severe head injury. *Surgical Forum, 26*, 484–486.

Greenberg, R.P., Becker, D.P., Miller, J.P., and Mayer, D.J. (1977). Evaluation of brain function in severe human head trauma with multimodal evoked potentials. Part 2: Localization of brain dysfunction and correlation with posttraumatic neurological conditions. *Journal of Neurosurgery, 47*, 163–177.

Guidelines for the determination of death. (1981). Report of the medical consultants on the diagnosis of death to the President's Commission for the Study of Ethical Problems in Medicine and Biomedical and Behavioral Research. *Journal of American Medical Association, 246*, 2184–2186.

Hagen, C., Malkmus, D., and Durham, P. (1979). Measures of cognitive functioning in the rehabilitation facility. In *Rehabilitation of head injured adults: Comprehensive physical management*. Downey, CA: Professional Staff Association of the Rancho Los Amigos Hospital.

Hall, J.W. III. (1988). Auditory evoked responses in acute brain-injured children and adults. *American Journal of Otology, 9 (supplement)*, 36–46.

Hall, J.W. III. (1985). The effects of high-dose barbiturates on the acoustic reflex and auditory evoked responses: Two case reports. *Acta Otolaryngologica (Stockholm), 100*, 387–398.

Hall, J.W. III. (1992). *Handbook of auditory evoked responses*. Needham, MA: Allyn & Bacon.

Hall, J.W. III, Brown, D.P., and Mackey-Hargadine, J. (1985). Pediatric applications of serial auditory brainstem response measurements. *International Journal of Pediatric Otorhinolaryngology, 9*, 201–218.

Hall, J.W. III, Bull, J., and Cronau, L. (1988). The effect of hypo- vs. hyperthermia on auditory brainstem response: Two case reports. *Ear and Hearing, 9*.

Hall, J.W. III, Fletcher, S.A., and Winkler, J.B. (1987). Pediatric auditory brainstem responses in intensive care units. *Seminars in Hearing, 8*, 103–114.

Hall, J.W. III and Hargadine, J.R. (1986). Sensory evoked potentials in the diagnosis of brain death. In Miner, M.E. and Wagner, K.A. (eds.), *Neurotrauma: Treatment, rehabilitation and related issues*, pp. 133–153. Stoneham, MA: Butterworth Publishers.

Hall, J.W. III, Hargadine, J.R., and Allen, S.J. (1985). Monitoring neurologic status of comatose patients in the intensive care unit. In Jacobson, J.T. (ed), *The auditory brainstem response*, pp. 253–283. San Diego, CA: College-Hill Press.

Hall, J.W. III, Huangfu, M., and Gennarelli, T.A. (1982). Auditory function in acute head injury. *The Laryngoscope, 93*, 383–390.

Hall, J.W. III, Huangfu, M., Gennarelli, T.A., Dolinskas, C.A., Olson, K., and Berry, G.A. (1983). Auditory evoked response, impedance measures and diagnostic speech audiometry in severe head injury. *Otolaryngology—Head and Neck Surgery, 91*, 50–60.

Hall, J.W. III, Mackey-Hargadine, J., and Kim, E.E. (1985). Auditory brainstem response in determination of brain death. *Archives of Otolaryngology, 111*, 613–620.

Hall, J.W. III, Morgan, S.H., Mackey-Hargadine, J., Aquilar, E.A. III, and Jahrsdoerfer, R.A. (1984). Neuro-otologic applications of simultaneous multi-channel auditory evoked response recordings. *The Laryngoscope, 94*, 883–889.

Hall, J.W. III and Tucker, D.A. (1986). Sensory evoked responses in the intensive care unit: A tutorial. *Ear and Hearing, 7*, 200–232.

Hall, J.W. III, Tucker, D.A., Fletcher, S.J., and Habersang, R. (1989). Auditory evoked responses in the management of head-injured children. In Miner, M.E. and Wagner, K.A. (eds.), *Neurotrauma: Treatment, rehabilitation and related issues* (2nd ed). Stoneham, MA: Butterworth Publishers.

Hall, J.W. III, Winkler, J.B., Herndon, D.N., and Gary, L.B. (1987). Auditory brainstem response in auditory assessment of acute severely burned children. *Journal of Burn Care and Rehabilitation, 8*, 195–198.

Hall, J.W. III, Winkler, J.B., Herndon, D.N., and Gary, L.B. (1986). Auditory brainstem response in young burn wound patients treated with ototoxic drugs. *International Journal of Pediatric Otorhinolaryngology, 12*, 187–203.

Hansen, J.C. and Hillyard, S.A. (1980). Endogenous potentials associated with selective auditory attention. *Electroencephalography and Clinical Neurophysiology, 49*, 277–290.

Harris, D.P. (1989). Comparisons between central auditory test results and topographic maps of brain injury. A paper presented at the 16th annual meeting of the American Auditory Society, New Orleans.

Harris, D. and Hall, J.W. III. (1990). Feasibility of auditory event-related potential measurement in brain injury rehabilitation patients, *Ear and Hearing, 11*, 340–350.

Hillyard, S.A., Hink, R.F., Schwent, V.L., and Picton, T.W. (1974). Electrical signs of selective attention in the human brain. *Science, 182*, 177–179.

Hirose, G., Chujo, T., Kataoka, S., Kawada, J., and Yoshioki. (1990). Acute effects of anticonvulsants on brain-stem auditory evoked potentials. *Electroencephalography and Clinical Neurophysiology, 75*, 543–547.

Jacobson, G.P. and Newman, C.W. (1990). The decomposition of the middle latency auditory evoked potential (MLAEP) Pa component into superficial and deep source contributions. *Brain Topography, 2*, 229–236.

Jacobson, G.P., Newman, C.W., Privitera, M., and Grayson, A.S. (1991). Differences in superficial and deep source contributions to middle latency auditory evoked potential Pa component in normal subjects and patients with neurologic disease. *Journal of American Academy of Audiology, 2*, 7–17.

Jacobson, J.T., Hall, J.W. III, Bull, J., and Mackey-Hargadine, J. (1991). Hyperthermia effects in multimodality evoked potentials. Presented at American Auditory Society 18th Annual Meeting, Kansas City, MO.

Jennett, B. and Teasdale, G. (1981). *Management of head injuries*. Philadelphia, PA: F.A. Davis.

Karnaze, D.S., Marshall, L.F., McCarthy, C.S., Klauber, M.R., and Bickford, R.G. (1982). Localizing and prognostic value of auditory responses in coma after closed head injury. *Neurology, 32*, 299–302.

Katz, J. (1962). The use of staggered spondaic words for assessing the integrity of the central auditory nervous system. *Journal of Audiology Research, 2*, 327–337.

Kileny, P.R., Paccioretti, D., and Wilson, A.F. (1987). Effects of cortical lesions on middle-latency auditory evoked responses (MLR). *Electroencephalography and clinical Neurophysiology, 66*, 108–120.

Klockoff, I., Anggard, G., and Anggard, L. (1966). Recording of cranio-labyrinthine pressure transmission in man by acoustic impedance method. *Acta Otolaryngologica, 61*, 361–370.

Korein, J. (1984). The diagnosis of brain death. *Seminars in Neurology, 4,* 52–72.

Kohrman, M.H. and Spivack, B.S. (1990). Brain death in infants: Sensitivity and specificity of current criteria. *Pediatric Neurology, 6,* 47–50.

Kraus, N., Smith, D.I., and McGee, T. (1988). Midline and temporal lobe MLRs in the guinea pig originate from different generator systems: A conceptual framework for new and existing data. *Electroencephalography and Clinical Neurophysiology, 70,* 541–558.

La Puma, J., Schiedermayer, M.D., Gulyas, A.F., and Siegler, M. (1988). Talking to comatose patients. *Archives of Neurology, 45,* 20–22.

Lee, Y.S., Lueders, H., Dinner, D.S., Lesser, R.P., Hahn, J., and Klem, G. (1984). Recording of auditory evoked potentials in man using chronic subdural recordings. *Brain, 107,* 115–131.

Lesnick, J.E., Michele, J.J., Simeone, F.A., DeFeo, S., and Welsh, F.A. (1984). Alteration of somatosensory evoked potentials in response to global ischemia. *Journal of Neurosurgery, 60,* 490–494.

Levin, H.S. (1985). Part II: Neurobehavioral recovery. In Becker, D.P. and Povlishock, J.T. (eds.) *Central nervous system trauma status report,* pp. 281–299. Bethesda, MD: National Institute of Neurological and Communicative Disorders and Stroke, National Institutes of Health.

Levin, H.S., Benton, A.L., and Grossman, R.G. (1982). *Neurobehavioral consequences of closed head injury.* New York: Oxford University Press.

Liegeois-Chauvel, C., Musolino, A., and Chauvel, P. (1991). Localization of the primary auditory area in man. *Brain, 114,* 139–153.

Lindsay, K.W., Carlin, J., Kennedy, I., Fry, J., and McInnes, A. (1981). Evoked potentials in severe head injury—analysis and relation to outcome. *Journal of Neurology, Neurosurgery, and Psychiatry, 44,* 796–802.

Mackey-Hargadine, J.R. and Hall, J.W. III. (1985). Sensory evoked responses in head injury. *Central Nervous System Trauma, 2,* 187–206.

Matzker, J. (1959). Two new methods for the assessment of central auditory functions in cases of brain disease. *Annals of Otology, Rhinology, and Laryngology, 68,* 1185–1187.

McGraw, C.P. and Cindall, G.T. (1974). Cardio-respiratory alterations in head injury: Patient's response to stimulation. *Neurological Surgery, 2,* 263–266.

Michalewski, H.J., Prasher, D.K., and Starr, A. (1986). Latency variability and temporal interrelationships of the auditory event-related potentials (N1, P2, N2, and P3) in normal subjects. *Electroencephalography and Clinical Neurophysiology, 65,* 59–71.

Musiek, F.E. (1983). Assessment of central auditory dysfunction: The dichotic digit test revisited. *Ear and Hearing, 4,* 79–83.

Musiek, F.E. (1989). Probing brain function with acoustic stimuli. *ASHA, 31(8),* 100–106.

Narayan, R.K., Greenberg, R.P., Miller, J.D., and Becker, D. (1981). Improved confidence of outcome prediction in serve head injury. A comparative analysis of the clinical examination, multimodality evoked potentials, CT scanning, and intracranial pressure. *Journal of Neurosurgery, 54,* 751–762.

Newlon, R.G. and Greenberg, R.P. (1983). Assessment of brain function with multimodality evoked potentials. In Rosenthal, M., Griffith, E.R., Bond, M.R., and Miller, J.D. (eds.) *Rehabilitation of the head injured adult,* pp. 75–95. Philadelphia, PA: F.A. Davis.

Newlon, R.G., Greenberg, R.P., Hyatt, M.S., Enas, G.G., and Becker, D.P. (1982). The dynamics of neuronal dysfunction and recovery following severe head injury assessed with serial multimodal evoked potentials. *Journal of Neurosurgery, 57,* 168–177.

Nuwer, M.R. (1989). Assessment: EEG brain mapping—report of the American Academy of Neurology, Therapeutics and Technology Assessment Subcommittee. *Neurology, 39,* 1100–1101.

Oken, B.S. and Chiappa, K.H. (1985). Electroencephalography and evoked potentials in head trauma. In Becker, D.P. and Povlishock, J.T. (eds.) *Central nervous system trauma status report,* pp. 177–185. Bethesda MD: National Institute of Neurological and Communicative Disorders and Stroke, National Institutes of Health.

Oken, B.S. and Chiappa, K.H. (1986). Statistical issues concerning computerized analysis of brainwave topography. *Annals of Neurology, 19,* 493–494.

Papanicolaou, A.C., Loring, D.W., Eisenberg, H.M., Raz, N., and Contreras, F.L. (1986). Auditory brain stem evoked responses in comatose head-injured patients. *Neurosurgery, 18,* 173–175.

Piatt, J.H. Jr. and Schiff, S.J. (1984). High dose barbiturate therapy in neurosurgery of intensive care. *Neurosurgery, 15,* 427–444.

Polich, J. (1986). Normal variation of P300 auditory stimuli. *Electroencephalography and Clinical Neurophysiology, 65,* 236–240.

Pritchard, W.S. (1981). Psychophysiology of P300. *Psychological Bulletin, 90,* 506–540.

Raimondi, A.J. and Hirschauer, J. (1984). Head injury in the infant and toddler: Coma scoring and outcome scale. *Child's Brain, 11,* 12–35.

Rappaport, M., Hall, K.M., Hopkins, K., Belleza, T., Berrol, S., and Reynolds, G. (1977). Evoked brain potentials and disability in brain-damaged patients. *Archives of Physical and Medical Rehabilitation, 58,* 333–338.

Rappaport, M., Hall, K.M., Hopkins, K., Belleza, T., and Cope, D.N. (1982). Disability rating scale for severe head trauma: Coma to community. *Archives of Physical and Medical Rehabilitation, 63,* 118–123.

Reid, A., Marchbanks, R.J., Burge, D.M., Martin, A.M., Bateman, D.E., Pickard, J.D., and Brightwell, A.P. (1990). The relationship between intracranial pressure and tympanic membrane displacement. *British Journal of Audiology, 24,* 123–129.

Reuter, B.M. and Linke, D.B. (1989). P300 and coma. In Maurer, K. (ed.), *Topographic brain mapping of EEG and evoked potentials.* Berlin: Springer-Verlag.

Rosen, C.D. and Gerring, J.P. (1986). *Head trauma: Educational reintegration,* pp. 25–66. San Diego, CA: College Hill Press.

Rosenberg, C., Wogensen, K., and Starr, A. (1984). Auditory brainstem and middle and long-latency evoked potentials in coma. *Archives and Neurology, 41,* 835–838.

Scherg, M. and Von Cramon, D. (1988). Evoked potential source potentials of the human auditory cortex. *Electroencephalography and Clinical Neurophysiology, 63,* 344–360.

Seales, D.M., Rossiter, V.S., and Weinstein, M.E. (1979). Brainstem auditory evoked responses in patients comatose as a result of blunt head trauma. *Journal of Trauma, 19,* 347–353.

Shin, D.Y., Ehrenberg, B., Whyte, J., Bach, J., and DeLisa, J.A. (1989). Evoked potential assessment: Utility in prognosis of chronic head injury. *Archives of Physical and Medical Rehabilitation, 70,* 189–193.

Sklare, D.A. and Lynn, G.E. (1984). Latency of the P3 event-related potential: Normative aspects and within-subject variability. *Electroencephalography and Clinical Neurophysiology, 59,* 420–424.

Snyder, E. and Hillyard, S.A. (1976). Long-latency evoked potentials to irrelevant, deviant stimuli. *Behavoral Biology, 16,* 319–331.

Sohmer, H., Gafni, M., Goitein, K., and Fainmesser, P. (1983). Auditory nerve brainstem evoked potentials in cat during manipulation of cerebral perfusion pressure. *Electroencephalography and Clinical Neurophysiology, 55,* 198–202.

Sohmer, H. and Goitein, K. (1988). Auditory brain-stem (ABP) and somatosensory evoked potentials (SEP) in an animal model of a synaptic lesion: Elevated plasma barbiturate levels. *Electroencephalography and Clinical Neurophysiology, 71,* 382–388.

Sohmer, H., Gold, S., Cahani, M., and Attias, J. (1989). Effects of hypothermia on auditory brain-stem and somatosensory evoked responses: A model of synaptic and axonal lesion. *Electroencephalography and Clinical Neurophysiology, 74,* 50–57.

Sohmer, H., Freeman, S., and Schmuel, M. (1989). ABR threshold is a function of oxygen level. *Hearing Research, 40,* 87–92.

Speaks, C. and Jerger, J. (1965). Method for measurement of speech identification. *Journal of Speech and Hearing Research, 8,* 185–194.

Tandon, P.N., Sinha, A., Kacker, S.K., Saxena, R.K., and Singh, K. (1973). Auditory function in raised intracranial pressure. *Journal of Neurological Sciences, 18,* 455–467.

Toffol, G.J., Lansky, L.L., Hughes, J.R., Blend, M.J., Pavel, D.G., Kecskes, S.A., Ortega, R.E., and Tan, W.S. (1987). Pitfalls in diagnosing brain death in infancy. *Journal of Child Neurology, 2,* 134–138.

Toutan, S.M., Klauber, M.R., Marshall, L.F., Toole, B.M., Bowers, S.A., Seelig, J.M., and Varnell, J.B. (1984). Absent or compressed basal cisterns on first CT scan: Ominous predictors of outcome in severe head injury. *Journal of Neurosurgery, 61,* 691–694.

Walker, M.L., Mayer, T.A., Storrs, B.B., and Hylton, P.D. (1985). Pediatric head injury—Factors which influence outcome. *Concepts in Pediatric Neurosurgery, 6,* 84–97.

Willeford, J. (1977). Assessing central auditory behavior in children: A test battery approach. In Keith, R. (ed.), *Central auditory dysfunction.* New York: Grune & Stratton.

Yingling, C.D., Hosobuchi, Y., and Harrington, M. (1990). P300 as a predictor of recovery from coma. *Lancet, 336,* 873.

Zuccarello, M., Fiore, D.L., Pardatscher, K., Martini, A., Paolin, A., Trincia, G., and Andrioli, G.C. Importance of auditory brainstem responses in the CT diagnosis of traumatic brainstem lesions. *American Journal of Neuroradiology, 4,* 481–483.

CHAPTER 20

BRAIN MAPPING OF AUDITORY EVOKED POTENTIALS

GARY P. JACOBSON

Conventional clinical techniques that are used to record auditory evoked potentials (AEPs) permit the visualization of a waveform that varies in voltage as a function of time. Multichannel evoked potential recordings have flourished with the advent of more sophisticated computers that are capable of acquiring and analyzing large quantities of data. Today it is not uncommon to see clinical investigators routinely recording four channels of auditory brainstem response (ABR) data whereas 15 years ago it was common for investigators to record one channel of data. The change in technique was precipitated by the knowledge that more clinical information could be derived from multichannel data (Hall et al., 1984). However, the desire to view the scalp voltage field in its entirety has led to the development of topographic methods to represent this electrical activity. The common term for describing computerized evoked potential topography is *brain mapping*. The interest in brain mapping has grown in the past decade. Interest in computerized analysis techniques has occurred due to a feeling that there is more information present in the multichannel EP record than can be appreciated through conventional single or dual channel waveform analysis, and due to the seductiveness of color pictures.

At the time of this writing (1990) there are 10 commercial manufacturers that produce brain mapping instrumentation, a new journal called *Brain Topography* that was developed to address issues pertinent to functional brain imaging and, an organization of brain mapping practitioners called the International Society for Brain Electromagnetic Topography (ISBET) has been established. Additionally, for the first time, audiologists are beginning to show interest in this technology (Jacobson and Grayson, 1988; Finitzo and Freeman, 1989; Finitzo et al., 1987; Maurer, 1989; Kraus and McGee, 1988; Kraus et al., 1985). For a general overview of the areas of computerized EEG and EP topography, the interested reader is directed to the excellent review by Nuwer (1988a,b) and the edited works of Duffy (1986), and Maurer (1989). Although it has been suggested that AEP mapping might be useful for the identification (and subtyping) of dyslexic children, schizophrenics, patients with epilepsy, patients with affective disorders, and patients with cerebral infarcts and brain tumors, the diagnostic capabilities of brain mapping have not been demonstrated convincingly and, to date, brain mapping remains a "tool" rather than a "test." At present AEP mapping is an investigational technique that is being used to understand the underlying origins of scalp recorded EPs and central nervous system (CNS) diseases. The purpose of the present chapter will be to introduce the reader to AEP brain mapping, its history, recording and analysis techniques, the normal appearance of AEP component maps, diagnostic possibilities, and future applications of this technology.

HISTORY

The history of EP topography begins with the pioneering work of Remond and Lesevre (1965) who developed a technique known as "chronotopography." This technique was used to visualize the peaks and troughs in multichannel visual evoked potential (VEP) data that was collected from electrodes that were placed over the occipital cortex. An example of this technique

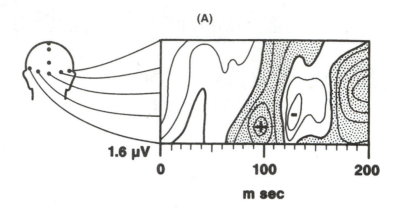

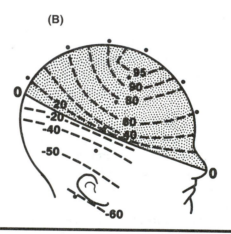

FIGURE 20.1. (A) Chronotopograph of a visual evoked potential following hemifield checkerboard stimulation (adapted from Remond and Lesevre, 1965). In this figure time is depicted on the "X" axis, and space over the occipital scalp (i.e., where the electrodes were placed) is depicted on the "Y" axis. The "Z" axis (i.e., rising out of the page) is the scalp voltage with negative voltages being represented by black and positive voltages being represented by white. Concentric ovoids represent mountains in the voltage "landscapes" or topographs. The peaks are represented by the smallest circles. (B) Isopotential contour curves for auditory evoked potential component P200 (adapted from Vaughan and Ritter, 1970). A description of isopotential contour curves are provided in the text.

is illustrated in Figure 20.1A. The X axis represents time and the Y axis represents a restricted area of the occipital scalp where the electrodes were placed. The Z axis (i.e., the axis extending out of the page toward the reader) represents the amplitude of the various VEP components. The light area represents upward deflec- tions from baseline (i.e., positive scalp voltages or peaks) and the dark area represents downward deflec- tions from baseline (i.e., negative scalp voltages or troughs). These pictures made it possible to view changes in scalp voltages that occurred over time, al- though the technique was difficult to interpret.

Vaughan et al. (1969) and Goff et al. (1969) introduced a "relative" or "normalized" method of depicting multichannel AEP data. These representations are called isopotential (i.e., one voltage) contour curves.[1] Examples of AEP maps that have been generated using this technique are illustrated in Figure 20.1B. In this technique multichannel data is recorded and the site of the maximum EP voltage is identified. A line is drawn encompassing that area of the scalp wherein the EP is recorded at its maximum amplitude (i.e., 100% amplitude). A second line is drawn encompassing the area enclosed by the first and including (for example) the area of the scalp wherein the EP is recorded at 90 percent of its maximum amplitude. This procedure is followed for the 80 percent to 0 percent contour curves. The curves can define 5 percent of maximum areas instead of 10 percent areas and can represent positive and negative voltages. The technique is called a "relative" or "normalized" mapping method because actual values (voltages) are not shown in the pictures. Only relative values with reference to the maximum voltage were depicted.

The most recent innovation in EP topography was developed by Duffy and his colleagues at Boston Children's Hospital and published in the journal *Neurology* (Duffy et al., 1979). This technique was called Brain Electrical Activity Mapping or "BEAM™." Using this technique, multichannel EP fields may be transformed into gradients of gray or multi-color images where each image represents a moment in time in the generation of an EP and where the display of colors (i.e., shades of gray, or, hues of red or blue) on a head diagram refers to a specific voltage value. These values (or images) may be compared to a set of reference (i.e., average of control group) data to determine whether there are scalp regions where a subject's EP data deviates significantly from that obtained from a normal group. The reader should be reminded that the term BEAM is a registered trademark (owned by Nicolet Biomedical) and describes a specific data acquisition and analysis brain mapping system that was developed by Duffy et al. (1979).

There are a number of issues to be considered in the generation of brain maps. These issues fall under the general headings of data acquisition, data analysis, and map generation. These areas will be addressed separately.

DATA ACQUISITION

Calibration

Calibration should be performed by routing a known electrical signal (i.e., usually a rectangular pulse) from the electrode junction box through the entire system. The resulting waveform should have an amplitude consistent with the level of amplification of the system and should have a duration consistent with the width of the pulse at the input. It would be ideal to route various calibrated sine waves through the system covering the frequency range of the spectrum of EPs of interest. In fact, however, for commercially available systems calibration is usually performed within the brain mapping machine, bypassing the electrode junction box. Adjusting the EEG amplifiers for calibration adjustments is usually difficult and requires manipulation of potentiometers contained on circuit boards within the computer.

Quantity of Electrodes

A substantially greater number of electrodes must be placed on the scalp for brain mapping than for clinical AEP testing. This is due to the need to describe the voltage field[2] adequately over the entire head. These electrodes are applied to the scalp using the International 10–20 coordinate system (Jasper, 1958). This system of electrode placement is illustrated in Figure 20.2A (see color plate). The 10–20 system gets its

---

[1]Isopotential contours are a method of spatially representing scalp voltages using relative scaling techniques (See Figure 20.1B). This method uses lines boundaries to illustrate areas of the scalp where like electrical potentials, or "isopotentials" (with reference to the maximum voltage of a given evoked potential) are recorded.

[2]Near-field and far-field evoked potentials are propagated from the brain through heterogeneous volume conductors including the cerebrospinal fluid, meninges, skull, and muscle to the scalp. These intervening structures serve to disperse brain potentials as they approach the scalp surface. The shape of the resulting voltage pattern is called the "voltage field."

name from the distance between adjacent electrodes. According to this system each electrode on the scalp is 10 percent or 20 percent of the distance between the nasion and inion, the pre-auricular point on the left to pre-auricular point on the right, or, circumference of the head measured around the nasion, pre-auricular points and inion. There are some who feel that EP voltages obtained from 16 electrodes are an insufficient number with which to infer the 4000+ values that are needed to make a color brain map. The failure to apply a sufficient number of electrodes to describe a voltage field is known as "spatial aliasing." The concept of "spatial aliasing" is akin to the concept of aliasing in the sampling of electrical activity by an averaging system.

In conventional EPs we choose a sampling rate for the computer that is roughly double the highest frequency of the EP spectrum. This is known as the Nyquist frequency. This allows high-frequency signals to be sampled frequently enough to depict the waveform accurately. In brain mapping we strive to represent accurately the topography of electrical events that occur in areas of the scalp where we have no electrodes. The number of electrodes that must be placed on the scalp depends upon the spatial frequency of the electrical event that is being represented pictorially. Spatial frequency is a somewhat esoteric term that is defined by the magnitude of change that occurs over a scalp area per unit time. In other words, EPs with topographies that are restricted to small circumscribed scalp regions, having large amplitudes, and that occur over a short time period are said to have high spatial frequencies. Alternately, EPs that have broad voltage fields with shallow voltage gradients may be said to be composed of lower spatial frequencies. The Nyquist distance describes the maximum distance that may exist between electrodes to describe the voltage field of an EP accurately. The fact that the Nyquist distance is critical for the accurate representation of scalp electrical fields has been acknowledged by a number of investigators (Gevins, 1984; Lopes da Silva, 1987), however, Spitzer et al. (1989) have described a method of determining the minimum interelectrode spacing for a particular EP of interest. This multi-step method requires that closely spaced electrodes be placed first over the area where the EP component is likely to occur.

Electrode Reference

Each of the 16–21 electrodes that are placed on the scalp is referenced to another electrode. The purpose of the reference site is to detect common electrical interference that is generated by the body (i.e., EKG) or is emanating from the environment (i.e., 60 Hz interference). Ideally, the magnitude and waveshape of this common activity is similar at the active and reference electrode locations and therefore is cancelled within the differential amplifier. For most sensory evoked potentials (SEPs) any location on the head is considered an "active" reference site since EP fields often spread out over the scalp, however, it is common to reference scalp electrodes to an ear lobe, mastoid, or nose. Though reference contamination is known to have a profound effect on the recording of time-voltage EP waveforms, it does not influence the shape of EP voltage landscapes since the reference electrode injects a constant voltage into each active electrode and, thus uniformly distributes this contamination (Lehmann and Skrandies, 1980). The absolute voltage values referenced to baseline will be influenced by the choice of the reference electrode site. It is best in doing all EP recordings to choose a non-cephalic reference site. The most popular reference sites are the throat, cervical vertebra, or the optimal balanced sterno-vertebral technique (Stephenson and Gibbs, 1951). The latter technique is not only non-cephalic but minimizes EKG interference. It is noteworthy that the capability of two additional "unbiased" or "reference-free" techniques reside within some mapping devices. One technique is called the common average reference, CAR (Offner, 1950; Lehmann et al., 1986). In the CAR the reference voltage for each electrode on the scalp at any moment during the averaging epoch is the average of voltages at all electrodes on the scalp at the same moment in time. The second type of unbiased reference is called the "source-derivation" reference (Hjorth, 1975, 1980) and will be considered later in this chapter.

Evoked Potential Recording

The patient is prepared for testing in the same manner as one would prepare a patient for conventional clinical EPs. Indeed, the stimulating and recording parameters are identical to those that are used for clinical testing. The principal difference is the larger number of channels that must be averaged simultaneously. The maximum stimulation rates depend on the speed of the computer processor and the number of memory locations that are available for each channel of data acquisition. The need for maintaining the alertness of the subject must be anticipated since cortically generated EPs are often affected by the level of arousal of the subject (Picton et al., 1974b). Different techniques have developed to insure attentiveness of patients. One simple method is to have the subject or patient count the number of stimuli that are presented during signal averaging. Additionally, since the eyes are dipoles that are positively charged at the cornea and negatively charged at the retina (due to the corneo-retinal potential) eye movements must be monitored during data collection. Electroculographic (EOG) contamination becomes particularly troublesome in the recording of late low frequency endogenous EPs such as the P300 or the contingent negative variation (CNV). A simple method of monitoring EOG activity is to place a pair of electrodes diagonally above (rostral to the outer canthus) and below (at the inner canthus) one eye. The level of activity from this recording derivation may be used to determine whether the incoming EEG should be rejected by the artifact rejection system in the computer.

Baseline Setting

A method must be used to determine where the zero voltage line runs through the EP tracings. Defining the scalp topography of a voltage field is of primary concern. This means that we are interested in accurately representing both positive and negative deflections of the waveform about a zero baseline. A number of baseline-setting schemes may be used. For instance, a baseline may be established by averaging the voltages at each point across the waveform. However, this assumes that there will be as many points above zero as below zero and this does not occur for many EPs (i.e., the P100 of the pattern-reversal VEP). A second and more historically accepted method involves setting baseline as the average of voltages that occur in a pre-

stimulus period. It is presumed that during this pre-stimulus period (i.e., normally at least $1/10$ the duration of the averaging epoch) that the baseline should be flat. Any perturbations that occur during this period should represent only unaveraged EEG or EMG activity. Since the averaged baseline period should be flat if the recording conditions are optimal, the pre-stimulus period also provides an estimate of the quality of data obtained during the recording session. This baseline setting technique is appropriate only if later components of a given SEP do not affect the voltage that accrues during the pre-stimulus baseline period. Lastly, a baseline for a given component may be set to the peak or trough of its preceding component.

Interpolation of Data Points

After data collection is completed the computer will have generated 16–21 single EPs, one EP for each acquisition channel (See Figure 20.2B, color plate). Each EP consists of a series of points (i.e., 256–512 points depending on the computer) that represent voltage values at each time point over the averaging epoch. Approximately 4000 values (picture units or pixels) are needed to construct a smooth contiguous map picture. Thus, actual voltage values are "known" for less than 1 percent of the scalp surface. This leaves 99 percent of the scalp surface for which voltage values are "unknown." These unknown voltage values must be obtained from scalp sites where no electrodes are present. These values may be predicted using a technique that is called interpolation. For example, we can take a small part of the scalp and construct a square; at each corner of the square place an electrode. If the topmost electrodes are assigned a value of 5 µV and the two bottom electrodes are assigned a value of 1 µV, we can estimate based on the distance between the top and bottom electrodes what values would fall along the lines that connect the top and bottom electrodes. The space in the center of the square can be filled in with estimated values by connecting, for example, the top left electrode with the bottom right electrode and interpolating the values between. Through the process of interpolation 4000+ estimated voltage values can be estimated from the 16–21 known observed values. An example of how interpolation can be used to construct a color map of the Pa component of the middle latency auditory evoked potential (MLAEP) is illustrated in Figure 20.2C (see color plate). Both three-point (i.e., interpolation is generated using three electrodes in a triangular format) and four-point (i.e., interpolation is generated using four electrodes in a square format) linear and curvilinear interpolation techniques are being utilized. In linear interpolation the head surface is considered flat and in curvilinear interpolation the head is considered a curved surface. Curvilinear interpolation generally yields smoother maps with less dramatic changes in color with increases in amplitude of the EP.

Representation of Data

The resulting numbers are converted to darkness (density) of gray (i.e., gray-scale maps) or colors. The most popular system is for scalp positive voltages to be represented by red colors and scalp negative voltages to be represented by blue colors.[3]

The simplest "real-world" analogy for brain mapping is the weather map of a country (i.e., the head in this analogy) where temperature (i.e., voltage) is represented by colors with red colors denoting warmer temperatures (greater positive voltages) and blue colors representing cooler temperatures (greater negative voltages). In fact, the same interpolation techniques are used to "color in" the weather map that is found in the newspaper. In this manner, temperatures may be predicted for areas where future temperatures are unknown from areas where future information is available. Weather maps may be viewed one day at a time (i.e., one ms at a time) or may be viewed in sequence (i.e., ms by ms) so that temperature changes (i.e., voltage changes) across the country might be observed. In the same manner, it is possible to view the voltage field map of the middle latency AEP (MLAEP) Pa component, or, one can rapidly view consecutive voltage field

---

[3]In contrast, Desmedt and Nguyen (1984; et al., 1987) who have contributed greatly to the understanding of mapping of the somesthetic cortex feel that positive voltages should be represented by cool colors (e.g., blues) and negative voltages should be represented by hotter colors (e.g., reds).

maps from 15–59 ms in a serial format. This method of viewing mapped EP data is referred to as "cartooning." The representation of data in a pictorial format whether as a bar graph or line chart is done to make this information easier to grasp. In the same manner the representation of voltage-varying EP data in a topographic format was developed to make the two-dimensional spatial properties of the EP field more accessible.

Just as it is possible to increase the size of an EP waveform that is displayed on an oscilloscope screen, it is possible to increase the size of the 16–21 channels of EPs in brain mapping. It is critical that the waveform data be viewed when this is being done to insure that the waveforms are not being overamplified. If this occurs, the entire scalp map will appear as the color of the maximum range positively or negatively (i.e., dark red or dark blue).

Collecting multichannel data creates a problem equal in magnitude to the amount of data that has been collected. First, agreement must be reached on methods of quantifying this data. Finally, methods of data analysis must be developed. These concerns will be addressed in the following section.

DATA ANALYSIS

Quantification of Data

The most conventional method for quantifying multichannel data is to measure the voltage value with reference to baseline at each moment in time for each electrode across the entire averaging epoch. Lehmann and Skrandies (1980) have asserted that it is most meaningful to analyze the EP fields at points in time when they are at their maxima and when the field pattern is most stable. The determination of at what latency EP peaks reach their maxima is a relatively easy task in conventional time-voltage analysis but is a far more difficult task in the measurement of multi-channel topographically recorded EPs. Lehmann and Skrandies (1980) developed a method called *global field power* (GFP) measurement that accomplishes the purpose of identifying time periods when EP fields reach their extremes and are most stable. Data is first re-referenced using the common average reference. For any time point the GFP consists of the root of the mean of the squared voltage deviations at all electrodes from the mean of all instantaneous voltages. This process is carried out at each time point across the averaging epoch. The result is a single waveform consisting of peaks and troughs. The peaks in this waveform correspond with points in time when scalp voltage field strength is at its greatest. It is at these time points that the measurement of amplitude (at each electrode), peak latency and overall scalp topography are recommended.

Another measurement technique is the relative magnitude of an EP with reference to its peak amplitude at differing scalp regions (isovoltage contour curves). The units of measurement in this technique are percentages with the scalp region where the maximum amplitude is located being designated 100%. Another measurement technique is percent left-right asymmetry to monaural or binaural stimulation.

Methods of Data Analysis

The most common analysis technique is the comparison of data obtained from a single subject with that obtained from a large group of normal subjects. There has been a trend for manufacturers of brain mapping instrumentation to either collect and distribute their own data bases for a given EP, or to support the development of a normative data base by users of a particular brand of brain mapping equipment. The latter method entails the distribution to users of specific protocols that must be adhered to rigidly. Normative data is forwarded by users to the manufacturer where a normative data base is established. The former model (that wherein the manufacturer develops and supplies a data base) was first used in the BEAM system. The latter model is the one most used by manufacturers in recent times.

Although analysis methods such as discriminant analysis, analysis of variance, multivariate analysis of variance, feature analysis, principal components analysis, singular value decomposition, and eigenfunction analysis have been used to help define features that can be used to best differentiate groups of subjects (or patients) the Z-transformation (Z-score) is the most common data analysis technique that has been imposed on

topographic EP data (Duffy, 1981, 1982, 1985; Duffy et al., 1981). In this analysis, a voltage value at a given moment in time at each electrode for a given subject (or patient) is compared to the mean voltage value for a "normal" control group for the equivalent electrode at the equivalent moment in time. Differences between the observed voltage values from the subject and the mean voltage values at each electrode location obtained from the control group are expressed as Z-scores (standard deviations) from the group mean. The numeric values (unit values of standard deviations) assigned to each electrode location for a given moment in the averaging epoch are interpolated using the same techniques that were utilized to create the voltage field map. The Z-score analysis results in a map where color does not represent voltage but instead represents the magnitude of difference between the observed voltage field data at a given time point and compared with that obtained from a normal group at the identical time point. In this case, red colors might represent positive standard deviations (i.e., number of standard deviations above the mean) and blue colors might represent negative standard deviations (i.e., number of standard deviations below the mean). These comparisons may be made on a time-point by time-point basis and, thus, Z-transformed maps may be "cartooned" so that a rapid assessment of the data can be derived. An example of Z-score maps for a normal subject during the time period from 5 ms before through 59 ms after click stimulus onset is shown in Figure 20.2D (see color plate). It is important to note that areas of the scalp where the deviation from the group data is greatest do not represent areas of *disease* but only represent regions where the subject's electrical activity differs most from the control group (Harner, 1986; Nuwer, 1988a). It is known that by chance it is possible that areas of significance will be found for one out of every 20 data points per map (i.e., 0.05 significance). Therefore, it is essential that these data meet three criteria before claims of significance can be supported. First the topographic significance must be "regional." The finding of a statistical significance at one focal scalp location at one moment in the averaging epoch is most likely artifactual in origin (i.e., due to a bad electrode). True abnormalities are usually regional in appearance (i.e., frontal, temporal, hemispheric). Additionally, scalp regions of statistical significance should persist for more than a few time points. Finally, the finding of statistical significance should be reproducible on repeated measurements. Topographically recorded EPs must be subjected to the same scrutiny as conventional clinical EP data. While Z-transformation techniques have been used to compare single subject data to group data, t-test techniques have been used to compare data at successive time points obtained from two groups of subjects (i.e., normal and Alzheimer's disease). In this case, color would not represent voltage or standard deviations from a mean, rather it would represent t-values or significance levels.

Several important factors limit the usefulness of Z-transformation and t-test techniques. The establishment of a normative data base for single subject comparisons is filled with problems related to subject selection. What constitutes a normal subject? Are normal subjects those individuals who do not smoke and drink, those who have never had a migraine and are not taking any medications? These *supernormal* subjects participated in the development of the normative data base for the BEAM system developed by Duffy et al. (1979). The trend in recent times has been to use "average" normal subjects. The subject selection criteria is not as strict in the definition of this group; however, these subjects are more representative of the general population. Another issue is that the use of Z-scores implies that the data is normally distributed. Kraus and McGee (1988) have illustrated that the distribution of amplitudes of the MLAEP Pa recorded from the Fz electrode and taken from a group of normal subjects is skewed. Thus, alternative methods must be used to either transform these data (i.e., log, square root, arctangent transformations) into a normal distribution prior to the establishment of a normal data base, or other analysis techniques must be used. Additionally, it is assumed when multiple t-tests are imposed on a set of data (i.e., the voltages for each electrode at successive time points) that these dependent variables (i.e., electrode variables at successive time points) are uncorrelated. In fact, the voltage points that comprise the EP waveform are highly correlated in time and space (i.e., the voltages for adjacent electrodes at a

given time point are predictable). These issues have been discussed in detail by Oken and Chiappa (1986), Duffy et al. (1986) and Nuwer (1988a,b). Finally, EP latency is the most commonly used quantification technique for clinical EP examinations. Absolute EP amplitude is known to be highly variable both within and between subjects. Yet it is absolute EP amplitude (the quantification method that is never used in the practice of clinical EPs) that is used to quantify topographically recorded EPs.

Limitations of Topographic Analysis Techniques

The ultimate objective of EP mapping is to make assertions regarding the anatomy underlying the generation an EP. These assertions may concern the predicted locations of the underlying neural generators (i.e., the inverse solution), or they may concern the physiological normalcy of brain regions. There are several factors that limit the ability to generalize from topographic data.

To make judgments about the intactness of a brain area from EP data, it must be assumed that single localized generators are responsible for these scalp-recorded electrical events. It is known that this is not true. The EP recorded from the scalp surface is the result of the algebraic summation of multiple concurrently active dipole sources. Some of these sources may be superficial (i.e., cortical) and some may be deep (i.e., brainstem) in origin. Additionally, the geometry of the dipoles may make some scalp regions appear active when the location of the generator may be centimeters distant. For instance, the MLAEP Pa component normally shows a symmetrical positive field in the frontal and central scalp regions and a symmetrical negative field in the occipital regions. The best available evidence suggests that Pa is generated in the temporal lobes and deep midline brainstem structures (Kraus et al., 1988). One must carefully interpret the finding of statistically significant lateralized frontal differences in a patient. Would these differences (compared to group normal values) indicate the presence of an ipsilateral frontal lobe abnormality, or, an ipsilateral temporal lobe abnormality?

In order to infer from scalp recorded activity the intactness of underlying brain structures, it must be accepted that the impedances of the scalp, skull, meninges, cerebrospinal fluid (CSF), and brain structures are homogenous and primarily resistive. If this were true, voltage fields would not be distorted as they were propagated from the brain to the scalp surface. It is known that these structures are heterogenous in their impedance characteristics. For instance, CSF has a low impedance and serves to shunt current. Accordingly, cortical activity that may be generated focally within the cortex "spreads out" at the scalp surface. Additionally, the openings in the skull for the eyes, ears, nose and mouth serve to affect the shape of the voltage field recorded from the scalp since these landmarks act as low impedance regions were current may be shunted.

Finally, in order to infer from scalp-recorded electrical events the intactness of the underlying brain structures, it must be accepted that scalp electrodes are placed accurately over the brain regions of interest. While an expert technologist using the 10–20 system can place scalp electrodes within a 1 cm tolerance, the intersubject variability in underlying brain anatomy and intrasubject brain asymmetries can be considerable and can confound the interpretation of this data (Homan et al., 1987; Coppola et al., 1987; Myslobodsky and Bar-Ziv, 1989).

Each deviation away from these assumptions limits greatly our ability to infer from surface recorded electrical activity the location and intactness of underlying brain structures. It is because of these inadequacies that neuromagnetic recording techniques (magnetic fields emitted by the brain are not affected by these constraints) have gained popularity in recent years.

Source Derivation

Scalp mapping techniques have been used in an attempt to derive information regarding the underlying sources of scalp recorded voltage fields. It is important to note that if one has knowledge of the strength, numbers, locations, and geometries of generators that lie within the brain, as well as the impedance characteristics of the structures that separate the generators from the recording electrodes, it is possible to predict with a high degree of accuracy the appearance of the scalp recorded voltage fields. This is called a *forward solution*. However, given a scalp field—for instance, the scalp voltage field at 32

ms following the onset of a 75 dB nHL click—there are numerous combinations of brain events that can produce identical evoked scalp fields. Thus, the *inverse solution* is much more tricky. The results of techniques that are used to form an inverse solution are partly based on a priori knowledge from depth recordings in animal investigations of the numbers, locations, and relative strengths of electrical generators that underlly the generation of a given EP component.

Techniques have evolved over the past 15 years that have been used with varying degrees of success to attempt an inverse solution to scalp surface recordings. These techniques have employed bipolar derivations of electrodes placed on the scalp using the conventional 10–20 system (Hjorth, 1975; Wallin and Stalberg, 1980), or other multielectrode configurations having uniform interelectrode distances (McKay, 1983; Srebro, 1985), or arbitrary interelectrode distances (Perrin et al., 1987; Pernier et al., 1988). The *source derivation* technique developed by Hjorth (1975) has been used to help derive the location of epileptogenic foci from the EEG records of seizure patients. The technique is both simple and elegant. The reference electrode for each electrode on the scalp is the weighted average of the voltages recorded from its eight nearest neighboring electrodes. The weighting values or the relative contributions to the average from each of the neighboring electrodes is determined by their distance from the central electrode. Those electrodes of the eight neighboring electrodes that are closer to the central electrodes have a higher weighting in the average than the more distant of the eight neighboring electrodes. The Hjorth source reference results in the scalp field becoming more circumscribed (i.e., the scalp field is more confined). Indeed, this reference technique which uses the Laplacian source operator may be used to obtain the second spatial derivative or current source density[4] from scalp electrical fields. Current source density maps consist of circumscribed

---

[4]Source current density (SCD) is a method of reducing the "spatial smearing" of an evoked potential field. The technique attempts to locate the scalp sites where local current flow emerges and re-enters the scalp. The midpoint between these sites provides an approximation of the location of the equivalent dipole source beneath the scalp.

positive and negative fields. The location of the positive field on the scalp represents the site of the *current source* and the location of the negative field on the scalp represents the site of the *current sink*.[5] The location and direction of the equivalent dipole is estimated by an arrow connecting the sink to the source. The source derivation techniques acts like a spatial high-pass filter. Thus, focal electrical activity that is generated in the superficial cerebral cortex is accentuated whereas broad electrical fields that emanate from the deeper cerebral cortex and subcortical areas, or far-fields that emanate from brainstem structures, are attenuated or cancelled entirely. It is known from dipole modeling studies that as the depth of a dipole generator is increased to one-half the radius of the skull, the source activity recorded from the scalp will approach zero. When the source of an EP can be modeled as a single dipole it is known that the equivalent electrical dipole is oriented orthogonal to the equivalent magnetic field dipole that is obtained from neuromagnetic field recordings (Pernier et al., 1988). Accordingly, there is concurrence in many situations between electrical recordings and neuromagnetic recordings of EPs. Therefore, source derivations techniques may be used to estimate (within limits) the location and provide gross information about the depth of AEP generators given the constraints and pitfalls of attempts to estimate an inverse solution using scalp recorded events.

AUDITORY BRAINSTEM RESPONSE (ABR) MAPPING

Background

The ABR is a far-field response, and as such, the latency and amplitude of the 5–7 components are relatively unaffected by changes in the location of a single

---

[5]The term *current source* refers to the site or sites on the scalp having a positive current density, denoting the presence of local radial current flow extending from the source intracranially to the scalp surface. The term *current sink* refers to the site or sites on the scalp having a negative current density indicating the presence of a local radial current flow from the scalp surface to the brain.

recording electrode. It is known that the wave I and wave II components of the response originate from the VIIIth nerve and cochlear nucleus (Møller et al., 1981b; Møller and Jannetta, 1985). ABR components waves III–V originate from within the pontine auditory system (Møller et al., 1981a; Møller and Jannetta, 1982; Møller and Jannetta, 1985). ABR components wave VI and wave VII may originate from the mesencephalic and diencephalic auditory system (Møller et al., 1981a; Møller and Jannetta, 1985).

ABR Mapping

The scalp topography of the ABR in the monkey was described by Legatt et al. (1986). These investigators reported that the voltage field of wave 1a (analogous to wave I of the human) was positive over the contralateral scalp and negative at or near the ipsilateral mastoid (i.e., ipsilateral to the ear receiving the click stimuli). These findings would suggest that the generator of wave I was a transverse dipole that was oriented in a lateral-medial direction consistent with the location of the auditory nerve in the head. The monkey wave 3 (analogous to human wave II) showed a broad scalp distribution with a shallow gradient and appeared largest in magnitude in the anterior scalp. The shallow voltage gradients suggested the presence of a deep generator (i.e., intracranial portion of auditory nerve). Waves 5 and 7 (analogous to human waves III and V) were largest at the scalp just posterior to the vertex. The voltage gradients were steep both anterior and posterior to this maxima. It was the impression of the researchers that these findings suggested that the generators of waves 5 and 7 were oriented vertically in the direction of the lateral lemnisci. It is interesting that the voltage field of wave 8 (analogous to human wave VI) peaked between the vertex and contralateral mastoid and was felt, therefore, to represent activity emanating from geniculocortical projections. This observation is consistent with that of Martin and Moore (1977).

The scalp distribution of the human ABR has been described by Shimizu and Hirasawa (1985) and Grandori (1986, 1989). Shimizu and Hirasawa (1985) reported the normal scalp topography of the ABR using 12 electrodes. The investigators reported that wave II was recorded with maximum amplitude at the contralateral occipital region. The voltage field of wave III was recorded maximally at the ipsilateral centroparietal region. The voltage field of wave V was recorded maximally in the central and central parietal regions. The scalp topography of wave V can be seen in Figure 20.3A (see color plate). These results suggested to the investigators that the generator of wave II was contralateral in origin and the generator of wave III was ipsilateral in origin. These findings have not to date been supported in animal or human studies.

Grandori (1986) has reported the scalp topography of the ABR using 31 electrodes. These recordings were initially referenced to a frontal electrode and were subsequently re-referenced off-line to a common average reference. These data were subsequently subjected to a dipole localization technique. The results of his investigation in large part mirror those reported by Legatt et al. (1986). Both waves I and III appeared as a positive fields in the contralateral posterior scalp and appeared as negative fields at (i.e., wave I), or below (i.e., wave III) the ear being stimulated. These findings suggested that these two components originated from structures in the ipsilateral auditory system (i.e., VIII N. and cochlear nuclei). The scalp field of wave V appeared positive at the vertex and slightly negative at the caudal portion of the occipital pole. The findings of Grandori (1986) have suggested that the equivalent dipole that explains the existence of wave V is located at the center of the head and may represent activity ascending from the superior olivary complex through the lateral lemniscus. These findings have supported the results of multichannel time-voltage recordings reported by Scherg and Von Cramon (1985a) that were subjected to dipole localization methods (DLM). To date, there have been no published investigations evaluating ABR maps in patients with neurologic disease.

Although a few investigators have shown interest in the scalp topography of short-latency, far-field recorded AEPs, the greatest interest has been shown in the description of the scalp distributions of middle and long latency stimulus related AEPs.

MIDDLE LATENCY AUDITORY EVOKED POTENTIAL AND 40 Hz STEADY-STATE RESPONSE MAPPING

Background

The scalp surface topography of the MLAEP has received little attention since the isopotential contour curves of Goff et al. (1969) and Vaughan (1969) were published. These investigators, and Picton et al. (1974a) reported that the Pa component of the MLAEP showed a broad scalp distribution and was maximal in amplitude in the frontal and central scalp regions (Picton et al., 1974a). Goff et al. (1977) reported the scalp topography of the AEP over an averaging epoch of 490 ms. The authors observed 22 discrete AEP components and described a positivity at about 35 ms that was of maximal amplitude in the frontal region that may have represented the Pa component. However, the authors stated that the P35 component had myogenic origins. Cohen et al. (1982) described the coronal scalp topography of the MLAEP. A string of seven electrodes were placed on a line anterior to Cz and approximately 2.5 cm apart. The authors were able to record a polarity reversal of the Pa component over the level of the superior temporal plane with a bipolar referencing technique using successive pairs of coronally placed electrodes. Wood and Wolpaw (1982) conducted a topographic study of the MLAEP recorded over one hemisphere (contralateral to the ear stimulated) using 20 closely spaced surface electrodes. This study was complicated by technical problems such as the use of overly restrictive bandpass filtering (0.1–300 Hz), and insufficient averaging to resolve a stable waveform (144 samples per EP tracing). However, the authors reported the presence of two distinct components within the time period between 28 and 35 ms. The investigators reported a maximum positivity centered at Fpz and a maximum negativity centered at approximately T6-Oz. Ozdamar and Kraus (1983), like Cohen et al. (1982), have described the coronal topography of the MLAEP using five active electrodes. The authors reported that the Pa amplitude was recorded largest at the vertex and showed amplitude decrements lateral to the vertex. Thus, previous descriptions of the scalp topography of the MLAEP have been limited to a few investigations that have used differing numbers of recording electrodes over differing regions of the scalp and very different stimulating techniques.

MLAEP Mapping

In recent years, multichannel topographic investigations of the MLAEP have been used to infer origins of the principal components Na and Pa in normal subjects using conventional recording methods and source derivation techniques. Additionally, multichannel MLAEP testing has been used to evaluate patients with well-defined brain lesions in an attempt to determine whether MLAEP mapping could be used for electrodiagnostic purposes.

The scalp topography of the MLAEP in animals has been studied extensively. The guinea pig and cat analogs of the human Pa component are recorded primarily from the contralateral temporal regions (Kaga et al., 1980; Kraus et al., 1985; Chen and Buchwald, 1986). This predictable lateralization of component Pa is not observed in humans (Deiber et al., 1988; Jacobson and Grayson, 1988; Kraus and McGee, 1988).

A number of investigators have recently described the scalp topography of the MLAEP in humans using both conventional cephalic references (i.e., linked ear lobe, Kraus and McGee, 1988) and using "unbiased" references such as the balanced sterno-vertebral reference (Deiber et al., 1988), cervical vertebral reference (Kraus and McGee, 1988) and the common average reference (Comacchio et al., 1988; Jacobson and Grayson, 1988). Kraus and McGee found no significant differences in the topography of the MLAEP when maps derived from earlobe references and cervical vertebral references were compared. Also, descriptions of the MLAEP have been consistent from study to study.

Scalp Topography of Component Na.   Deiber et al. (1988) have studied the scalp topography of the Na component. The investigators described the field maximum to occur in the midfrontal regions and to show a gradual decrease in amplitude from frontal to occipital regions. The widespread nature of the voltage field and its shal-

low voltage gradient suggested to the investigators that the generators were deeply placed subcortically. The same widespread distribution of the voltage field of Na was described by Kraus and McGee (1988)

Scalp Topography of Component Pa.   Maps illustrating the voltage field distribution of the Pa component following left and right ear click stimulation are illustrated in Figure 20.3B (see color plate). The maps are presented at the mean peak latency of the Pa component at the Cz electrode. The latency of the Pa component that is depicted in the figures has been uncorrected for a 0.86 ms acoustic transmission delay. This delay occurred because the click stimulus was presented to the listeners through a length of plastic tubing that terminated in a foam earplug. The peak of the Pa component in the Cz channel was chosen over other electrodes for purposes of map depiction since the amplitude of the Pa component was maximally recorded at that electrode location regardless of the ear stimulated.

The Pa component at Cz shows a mean peak latency of 29.89 ms following left ear stimulation and 29.14 ms following right ear stimulation. The isopotential contours are symmetrical and maximally recorded at Cz and Fz regardless of which ear was stimulated. There is a steep gradient away from this peak and the Pa component shows a polarity reversal between the T3 and F7, P3 and C3, Pz and Cz, P4 and C4, and T4 and F8 electrodes. A negative polarity voltage field is recorded posterior to this line that peaks in amplitude in the posterior temporal and occipital scalp regions (i.e., T5, O1, Oz, O2, T6). These findings are consistent with those of earlier investigators who utilized multichannel non-mapping recording techniques and are consistent with the hypothesis that the Pa component in part originates from a pair of tangential dipoles that are located in the auditory cortex.

It is interesting that the difference in the peak latency of Pa following left and right ear stimulation was statistically significant (indicating a right ear advantage?). This phenomenon had not previously been reported although a similar latency difference could be appreciated in the analysis of the mapped data presented in Table 1 by Deiber et al. (1988).

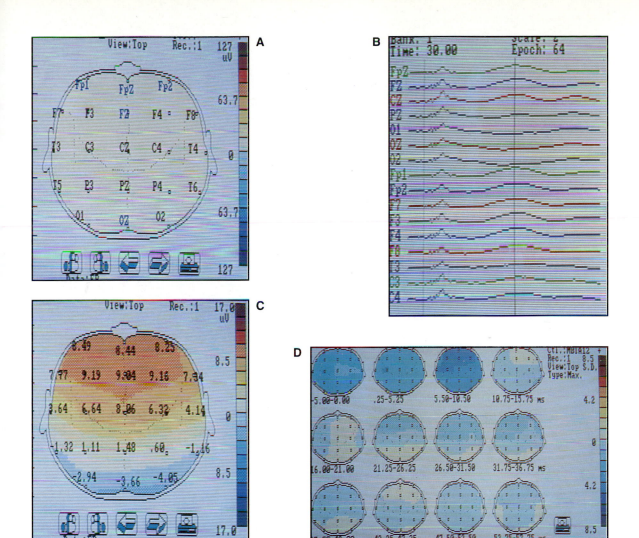

FIGURE 20.2. (A) The international 10-20 electrode system (Jasper, 1958). (B) Multichannel (16-channel) evoked potential recordings from which maps are constructed. The vertical cursor is placed at the peak latency of Pa. (C) Voltage values are present at each of the 21 channels at the peak latency of component Pa. A four-point linear interpolation has been employed to fill in the area where the actual voltage values are not known. The color bar on the right side of the figure is used to determine the voltage range assigned to each color. (D) An example of Z-score mapping for a normal individual. Color does not represent voltage; color represents numbers of standard deviations from the mean. Voltages have been integrated over 5 ms periods. Stimuli were clicks presented binaurally at 75 dB nHL at a stimulus rate of 2.3/sec. Data was filtered 10-1500 Hz. The linked earlobes were used as a reference. These maps represent the grand average of 15 normal-hearing, neurologically intact subjects. (Note: True voltages are 1/10 that presented in these and future MLAEP figures.)

The editor would like to acknowledge Bio-logic System Corp. for its support in the publication of these color brain mapping illustrations.

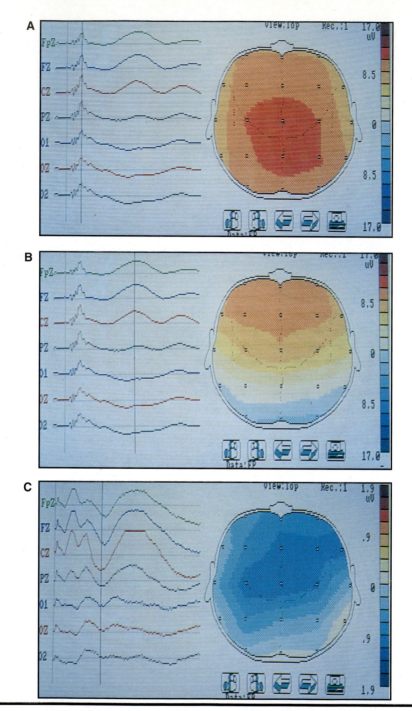

FIGURE 20.3. (A) The scalp topography of P5 of the ABR to binaural click stimulation. (B) The scalp topography of Pa of the MLAEP. (C) The scalp topography of the N1 component of the LLAEP. Stimulation and recording parameters were identical to those stated in Figure 20.1 for data depicted in Figures 20.3A and B. Stimuli were presented at a rate of 1.7 /sec at 85 dB nHL, and bioelectrical activity was bandpassed 0.3-30 Hz for data depicted in Figure 20.3C. A linked ear reference was used. This map represents the grand average of 20 normal-hearing, neurologically intact subjects. The data presented in Figure 20.3C were collected by George Lynn, Ph.D., and donated in his memory by Ernst Rodin, M.D., Wayne State University, Epilepsy Center, Detroit, MI.

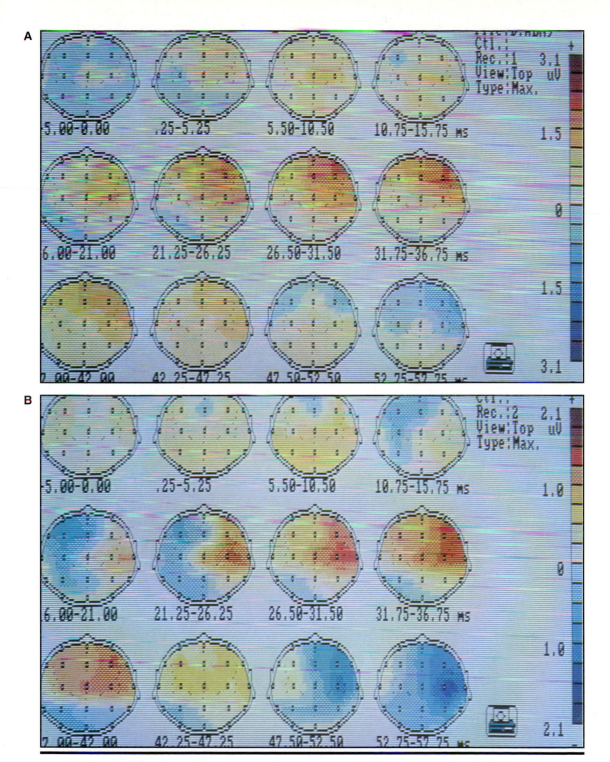

FIGURE 20.4. Scalp topography of component Pa (16-42 ms) for two patients with temporal lobe lesions. (A) This patient has sustained a left middle cerebral artery infarction involving the primary auditory cortex and deep white matter. (B) This patient has a mass lesion involving left deep temporal structures. Notice the lateralization of activity to the intact right hemisphere during this time period.

A

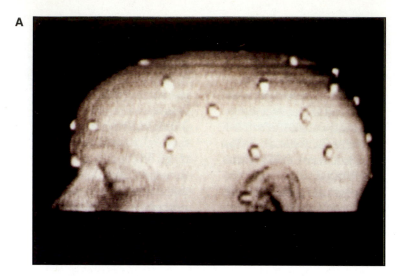

B

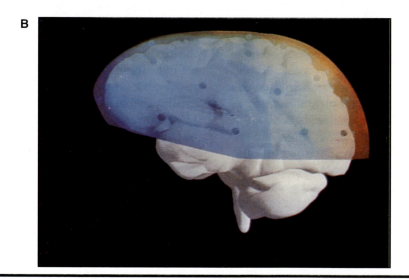

FIGURE 20.5. (A) 3D reconstruction of multislice MRI (partial saturation pulse sequence) with electrode markers shown on scalp. (B) 3D reconstruction of multislice MRI (partial saturation pulse sequence) with electrode markers shown over brain. Color-coded alpha activity was recorded from a normal male subject relaxing with eyes closed. Posterior red color represents about 50 uv of alpha, which was averaged from 30 seconds of artifact-free EEG. The subject was a 37-year-old right-handed male. The methods are described in the text. This figure was originally published in *Brain Topography, 1,* 170 (1989), and has been reprinted with the permission of the author (Dr. Torello) and the publisher (Human Sciences Press).

Decomposition of MLAEP into superficial and deep components. Mapping techniques combined with source derivation techniques also have been used recently to help validate the hypothesis that the Pa component is generated by two functionally independent systems (Kraus et al., 1988; Jacobson et al., in preparation). Evidence obtained from near-field intracranial EP studies in humans (Celesia, 1968; Lee et al., 1984), recordings obtained from patients with CT or MRI confirmed brain lesions (Kraus et al., 1982; Kileny et al., 1987, Scherg and Von Cramon, 1986), and neuromagnetic investigations of middle latency auditory evoked fields (Makela and Hari, 1987) have suggested that component Pa is generated bilaterally within the primary auditory cortices. However, mounting evidence obtained from human and animal investigations has suggested that component Pa is generated from both cortical and subcortical structures. For example, Parving et al. (1980), Rosati et al. (1982), and Woods et al. (1987) have reported patients who have sustained bilateral temporal lobe infarctions and have remained physiologically capable of generating a Pa component. Kraus et al. (1988) have described in elegant detail the dissociation between temporal lobe and midline recorded correlates of the Pa component in guinea pigs when temporal lobe activity is depressed transiently or permanently. Most recently, Deiber et al. (1989) have added support to the hypothesis of Kraus et al. (1988). Deiber et al. demonstrated that the scalp topography of Pa changes as a function of the depth of sleep. The investigators evaluated the scalp topography of the MLAEP in ten subjects during a night of sleep. The scalp topography of Pa was symmetrical prior to sleep following monaural stimulation. Deiber et al. reported that the amplitude of Pa was larger when recorded over the frontal scalp region contralateral to the ear stimulated during sleep stages II and III and during REM sleep. Therefore, the results appear to support the hypothesis that Pa is the product of a complex system of neural generators. Some of these generators are probably subcortical (possibly in the mesencephalic reticular formation, Kraus et al., 1988), are capable of affecting changes on the cortically generated responses that occur coincident in time with the subcortical re-

sponses (i.e., at the same time as Pa) and are affected by the level of arousal of the subject.

Jacobson and Newman (1989) have described a method for decomposing the MLAEP into superficial (i.e., cortical) and deep (i.e., subcortical) activity using source derivation techniques. These methods have been previously used with EEG data to successfully determine the depth of epileptiform brain discharges (Hjorth and Rodin, 1988). Briefly, the MLAEP map that has been created using source derivation techniques that are sensitive to generators in the cortical surface is subtracted from the same MLAEP map obtained using the CAR. The resultant map residual electrical activity present in the MLAEP that has a low spatial frequency. The results of this investigation have supported the contention that the MLAEP is generated by two neural systems, one in the auditory cortex bilaterally, and one deep midline system that is subcortical in nature.

Mapping of the MLAEP in the Presence of Neurologic Disease

Several investigators, using three-and four-channel recording techniques, have demonstrated that the MLAEP is affected by ipsilateral brain lesions. Kileny et al. (1987) reported their observations of 11 patients with temporal lobe lesions. The authors found significant reductions in the amplitudes of Na/Pa and of the absolute baseline-peak amplitude of Pa at the scalp overlying temporal lobes with lesions that affected the superior temporal gyrus. The sensitivity of the MLAEP component Pa to lesions that affect the primary auditory cortex has been reported by others (Kraus et al., 1982; Ozdamar et al., 1982).

However, several investigators have reported no ipsilateral MLAEP aberrations while others have reported the preservation of MLAEP despite the presence of bilateral temporal lobe injury (Parving et al., 1980; Rosati et al., 1982; Woods et al., 1987). There has been one report demonstrating ipsilateral enhancement of the Na/Pa amplitude following ipsilateral temporal lobectomy (Jacobson et al., in press). Despite the apparent interest in the effects of central auditory nervous system disease on multichannel MLAEP recordings, there has been only one mapping investigation of patients with these disorders. Pool et al. (1989) have published topographically recorded MLAEP data gathered from 6 patients with CT substantiated infarctions involving the left middle cerebral artery. The authors analyzed amplitude and latency differences at C3, Cz and C4 electrodes for the 28–48 msec time period (4 ms per data point) between the stroke patients and a group of 10 neurologically normal subjects. The left MCA infarction affected significant latency prolongations in component Pa for the patient group. The amplitude of Pa was greatest at Cz and C4 for the patient group. The group of normals showed a symmetrical voltage field with no significant amplitude differences at C3, Cz or C4 therefore, statistical mapping of the Pa component revealed a clear significance present at the C3 electrode. Statistical significance was defined as exceeding 3 standard deviations over 3 consecutive measurement points (i.e., 12 ms). These findings are consistent with those previously reported by Kraus et al. (1982) and Kileny et al. (1987) who used conventional clinical EP recording techniques. It is noteworthy that Kraus and McGee (1988) have reported that 15% of normal subjects did not demonstrate a Pa voltage field that conformed to the normal average template they derived from 40 normal hearing adults. The scalp topographies of AEPs from 1–59 ms (i.e., wave V, Na, Pa, Pb) following binaural click stimulation for two subjects with left middle cerebral artery infarctions are illustrated in Figures 20.4A and 20.4B (see color plate). A clear lateralization of activity to the scalp region overlying the intact right hemisphere during the development and decay of Pa may be observed.

Mapping of the 40 Hz Steady-State Potential

The 40 Hz steady-state potential has been hypothesized as being a rate-modulated MLAEP. However, unlike the MLAEP, the 40 Hz steady-state potential is attenuated by sleep and has been shown to be present in comatose patients (Firsching et al., 1987) and in patients with well-documented temporal lobe lesions (Spydell et al., 1985). Therefore, it has been hypothesized that the 40 Hz steady-state potential is probably generated subcortically in the midbrain reticular acti-

vating system. However, neuromagnetic recordings of the evoked magnetic field following auditory stimulation at 40 Hz has revealed that these responses are being generated cortically and demonstrate phase reversals above and below the primary auditory cortex (Hari et al., 1980). Mapping of the 40 Hz steady-state potential has yielded conflicting results. Kraus and McGee (1988) generally found little difference between the scalp topography of the MLAEP Pa component obtained at stimulation rates of 9/sec and the 40 Hz steady-state potential. When grand group average maps were created by averaging values obtained for each subject at each of the 256 time points across the averaging epoch, the 40 Hz steady-state potential consisted of a broad voltage field that had a maximum value recorded in the central and frontal scalp. When the group grand average maps were created by latency correcting the Pa components (i.e., latency shifting each individuals Pa component so that Pa peaks were aligned prior to group averaging) the scalp topography of the 40 Hz steady-state potential showed a peak only in the central and frontal polar central regions. Also, the amplitude of the 40 Hz steady-state potential was predictably larger than the Pa component of the MLAEP.

Alternately, Johnson et al. (1988) evaluated the scalp topography of the 40 Hz steady-state potential in young and old subjects using the source derivation technique described by Hjorth (1975, 1980) and found clear polarity reversals that occurred bilaterally over the temporal areas. There did not appear to be an age-related affect on the amplitude, phase, or scalp topography of the 40 Hz potential. The location of the phase reversals appeared to be appropriately orthogonal to the location of neuromagnetically recorded phase reversals when equivalent stimuli are utilized (Hari et al., 1980). Thus, there continues to be confusion with respect to the location of the underlying generators of the MLAEP and the 40 Hz steady-state potential.

LATE CORTICAL AUDITORY EVOKED POTENTIAL (LAEP) MAPPING

Background

There has been greater interest in recent years in the use of LAEP mapping for clinical electrodiagnostic purposes. The LAEP consists of three primary components, these are the P50 (P1), the N100 (N1) and the P200 (P2). The P1 is commonly felt to represent the Pb component of the MLAEP. Though higher level variables such as arousal state and selective attention are known to affect the amplitude, latency and overall waveform morphology of the LAEP, it is the later responses such as the P300 (Sutton et al. 1965) that are referred to as the endogenous EPs and are profoundly affected by the psychological state of the subject. Although these responses have been used extensively in topographic mapping studies to probe information processing, these EPs are not modality-specific (i.e., the EPs may be elicited by visual, somesthetic, or auditory stimulation) and therefore, will not be reviewed in this section on LAEP.

It is generally felt that the LAEPs are generated in part by the auditory cortex in the temporal lobe and frontal association cortex. It is known from the results of multichannel studies of the LAEP that the scalp topographies of P1, N1, and P2 are different and that multiple co-existing generator sources are responsible for the presence of N1 and P2 (Hansen and Hillyard, 1984; Woods et al., 1984; Sams et al., 1985; Giard et al., 1988). Support for a temporal lobe origin of N1 and P2 comes from 1) human multichannel electrode studies illustrating a polarity inversion of the N1 and P2 over the superior temporal plane (Vaughan and Ritter, 1970, Peronnet et al., 1974), 2) neuromagnetic auditory evoked cortical field (AECF) studies (Hari et al., 1980; Reite et al., 1982; Sams et al., 1985; Pantev et al., 1986a,b,c) which shown a polarity reversal of M90 (i.e., magnetic field response analogy for N100) and M200 fields in a direction orthogonal to that of the electrical potential field, and, 3) clinical studies that have demonstrated absent N1 and P2 components recorded from scalp regions overlying areas of temporal lobe infarction (Peronnet et al., 1974; Pool et al., 1989).

Results of multichannel electrode studies have shown: 1) that N1 and P2 are maximally recorded at the vertex (probably due to the fact that monaural stimulation activates both auditory cortices—Picton et al., 1974; Vaughan and Ritter, 1970; Goff et al., 1977); 2) that the voltage field maxima tend to be slightly larger over the scalp contralateral to the ear stimulated,

that the electrical responses are large in comparison to MLAEPs and therefore probably represent near-field events; 3) that a polarity reversal of the N1 and P2 may be observed at or about the T3 and T4 electrodes, suggesting that the N1 and P2 are at least partially generated within the temporal lobes; and 4) that a minimum of two overlapping source generators coexist during the generation of N1 and P2 and these generators are probably located in the secondary auditory cortex on the lateral surface of the temporal lobes and in the frontal association areas (Wolpaw and Penry, 1975; Wood and Wolpaw, 1982; Scherg and Von Cramon, 1985b).

Mapping of the LAEP

Brain mapping of the LAEP has supported the observations of those who conducted multichannel voltage studies of the LAEP (Goff et al., 1969; Vaughan et al., 1969; Picton et al., 1974a; Goff et al., 1977). These investigations have focused on the N1 component due to its relatively high amplitude. Tonnquist-Uhlen et al. (1989) and Perrin et al. (1989) both have described the scalp topography of N1. Component N1 consists of a broad fronto-central negativity. The maximum voltage is recorded anterior to the interaural line and appears slightly higher in amplitude contralateral to the ear being stimulated (Perrin et al., 1989; Tonnquist-Uhlen et al., 1989). The scalp topography of N1 is illustrated in Figure 20.3C (see color plate). When voltage field activity for component N1 is subjected to source current density (SCD) analysis (equivalent to source derivation), the resulting field shows a current source in the posterior temporal lobes bilaterally (i.e., T5, T6) but with greater amplitude contralateral to the ear being stimulated (Perrin et al., 1989). The current sinks are located in the left and right central regions (i.e., C3 and C4).

Effects of Age. The effects of aging on the LAEP have been examined. Duffy et al. (1984b) evaluated the effects of age on the mapped LAEP. The investigators found statistically significant, age-related differences that were greatest between the 30–40 and 50–59 year old groups. The AEP differences occurred during the 152–172 ms period in the left frontal polar region and during the 264–284 ms period in the right frontal-central-temporal region. These age-related findings were correlated with age-related changes in verbal memory. More recently, Borg (1988) evaluated differences in mapped LAEP between a group of children aged 8–12 years and adults aged 20–46 years. The investigators discovered that whereas adults demonstrated an N1 that consistently lateralized to the contralateral scalp, the N1 for children showed a focus that consistently localized to the right scalp regardless of the ear stimulated. The authors interpreted these age-related differences in scalp topography not to changes in central processing of sound but perhaps to maturational changes in the orientation of the generator of N1.

LAEP Mapping in Disease

Several investigators have reported changes in the LAEP that accompany diseases affecting the CNS.

Stroke, Tumor, Migraine and Epilepsy. Recently, Pool et al. (1989) have compared topographic long latency data obtained from six patients with CT demonstrated infarctions involving the left middle cerebral artery territory and 10 neurologically normal subjects. The authors analyzed between group differences in amplitude and latency at the C3, Cz and C4 electrodes for the 72–128 ms latency period (4 ms per data point). The results suggested that P1 was often absent at C3 (5/6 patients) in the left MCA infarction group. Additionally, the N1 potential was present over the damaged hemisphere with comparable latency and only slightly reduced amplitude over the ipsilateral affected hemisphere. Statistical mapping of N1 revealed that two broad scalp regions reached significance. These regions included the left central-frontal region, and the right central-frontal-temporal regions. The finding of abnormal LAEPs ipsilateral to the hemisphere damaged by stroke has been observed by other investigators in conventional clinical LAEP studies (Knight et al., 1980; Woods et al., 1984; Woods et al., 1987).

Case presentations of either low voltage, or high voltage and prolonged LAEPs have been reported in the literature (Duffy et al., 1979) however no detailed study of LAEP mapping in brain tumors has been conducted.

Epilepsy. Duffy (1982, 1985), utilizing the BEAM instrumentation, has reported the presence of increased EP activity (compared with normals) in patients with seizure disorders. This "hyperactivity" is explained by Duffy as being caused by the brain being more stimulable or "irritated" in the region of the seizure focus. There have been to date no detailed LAEP mapping studies in epilepsy. This is interesting given a report of a conventional LAEP study wherein components N1 and P2 were found to be present in partial and generalized seizure groups but that components P340 and P400 are absent only in the partial seizure group (Kowell et al., 1987).

Migraine. Kumar and Dobben (1988), using BEAM instrumentation, have recently reported a case study of a patient with dizziness and migraine where MRI and EEG were normal but where statistical mapping of the LAEP showed areas of suspicion. The authors showed regional abnormalities for this subject that were confined to the posterior right occipital region (76–112 ms) and bilateral occipital regions (336–372 ms).

Alzheimer's Disease. Duffy et al. (1984a) have demonstrated topographically confined areas of suspicion in the brain maps of patients with presenile and senile dementia of the Alzheimer's type. The authors found that the LAEP between 84 and 104 ms in the left anterior temporal region differentiated the presenile dementia patients from the control subjects. The authors reported that one "...feature derived from the mid latency period of the AEP was increased compared to control values." The investigators failed to specify further during which latency period and where topographically this abnormality was present. In general, the investigators found that EP data was not as useful as EEG data in differentiating normal subjects from patients with senile dementia. The authors also reported general problems with the identification of waveforms in the demented population that complicated the analysis of data.

Most recently, Buchwald et al. (1989) in a single channel voltage study, have reported their observations recording Pa of the MLAEP and P1 of LAEP in age-matched controls and in patients with Alzheimer's

Disease (AD). The authors discovered that whereas Pa was present in both groups, P1 was absent in the group with AD. It is believed that P1 is generated in the thalamus by a cholinergically mediated component that is located within the ascending reticular activating system. It was logical therefore to assume that a disease affecting the cholinergic system would affect changes in this component.

It is interesting that Duffy et al. (1984) and Buchwald et al. (1989) have identified differing epochs where LAEPs differ between normal and demented groups. This may mean that the generation of several components (or subcomponents) of the LAEP may be mediated by a cholinergic subsystem. Several investigators have demonstrated differences between flash and pattern reversal VEPs in normal and AD groups (Harding et al., 1985; Wright et al., 1984). Therefore, it is likely in the future that AEP mapping may be used to help identify patients with these neuro-degenerating diseases.

Schizophrenia.   LAEP abnormalities in patients with schizophrenia have been reported by Morhisa et al. (1983) and Morhisa and McAnulty (1985). The investigators reported significant differences in LAEPs when normals were compared to medicated and unmedicated schizophrenics, and when schizophrenics with normal frontal lobe anatomy were compared with schizophrenics with frontal lobe atrophy. Morhisa et al. (1983) reported regional differences in the LAEP between normals and unmedicated and medicated schizophrenic patients. These abnormalities occurred in the right central and temporal scalp regions between 104 and 124 ms for the unmedicated patients and between 112 and 132 ms for the medicated patients. These intervals represent the period from when N1 reaches its peak and returns to baseline. These findings were unusual since EEG and VEP abnormalities were observed over the left hemisphere in these groups. Morhisa and McAnulty (1985) have illustrated that schizophrenics with frontal lobe atrophy demonstrated regional LAEP abnormalities during the period of time when P300 occurs (260–296 ms and 348–384 ms) in the right hemisphere.

Recently Shenton et al. (1989) using an auditory "oddball" paradigm have demonstrated that the scalp topography of P200 (204–272 ms) for schizophrenic patients in the frequent-attend condition is significantly different than that of normal controls. The map of the integrated voltages during this period was larger on the right anterior temporal scalp (T4) for the schizophrenic group. The normals showed a voltage maximum at T3 during this period. What was interesting was the correlation between P200 amplitude and negative symptoms on formalized testing. The authors found that P200 in the infrequent-attend condition was larger in magnitude when subject's negative symptom scores increased.

The significance of all of these findings is not clear. Investigators have used differing instrumentation and paradigms and have arrived at differing results (i.e., differing LAEP epochs showing statistically significant differences). It is encouraging that there does appear to be a demonstrable association between behavior and brain electrophysiology in schizophrenia.

Spastic Dysphonia.   Finitzo and colleagues, using BEAM instrumentation, have provided information about spastic dysphonia (SD), a disorder that has been felt to be of psychogenic origin. Finitzo et al. (1987) provided MRI, SPECT, CT, ABR, and BEAM LAEP data for 3 of 7 patients who were involved in motor vehicle accidents and who later developed SD. On statistical mapping two patients demonstrated left temporal abnormalities (one frontal-temporal and the other posterior-temporal) the third patient demonstrated a regional difference in the right temporal-posterior parietal region. Unfortunately, latency values were not provided and therefore it is not possible to determine whether these regional differences were present during the development, or decay of LAEP components. Additionally, there was great disparity in the locations of these regional abnormalities from patient to patient which makes it difficult to determine a common underlying system that was disrupted by the motor vehicle accident that may have caused the SD. One could argue that the head trauma associated with the accident may have caused the electrophysiologic abnormalities seen in these patients and that the association between SD and the electrophysiological abnormalities in these patients was coincidental. It is clear that physiologic correlations are impossible to predict given a small subject sample and the current status of test interpretation.

Most recently Finitzo and Freeman (1989) have presented an extensive report of their research into electrophysiologic mechanisms underlying SD. Specific to brain mapping the authors presented LAEP evidence obtained from 75 patients with SD. The authors found LAEP abnormalities in 56% of their subjects. Most subjects demonstrated statistically significant mapping abnormalities in more than one region. An abnormality in mapping was defined as a region showing more than 3 standard deviations from the mean over a minimum of three consecutive time points. The regions commonly affected were the medial frontal central scalp, right parietal and posterior temporal scalp and left temporal scalp. The most common area of EP abnormality was the paramedian frontal central cortex. It is important to note that neither waveform nor latency periods were specified wherein the mapping abnormalities occurred. It was the authors impression that multiple lesions in various locations and severities may interact and result in SD. There is anecdotal evidence (Goldsmith, 1989) that the same group of investigators have demonstrated abnormalities in the LAEP of stuttering patients.

Dyslexic and Learning Disabled Children. Duffy and colleagues (1980*a,b,* 1988) have evaluated children with diagnoses of dyslexia. The investigators have used LAEP mapping to help differentiate children with "pure" dyslexia from normal age-matched controls. Statistical analysis demonstrated significant differences in the LAEP between 108–120 ms (during the generation of N1), 192–204 ms (during the generation of P2), and during 336–348 ms. The abnormalities were confined to the left posterior temporal-occipital regions. The authors have suggested that these findings may reflect an abnormality in the auditory association cortex.

Recently, Borg et al. (1987) evaluated the mapped LAEP in 14 speech-delayed children. They found no cortical response in two subjects. They found abnormal localization of the response (i.e., normally localized to the contralateral scalp) or abnormalities in EP polarity in six subjects and a normal response in the remaining six subjects.

MAPPING OF AUDITORY EVENT-RELATED DESYNCHRONIZATION (ERD) OF EEG

Grillon and Buchsbaum (1986) have attempted to demonstrate that auditory system stimulation could result in a regional desynchronzation (i.e., attenuation) of the EEG. This ERD is conventionally elicited by having a subject perform a motor task such as clenching and unclenching the fist. This usually results in a desynchronization of the EEG over the contralateral motor cortex (Pfurtsheller and Aranibar, 1977). Grillon and Buchsbaum (1986) presented a 200 Hz tone in the sound-field at intensities of 50, 70, 80, and 90 dB SPL for 10 seconds and concurrently recorded the EEG using brain mapping techniques. The authors found that tonal presentation resulted in EEG changes that were most evident in the theta and alpha frequency bands. The greatest ERD occurred at Pz, P3, and Po (parietal-occipital midline junction) electrodes in the alpha band, in the occipital electrodes for the theta/alpha transition frequencies (i.e., 7–9 Hz) and in the occipital and temporal regions in theta band. The observed effects increased with stimulus intensity.

SUMMARY

The student and beginning practitioner of brain mapping must be a critical reader of the emerging literature. The reader must realize that regional comparisons between brain-mapped EP data (or EEG data) and CT or MRI studies are inappropriate. The latter two techniques derive images from "real" data, whereas, brain-mapped data is largely interpolated. Additionally, there has been a conspicuous absence of waveform data (from whence the EP maps were generated) in the mapping literature. Thus, the reader has been deprived of an evaluation of the raw data and has had to accept the quality of the raw data on faith alone. Finally, many of the reported investigations have been retrospective (or exploratory) in nature. These studies have evaluated EP data collected from patient groups in an attempt to define features that are characteristic of these patient groups and uncharacteristic of normal groups. There have been few prospective (or confirmatory) investigations to validate the usefulness of these discriminant variables. Additionally, there have been no investigations to determine whether brain mapping of EPs adds anything to the diagnostic effectiveness of conventional EP techniques (Hachinski, 1989). Until these prospective studies are performed, reviewed and published the aforementioned *observations* must be considered only *observations*.

There have been heated exchanges within the covers of the neurological and clinical neurophysiologic journals in the past few years. These exchanges have involved investigators who employ topographic techniques for clinical purposes. The basis of these arguments is that there are investigators who feel that it is possible to classify or diagnose patients who have differing types of perceptual or psychiatric disease on the basis of statistical comparisons of their data with that of group data (i.e., either normal group or patient group data—Duffy et al., 1986; John, 1989). Those who strongly disagree with these investigators cite issues such as the lack of prospective investigations, or confirmatory findings by other independent investigators, the use of inadequate or misleading statistical techniques that increase the possibility of finding statistically significance due to the sheer numbers of correlated variables that are being analyzed (Oken and Chiappa, 1986; Fisch and Pedley, 1989; Duffy, 1989; Nuwer, 1989). These communications prompted one journal editor to employ a statistician to assist in a review of experimental papers (Asbury, 1986).

It is clear that at present EP topography or "brain mapping" is a tool and *not* a diagnostic test. This highly sophisticated tool has enabled us to view evoked potential data in an entirely new dimension that being the spatial dimension. As with all new technologies that are developed, there is an interval of time that must pass before we can determine how this tool can be used to our best advantage. It is hoped that during this time clinical investigators will use this new technology wisely and with the best interests of the patient kept foremost in mind. It is also hoped that fundamental issues regarding appropriate methods for the quantification and analysis of data will be solved. It is certain that for the present time, consistent with the position statement of the American Encephalographic Society (1987), that brain mapping techniques must be considered only adjunctive methods for conventional EP investigations.

Most recently, Torello et al. (1987) at Ohio State University have demonstrated how both structural and functional imaging technology can be combined to provide new and exciting information about the brain. The investigators conducted magnetic resonance imaging (MRI) and EEG brain mapping studies on a 37-year-old, right-handed, male subject. Prior to beginning the MRI, 28 oil-filled capsules (vitamin E capsules) were affixed to the subject's scalp using the 10–20 co-ordinate system. These capsules may be visualized during MRI investigations using the partial saturation sequence. Following the MRI study the EEG was conducted with scalp electrodes replacing the sites where the capsules were placed. The MRI and EEG mapping data were manipulated off-line by the Ohio State University Computer Graphics Group. This post-processing enabled the investigators to reconstruct in 3 dimensions the subject's head (with electrode markers in place) and the subject's brain. The color brain-mapped EEG data was then superimposed and made semi-transparent (See Figure 20.5, color plate). The resulting image is startling in its detail and clarity. Although this investigation was conducted in an attempt to determine the capabilities of advanced computer graphic techniques, the results have demonstrated the natural evolution of brain mapping. It is certain that within the near future *functional* voltage or current brain mapping will be combined with *structural* brain imaging techniques to provide complementary types of diagnostic information to neurodiagnosticians.

REFERENCES

American Encephalographic Society. (1987). Statement on clinical use of quantitative EEG. *Journal of Clinical Neurophysiology, 4,* 75.

Asbury, A.K. (1986). Statistical issues concerning computerized analysis of brainwave topography: An editorial comment. *Annals of Neurology, 19,* 497.

Borg, E., Spens, K.E., and Tonnquist, I. (1988). Auditory brain map, effects of age. *Scandinavian Audiology, (Suppl.) 30,* 161–164.

Borg, E., Spens, K.E., Tonnquist., I., and Rosen, S. (1987). Brain map. New possibilities in diagnosis of central auditory disorders? *Acta Otolaryngologica, 103,* 612.

Buchwald, J.S., Erwin, R.J., Read, S., Van Lancker, D., and Cummings, J.L. (1989). Midlatency auditory evoked responses: Differential abnormality of P1 in Alzheimer's disease. *Electroencephalography and Clinical Neurophysiology, 74,* 378–384.

Celesia, G.C., Broughton, R.J., Rasmussen, R., and Brach, C. (1968). Auditory evoked responses from the exposed human cortex. *Electroencephalography and Clinical Neurophysiology, 84,* 458–466.

Chen, B.M. and Buchwald, J.S. (1986). Midlatency auditory evoked responses: Differential effects of sleep in the cat. *Electroencephalography and Clinical Neurophysiology, 65,* 373–382.

Cohen, M.M. (1982). Coronal topography of the middle latency auditory evoked potentials (MLAEPs) in man. *Electroencephalography and Clinical Neurophysiology, 53,* 231–236.

Comacchio, F., Grandori, F., Magnavita, V., and Martini, A. (1988). Topographic brain mapping of middle latency auditory evoked potentials in normal subjects. *Scandinavian Audiology, (Suppl.), 30,* 165–172.

Coppola, R., Karson, C., Daniel, D., and Myslobodsky, M. (1987). EEG asymmetry in relation to skull asymmetry. *Journal of Clinical Neurophysiology, 4,* 282–283.

Deiber, M.P., Ibanez, V., Bastuji, H., Fischer, C., and Mauguiere, F. (1989). Changes of middle latency auditory evoked potentials during natural sleep in humans. *Neurology, 39,* 806–813.

Deiber, M.P., Ibanez, V., Fischer, C., Perrin, F., and Mauguiere, F. (1988). Sequential mapping favours the hypothesis of distinct generators for Na and Pa middle latency evoked potentials. *Electroencephalography and Clinical Neurophysiology, 71,* 187–197.

Desmedt, J.E. and Nguyen, T.H. (1984). Bit-mapped colour imaging of the potential fields of propagated and segmental subcortical components of somatosensory evoked potentials in man. *Electroencephalography and Clinical Neurophysiology, 58,* 481–497.

Desmedt, J.E., Nguyen, T.H., and Bourguet, M. (1987). Bit-mapped color imaging of human evoked potentials with reference to the N20, P22, P27 and N30 somatosensory responses. *Electroencephalography and Clinical Neurophysiology, 68,* 1–19.

Duffy, F.H. (1981). Brain electrical activity mapping (BEAM): Computerized access to complex brain function. *International Journal of Neuroscience, 13,* 55–65.

Duffy, F.H. (1989). Clinical value of topographic mapping and quantified neurophysiology. *Archives of Neurology, 46,* 1133–1134.

Duffy, F.H. (1985). The BEAM method for neurophysiological diagnosis. *Annals of the New York Academy of Science, 457,* 19–34.

Duffy, F.H. (1982). Topographic display of evoked potentials: Clinical applications of brain electrical activity mapping (BEAM). *Annals of the New York Academy of Science, 388,* 183–196.

Duffy, F.H. (1986). *Topographic mapping of brain electrical activity.* Stoneham, MA: Butterworth.

Duffy, F.H., Albert, M.S., and McAnulty, G. (1984*a*). Brain electrical activity in patients with presenile and senile dementia of the Alzheimer type. *Annals of Neurology, 16,* 439–448.

Duffy, F.H., Albert, M.S., McAnulty, G., and Garvey, A.J. (1984*b*). Age-related differences in brain electrical activity of healthy subjects. *Annals of Neurology, 16,* 430–438.

Duffy, F.H., Bartels, P.H., and Burchfiel, J.L. (1981). Significance probability mapping: An aid in the topographic analysis of brain electrical activity. *Electroencephalography and Clinical Neurophysiology, 51,* 455–462.

Duffy, F.H., Bartels, P.H., and Neff, R. (1986). A response to Oken and Chiappa. *Annals of Neurology, 19,* 494–496.

Duffy, F.H., Burchfiel, J.L., and Lombroso, C.T. (1979). Brain electrical activity mapping (BEAM): A method for extending the clinical utility of EEG and evoked potential data. *Annals of Neurology, 5,* 309–321.

Duffy, F.H., Denckla, M.B., Bartels, P.H., and Sandini, G. (1980*a*). Dyslexia: Regional differences in brain electrical activity by topographic mapping. *Annals of Neurology, 7,* 412–420.

Duffy, F.H., Denckla, M.B., Bartels, P.H., Sandini, G., and Keissling, L.S. (1980*b*). Dyslexia: Automated diagnosis by computerized classification of brain electrical activity. *Annals of Neurology, 7,* 421–428.

Duffy, F.H., Denckla, M.B., McAnulty, G.B., and Holmes, J.A. (1988). Neurophysiological studies in dyslexia. *Res. Publ. Assoc. Res. Nerv. Ment. Dis., 66,* 149–170.

Finitzo, T. and Freeman, F. (1989). Spasmodic dysphonia, whether and where: Results of seven years of research. *Journal of Speech and Hearing Research, 32,* 541–555.

Finitzo, T., Pool, K.D., Freeman, F.J., Cannito, M.P., Schaefer, S.D., Ross, E.D., and Devous, M.D. (1987). Spasmodic dysphonia subsequent to head trauma. *Ar-*

chives of Otolaryngology—Head and Neck Surgery, 113, 1107–1110.

Firsching, R., Luther, J., Eidelberg, E., Brown, W.E., Story, J.L., and Boop, F.A. (1987). 40 Hz middle latency auditory evoked response in comatose patients. *Electroencephalography and Clinical Neurophysiology, 67,* 213–216.

Fisch, B.J. and Pedley, T.A. (1989). The role of quantitative topographic mapping or 'neurometrics' in the diagnosis of psychiatric and neurological disorders: The cons. *Electroencephalography and Clinical Neurophysiology, 73,* 5–9.

Gevins, A.S. (1984). Analysis of electromagnetic signals of the human brain: Milestones, obstacles, and goals. *IEEE Biomedical Engineering, BME-31,* 833–850.

Giard, M.H., Perrin, F., Pernier, J., and Peronnet, F. (1988). Several attention-related wave forms in auditory areas: A topographic study. *Electroencephalography and Clinical Neurophysiology, 69,* 371–384, .

Goff, W.R., Matsumiya, Y., Allison, T., and Goff, G.D. (1969). Cross-modality comparisons of averaged evoked potentials. In Donchin, E. and Lindsley, D.B. (eds.), *Average evoked potentials,* pp. 95-141. Washington, DC: NASA, SP-191.

Goff, G.D., Matsumiya, Y., Allison, T., and Goff, W.R. (1977). The scalp topography of human somatosensory and auditory evoked potentials. *Electroencephalography and Clinical Neurophysiology, 42,* 57–76.

Goldsmith, M.F. (1989). Brain studies may alter long-held concepts about likely causes of some voice disorders. *Journal of the American Medical Association, 261,* 964–965.

Grandori, F. (1986). Field analysis of auditory evoked brainstem potentials. *Hearing Research, 21,* 51–58.

Grandori, F. (1989). Surface maps and generators of brainstem auditory evoked potential waves I, III and V. In Maurer, K. (ed.), *Topographic mapping of EEG and evoked potentials,* pp. 407-411. Berlin: Springer-Verlag.

Grillon, C. and Buchsbaum, M.S. (1986). Computed EEG topography of response to visual and auditory stimuli. *Electroencephalography and Clinical Neurophysiology, 63,* 42–53.

Hachinski, V. (1989). Brain mapping. *Archives of Neurology, 46,* 1136.

Hall, J.W., Morgan, S.H., Mackey-Hargadine, J., Aguilar, E.A., and Jahrsdoerfer, R.A. (1984). Neuro-otologic applications of simultaneous multi-channel auditory response recordings. *Laryngoscope, 94,* 883–889.

Hansen, J.C. and Hillyard, S.A. (1984). Endogenous brain potentials associated with selective auditory attention. *Psychophysiology, 21,* 394–405.

Harding, G.F.A., Wright, C.E., and Orwin, A. (1985). Primary presenile dementia: The use of the visual evoked potential as a diagnostic indicator. *British Journal of Psychiatry, 147,* 532–539.

Hari, R., Aittoniemi, K., Jarvinen, M-L., Katila, T., and Varpula, T. (1980). Auditory evoked transient and sustained magnetic fields of the human brain. *Experimental Brain Research, 40,* 237–240.

Harner, R. (1986). Clinical application of computed EEG topography. In Duffy, F. (ed.), *Topographic mapping of brain electrical activity,* pp. 347-356. Boston, MA: Butterworth.

Hjorth, B. (1975). An on-line transformation of EEG scalp potentials into orthogonal source derivations. *Electroencephalography and Clinical Neurophysiology, 39,* 526–530.

Hjorth, B. (1980). Source derivation simplifies topographical EEG interpretation. *American Journal of EEG Technology, 20,* 121–132.

Hjorth, B. and Rodin, E. (1988). Extraction of "deep" components from scalp EEG. *Brain Topography, 1,* 65–69.

Homan, R.W., Herman, J., and Purdy, P. (1987). Cerebral location of international 10–20 system electrode placement. *Electroencephalography and Clinical Neurophysiology, 66,* 376–382.

Jacobson, G.P. and Grayson, A.S. (1988). The normal scalp topography of the middle latency auditory evoked potential Pa component following monaural click stimulation. *Brain Topography, 1,* 29–36.

Jacobson, G.P. and Newman, C.W. (1990). The decomposition of middle latency response component Pa into superficial and deep source contributions. *Brain Topography, 2,* 229–236.

Jasper, H.H. (1958). Report of Committee on Methods of Clinical Examination in Electroencephalography. *Electroencephalography and Clinical Neurophysiology, 10,* 370–375.

John, E.R. (1989). The role of quantitative EEG topographic mapping or 'neurometrics' in the diagnosis of psychiatric and neurological disorders: The pros. *Electroencephalography and Clinical Neurophysiology, 73,* 2–4.

Johnson, B.W., Weinberg, H., Ribary, U., Cheyne, D.O., and Ancill, R. (1988). Topographic distribution of the 40 Hz auditory evoked event-related potential in normal and aged subjects. *Brain Topography, 1,* 117–121.

Kaga, K., Hink, R.F., Shinoda, Y., and Suzuki, J. (1980). Evidence for a primary cortical origin of a middle latency auditory evoked potential in cats. *Electroencephalography and Clinical Neurophysiology, 50,* 254–266.

Kileny, P., Paccioretti, D., and Wilson, A.F. (1987). Effects of cortical lesions on middle-latency auditory evoked responses. *Electroencephalography and Clinical Neurophysiology, 66,* 108–120.

Knight, R.T., Hillyard, S.A., Woods, D.L., and Neville, H.J. (1980). The effects of frontal and temporal-parietal lesions on the auditory evoked potential in man. *Electroencephalography and Clinical Neurophysiology, 50,* 112–124.

Kowell, A.P., Reveler, M.J., and Nuwer, M.R. (1987). Topographic mapping of EEG and evoked potentials in epileptic patients. *Journal of Clinical Neurophysiology, 4,* 233–234.

Kraus, N. and McGee, T. (1988). Color imaging of the human middle latency response. *Ear and Hearing, 9,* 159–167.

Kraus, N., Ozdamar, O., Hier, D., and Stein, L. (1982). Auditory middle latency responses (MLRs) in patients with cortical lesions. *Electroencephalography and Clinical Neurophysiology, 54,* 275–287.

Kraus, N., Smith, D.I., and Grossman, J. (1985). Cortical mapping of the auditory middle latency response in the unanesthetized guinea pig. *Electroencephalography and Clinical Neurophysiology, 62,* 219–226.

Kraus, N., Smith, D.I., and McGee, T. (1988). Midline and temporal lobe MLR's in the guinea pig originate from different generator systems: A conceptual framework for new and existing data. *Electroencephalography and Clinical Neurophysiology, 70,* 541–558.

Kumar, A. and Dobben, G.D. (1988). Central auditory and vestibular pathology. *Otolaryngology Clinics of North America, 21,* 377–389.

Lee, Y.S., Lueders, H., Dinner, D.S., Lesser, R.P., Hahn, J., and Klem, G. (1984). Recording of auditory evoked potentials in man using chronic subdural electrodes. *Brain, 107,* 115–131.

Legatt, A.D., Arezzo, J.C., and Vaughan, H.G. (1986). Short-latency auditory evoked potentials in the monkey. I. Waveshape and surface topography. *Electroencephalography and Clinical Neurophysiology, 64,* 41–52.

Lehmann, D. and Skrandies, W. (1980). Reference-free identification of components of checkerboard-evoked multichannel potential fields. *Electroencephalography and Clinical Neurophysiology, 48,* 609–621.

Lehmann, D., Ozaki, H., and Pal, I. (1986). Averaging of spectral power and phase via vector diagram best fits without reference electrode or reference channel. *Electro-*

encephalography and Clinical Neurophysiology, 64, 350–363.

Lopes da Silva, F.H. (1987). Computerized EEG analysis: A tutorial overview. In Halliday, A.M., Butler, S.R., and Paul, R. (eds.), *A textbook of clinical neurophysiology,* pp. 85-87. New York: John Wiley.

Makela, J.P. and Hari, R. (1987). Evidence for cortical origin of the 40 Hz auditory evoked response in man. *Electroencephalography and Clinical Neurophysiology, 66,* 539–546.

Maurer, K. (ed.) (1989). *Topographic brain mapping of EEG and evoked potentials.* Berlin: Springer-Verlag.

McKay, D.M. (1983). On-line source density computation with a minimum of electrodes. *Electroencephalography and Clinical Neurophysiology, 56,* 696–698.

Møller, A.R. and Jannetta, P.J. (1982). Evoked potentials from the inferior colliculus in man. *Electroencephalography and Clinical Neurophysiology, 53,* 612–620.

Møller, A.R. and Jannetta, P.J. (1985). Neural generators of the auditory brainstem response. In Jacobson, J. (ed.), *The auditory brainstem response,* pp. 13-31. San Diego, CA: College-Hill.

Møller, A.R., Jannetta, P.J., and Møller, M.B. (1981*a*). Neural generators of brainstem evoked potentials. Results from human intracranial recordings. *Annals of Otology, 90,* 591–596.

Møller, A.R., Jannetta, P., Bennett, M., and Møller, M.B. (1981*b*). Intracranially recorded responses from the human auditory nerve: New insights into the origin of brain stem evoked potentials (BSEPs). *Electroencephalography and Clinical Neurophysiology, 52,* 18–27.

Morhisa, J.M. and McAnulty, G.B. (1985). Structure and function: Brain electrical activity mapping and computed tomography in schizophrenia. *Biology of Psychiatry, 20,* 3–19.

Morhisa, J.M., Duffy, F.H., and Wyatt, R.J. (1983). Brain electrical activity mapping (BEAM) in schizophrenic patients. *Archives of General Psychiatry, 40,* 719–727.

Myslobodsky, M.S. and Bar-Ziv, J. (1989). Locations of occipital EEG electrodes verified by computed tomography. *Electroencephalography and Clinical Neurophysiology, 72,* 362–366.

Nuwer, M.R. (1988*b*). Quantitative EEG 2. Frequency-analysis and topographic mapping in clinical settings. *Journal of Clinical Neurophysiology, 5,* 45–85.

Nuwer, M.R. (1988*a*). Quantitative EEG. 1. Techniques and problems of frequency-analysis and topographic mapping. *Journal of Clinical Neurophysiology, 5,* 1–43.

Nuwer, M.R. (1989). Uses and abuses of brain mapping. *Archives of Neurology, 46,* 1134–1136.

Offner, F.F. (1950). The EEG as potential mapping: The value of the average monopolar reference. *Electroencephalography and Clinical Neurophysiology, 2,* 215–216.

Oken, B.S. and Chiappa, K.H. (1986). Statistical issues concerning computerized analysis of brainwave topography. *Annals of Neurology, 19,* 493–494.

Ozdamar, O. and Kraus, N. (1983). Auditory middle latency responses in humans. *Audiology, 22,* 34–49.

Ozdamar, O., Kraus, N., and Curry, F. (1982). Auditory brain stem and middle latency responses in a patient with cortical deafness. *Electroencephalography and Clinical Neurophysiology, 53,* 224–230.

Pantev, C., Hoke, M., and Lehnertz, K. (1986a). Randomized data acquisition paradigm for the measurement of auditory evoked magnetic fields. *Acta Otolaryngologica, Suppl., 432,* 21–25.

Pantev, C., Hoke, M., Lutkenhoner, B., Lehnertz, K., and Spittka, J. (1986b). Causes of differences in the input-output characteristics of simultaneously recorded auditory evoked magnetic fields and potentials. *Audiology, 25,* 263–276.

Pantev, C., Lutkenhoner, B., Hoke, M., and Lehnertz, K. (1986c). Comparison between simultaneously recorded auditory-evoked magnetic fields and potentials elicited by ipsilateral, contralateral and binaural tone burst stimulation. *Audiology, 25,* 54–61.

Parving, A., Salomon, G., Elberling, C., Larsen, B., and Lassen, N.A. (1980). Middle components of the auditory evoked response in bilateral temporal lobe lesions. *Scandinavian Audiology, 9,* 161–167.

Pernier, J., Perrin, F., and Bertrand, O. (1988). Scalp current density fields: Concept and properties. *Electroencephalography and Clinical Neurophysiology, 69,* 385–389.

Peronnet, F., Michel, F., Echallier, J.F., and Girod, J. (1974). Coronal topography of human auditory evoked responses. *Electroencephalography and Clinical Neurophysiology, 37,* 225–230.

Perrin, F., Bertrand, O., and Pernier, J. (1989). Early cortical somatosensory and N1 auditory evoked responses: Analysis with potential maps, scalp current density maps and three-concentric-shell head models. In Maurer, K. (ed.), *Topographic brain mapping of EEG and evoked potentials,* pp. 390-395. Heidleberg: Springer-Verlag.

Perrin, F., Bertrand, O., and Pernier, J. (1987). Scalp current density mapping: Value and estimation from potential data. *IEEE Trans. Biomedical Engineering, 34,* 283–288.

Pfurtscheller, G. and Aranibar, A. (1977). Event-related cortical desynchronization detected by power measurement of scalp EEG. *Electroencephalography and Clinical Neurophysiology, 42,* 817–826.

Picton, T.W. and Hillyard, S.A. (1974b). Human AEPs. II. Effect of attention. *Electroencephalography and Clinical Neurophysiology, 36,* 191–199.

Picton, T.W., Hillyard, S.A., Krausz, H.I., and Galambos, R. (1974a). Human auditory evoked potentials. I. Evaluation of components. *Electroencephalography and Clinical Neurophysiology, 36,* 179–190.

Pool, K.D., Finitzo, T., Tzong-Hong, C., Rogers, J., and Pickett, R.B. (1989). Infarction of the superior temporal gyrus: A description of auditory evoked potential latency and amplitude topology. *Ear and Hearing, 10,* 144–152.

Reite, M., Zimmerman, J.T., and Zimmerman, J.E. (1982). MEG and EEG auditory responses to tone, click and white noise stimuli. *Electroencephalography and Clinical Neurophysiology, 53,* 643–651.

Remond, A. and Lesevre, N. (1965). Distribution topographique des potentiels evoques occipitaux chez l'homme normal. *Rev. Neurol., 112,* 317–330.

Rosati, G., Bastiani, P.D., Paolino, E., Prosser, A., Arslan, E., and Artioli, M. (1982). Clinical and audiological findings in a case of auditory agnosia. *Journal of Neurology, 227,* 21–27.

Sams, M., Hamalainen, M., Antervo, A., Kaukoranta, E., Reinikainen, K., and Hari, R. (1985). Cerebral neuromagnetic responses evoked by short auditory stimuli. *Electroencephalography and Clinical Neurophysiology, 61,* 254–266.

Scherg, M. and Von Cramon, D. (1985a). A new interpretation of the generators of BAEP waves I–V: Results of a spatio-temporal dipole model. *Electroencephalography and Clinical Neurophysiology, 62,* 290–299.

Scherg, M. and Von Cramon, D. (1985b). Two bilateral sources of the late AEP as identified by a spatio-temporal dipole model. *Electroencephalography and Clinical Neurophysiology, 62,* 32–44.

Scherg, M. and Von Cramon, D. (1986). Evoked dipole source potentials of the human auditory cortex. *Electroencephalography and Clinical Neurophysiology, 65,* 344–360.

Shenton, M.E., Faux, S.F., McCarley, R.W., Ballinger, R., Coleman, M., and Duffy, F.H. (1989). Clinical correlations of auditory P200 topography and left temporo-central deficits in schizophrenia: A preliminary study. *Journal of Psychiatric Research, 23,* 13–34.

Shimizu, N. and Hirasawa, K. (1985). Topographic mapping of brainstem auditory evoked responses in humans (The second report). *Brain Development, 7,* 145.

Simson, R., Vaughan, H.G., and Ritter, W. (1976). The scalp topography of potentials associated with missing visual or auditory stimuli. *Electroencephalography and Clinical Neurophysiology, 40,* 33–42.

Spitzer, A.R., Cohen, L.G., Fabrikant, J., and Hallet, M. (1989). A method for determining optimal interelectrode spacing for topographic mapping. *Electroencephalography and Clinical Neurophysiology, 72,* 355–361.

Spydell, J.D., Pattee, G., and Goldie, W.D. (1985). The 40 Hertz event-related potential: Normal values and effects of lesions. *Electroencephalography and Clinical Neurophysiology, 62,* 193–202.

Srebro, R. (1985). Localization of visually evoked cortical activity in humans. *Journal of Physiology, 360,* 233–246.

Stephenson, W.A. and Gibbs, F.A. (1951). A balanced noncephalic reference electrode. *Electroencephalography and Clinical Neurophysiology, 3,* 237–240.

Sutton, S., Tueting, P., Zubin, J., and John, E.R. (1965). Evoked potential correlates of stimulus uncertainty. *Science, 150,* 1187–1188.

Tonnquist-Uhlen, I., Borg, E., and Spens, K-E. (1989). Auditory stimulation brain map. *Scandinavian Audiology, 18,* 3–12.

Torello, M.W., Phillips, T., Hunter, W.W., and Csuri, C.A. (1987). Combinational imaging: Magnetic resonance imaging and EEG displayed simultaneously. *Journal of Clinical Neurophysiology, 4,* 274–275.

Vaughan, H.G. (1969). The relationship of brain activity to scalp recordings of event-related potentials. In Donchin, E. and Lindsley, D.B. (eds.) *Average evoked potentials,* pp. 45–94. Washington, DC: NASA, SP-191.

Vaughan, H.G., Jr. and Ritter, W. (1970). The sources of auditory evoked responses recorded from the human scalp. *Electroencephalography and Clinical Neurophysiology, 28,* 360–367.

Wallin, G. and Stalberg, E. (1980). Source derivation in clinical routine EEG. *Electroencephalography and Clinical Neurophysiology, 50,* 282–292.

Wolpaw, J.R. and Penry, J.K. (1975). A temporal component of the auditory evoked response. *Electroencephalography and Clinical Neurophysiology, 39,* 609–620.

Wood, C.C. and Wolpaw, J.R. (1982a). Scalp distribution of human auditory evoked potentials. I. Evaluation of reference electrode site. *Electroencephalography and Clinical Neurophysiology, 54,* 15–24.

Wood, C.C. and Wolpaw, J.R. (1982b). Scalp distribution of human auditory evoked potentials. II. Evidence for overlapping sources and involvement of the auditory cortex. *Electroencephalography and Clinical Neurophysiology, 54,* 25–38.

Woods, D.L., Clayworth, C.C., Knight, R.T., Simpson, G.V., and Naeser, M.A. (1987). Generators of middle- and long-latency auditory evoked potentials: Implications from studies of patients with bitemporal lesions. *Electroencephalography and Clinical Neurophysiology, 68,* 132–148.

Woods, D.L., Knight, R.T., and Neville, H.J. (1984). Bitemporal lesions dissociate evoked potentials and perception. *Electroencephalography and Clinical Neurophysiology, 57,* 208–220.

Wright, C.E., Harding, G.F.A., and Orwin, A. (1984). Presenile dementia—the use of flash and pattern VEP in diagnosis. *Electroencephalography and Clinical Neurophysiology, 57,* 405–415.

CHAPTER 21

AUDITORY EVOKED POTENTIAL TESTING STRATEGIES

BRAD A. STACH
JAMES F. JERGER
TERREY OLIVER PENN

Ideally it would be desirable to list a single, universal test procedure for every auditory evoked potential (AEP) examination. But differing problems encountered in the clinical situation dictate the need for a variety of testing strategies. These strategies may vary within each of the types of AEPs, the auditory brainstem response (ABR), the middle latency response (MLR), and the late vertex response (LVR), and they may vary across AEP types. The most important factors in determining appropriate strategies include the nature of the AEP application, and, within an application, the ubiquitous trade-off between frequency specificity and subject state and the dependence of results on degree of peripheral hearing loss.

FACTORS THAT INFLUENCE AEP STRATEGIES

Nature of the AEP Application

The specific AEP application impacts, to a great extent, the optimal testing strategy. We can distinguish three fundamental clinical applications of AEPs:

1. neonatal hearing screening;
2. hearing threshold prediction in infants, young children, and adults with nonorganic hearing loss; and
3. diagnostic applications.

In neonatal screening, the goal is simply to categorize auditory function as either normal or abnormal in order to identify babies in need of subsequent follow-up. The focus is to provide both an estimate of overall peripheral sensitivity and an estimate of central auditory status. An efficient testing strategy must provide data directed to these two fundamental questions in a manner that maximizes the correct identification, or "hit" rate, while minimizing the incorrect identification, or "false-alarm" rate.

In the evaluation of patients who cannot or will not cooperate during behavioral testing, however, the goal is usually more detailed. Here, the typical concern is to obtain as much information as possible about the degree of loss, the nature of the audiometric contour, and the extent of interaural asymmetry. An effective testing strategy must, therefore, not only estimate overall degree of loss but also provide frequency-specific information about shape of loss, an estimate of which is the better ear, and an estimate of how much it differs from the poorer ear.

In diagnostic applications, still another goal is pursued. Here, the aim is to explore the exact morphology of the AEP waveforms, to document the presence of all component waves, and to measure both absolute and relative latencies of the various component peaks. Thus, the optimal testing strategy will concentrate on suprathreshold measures designed to enhance all components of the AEPs.

The differing demands of these three principal applications of AEPs have led to specific strategies unique to each application.

Frequency Specificity versus Subject State

One very important factor in developing AEP strategies, particularly regarding the prediction of hearing loss, is the tradeoff between the frequency specificity of a particular AEP and the AEP's relative immunity to physiologic state of the subject. Figure 21.1 illustrates this tradeoff. Frequency specificity, or the extent to which a response represents a specific frequency region, varies as a function of the stimulus that is required to evoke a particular AEP. Because ABR requires a high degree of neural synchrony, a rapid-onset click stimulus, with its broad frequency spectrum, must be used. Because of the broad spectrum of the stimulus, frequency specificity is relatively poor. Thus, threshold prediction by click-evoked ABR reflects hearing only over a broad range of frequencies from 1000 to 4000 Hz. In contrast, the LVR can be elicited with any auditory stimulus, including a pure tone. Consequently, it can evoke a relatively more frequency specific response than a click. The MLR lies somewhere between the ABR and LVR on the continuum, since it can be elicited with tone pips that are not as frequency specific as longer tone bursts but are more frequency specific than clicks.

If the goal of AEP threshold testing were the prediction of the degree and audiometric configuration of the hearing loss, then the LVR would be the clear choice, were it not for the influence of physiologic state. The ABR is quite immune to the influence of physiologic

state and can even be measured in patients who are in coma (Starr, 1976). Conversely, the LVR requires the active attention of the patient and will seldom be recordable during sleep. Once again, the MLR falls between the ABR and LVR on the continuum of immunity to physiologic state.

In the testing of infants and young children, AEP recording is best accomplished during sleep or under sedation, which requires use of the ABR. But use of the ABR limits prediction of audiometric configuration because of its lack of frequency specificity.

Dependence on Degree of Loss

The extent to which various ABR measures can be effectively interpreted diagnostically depends, to a great extent, on the degree of peripheral sensitivity loss, especially in the critical 1000 to 4000 Hz frequency range. Any effective diagnostic testing strategy must take this critical hearing-loss dependence into account.

In the following sections, we list the various testing strategies that have been proposed for each of the three basic clinical applications for each of the three AEPs, discuss their strengths and weaknesses, and suggest a single recommended test strategy for each AEP application.

NEONATAL SCREENING

Neonatal screening by ABR, first proposed by Galambos (1978), has since been initiated by a number of investigators in a variety of settings. Proposed testing strategies are, however, remarkably uniform (Hall, Kripal, and Hepp, 1988). The majority of centers engaged in neonatal screening continue to use the test parameters first suggested by Galambos and his associates. They suggested that click presentation levels be 30 and 60 dB nHL, the click rate be 37/s, EEG filters be set to pass a band from 150 to 3000 Hz, 2048 responses be averaged, and that each ear be tested separately by air conduction only (Schulman-Galambos and Galambos, 1979). Only minor variations on this consistent theme have been proposed. In an effort to reduce the false-positive rate, it has been suggested that the 30 dB test level be raised to 35 or 40 dB (Alberti, Hyde, Riko, Corbin, and Abramovich, 1983; Dennis, Sheldon,

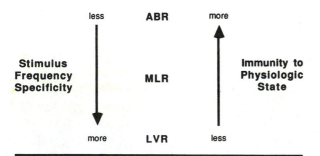

FIGURE 21.1. Representation of the tradeoff between frequency specificity and immunity to physiologic state for the auditory brainstem response (ABR), the middle latency response (MLR), and the late vertex response (LVR).

Toubas, and McCaffee, 1984), that the rate be lowered to 21 (Dennis et al., 1984; Stein, Özdamar, Kraus, and Paton, 1983) or even 10/s (Jacobson, Seitz, Mencher, and Parrott, 1980), that the EEG passband be lowered to 30 Hz (Stapells, 1989), and the number averaged be increased to 4000 (Alberti et al., 1983). In general, however, there is reasonably good agreement on how to carry out the actual screening test procedure.

In recent years, algorithms have been developed for machine scoring of the ABR (Özdamar, Delgado, Eilers, and Widen, 1990; Peters, 1986). Instruments have been developed that present stimuli, record and average EEG, and then compare the averaged waveform to pre-existing templates in an effort to determine the presence of an ABR. One instrument that has proven to be a successful screener is the ALGO device (Jacobson, Jacobson, and Spahr, 1990; Kileny, 1988). As computer algorithms improve, automated screeners will likely replace more conventional screening strategies.

Most investigators will agree that a crucial issue confronting neonatal screeners is the high failure rate typically observed when a series of infants is screened in the ICU and the subsequent apparent resolution of many of the initial failures. Galambos, Hicks, and Wilson (1984) note, for example, that in their experience, 16% of infants in the neonatal ICU will fail the initial screen, but as many as one-third of these babies will pass a retest administered 6 to 8 weeks after the initial test.

Most investigators agree that such apparently resolving loss is due to middle ear disorder on the first test, which then resolves before the 6 to 8 week retest (Cevette, 1984; Finitzo-Hieber, 1982; Hecox, 1984; Stein, 1984), but no one can be sure of the exact numbers involved. Other possibilities that must be entertained, however, include maturation of the ABR response during the first month of life (Hooks and Weber, 1984; Roberts, Davis, Phon, Reichert, Sturtevant, and Marshall, 1982; Starr, Amlie, Martin, and Sanders, 1977), wakefulness of the neonates (McCall and Ferraro, 1991), and simple failure of the screening instrument in a certain percentage of cases due to ambient acoustic and electrical noise in the testing environment.

Nevertheless, much of the continuing controversy over the desirability of neonatal screening (Cevette, 1984; Downs, 1982; Jacobson et al., 1980; Roberts et al., 1982) centers on this relatively high false-positive rate. Whether one regards them as the fruit of test flaws, the results of late maturation, or the consequence of subsequently resolving middle-ear disease, there is general agreement that such screening failures are undesirable concomitants of the search for significant permanent sensorineural hearing loss. Many feel that unless this false-positive rate can be kept to an acceptable minimum, neontal screening for hearing loss cannot be cost-effective. Others point out, however, that even a relatively high false-positive rate is a small price to pay for the identification of even a small number of children with handicapping hearing loss at so early an age (Northern and Downs, 1974, p. 99).

What may prove to be a useful strategy for minimizing the false-positive rate due to resolving middle-ear disorder was first proposed by Weber (1983) and later elaborated by Hooks and Weber (1984). They reasoned that, if conductive hearing loss due to middle-ear disease leads to an undesirable screening "fail," then an effective strategy might be to test only by bone conduction (BC). If the click is introduced directly to the infant's skull via a bone-conduction transducer, then the confounding effect of conductive hearing loss would be effectively bypassed. So long as the sensorineural system is intact, the infant should pass the screen in spite of temporary conductive loss.

The presence of a normal ABR response at a BC hearing level (HL) or 30–40 dB would not, of course, ensure normal hearing in both ears. The BC response would reflect only the sensitivity of the better cochlea. Thus, significant interaural asymmetries in sensorineural sensitivity level would be missed by such a procedure. However, if the principal goal of neonatal screening is to identify handicapping hearing loss at the earliest possible age, so that remediation may be introduced according to an optimal schedule, then failure to identify unilateral loss in a child with normal hearing in one ear cannot be regarded as a serious flaw in the strategy.

On the positive side, such a strategy would, in theory at least, virtually eliminate the problem of false-positive results due to resolving middle ear disease in infants. Although there are some additional problems inherent in the measurement of an ABR by bone con-

TABLE 21.1.   Strategy for Neonatal ABR Screening

Test Parameter		Test Procedure
Signal:	click	1. Present signal by earphone to each ear separately or by BC transducer on forehead
Rate:	20–30/s	
Level:	30–40 dB nHL	2. Present signal at 30–40 dB nHL and 60–70 dB nHL
	60–70 dB nHL	3. If ABR response at 30–40 dB nHL is normal, pass
Filter passband:	100–3000 Hz	
Number averaged:	2,048	4. If ABR response at 30–40 dB nHL is abnormal, raise level to 60–70 dB nHL and retest.
		5. If ABR response at 60–70 dB nHL is normal, refer for follow-up exam to investigate possibility of mild-moderate loss.
		6. If ABR response at 60–70 dB nHL is abnormal, refer for follow-up exam to investigate possibility of severe-profound loss.

duction (Kavanagh and Beardsley, 1979; Mauldin and Jerger, 1979), and although these problems may be exacerbated in small infants, the proposed BC strategy seems promising (Stapells and Ruben, 1989).

Based on the foregoing observations, Table 21.1 summarizes a recommended neonatal ABR screening strategy.

In connection with neonatal screening, it is important to remember that:

A. The click response only reflects sensitivity in the 1000 to 4000 Hz region of the audiogram.
B. The false-positive rate for this test is going to be high, especially if testing by air conduction only.
C. The "yield" (correct identification of significant permanent sensorineural loss) will depend on the population being screened. Even when screening is confined to high-risk groups, however, the yield may not exceed 1.5–3.5% of infants evaluated (Cox, Hack, and Metz, 1981).

THRESHOLD PREDICTION BY AEPS

Infants and Young Children

Evaluation of infants and young children is best accomplished with use of the ABR, because the MLR and LVR are so sensitive to physiologic state. ABR testing of very young infants can usually be carried out in natural sleep. But in older infants and young children, especially in the 12- to 36-month range, it is usually necessary to sedate or anesthetize the child (Jerger, Hayes, and Jordan, 1980). This usually introduces a time constraint into the clinical evaluation. Depending on the sedative, barbiturate, or anesthetic agent used, the child may be sufficiently immobilized for only a finite period, usually 30–45 minutes.

Within this timeframe, the clinician must explore overall sensitivity, audiometric contour, and interaural asymmetry. A typical strategy in such a situation is to gather all data on one ear, then switch to the other ear and gather similar data. However, there is a very real danger in such a strategy. If the sedation wears off and the child wakes up after one ear has been tested, but before testing can be carried out on the other ear, then the clinician is in the unenviable position of knowing all about the hearing on one ear but not knowing whether this happens to be the better ear, the poorer ear, or a good representation of both ears. There is no choice but to reschedule the child for another evaluation.

Binaural Strategy.   To meet the challenge of this situation, we have evolved, in our own clinical testing

ABR Binaural Strategy

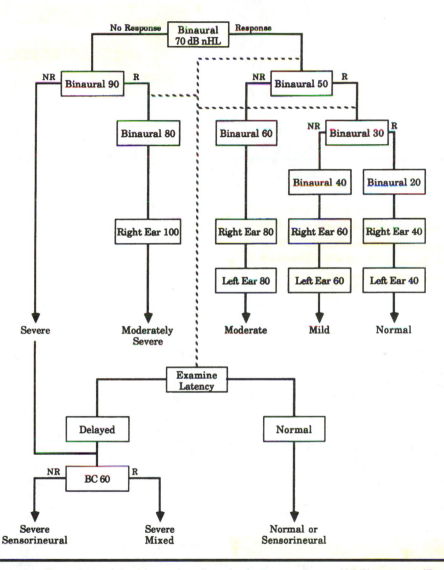

FIGURE 21.2.   Flow chart of the binaural auditory brainstem response (ABR) strategy (R = response; NR = no response; BC = bone conduction).

of children, an alternative approach that we refer to as the binaural strategy. Figure 21.2 is a flow-chart of the procedure. The essence of the binaural strategy is to initiate testing with the click presented to both ears simultaneously (binaural mode). The clinician then seeks "threshold" in the conventional manner by systematically lowering signal intensity level until the lowest level at which the ABR response can be observed is defined. In the binaural strategy, this initial threshold seeking yields the binaural threshold, that is, the threshold level for a binaural signal. After this binaural threshold has been defined, the clinician checks for binaural symmetry by testing monaurally in each ear at a level 20 dB above the previously defined binaural threshold. If the two monaural responses are approximately equal, the clinician may sagely conclude that sensitivity is about the same in the two ears, and testing is complete. If, on the other hand, the two monaural responses are substantially different, then the clinician pursues monaural threshold on the apparently poorer ear. There is no need for further testing of the better ear since, in the case of asymmetry, it may be safely concluded that the binaural response is an accurate test of the better ear.

The rationale for the binaural strategy is that, when testing time may be limited and full evaluation curtailed, it is more important to define sensitivity in the better ear, even if it is not known which ear that is, than to obtain detailed information on the right ear but not know what sensitivity is like in the left ear.

If there is only time to complete one threshold run before the child wakes up, then, if that defined threshold is the binaural threshold, at least hearing on the better ear is known, and a reasonably appropriate intervention strategy can be planned without further information. For example, if the binaural threshold is normal, there is no need to be concerned about the presence of a handicapping loss even if there is substantial loss in one ear. Conversely, if the binaural threshold is elevated, early appropriate intervention can be planned without further information about the status of individual ears. With an experimental binaural hearing aid fitting, for example, optimal stimulation for the ear most likely to benefit from amplification will be guaranteed.

In effect, the binaural strategy is based on the following considerations:

1. There are only two possibilities:
   a. hearing sensitivity is the same in both ears, or
   b. hearing sensitivity is different in the two ears.
2. If sensitivity is the same in both ears, then the binaural threshold is an accurate representation of either ear and there is no need for further, ear-specific, testing.
3. If sensitivity is different in each ear, then the binaural threshold is an accurate representation of the better ear, and only the poorer ear needs further exploration.
4. If the sensitivity level of a child's better ear is known, a useful and meaningful intervention strategy can be initiated without further, ear-specific information, if such information is not easily obtainable.

Clearly, the validity of the binaural strategy rests on the assertion that the binaural threshold always reflects sensitivity of the better ear. It is possible, however, that the ABR response could be normal in each ear separately, but abnormal to binaural stimulation. We know of no such reports in the world's literature. On the contrary, it has been repeatedly observed (Blegvad, 1975; Gerull and Mrowinski, 1984) that at equivalent sensation levels the binaural response is always at least as large as, and usually larger than, either monaural response. Suppose, however, that a child has brainstem disorder affecting the ABR response. Could this invalidate the binaural strategy by predicting loss when sensitivity was in fact normal in both ears? If the effect on ABR were unilateral, then the binaural response would be normal and prediction of normal sensitivity in at least one ear would continue to hold, and an erroneous prediction of significant peripheral hearing loss would not occur. If the brainstem disorder affected the ABR response bilaterally, then the binaural ABR response would, in all likelihood, be abnormal and might lead to the erroneous prediction of significant peripheral hearing loss. But it would be in this respect, no different from the two abnormal monaural responses, each of which would also erroneously predict significant peripheral loss. Thus, the use of the binaural strategy in no way increases the likelihood of this kind of error.

In our extensive clinical experience with the binaural strategy, we have encountered only one case in which the binaural threshold was poorer than the monaural threshold. The child had a unilateral conductive hearing loss that prolonged the latency of ABR wave V just enough to be out of phase with the ABR from the other ear. The sum of the two ABRs during binaural testing predicted a threshold that was approximately 10 dB poorer than the better-ear threshold. Use of the second part of the binaural strategy, that is, testing each ear independently at 20 dB above the binaural threshold, led the clinician to discover the ear difference and seek thresholds for each ear independently. Because of the rarity of this case, and because continuation of the binaural strategy detected the problem, we continue to use the strategy with confidence that this kind of error would be unlikely to be of consequence.

Frequency Specificity. While the binaural click threshold yields a satisfactory estimate of sensitivity in the 1000 to 4000 Hz region of the audiogram, it fails to provide crucial information on audiometric contour. A click threshold in the region of 70 dB HL, for example, is consistent with either a flat loss at 70 dB HL across the frequency range or a steeply sloping contour with normal sensitivity at 500 Hz, but with a contour sharply dropping to 60 to 80 dB at 2000 and 4000 Hz. Audiologists do not need to be reminded that intervention strategies would, ideally, be quite different in these two cases. Thus, frequency-specific information about audiometric contour, especially in the 500 Hz region, is highly desirable in the evaluation of infants and children.

Since the click response does not provide such information, it is necessary to employ more frequency-specific test signals. But here is encountered an inevitable interaction between frequency specificity of the test signal and quality of the ABR response (Davis, Hirsh, Popelka, and Formby, 1984). In general, the more energy is confined to a narrow, low-frequency region, the poorer is the "early" evoked response (Klein and Teas, 1978) and, consequently, the less satisfactory is its value as a threshold predictor. Nevertheless, for infants and young children, use of the ABR evoked by tone bursts (usually tone pips with two-cycle rise, one cycle at maximum amplitude, and a two-cycle fall: 2-1-2) remains the method of choice for prediction of low-frequency sensitivity. ABRs to 500 Hz tone bursts can usually be detected to within 30 dB of actual threshold (Hayes and Jerger, 1982; Stapells, 1989). While such a prediction is clearly crude, nevertheless it provides a general estimate of the low frequency sensitivity and assists in defining audiometric contour.

Other approaches that have been taken to predict threshold in children include the SN-10 response (Davis and Hirsh, 1976; Suzuki, Hirai, and Horiuchi, 1977), the steady-state evoked potential (SSEP) or 40 Hz event-related potential (Galambos, Makeig, and Talmachoff, 1981), and the use of conventional MLR (Goldstein and McRandle, 1976) and LVR (Davis, Hirsh, Shelnutt, and Bowers, 1967) measurements. Each of these approaches has characteristic advantages and disadvantages. The SN10 response is presumably less influenced by state variables than the relatively longer latency SSEP (but see Klein, 1983), but it tends to be difficult to detect at low levels of low-frequency tone pips, and the accuracy of its predictions has been questioned (Hayes and Jerger, 1982). The SSEP, on the other hand, tends to be well-defined even at very low signal levels (Galambos et al., 1981). It seems to work as well, or even better, at low frequencies than at high frequencies. Unfortunately, it does not appear to exist in babies or young children (Jerger, Chmiel, Glaze, and Frost, 1987; Stapells, Galambos, Costello, and Makeig, 1988), the very population for which it is needed. With regard to conventional MLR and LVR, failure in these young populations results from the fluctuating effects of physiologic state variables (Brown and Shallop, 1982; Ornitz, Ritvo, Carr, Panman, and Walter, 1967; Shallop and Osterhammel, 1983; Skinner and Shimoto, 1975). In particular, amplitude declines substantially in sleep (Mendel and Goldstein, 1971; Kraus, McGee, and Comperatore, 1989) and under sedation (Hume and Cant, 1977; Suzuki, 1973).

In general, the use of either clicks or tone pips presented either binaurally or monaurally follows traditional methodology for threshold prediction. Signal intensity is varied systematically while the evoked response threshold, that is, the lowest level of the signal producing a recognizable and repeatable electrophysiological response, is sought. In the case of click-elicited ABRs, this approach has been generally quite successful. In the case of tone pip-elicited responses, however, threshold accuracy remains less than desirable (Davis and Hirsh, 1976; McDonald and Shimizu, 1981).

Nevertheless, there can be no doubt that useful information about audiometric contour can be derived from tone-pip responses (Brown and Shallop, 1982;

TABLE 21.2. Strategy for ABR Testing of Infants and Children

Test Parameter		Test Procedure
Signal:	click and 500-Hz tone pip (2-1-2)	**Click Phase** 1. Use binaural strategy to define binaural click threshold.
Rate:	20–30/s	2. Test monaurally at binaural threshold + 20 dB.
Level:	varied to seek threshold	3. If monaural responses are not equivalent, seek threshold of poorer ear.
Filter passband:	100–3000 Hz	4. If monaural responses are equivalent, move to tone-pip phase.
Number averaged:	2,048	**Tone-Pip Phase** 1. Use monaural strategy to define 500-Hz tone-pip threshold on each ear.

Hawes and Greenberg, 1981; Shallop and Osterhammel, 1983; Stapells, 1989). Some form of the response to tone pips should be an integral part of the ABR examination of all infants and young children.

Based on the foregoing observations, Table 21.2 presents a strategy for the evaluation of older infants and young children.

In the use of this strategy, it is important to remember that:

1. If the sensitivity of the better ear is known, intervention can proceed appropriately.
2. Click thresholds do not tell all there is to know about shape of audiogram. Knowledge of sensitivity at 500 Hz is very important for appropriate intervention.

Threshold Prediction in Adults

Frequency-specific electrophysiologic prediction of auditory thresholds is much more easily attainable in adults than in children. Here, because testing can be carried out while the patient is awake, the later evoked potentials, such as the MLR, its variant the SSEP, and the LVR, can be brought to bear on the question of threshold prediction.

The MLR and the SSEP have been shown to be accurate predictors of sensitivity in adults (Dauman, Szyfter, Charlet de Sauvage, and Cazals, 1984;

Goldstein and Rodman, 1967; Kileny and Shea, 1986; Lenarz, Gülzow, Grözinger, and Hoth, 1986; Lynn, Lesner, Sandridge, and Daddario, 1984; Musiek and Geurnink, 1981). Constraints upon their use are twofold. First, their amplitude varies with sleep (Jerger, Chmiel, Frost, and Coker, 1986; Jones and Baxter, 1988; Linden, Campbell, Hamel, and Picton, 1985; Mendel and Goldstein, 1971), which tends to reduce the accuracy of threshold prediction. Maintenance of subject vigilance to the listening task is often difficult, because the rate of stimulus presentation is sufficiently fast that it precludes having the patient count stimuli. Consequently, sleep is a typical alternative. Second, frequency specificity is not as precise in these responses as in the LVR. Therefore, given none of the restraints of physiologic state, the choice of a response that is less frequency specific has little rational basis.

One advantage that the SSEP may have over the MLR or the LVR is that its presence can be measured objectively, within limits, by Fourier analysis (Stapells, Makeig, and Galambos, 1985). If the variability of phase of the Fourier component over successive trials is measured, this objective assessment of the SSEP can be a sensitive predictor of threshold and, at the same time, immune to the effects of physiologic state (Jerger et al., 1986).

The LVR is the current method of choice for electrophysiologic prediction of low-frequency hear-

TABLE 21.3.   Strategy for Threshold Prediction in Adults

Test Parameter		Test Procedure
Signal:	ABR— click	**ABR Phase**
	LVR— 0.5-4 KHz tone bursts	1. Use binaural strategy to define binaural click threshold.
Rate:	ABR— 20–30/s	
	LVR— 0.5/s	2. Test monaurally at binaural threshold + 20 dB.
Level:	varied to seek threshold	3. If monaural responses are not equivalent, seek threshold of poorer ear.
Filter passband:	ABR— 100–3000	
	LVR— 1–100 Hz	4. If monaural responses are equivalent, move to LVR phase.
Number averaged:	ABR— 2,048	**LVR Phase**
	LVR— 64	1. Use monaural strategy to define tone-burst thresholds at frequencies of interest on each ear.

ing sensitivity in adults (Hyde, Alberti, Matsumoto, and Li, 1986; Suzuki, Yamamoto, Taguchi, and Sakabe, 1976). The procedure for measuring the LVR requires the patient to count stimuli as they are presented, thereby assuring vigilance to the task. Thus, although highly sensitive to physiologic state, the threshold of the LVR can be determined effectively in adult patients. The strategy for obtaining LVR threshold follows conventional methodology. Signal intensity is varied systematically, while the LVR threshold is sought. Testing parameters are delineated in Table 21.3. The LVR can be used in one of two ways for threshold prediction: 1) as a predictor of threshold across the frequency range; or 2) as a low-frequency supplement to ABR prediction of higher frequencies. Use of the LVR for threshold prediction can be rather time-consuming, especially if used across the frequency range. While this type of accuracy may be important for medical-legal purposes, often the clinical question is sufficiently general that a prediction of high-frequency sensitivity can be made with ABR and a prediction of low-frequency sensitivity with LVR.

DIAGNOSTIC APPLICATIONS

Recommended stimulus and recording parameters for the diagnostic applications of the ABR, MLR, and LVR are delineated in Table 21.4. These parameters are generally agreed upon and are based on the nature of the AEP being recorded. They are recommended as starting parameters, with the understanding that they often need to be altered depending on the nature of the patient, testing environment, etc. With regard to the stimulus, ABR requires greatest synchrony of neural firing and is thus most easily recordable in response to a click stimulus. The MLR requires less synchrony and can be elicited by a 2-1-2 tone pip (two-cycle rise and fall and a one-cyle plateau). The LVR requires even less synchony and can be elicited with a tone burst that has a rise-decay time of sufficient duration to avoid an audible click. Although all three AEP types could be recorded with very slow stimulus rates, the ABR requires a large number of sweeps, and faster rates are more efficient. For the MLR, rates should be as slow as efficiently possible, and, for the LVR, the rate must be slow enough to allow the patient to count stimuli. The ABR and MLR are best recorded at higher intensity levels, while the LVR can be recorded at lower intensity levels due to the longer stimulus duration.

Since the ABR waveform has its main frequency components at approximately 500 and 1000 Hz, filter passbands must be sufficiently wide to record the response. The main frequency component of the MLR is approximately 40 Hz and of the LVR is approximately 5 to 10 Hz. Filter passbands must be set accordingly.

TABLE 21.4. Typical Evoked Potential Signal and Recording Parameters for Diagnostic ABR, MLR, and LVR

	Auditory Evoked Potential		
	ABR	MLR	LVR
Stimulus Parameters			
Signal type	click	tone burst	tone burst
Duration (ms)	0.1	10	100
Rate (per sec)	21.1 and 81.1	2.2	0.5
Intensity (dB nHL)	70	70	50
Recording parameters			
Epoch (ms)	10	100	500
Number averaged	2,048	1,024	64
Filter passbands (Hz)			
High pass	150	10	1
Low pass	3,000	1,000	100

ABR Diagnostic Strategies

The diagnostic value of the ABR depends, to a great extent, on the identification of component waves, evaluation of waveform morphology, and the accurate measurement of both absolute and interwave latencies. The optimization of these various measures requires careful consideration of six specific parameters of the test situation.

1. Test level
2. Test mode
3. Click rate
4. Click polarity
5. Filter passband
6. Interpretive strategy

In the following sections each of these factors is considered in turn.

Test Level.   Best results are achieved when the signal intensity is sufficient to elicit a well-defined waveform including, at minimum, identifiable waves I, III, and V. In the ear with normal hearing, this usually requires an intensity level of at least 60 dB nHL. Thus, diagnostic

ABR testing is best carried out at relatively high signal levels, usually in the range of 60–80 dB nHL. However, there is some hazard in setting the intensity level too high. Hecox (1983), for example, has pointed out that amplitude relations among component waves, especially the I/V amplitude ratio, may be distorted at very high signal levels (80–100 dB). These considerations suggest that the optimal signal level would be about 70 dB nHL (or approximately 100 dB peSPL). And, indeed, many laboratories use 70 dB as the standard signal level for diagnostic ABR testing.

If all patients we test had normal peripheral hearing, there would be no need for further discussion of appropriate test levels. But, unfortunately, a substantial number of patients for whom ABR is a useful diagnostic test have some degree of peripheral hearing loss (Hayes, 1980), especially in the high-frequency region of the audiogram that is so important for mediation of the click response. If there is even moderate high-frequency loss, however, the 70 dB nHL test level may no longer be sufficient to elicit an ideal ABR waveform. If the sensation level of the test signal is not sufficient, then all component waves may not be identifiable, especially the important landmark, wave I. A first inclination in this case might be to raise the test level by an amount equal to the sensitivity loss in the critical high-frequency region (1–4 kHz); in other words, to maintain a constant 70 dB sensation level. Anyone familiar with the suprathreshold characteristics of the ear with cochlear impairment, however, already knows that this approach will not work. Because of suprathreshold distortions in these ears (e.g., "loudness recruitment"), such an approach would be neither desirable nor practical. If the loss in the 1000 to 4000 Hz region were 40 dB, for example, the constant 70 dB sensation level would be achieved at 110 dB nHL. However, this level would almost certainly be extremely unpleasant for the patient with cochlear hearing loss and, as noted above, might distort interwave amplitude relationships. Fortunately, such a high level is not necessary to observe the optimal waveform obtainable from this ear. In fact, a level of 80 to 90 dB nHL would probably be sufficient to observe the best waveform that the ear is capable of producing. But, even at this optimal level, the response may not show a wave I as well defined as one would expect to see in the response from a normal ear. As the degree of high-frequency hearing loss increases, all of the early waves (I, II, and III), but especially wave I, become increasingly difficult to identify (Hecox and Galambos, 1974). From the standpoint of test strategy, then, the problem is to find the test level that has the best probability of yielding identifiable early waves but that remains within the range of intensities acceptable to the patient. A useful strategy, therefore, is to first examine the pure tone audiometric thresholds in the 1000 to 4000 Hz region. If the average of the three thresholds at 1000, 2000, and 4000 Hz (pure tone average; PTA 2) falls in the 0 to 19 dB range, then it is probably safe to use a standard test level of 70 dB nHL. If the PTA 2 is in the range from 20 to 39 dB, however, the level should be raised to 80 dB nHL. For PTA 2 in the range from 40 to 59 dB, the test level should be 90 dB nHL, and for PTA 2 in the range from 60 to 79 dB, the test level should be 100 dB nHL. For PTA 2 greater than 79 dB, it may be desirable to raise the level an additional 5 dB, although many commercial ABR systems are not capable of delivering clicks at such high intensity levels.

Test Mode.   In diagnostic evaluation, it is customary to test only in the monaural mode. Since the binaural ABR reflects only the response from the better ear, it is a more efficient use of time to test the two ears separately and compare the two monaural responses for symmetry. It should be noted, however, that Dobie and Berlin (1979) have proposed a procedure for comparing the binaural response with the sum of the two monaural responses in order to derive a difference measure thought to be sensitive to certain forms of central disorder. Apart from this unique application, however, common diagnostic evaluation typically proceeds by testing the two ears separately and examining each monaural response for normalcy of waveform, absolute and interwave latencies, and amplitude ratios. Diagnostically significant abnormalities take the form of degraded morphology, absence of component waves, delayed absolute or interwave latencies or both, and abnormal amplitude ratios (Hecox, Cone, and Blaw, 1981; Starr and Achor, 1975; Starr and Hamilton, 1976; Stockard and Rossiter, 1977).

Click rate.   Click rate is an important variable in diagnostic evaluation (Gerling and Finitzo-Hieber, 1983; Hecox, 1983). It is usually desirable to set the click rate low enough to ensure observation of all component waves. Commonly a rate in the vicinity of 10–20 clicks/s is appropriate for this task. At this point, the examiner evaluates the response carefully. If the morphology is relatively good, all essential component waves can be observed, and latencies seem reasonably normal, then it may be desirable to stress the mechanism by retesting at a higher click rate (Pratt, Ben-David, Peled, Podoshin, and Scharf, 1981). Some investigators will routinely raise the click rate to 80 clicks/s and retest. Other investigators may take the time to generate an entire rate function by retesting at rates of 40, 60, and 80 clicks/s, or even at smaller intervals. It is sometimes the case that responses appearing to be reasonably normal at click rates of 10–20/s will show some pathologic degradation at high click rates, suggesting retrocochlear disorder (Shanon, Gold, and Himmelfarb, 1981; Zöllner and Eibach, 1981).

If the morphologic characteristics of the response to clicks at 10–20/s are decidedly abnormal, then the appropriate strategy is to decrease the click rate in order to probe for a more well-defined response. In the case of high-frequency peripheral hearing loss, for example, wave I may not be indentifiable at a click rate of 20/s but may appear if the click rate is lowered to 10 or 5/s. The strategy for varying click rate, therefore, should be to increase the rate when the response at the standard rate is well defined and to decrease rate when the response at the standard rate is not.

Click Polarity.   Click polarity, in diagnostic ABR evaluation, is still a matter of some dispute. Arguments have been made in support of condensation only, rarefaction only, and alternation of polarity. Perhaps the most persuasive data bearing on this issue have been provided by Salt (1982). Using an ear canal probe-microphone technique, this investigator showed that what begins electrically as a condensation click actually turns out to be an acoustic condensation in the real ear canal in only about 60% of subjects. In the remaining 40%, the acoustic properties of the ear canal actually reverse the polarity at the ear drum. In this circumstance, the best strategy would appear to be use of alternating clicks in order to maintain a signal constancy from patient to patient. In some patients with steeply sloping high frequency sensorineural loss, however, there may be marked differences in responses to condensation and rarefaction clicks (Borg and Löfqvist, 1981, 1982) arguing for testing both responses separately as well as in the alternating condition.

Since sensitivity to polarity differences may be an indication of neural pathology, the argument is an important one. One viable approach to this problem is to record half of the sweeps with condensation clicks, record the other half with rarefaction clicks, and add them together for the final waveform. Another strategy is to use alternating polarity routinely, and employ condensation and rarefaction averages only if the alternating-polarity waveform is abnormal. Evaluating responses to condensation and rarefaction clicks is particularly enlightening in those patients with a loss of later ABR waveform components due to phase differences in the waveforms that result from sensitivity to click-polarity differences.

Filter Passband.   Filter passband is another issue that has been debated over the years. Early in the history of ABR testing, some investigators advocated use of a narrow band from 300 to 3000 Hz in order to minimize low-frequency artifact from the ongoing EEG. Other investigators, however, felt that a good deal of useful information lay in the region from 50 to 300 Hz and should not be discarded. A reasonable compromise between these two positions now seems to have been achieved with a fairly universally accepted passband from 100 to 3000 Hz.

Interpretive Strategy.   Over the years, several strategies have been proposed for evaluating the diagnostic significance of ABR waveforms. The various proposed indices of abnormality include

1. absolute latency of wave V,
2. wave V interaural difference,
3. I–V interwave interval,
4. interaural difference in I–V interwave intervals,
5. I/V amplitude ratio,
6. interaural difference in I/V amplitude ratios,
7. selective loss of late waves, and
8. grossly degraded waveform morphology.

The last two indices, selective loss of late waves and grossly degraded waveform morphology, while less objective that the first six, tend to be fairly obvious and dramatic when they do occur. But abnormality in the various latency and amplitude measures is not always so obvious and dramatic. In some early cases of acoustic tumor, for example, waveform morphology may be very good on both ears, the abnormality on the tumor ear being confined to a 0.4 to 0.5 ms interaural difference in the I–V interpeak interval. In these latter cases, there has been some disagreement as to the best strategy for taking normal variability into account in diagnostic evaluation. The conventional notion of defining normal limits as a band, plus or minus two standard deviations, around the normal mean is compelling but fails to deal with three important related issues:

1. Is the underlying distribution truly normal or even symmetric?

2. Is 5% actually the appropriate risk of alpha error in the typical diagnostic evaluation?
3. How should one weigh abnormalities revealed by the various indices? Are some abnormalities more significant that others?

We have fairly good evidence on the first question. Stockard, Stockard, and Coen (1983) and Klein and Teas (1978) have shown that indices like absolute and interwave intervals are indeed normally and symmetrically distributed and with remarkably constant standard deviations. It is not, therefore, unreasonable to define normal variability as a range of values encompassing a given number of standard deviations around the arithmetic mean. For example, the latency of the I–V interpeak interval is a well-defined 4.0 ms, with a 0.2 ms standard deviation. Therefore, a I–V interval of more than 4.4 ms falls outside the boundary of two standard deviations and exceeds the 5% confidence level.

Not so straightforward, however, is this tacit adoption of a 5% alpha error level by adopting the two-standard deviations (more appropriately 1.96 SD) boundary. In so doing we are, in effect, saying that we are willing to be wrong on 5% of the occasions in which we identify an ABR measure as abnormal. Is this acceptable? Is the value of a correct identification sufficient to justify a 5% false-alarm rate? A strong argument can be made for an affirmative answer to such a question. In fact, one could argue that an even higher alpha error is desirable. If, goes the argument, one purpose of the ABR test is to act as a screen to identify patients with potentially life-threatening diseases (e.g., intra- or extra-axial brain tumors), and the consequence of an abnormal finding is simply further testing, usually by sophisticated radiographic imaging techniques to confirm the presence of a lesion, then a relatively high alpha error level is tolerable. The value of correct identification, especially to the patient, is high, and the cost of a false alarm is no more than the cost and inconvenience of further testing. In this circumstance, one could argue for an alpha level of 10 or even 20%. There is, indeed, nothing magical about the 5% level of confidence in this example. Yet, 5% limits are so ingrained in our thinking that it would be very difficult to find acceptance for higher levels of

alpha error. However, a more sophisticated approach to the problem of selecting an appropriate confidence level would be to base such selection on a careful analysis of relative costs and values associated with the various possible correct and incorrect outcomes rather than on appeal to tradition.

We still lack sufficient data to assign relative weights to the various indices of abnormality. Many investigators would readily rank order at least some of the indices, placing least weight on amplitude ratios (see, however, Musiek, Kibbe, Rackliff, and Weider, 1984), somewhat more weight on absolute latencies, and even more weight on interpeak intervals. And, there is strong support for weighting interaural differences higher than ear-specific measures. We still do not have enough data, however, to tell us exactly how much these various weights should be in a quantitative sense. The issue is further complicated by the fact that all possible indices are not always available for each patient. The most valuable indices, those based on interwave intervals, for example, cannot be computed if wave I is not identifiable, a circumstance that arises often when there is substantial high-frequency hearing loss in the ear under test.

In our experience, emphasis is most often placed on two relative measures, the I–V interval and the I–V interaural difference. If neither of these measures exceed the 5% level, then the interpretation is that the ABR is normal, regardless of what the absolute latency might be. If, on the other hand, the I–V interval cannot be defined due to absence or ambiguity of wave I, then absolute latency of wave V is scrutinized. We analyze absolute wave V latency by comparing it to the boundaries shown in Figure 21.3 (Jerger and Johnson, 1988). These boundaries were established separately for males and females as a function of "effective click level." Effective click level was defined as the difference (in dB) between the actual click level (in dB nHL) and the patient's behavioral threshold at 4000 Hz. Boundaries were drawn to encompass 99% of all wave V latencies in patients with cochlear hearing loss. If an absolute latency falls outside of the boundary, it is considered to be abnormal.

Based on the foregoing observations, Table 21.5 presents a strategy for diagnostic evaluation. In the use

(A)

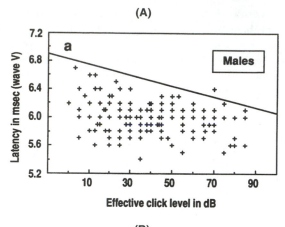

(B)

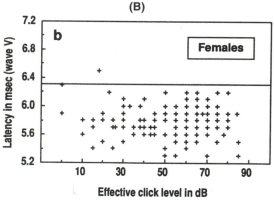

FIGURE 21.3.   Scattergrams of wave V latency as a function of effective click level. Boundary line encompasses 99% of wave V latencies in cochlear hearing loss. (A) Males; (B) females (From Jerger, J. and Johnson, K., Interactions of age, gender, and sensorineural hearing loss on ABR latency. *Ear and Hearing, 9,* 168–176. © Williams & Wilkins, 1988; with permission).

of this strategy it is important to remember the following points:

A. Do not lose sight of the forest for the trees. Before dwelling on the fine grain of tenths of milliseconds of interwave intervals, it is well to ask the basic questions:

1. Is the ABR waveform morphology obviously abnormal?

2. Is the ABR abnormality consistent with the configuration of the audiogram?

3. Can an ABR interaural difference be explained by the audiometric interaural difference?

In a fairly large share of patients with retrocochlear disorder, answers to these fundamental questions are straightforward and obviate the necessity for anguishing over the precise identification of component waves or the exact measurements of either absolute or relative latencies.

B. When in doubt, slow up. There is nothing magical about a click rate of 20/s. It is simply a compromise between the desire for a well-defined waveform and the desire to keep testing time to a minimum. If anything about the ABR response to a relatively fast rate like 20/s appears to be suspicious, the best strategy is to retest at a slower rate (10/s or even 5/s) in order to achieve better waveform definition, especially of wave I.

MLR Diagnostic Strategies

The diagnostic value of MLR depends, to a great extent, on identification of the latency and inter-ear and inter-hemisphere morphology of component Pa. The MLR is a difficult response to record and seems particularly susceptible to a variety of parametric and state variables that do not affect the ABR and seem to have less of an affect on the LVR. Detectability of the MLR depends most importantly on the following testing parameters: subject state, stimulus rate, recording site, filter passband, and interpretive strategy.

Subject State.   Amplitude of the MLR can vary considerably as a result of physiologic state of the individual being tested (Deiber, Ibañez, Bastuji, Fischer, and Mauguiere, 1989; Jones and Baxter, 1988; Mendel and Goldstein, 1971). Detectability of the response has even been shown to vary as a function of stage of sleep (Kraus et al., 1989). Because of these factors, interpretation of the MLR depends on either knowledge of the state or control over the state of the individual under test. Ideally, all MLR testing would be carried out with EEG monitoring for classifying sleep stage, and the

TABLE 21.5.   Strategy for Diagnostic ABR Evaluation

Test Parameter	Test Procedure

Signal: click
 	
Polarity: alternating and/or condensations and rarefactions separately
 	
Rate: adjustable
 	
  1. Begin at 20/s
 	
  2. Follow with 80/s
 	
  3. If neither yields a satisfactory waveform, slow rate to 10 or 5/s
 	
Level: adjust according to PTA2
	Examine waveforms for adequacy of morphology and presence of component waves. If these criteria are met, examine the following:
	
	1. I-V interwave interval on each ear
	
	2. Interaural difference in I-V interwave interval
	
	3. Absolute latency of wave V on each ear
	
	4. Interaural difference in wave V latency

PTA2 (dB)	Test Level (dB nHL)
0–19	70
20–39	80
40–59	90
60–79	100
≥80	105

Filter passband: 100–3000 Hz
Number averaged: 2,048

response would be interpreted in light of such classification. Practically, such an analysis is rarely an option. An alternative is to assure that the patient is awake and alert throughout MLR testing. One strategy that has been effective is to begin AEP testing with the MLR while the patient is as alert as possible. Waiting to carry out MLR testing until after a patient has slept through ABR testing enhances the likelihood that subject state will interfere with interpretation. Another strategy is to introduce periods of silence throughout the recording period and to ask the patient to count the silent intervals. Such a procedure encourages alertness and vigilance to the listening task.

Stimulus Rate.   Morphology of the MLR and, consequently, detectability, depend substantially on the rate of stimulus presentation. Although early studies concluded that there was little effect of rate on the MLR (Goldstein, Rodman, and Karlovich, 1972; Goldstein and McRandle, 1976), later studies found rate to be a significant factor (Suzuki and Kobayashi, 1984; Jerger

et al., 1987; Kraus, Smith, and McGee, 1987). It appears now that, while rate does not appear to have much of an effect on MLR amplitude in young adults, it does affect amplitude in infants and the elderly (Jerger, Oliver, and Chmiel, 1988). The effect is one of a reduction in amplitude at higher stimulus rates. Maximum amplitudes can usually be observed at rates of 2/s, whereas rates of 10/s can have a detrimental effect on MLR amplitude. Although waveform amplitude and morphology may be enhanced at even slower rates, clinical efficiency issues would probably preclude such testing.

Recording Site.   The MLR, like the ABR, is conventionally recorded with the active electrode located at the vertex. Recent evidence suggests that additional diagnostic information may be gleaned from recording at different electrode sites. For example, Marvel, Jerger, and Lew (1992) showed, with topographic brain mapping, that the distribution of MLR activity across the head was different in a group of elderly subjects that had auditory processing disorder as opposed to an elderly group that did not. One implication of these results is that the diagnostic utility of MLR is likely to be enhanced by assessment of topography of the response. In addition, various anecdotal reports have suggested that Pa of the MLR can be present at electrodes placed near the temporal lobes and absent at the vertex electrode, and vice versa. Also, two-channel recordings from vertex to each earlobe provide information about both ear effects and hemisphere effects, which may prove to be another way to enhance the diagnostic utility of the MLR. The best strategy, then, is probably to record from as many electrode sites as possible. Clinical constraints, however, often limit the ability to do so and, consequently, reduce the diagnostic sensitivity of the MLR procedure.

Filter Passband.   Controversy about filter passband surrounds no response more than the MLR. Results from early studies that used very narrow passbands have been challenged more recently by investigators using broader passbands (Kileny, 1983; Jerger et al., 1987). Since the major energy component of the MLR waveform is approximately 40 Hz in adults and 20 Hz in children, filter passbands must be sufficiently broad to pass these frequencies and not temporally distort the waveform. Currently, the recommended passband is from 10 to 1000 Hz. Although the high-frequency cut-off may be lowered somewhat for practical reasons in the clinic, the low-frequency cut-off can affect detectability of the response, which is, for example, better at 15 Hz than at 3 Hz (Kraus, Reed, Smith, Stein, and Cartee, 1987).

Interpretive Strategy.   Criteria for interpretation of the MLR are not well established. Those criteria that have been used generally specify the Pa component as the main response to be measured. In our own work (Stach and Hudson, 1990), we have found the following criteria to be useful. For a response to be considered normal, it must have an identifiable, repeatable, vertex-positive wave, with a visible positive rise and negative fall, that occurs between 21 and 38 ms following stimulus onset. Interpretation of the MLR is based on presence of a response and ear symmetry of amplitude, latency, and morphology. Although amplitude and morphology of the MLR are variable, when asymmetries do exist, they tend to be fairly obvious and dramatic. While this is less objective than we would prefer, our current level of understanding precludes more specific interpretive strategies.

Interpretation of the MLR can be made not only from differences between ears, but also from differences between hemispheres. In some patients with neurologic disorder, the MLR is absent when recorded from one hemisphere, regardless of ear stimulated, but not the other. For example, in a patient with a right cerebral vascular accident, we observed an MLR when recording from the vertex-to-left-earlobe electrodes whether the stimulus was presented to the right ear or the left ear. In contrast, no MLR could be recorded from the vertex-to-right-earlobe electrodes, regardless of which ear was stimulated. While this certainly is no substitute for topographic mapping, nevertheless, the use of two channel recordings to observe hemisphere effects may prove to be a valuable diagnostic approach.

LVR Diagnostic Strategies

The diagnostic value of the LVR depends on identification of the latency and inter-ear and inter-hemisphere morphology of components N1 and P2. The LVR is a very robust response and can be recorded reliably from awake adults. Successful recording of the LVR depends most importantly on the following testing parameters: subject state, stimulus rate, and interpretive strategy.

Subject State.   The LVR is highly vulnerable to physiologic state of the patient being tested. For that reason, the response is best recorded and interpreted only in awake patients who are attending to the auditory stimuli. To enhance vigilance to the stimuli, the patient is typically asked to count the number of stimuli presented during each trial.

Stimulus Rate.   If for no other reason than the fact that the patient needs to count stimuli, a slow rate of stimulus presentation is required. Typical stimulus rate is 0.5/s.

Interpretive Strategy.   Similar to the MLR, criteria for interpretation of the LVR are not well established. Those criteria that have been used generally assess a negative peak occurring at about 90 ms (N1) and a positive peak occurring at about 180 ms (P2). In our own work (Stach and Hudson, 1990), we have found the following criteria to be useful. For a response to be considered normal, it must have an identifiable, repeatable, vertex-negative N1 peak that occurs between 59 and 139 ms following stimulus onset. It must also have a vertex-positive P2 peak that occurs between 125 and 208 ms. These boundaries represent 3 standard deviations around the mean latency. Interpretation of the LVR is based on presence of a response and ear symmetry of amplitude, latency, and morphology. Again, as is the case with the MLR, when asymmetries do exist, they tend to be fairly obvious and dramatic. In addition, the use of two-channel recording to observe hemisphere effects is to be encouraged.

CONCLUSION

We have attempted to present relatively specific test strategies for the three fundamental clinical applications of AEPs. Inevitably, in such an ambitious undertaking, there must be some compromise to resolve the range of approaches taken by different investigators. Throughout the chapter, therefore, we have attempted to reflect not only those aspects of testing where consistency is the rule, but also those aspects where opinion is still divergent.

Our sole purpose in presenting these specific test strategies is to distill the wide range of experiences of various investigators into a set of procedures in which the clinician may have confidence. But we do not advocate that any of these recommendations become fixed and immutable. Instead, we recommend continued flexibility in our approach to the test situation and a continuing willingness to modify our approach as new evidence warrants such change.

REFERENCES

Alberti, P. W., Hyde, M. L., Riko, K., Corbin, H., and Abramovich, S. (1983). An evaluation of BERA for hearing screening in high-risk neonates. *Laryngoscope*, *93*, 1115–1121.

Blegvad, B. (1975). Binaural summation of surface-recorded electrocochleographic responses. *Scandinavian Audiology*, *4*, 233–238.

Borg, E. and Löfqvist, L. (1981). Auditory brainstem response (ABR) to rarefaction and condensation clicks in normal and steep high-frequency hearing loss. *Scandinavian Audiology*, *10* (Supplement 13), 99–101.

Borg, E. and Löfqvist, L. (1982). Auditory brainstem response (ABR) to rarefaction and condensation clicks in normal and abnormal ears. *Scandinavian Audiology*, *11*, 227–235.

Brown, D. D. and Shallop, J. K. (1982, fall). A clinically useful 500 Hz evoked response. *Nicolet Potentials*, *1*, 9–12.

Cevette, M. J. (1984). Auditory brainstem response testing in the intensive care unit. *Seminars in Hearing*, *5*, 57–69.

Cox, C., Hack, M., and Metz, D. (1981). Brainstem-evoked response audiometry: Normative data from the preterm infant. *Audiology*, *20*, 53–64.

Dauman, R., Szyfter, W., Charlet de Sauvage, R., and Cazals, Y. (1984). Low frequency thresholds assessed with 40 Hz MLR in adults with impaired hearing. *Archives of Oto-Rhino-Laryngology*, *240*, 85–89.

Davis, H. and Hirsh, S. K. (1976). The audiometric utility of brain stem responses to low-frequency sounds. *Audiology*, *15*, 181–195.

Davis, H., Hirsh, S. K., Popelka, G. R., and Formby, C. (1984). Frequency selectivity and thresholds of brief stimuli suitable for electric response audiometry. *Audiology*, *23*, 59–74.

Davis, H., Hirsh, S. K., Shelnutt, J., and Bowers, C. (1967). Further validation of evoked response audiometry (ERA). *Journal of Speech and Hearing Research*, *10*, 717–732.

Deiber, M.P., Ibañez, V., Bastuji, H., Fischer, C., and Mauguière, F. (1989). Changes of middle latency auditory evoked potentials during natural sleep in humans. *Neurology*, *39*, 806–813.

Dennis, J. M., Sheldon, R., Toubas, P., and McCaffee, M. A. (1984). Identification of hearing loss in the neonatal intensive care unit population. *The American Journal of Otology*, *5*, 201–205.

Dobie, R. A. and Berlin, C. I. (1979). Binaural interaction in brainstem-evoked responses. *Archives of Otolaryngology*, *105*, 391–398.

Downs, D. W. (1982). Auditory brainstem response testing in the neonatal intensive care unit: A cautious response. *Asha, 24,* 1009–1015.

Finitzo-Hieber, T. (1982). Auditory brainstem response: Its place in infant audiological evaluations. *Seminars in Speech, Language and Hearing, 3,* 76–87.

Galambos, R. (1978). Use of the auditory brainstem response (ABR) in infant hearing testing. In Gerber, S.E. and Mencher, G.T. (eds.), *Early diagnosis of hearing loss.* New York: Grune & Stratton.

Galambos, R., Hicks, G.E., and Wilson, M.J. (1984). The auditory brainstem response reliably predicts hearing loss in graduates of a tertiary intensive care nursery. *Ear and Hearing, 5,* 254–260.

Galambos, R., Makeig, S., and Talmachoff, P.J. (1981). A 40 Hz auditory potential recorded from the human scalp. *Proceedings of National Academy of Science USA, 78,* 2643–2647.

Gerling, I. J. and Finitzo-Hieber, T. (1983). Auditory brainstem response with high stimulus rates in normal and patient populations. *Annals of Otology, Rhinology and Laryngology, 92,* 119–123.

Gerull, G. and Mrowinski, D. (1984). Brain stem potentials evoked by binaural click stimuli with differences in interaural time and intensity. *Audiology, 23,* 265–276.

Goldstein, R. and McRandle, C.C. (1976). Middle components of the averaged electroencephalic response to clicks in neonates. In Hirsh, S.K., Eldredge, D.H., Hirsh, I.J., and Silverman, S.R. (eds.), *Hearing and Davis: Essays honoring Hallowell Davis.* St. Louis: Washington University Press.

Goldstein, R. and Rodman, L.B. (1967). Early components of averaged evoked responses to rapidly repeated auditory stimuli. *Journal of Speech and Hearing Research, 10,* 697–705.

Goldstein, R., Rodman, L.B., and Karlovich, R. (1972). Effects of stimulus rate and number on the early components of the averaged electroencephalic response. *Journal of Speech and Hearing Disorders, 15,* 559–566.

Hall, J.W., Kripal, J.P., and Hepp, T. (1988). Newborn hearing screening with auditory brainstem response: Measurement problems and solutions. *Seminars in Hearing, 9,* 15–33.

Hawes, M.D. and Greenberg, H. J. (1981). Slow brain stem responses (SN10) to tone pips in normally hearing newborns and adults. *Audiology, 20,* 113–122.

Hayes, D. (1980). Effect of degree of hearing loss on diagnostic audiometric tests. *American Journal of Otology, 2,* 91–96.

Hayes, D. and Jerger, J. (1982). Auditory brainstem response (ABR) to tone-pips: Results in normal and hearing-impaired subjects. *Scandinavian Audiology, 11,* 133–142.

Hecox, K. E. (1983, spring). Brainstem auditory evoked responses: Technical factors. Part I. *Nicolet Potentials, 2,* 19–22; 24.

Hecox, K. E. (1984, spring). Auditory evoked response: Audiologic applications. Part II. *Nicolet Potentials, 3,* 39–41; 47.

Hecox, K. E., Cone, B., and Blaw, M.E. (1981). Brainstem auditory evoked response in the diagnosis of pediatric neurologic diseases. *Neurology, 31,* 832–840.

Hecox, K. and Galambos, R. (1974). Brain stem auditory evoked responses in human infants and adults. *Archives of Otolaryngology, 99,* 30–33.

Hooks, R. G. and Weber, B.A. (1984). Auditory brain stem responses of premature infants to bone-conducted stimuli: A feasibility study. *Ear and Hearing, 5,* 42–46.

Hume, A.L. and Cant, B.R. (1977). Diagnosis of hearing loss in infancy by electric response audiometry. *Archives of Otolaryngology, 103,* 416–418.

Hyde, M., Alberti, P., Matsumoto, H., and Li, Y. (1986). Auditory evoked potentials in audiometric assessment of compensation and medicolegal patients. *Annals of Otology Rhinology and Laryngology, 95,* 514–519.

Jacobson, J.T., Jacobson, C.A., and Spahr, R.C. (1990). Automated and conventional ABR screening techniques in high-risk infants. *Journal of the American Academy of Audiology, 1,* 187–195.

Jacobson, J. T., Seitz, M. R., Mencher, G. T., and Parrott, V. (1980). Auditory brainstem response: A contribution to infant assessment and management. In Mencher, G.T. and Gerber, S.E. (eds.), *Early management of hearing loss.* New York: Grune & Stratton.

Jerger, J., Chmiel, R., Frost, J.D., and Coker, N. (1986). Effect of sleep on the auditory steady state evoked potential. *Ear and Hearing, 7,* 240–245.

Jerger, J., Chmiel, R., Glaze, D., and Frost, J.D. (1987). Rate and filter dependence of the middle-latency response in infants. *Audiology, 26,* 269–283.

Jerger, J., Hayes, D., and Jordon, C. (1980). Clinical experience with auditory brainstem response audiometry in pediatric assessment. *Ear and Hearing, 1,* 19–25.

Jerger, J. and Johnson, K. (1988). Interactions of age, gender, and sensorineural hearing loss on ABR latency. *Ear and Hearing, 9,* 168–176.

Jerger, J., Oliver, T., and Chmiel, R. (1988). Auditory middle latency response: A perspective. *Seminars in Hearing, 9,* 75–86.

Jones, L.A. and Baxter, R.J. (1988). Changes in the auditory middle latency responses during all-night sleep recording. *British Journal of Audiology*, *22*, 279–285.

Kavanagh, K. T. and Beardsley, J.V. (1979). Brain stem auditory evoked response. *Annals of Otology, Rhinology and Laryngology*, *88* (Supplement 58), 1–28.

Kileny, P. (1983). Auditory evoked middle latency responses: Current issues. *Seminars in Hearing*, *4*, 403–413.

Kileny, P. (1988). New insights on infant ABR hearing screening. *Scandinavian Audiology Supplement*, *30*, 81–88.

Kileny, P. and Shea, S.L. (1986). Middle-latency and 40-Hz auditory evoked responses in normal-hearing subjects: Click and 500-Hz thresholds. *Journal of Speech and Hearing Research*, *29*, 20–28.

Klein, A. J. (1983). Properties of the brain-stem response slow-wave component: I. Latency, amplitude, and threshold measurement. *Archives of Otolaryngology*, *109*, 6–12.

Klein, A. J. and Teas, D.C. (1978). Acoustically dependent latency shifts of BSER (wave V) in man. *Journal of the Acoustical Society of America*, *63*, 1887–1895.

Kraus, N., McGee, T., and Comperatore, C. (1989). MLRs in children are consistently present during wakefulness, stage 1, and REM sleep. *Ear and Hearing*, *10*, 339–345.

Kraus, N., Reed, N., Smith, D.I., Stein, L., and Cartee, C. (1987). High-pass filter settings affect the detectability of MLRs in humans. *Electroencephalography and Clinical Neurophysiology*, *68*, 234–236.

Kraus, N., Smith, D.I., and McGee, T. (1987). Rate and filter effects on the developing middle-latency response. *Audiology*, *26*, 257–268.

Lenarz, T., Gülzow, J., Grözinger, M., and Hoth, S. (1986). Clinical evaluation of 40 Hz middle-latency responses in adults: Frequency specific threshold estimation and suprathreshold amplitude characteristics. *ORL*, *48*, 24–32.

Linden, R.D., Campbell, K.B., Hamel, G., and Picton, T.W. (1985). Human auditory steady state potentials during sleep. *Ear and Hearing*, *6*, 167–174.

Lynn, J.M., Lesner, S.A., Sandridge, S.A., and Daddario, C.L. (1984). Threshold prediction from the auditory 40 Hz evoked potential. *Ear and Hearing*, *5*, 366–370.

Marvel, J.B., Jerger, J.F., and Lew, H. (1992). Asymmetries in topographic brain maps of auditory evoked potentials in the elderly. *Journal of the American Academy of Audiology*, *3*, 361-368.

Mauldin, L. and Jerger, J. (1979). Auditory brain stem evoked responses to bone-conducted signals. *Archives of Otolaryngology*, *105*, 656–661.

McCall, S. and Ferraro, J.A. (1991). Pediatric ABR screening: Pass-fail rates in awake versus asleep neonates. *Journal of the American Academy of Audiology*, *2*, 18–23.

McDonald, J.M. and Shimizu, H. (1981). Frequency specificity of the auditory brain stem response. *American Journal of Otolaryngology*, *2*, 36–42.

Mendel, M.I. and Goldstein, R. (1971). Early components of the averaged electroencephalic response to constant level clicks during all-night sleep. *Journal of Speech and Hearing Research*, *14*, 829–840.

Musiek, F.E. and Geurnink, N. (1981). Auditory brainstem and middle latency evoked response near threshold. *Annals of Otology, Rhinology, and Larynogology*, *90*, 236–240.

Musiek, F. E., Kibbe, K., Rackliffe, L., and Weider, D. J. (1984). The auditory brain stem response I–V amplitude ratio in normal, cochlear, and retrocochlear ears. *Ear and Hearing*, *5*, 52–55.

Northern, J. L. and Downs, M.P. (1974). *Hearing in children*. Baltimore: Williams & Wilkins.

Ornitz, E.M., Ritvo, E.R., Carr, E.M., Panman, L.M., and Walter, R.D. (1967). The variability of the auditory averaged evoked response during sleep and dreaming in children and adults. *Electroencephalography and Clinical Neurophysiology*, *22*, 514–524.

Özdamar, Ö., Delgado, R.E., Eilers, R.E., and Widen, J.E. (1990). Computer methods for on-line hearing testing with auditory brain stem responses. *Ear and Hearing*, *11*, 417–429.

Peters, J.G. (1986). An automated infant screener using advanced evoked response technology. *Hearing Journal*, *39*, 25–30.

Pratt, H., Ben-David, Y., Peled, R., Podoshin, L., and Scharf, B. (1981). Auditory brain stem evoked potentials: Clinical promise of increasing stimulus rate. *Electroencephalography and Clinical Neurophysiology*, *51*, 80–90.

Roberts, J. L., Davis, H., Phon, G. L., Reichert, T. J., Sturtevant, E. M., and Marshall, R. E. (1982). Auditory brainstem responses in preterm neonates: Maturation and follow-up. *Journal of Pediatrics*, *101*, 257–263.

Salt, A. (1982). Presentation on ear canal probe microphone measurements of click polarity. Paper presented at the 1st International Conference on Standards for Auditory Brainstem Response Measurement, Laguna Beach, CA, February.

Schulman-Galambos, C. and Galambos, R. (1979). Brainstem evoked response audiometry in newborn hearing screening. *Archives of Otolaryngology*, *105*, 86–90.

Shallop, J.K. and Osterhammel, P.A. (1983). A comparative study of measurements of SN10 and the 40/sec middle latency responses in newborns. *Scandinavian Audiology, 12,* 91–95.

Shanon, E., Gold, S., and Himmelfarb, M. (1981). Assessment of functional integrity of brain stem auditory pathways by stimulus stress. *Audiology, 20,* 65–71.

Skinner, P. and Shimoto, J. (1975). A comparison of the effects of sedatives on the auditory evoked cortical response. *Journal of the American Audiology Society, 1,* 71–78.

Stach, B.A. and Hudson, M. (1990). Middle and late auditory evoked potentials in multiple sclerosis. *Seminars in Hearing, 11,* 265–275.

Stapells, D.R. (1989). Auditory brainstem reponse assessment of infants and children. *Seminars in Hearing, 10,* 229–251.

Stapells, D.R., Galambos, R., Costello, J.A., and Makeig, S. (1988). Inconsistency of auditory middle latency and steady-state responses in infants. *Electroencephalography and Clinical Neurophysiology, 71,* 289–295.

Stapells, D.R., Makeig, S., and Galambos, R. (1985). Studies of the auditory steady-state response. III. Threshold estimation. *Journal of the Acoustical Society of America, 77,* S66.

Stapells, D.R. and Ruben, R.J. (1989). Auditory brain stem responses to bone-conducted tones in infants. *Annals of Otology, Rhinology, and Laryngology, 98,* 941–949.

Starr, A. (1976). Auditory brain stem responses in brain death. *Brain, 99,* 543–554.

Starr, A. and Achor, L. J. (1975). Auditory brainstem responses in neurological disease. *Archives of Neurology, 32,* 761–768.

Starr, A., Amile, R. N., Martin, W. H., and Sanders, S. (1977). Development of auditory function in newborn infants revealed by auditory brainstem potentials. *Pediatrics, 60,* 831–839.

Starr, A. and Hamilton, A. E. (1976). Correlation between confirmed sites of neurological lesions and abnormalities of far-field auditory brainstem responses. *Electroencephalography and Clinical Neurophysiology, 41,* 595–608.

Stein, L.K. (1984). Evaluating the efficiency of auditory brainstem response as a neonatal hearing screening test. *Seminars in Hearing, 5,* 71–77.

Stein, L. K., Özdamar, Ö., Kraus, N., and Paton, J. (1983). Follow-up of infants screened by auditory brainstem response in the neonatal intensive care unit. *Journal of Pediatrics, 103,* 447–453.

Stockard, J. and Rossiter, V. (1977). Clinical and pathologic correlates of brainstem auditory response abnormalities. *Neurology, 27,* 316–325.

Stockard, J.E., Stockard, J. J., and Coen, R. W. (1983). Auditory brainstem response variability in infants. *Ear and Hearing, 4,* 11–23.

Suzuki, T. (1973). Problems in electric response audiometry (ERA) during sedation. *Audiology, 12,* 129–136.

Suzuki, T., Hirai, Y., and Horiuchi, K. (1977). Auditory brainstem responses to pure-tone stimuli. *Scandinavian Audiology, 6,* 51–56.

Suzuki, T. and Kobayashi, K. (1985). An evaluation of 40-Hz event-related potentials in young children *Audiology, 23,* 599–604.

Suzuki, T., Yamamoto, K., Taguchi, K., and Sakabe, N. (1976). Reliability and validity of late vertex-evoked response audiometry. *Audiology, 15,* 357–369.

Weber, B. A. (1983). Masking and bone conduction testing in brainstem response audiometry. *Seminars in Hearing, 4,* 343–352.

Zöllner, C. and Eibach, H. (1981). Can the differential diagnosis cochlear-retrocochlear disorder be improved using the brainstem potentials with changing stimulus repetition rates? *HNO, 29,* 240–245.